Lecture Notes in Artificial Intelligence   5139

Edited by R. Goebel, J. Siekmann, and W. Wahlster

Subseries of Lecture Notes in Computer Science

Changjie Tang   Charles X. Ling
Xiaofang Zhou   Nick J. Cercone   Xue Li (Eds.)

Advanced Data Mining and Applications

4th International Conference, ADMA 2008
Chengdu, China, October 8-10, 2008
Proceedings

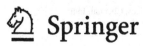 Springer

Series Editors

Randy Goebel, University of Alberta, Edmonton, Canada
Jörg Siekmann, University of Saarland, Saarbrücken, Germany
Wolfgang Wahlster, DFKI and University of Saarland, Saarbrücken, Germany

Volume Editors

Changjie Tang
Sichuan University, Computer School
Chengdu 610065, China
E-mail: tangchangjie@cs.scu.edu.cn

Charles X. Ling
The University of Western Ontario, Department of Computer Science
Ontario N6A 5B7, Canada
E-mail: cling@csd.uwo.ca

Xiaofang Zhou
Xue Li
The University of Queensland, School of Information Technology and
Electrical Engineering, Brisbane QLD 4072, Queensland, Australia
E-mail: {xueli; zxf}@itee.uq.edu.au

Nick J. Cercone
York University, Faculty of Science & Engineering
Toronto M3J 1P3 Ontario, Canada
E-mail: ncercone@yorku.ca

Library of Congress Control Number: Applied for

CR Subject Classification (1998): I.2, H.2, H.2.8, H.3-4, K.4.4, J.3, I.4, J.1

LNCS Sublibrary: SL 7 – Artificial Intelligence

ISSN 0302-9743

ISBN 978-3-540-88191-9 Springer Berlin Heidelberg New York

Springer is a part of Springer Science+Business Media

springer.com

© Springer-Verlag Berlin Heidelberg 2008

Typesetting: Camera-ready by author, data conversion by Scientific Publishing Services, Chennai, India
Printed on acid-free paper   SPIN: 12539390   06/3180   5 4 3 2 1 0

Preface

The Fourth International Conference on Advanced Data Mining and Applications (ADMA 2008) will be held in Chengdu, China, followed by the last three successful ADMA conferences (2005 in Wu Han, 2006 in Xi'an, and 2007 Harbin). Our major goal of ADMA is to bring together the experts on data mining in the world, and to provide a leading international forum for the dissemination of original research results in data mining, including applications, algorithms, software and systems, and different disciplines with potential applications of data mining. This goal has been partially achieved in a very short time despite the young age of the conference, thanks to the rigorous review process insisted upon, the outstanding list of internationally renowned keynote speakers and the excellent program each year. ADMA is ranked higher than, or very similar to, other data mining conferences (such as PAKDD, PKDD, and SDM) in early 2008 by an independent source: cs-conference-ranking.org.

This year we had the pleasure and honor to host illustrious keynote speakers. Our distinguished keynote speakers are Prof. Qiang Yang and Prof. Jiming Liu. Prof. Yang is a tenured Professor and postgraduate studies coordinator at Computer Science and Engineering Department of Hong Kong University of Science and Technology. He is also a member of AAAI, ACM, a senior member of the IEEE, and he is also an associate editor for the IEEE TKDE and IEEE Intelligent Systems, KAIS and WI Journals. Since 2002, he has published 27 journal papers and 53 conference papers including 8 top conferences such as AAAI, KDD, SIGIR, etc. Prof. Liu is Professor and Head of Computer Science Department at Hong Kong Baptist University. He was a tenured Professor and Director of School of Computer Science at University of Windsor, Canada. He has published over 200 research articles in refereed international journals and conferences, and a number of books. Prof. Liu has served academic and professional communities in various capacities, e.g., presently as Editor-in-Chief of Web Intelligence and Agent Systems, Associate Editor of IEEE Transactions on Knowledge and Data Engineering and Computational Intelligence, etc.

This year ADMA received totally 304 paper submissions from 21 different countries, making it, yet again, a truly international conference. A rigorous process of pre-screening and review involved 89 well-known international program committee members and 2 program co-chairs, in addition to numerous external reviewers. This screening process yielded the remarkable papers organized in these proceedings with 35 regular papers and 43 short papers, bearing a total acceptance rate of 25.6%.

Earthquakes on May 12th, 2008 changed the original schedule but never changed the authors' great support and the organizers' huge efforts to make ADMA succeed. During the hard days, we received numerous emails or calls asking and consoling about our situation. And the steering committee has given us enormous help and guidance. We have resumed work only days after the earthquake. With the help, consideration and hard work of all organizers, authors, and conference attendees, ADMA 2008 will become another successful international conference in the data mining community.

July 2008   Changjie Tang
                                                                Charles X. Ling
                                                                Nick Cercone
                                                                Xiaofang Zhou
                                                                Xue Li

Organization

ADMA 2008 was organized by Sichuan University, China.

Steering Committee Chair

Xue Li   University of Queensland (UQ), Australia

General Co-chairs

Nick Cercone   York University, Canada
Xiaofang Zhou   Queensland University, Australia

Program Co-chairs

Changjie Tang   Sichuan University, China
Charles Ling   University of Western Ontario, Canada

Local Arrangements Co-chairs

Jiliu Zhou   Sichuan University, China
Chuan Li   Sichuan University, China

Publicity Co-chairs

Tao Li   Florida University, USA, UK
Xingshu Chen   Sichuan University, China

Finance Co-chairs

Guirong Xue   Shanghai Jiaotong University, China
Dou Shen   Microsoft Redmond AdLab

Registration Chair

Mei Hong   Sichuan University, China
Meiqi Liu   Sichuan University, China

Web Co-masters

Chunqiu Zeng   Sichuan University, China
Yue Zhang   Sichuan University, China

Steering Committee

Xue Li, University of Queensland, Australia
Email: xueli@itee.uq.edu.au
URL: http://www.itee.uq.edu.au/~xueli

Qiang Yang, Hong Kong University of Science and Technology, China
Email:qyang@cse.ust.hk
URL: http://www.cse.ust.hk/~qyang/

Whang, Kyu-Young, Korea Advanced Institute of Science and Technology, Korea
E-mail: kywhang@cs.kaist.ac.kr
URL: http://dblab.kaist.ac.kr/Prof/main_eng.html

Osmar R. Zaïane, University of Alberta, Canada
E-mail: zaiane@cs.ualberta.ca
URL: http://www.cs.ualberta.ca/~zaiane/

Chengqi Zhang, University of Technology, Sydney, Australia
E-mail: chengqi@it.uts.edu.au
URL: http://www-staff.it.uts.edu/~chengqi

Program Committee

Hassan Abolhassabni   Sharif University of Technology, Iran
Reda Alhajj   University of Calgary, Canada
James Bailey   University of Melbourne, Australia
Michael R. Berthold   University of Konstanz, Germany
Fernando Berzal   University of Granada, Spain
Jeremy Besson   Insa-Lyon, France
Francesco Bonchi   KDD Laboratory–ISTI CNR Pisa, Italy
Rui Camacho   University of Porto, Portugal
Nick Cercone   York University, Canada
Yu Chen   Sichuan University, China
Frans Coenen   University of Liverpool, UK
Alfredo Cuzzocrea   University of Calabria, Italy
Xiangjun Dong   Shandong Institute of Light Industry, China
Zhaoyang Dong   University of Queensland, Australia
Xiaoyong Du   Renmin University, China
Mohammad El-Hajj   University of Alberta, Canada

Ming Fan	Zhengzhou University, China
Yi Feng	Zhejiang University, China
Joao Gama	University of Porto, Portugal
Jean-Gabriel G. Ganascia	LIP6 - University Paris
Hong Gao	Harbin Institute of Technology, China
Junbin Gao	University of New England, Australia
Yu Ge	North East University, China
Peter Geczy	National Institute of Advanced Industrial Science and Technology (AIST), Japan
Christophe Giraud-Carrier	Brigham Young University
Vladimir Gorodetsky	Intelligent System Lab, Russian Academy of Science, Russia
Bing Guo	Sichuan University, China
Jimmy Huang	York University, Canada
Alfred Hofmann	Springer Verlag, Germany
Shengyi Jiang	GuangDong University of Foreign Studies
Yulan Ju	Chief Editor and Standing Deputy Editor-in-Chief of *Journal of Frontiers of Computer Science and Technology* (FCST)
Dimitrios Katsaros	Aristotle University, Greece
Mehmet Kaya	Firat University, Turkey
Adam Krzyzak	Concordia University, Montreal/Canada
Andrew Kusiak	University of Iowa, USA
Longin Jan Latecki	Temple University Philadelphia, USA
Gang Li	Deakin University, Australia
Yingshu Li	Georgia State University, USA
Zhanhuai Li	Northwest Polytechnical University, China
Chuan Li	Sichuan University, China
Xue Li	University of Queensland (UQ), Australia
Charles Ling	University of Western Ontario, Canada
Wanquan Liu	Curtin University of Technology, Australia
Jing Liu	Xidian University, China
Giuseppe Manco	National Research Council of Italy, Italy
Nasrullah Memon	Aalborg University, Denmark
Xiaofeng Meng	School of Information, Renmin University of China, China
Weiyi Meng	State University of New York at Binghamton, USA
Juggapong Natwichai	Chiang Mai University, Chiang Mai, Thailand
Daniel C. Neagu	University of Bradford, UK
Tansel Ozyer	TOBB University, Turkey
Deepak S. Padmanabhan	IBM India Research Lab
Jian Peng	Sichuan University, China
Yonghong Peng	University of Bradford, UK
Mithun Prasad	Rensselaer Polytechnic Institute, USA
Naren Ramakrishnan	Virginia Tech, USA
Zbigniew W. Ras	University of North Carolina, USA
Jan Rauch	University of Economics, Prague, Czech Republic

Raul Giraldez Rojo	Pablo de Olavide University, Spain
Ashkan Sami	Shiraz University, Iran
Giovanni Semeraro	University of Bari, Italy
Shengfei Shi	Harbin Institute of Technology, China
Carlos Soares	University of Porto, Portugal
Jaideep Srivastava	University of Minnesota, USA
Simsek Sule	University of Missouri-Rolla, USA
Kay Chen Tan	National University of Singapore, Singapore
Ah-Hwee Tan	Nanyang Technological University, Singapore
Changjie Tang	Sichuan University, China
Arthur Tay	National University of Singapore, Singapore
Luis Torgo	University of Porto, Portugal
Grigorios Tsoumakas	Aristotle University, Greece
Ricardo Vilalta	University of Houston, USA
Paul Vitanyi	CWI, The Netherlands
Wei Wang	Fudan University, China
Guoren Wang	NorthEast University, China
Shuliang Wang	Wuhan University, China
Desheng Dash Wu	University of Toronto, Canada
Zhipeng Xie	Fudan University, China
Qiang Yang	Hong Kong University of Science and Technology, Hong Kong
JingTao Yao	University of Regina, Canada
Jeffrey Xu Yu	Chinese University of Hong Kong, Hong Kong, China
Sarah Zelikovitz	College of Staten Island, NY, USA
Jianzhou Zhang	Sichuan University, China
Shichao Zhang	University of Technology, Sydney, Australia
Yang ZHANG	Northwest A&F University, China
Aoying Zhou	East China Normal University, China
Shuigeng Zhou	Fudan University, China
Xiaofang Zhou	University of Queensland (UQ), Australia

Sponsoring Institutions

National Science Foundation of China
WiseSoft Company Limited, Sichuan University

Table of Contents

Keynotes

Regular Papers

Short Papers

An Introduction to Transfer Learning[*]

Qiang Yang

Dept. of Computer Science, Hong Kong University of Science and Technology, Clearwater
Bay, Kowloon, Hong Kong
qyang@cse.ust.hk
http://www.cse.ust.hk/~qyang

Abstract. Many existing data mining and machine learning techniques are
based on the assumption that training and test data fit the same distribution.
This assumption does not hold, however, as in many cases of Web mining and
wireless computing when labeled data becomes outdated or test data are from a
different domain with training data. In these cases, most machine learning
methods would fail in correctly classifying new and future data. It would be
very costly and infeasible to collect and label enough new training data. Instead,
we would like to recoup as much useful knowledge as possible from the old
data. This problem is known as transfer learning. In this talk, I will give an
overview of the transfer learning problem, present a number of important directions in this research, and discuss our own novel solutions to this problem.

---

[*] A Keynote Talk presented at the Fourth International Conference on Advanced Data Mining
and Applications (ADMA'08), Chengdu, China, October 8-10, 2008.

Autonomy-Oriented Computing (AOC), Self-organized Computability, and Complex Data Mining*

Jiming Liu

Department of Computer Science, Hong Kong Baptist University,
Kowloon Tong, Hong Kong
jiming@comp.hkbu.edu.hk
http://comp.hkbu.edu.hk/~jiming

Abstract. Future data-mining challenges will lie in the breakthroughs in new computational paradigms, models, and tools that can offer scalable and robust solutions to complex data-mining problems. The problems of such a nature can be: (1) *petabyte-scale* (e.g., mining Google books or social networks), (2) *dynamically-evolving* (e.g., detecting air traffic patterns, market trends, and social norms), (3) *interaction-rich* as well as *trans-disciplinary* (e.g., predicting and preventing world economic and/or ecological crisis), and/or (4) *highly-distributed* (e.g., security and adaptive computing, such as community evolution, in pervasive environments). Toward this end, various computing ideas and techniques have been proposed and explored that explicitly utilize the models of *computational autonomy* as inspired by nature. This talk focuses on one of such research initiatives, which concerns the development of an unconventional computing paradigm, called *Autonomy-Oriented Computing (AOC)*. In general, AOC tackles a complex computing problem by defining and deploying a system of local autonomy-oriented entities. The entities spontaneously interact with their environments and operate based on their behavioral rules. They self-organize their structural relationships as well as behavioral dynamics, with respect to some specific forms of interactions and control settings. Such a capability is referred to as the *self-organized computability* of autonomous entities. In this talk, we will examine basic concepts and principles in the development of an AOC system, and present some related data-mining examples in the area of complex networks, e.g., unveiling community structures, characterizing the empirical laws of WWW user behavior, and/or understanding the dynamic performance of social networks.

---

* A Keynote Talk presented at the Fourth International Conference on Advanced Data Mining and Applications (ADMA'08), Chengdu, China, October 8-10, 2008.

C. Tang et al. (Eds.): ADMA 2008, LNAI 5139, p. 2, 2008.

Improving Angle Based Mappings

Frank Rehm[1] and Frank Klawonn[2]

[1] German Aerospace Center
frank.rehm@dlr.de
[2] University of Applied Sciences Braunschweig/Wolfenbuettel
f.klawonn@fh-wolfenbuettel.de

Abstract. Visualization of high-dimensional data is an important issue in data mining as it enhances the chance to selectively choose appropriate techniques for analyzing data. In this paper, two extensions to recent angle based multi-dimensional scaling techniques are presented. The first approach concerns the preprocessing of the data with the objective to lower the error of the subsequent mapping. The second aims at improving differentiability of angle based mappings by augmenting the target space by one additional dimension. Experimental results demonstrate the gain of efficiency in terms of layout quality and computational complexity.

1 Introduction

Many branches of industry, commerce and research put great efforts in collecting data with the objective to describe and predict customer behavior or both technical and natural phenomena. Besides the size of such datasets, which make manual analysis impractical, data analysis becomes challenging due to a large number of attributes describing a data object. As a very first step in the chain of data mining, visualization is very helpful to understand some properties of multivariate data. Sophisticated techniques then are needed to project (or map) such high-dimensional data on a plane or in a 3D space. This paper adresses the domain of data visualization.

Multi-dimensional scaling (MDS) is a family of methods that seek to present important structures of the original data in a reduced number of dimensions. Commonly, distances between pairs of objects are tried to preserve, when finding these mappings. Recently, two new techniques - MDS_{polar}[1] and POLARMAP[2] - have been published which produce 2D-layouts while trying to preserve pairwise angles between data objects. This approach allows easily to apply binning strategies that reduce computational complexity drastically.

In this paper, we present some improvements concerning angle based projections. Thus, an extension will be proposed that compensates the limitations of angle based mappings, by arranging these layouts in three dimensions performing an additional step. Further, we propose some suitable preprocessing strategies that can improved the layout quality considerably.

The rest of the paper is organized as follows. In section 2 we describe the idea of angle based multi-dimensional scaling. Section 3 describes a new data preprocessing step. Section 4 presents the 3D-extension to angle based mapping and section 5 shows results. Finally, we conclude with section 6.

C. Tang et al. (Eds.): ADMA 2008, LNAI 5139, pp. 3–14, 2008.

2   Angle Based Mappings

When analyzing high-dimensional data, one is typically interested in visualizing the data. A general overview of the data structure often excludes some hypothesis and helps to follow other. Unfortunately it is not possible to visualize directly data that comprise more than three attributes. A very common technique – multi-dimensional scaling – provides dimension reduction without simply cutting away one ore more dimensions. Instead, it arranges the data in a lower dimensional space, while trying to keep original properties of the data. Usually, such methods try to preserve distances, i.e. dissimilarities, between pairs of objects. Many applications have shown that MDS works adequately. However, it is a matter of fact that, due to its quadratic character of distance considerations, distance based MDS techniques suffer under high computational cost. This is why many research focused on the improvement of multi-dimensional scaling [3, 4, 5, 6, 7].

In this section we briefly describe two angle based mapping techniques that speed-up the mapping procedure but having another optimization criterion, namely preserving angles between pairs of objects. Both techniques have in common that the length of each data vector will be preserved exactly and only angles need to be optimized. This approach reduces the number of variables to optimize by half for 2D mappings. One disadvantage of angle based mapping is the limitation to 2D. This issue will be addressed after the following description of MDS_{polar} and POLARMAP.

2.1 MDS_{polar}

For a p-dimensional dataset $X = \{x_1, \dots, x_n\}$, MDS_{polar} determines a 2-dimensional representation in polar coordinates $Y = \{(l_1, \varphi_1), \dots, (l_n, \varphi_n)\}$, where the length l_k of the original vector x_k is preserved and only the angle φ_k has to be optimized. This solution is defined to be optimal, if all angles between pairs of data objects in the projected dataset Y coincide as good as possible with the angles in the original feature space X.

A straight forward definition of an objective function to be minimized for this problem, taking all angles into account, would be

$$E = \sum_{k=2}^{n} \sum_{i=1}^{k-1} (|\varphi_i - \varphi_k| - \psi_{ik})^2 \qquad (1)$$

where φ_k is the angle of y_k, ψ_{ik} is the positive angle between x_i and x_k, $0 \leq \psi_{ik} \leq \pi$. E is minimal, if the difference of the angle of each pair of vectors of dataset X and the corresponding two vectors in dataset Y is zero. The absolute value is chosen in equation (1) because the order of the minuends can have an influence on the sign of the resulting angle. As discussed in [1] equation (1) is not suitable for finding an analytical solution or a gradient descent technique, since functional E is not differentiable in all points. Instead, is it appropriate to optimize the following function

$$E = \sum_{k=2}^{n} \sum_{i=1}^{k-1} (\varphi_i - \varphi_k - \psi_{ik})^2. \qquad (2)$$

which is easily differentiable. Disadvantageously, minimization of equation (2) would not lead to acceptable results, because an angle between y_i and y_k, that might perfectly match the angle ψ_{ik}, $\varphi_i - \varphi_k$ can either be ψ_{ik} or $-\psi_{ik}$. Therefore, when minimizing functional (2) in order to actually minimize functional (1), one can take the freedom to choose whether to be the term $\varphi_i - \varphi_k$ or the term $\varphi_k - \varphi_i$ to appear in equation (2).

Being free to choose between $\varphi_i - \varphi_k$ and $\varphi_k - \varphi_i$ in equation (2), one needs to take the following into account

$$(\varphi_k - \varphi_i - \psi_{ik})^2 = (-(\varphi_k - \varphi_i - \psi_{ik}))^2 = (\varphi_i - \varphi_k + \psi_{ik})^2.$$

Therefore, instead of exchanging the order of φ_i and φ_k, one can choose the sign of ψ_{ik}, leading to

$$E = \sum_{k=2}^{n} \sum_{i=1}^{k-1} (\varphi_i - \varphi_k - \theta_{ik}\psi_{ik})^2 \qquad (3)$$

with $\theta_{ik} = \{-1, 1\}$. In order to solve this modified optimization problem of equation (3) it is to take the partial derivatives of E, yielding

$$\frac{\partial E}{\partial \varphi_k} = -2 \sum_{i=1}^{k-1} (\varphi_i - \varphi_k - \theta_{ik}\psi_{ik}). \qquad (4)$$

To fulfil the necessary condition for a minimum one sets equation (4) equal to zero and solves it for the φ_k-values, which leads to

$$\varphi_k = \frac{\sum_{i=1}^{k-1} \varphi_i - \sum_{i=1}^{k-1} \theta_{ik}\psi_{ik}}{k-1}. \qquad (5)$$

Primarely, the solution is described by a system of linear equations. However, still the signs in form of the θ_{ik}-values need to be determined, which is usually done by an interative algorithm that greedily changes stress diminishing signs θ_{ik}.

2.2 POLARMAP

As for MDS$_{polar}$ also POLARMAP maps p-dimensional data onto the plane with the objective to preserve pairwise angles ψ_{ij} between data objects (x_i, x_j) as accurate as possible. Vector lengths l_k are preserved exactly. As an extension of MDS$_{polar}$, POLARMAP learns a function f that provides for any p-dimensional feature vector x_k the corresponding angle φ_k that is needed to map the feature vector to a 2-dimensional feature space.

Analogous to functional (1), intuitively one would define the objective function E as follows:

$$E = \sum_{i=1}^{n-1} \sum_{j=i+1}^{n} \left(|f(x_i) - f(x_j)| - \psi_{ij} \right)^2. \qquad (6)$$

E is minimal, if, for each pair of feature vectors, the difference of the two angles, which are computed by the respective function f is equal to the measured angle ψ_{ij} of the two vectors in the original space. Since functional (6) is not differentiable, again, it is reasonable to consider the following function

$$E = \sum_{i=1}^{n-1} \sum_{j=i+1}^{n} \left(f(x_i) - f(x_j) - \psi_{ij} \right)^2. \tag{7}$$

while handling the thusly arising sign problem separately. Function f might be any function, in the simplest case it is

$$f(x) = a^T \cdot \tilde{x} \tag{8}$$

where a is vector whose components are the parameters to be optimized and $\tilde{x}$ is the feature vector x itself or a modification of x. In the simplest case

$$\tilde{x} = x \tag{9}$$
$$a = (a_1, a_2, \dots, a_p)^T$$

will be used, where f describes in fact the linear combination of the components of x. Replacing term f by the respective function

$$E = \sum_{i=1}^{n-1} \sum_{j=i+1}^{n} \left(a^T \tilde{x}_i - a^T \tilde{x}_j - \psi_{ij} \right)^2 \tag{10}$$

$$= \sum_{i=1}^{n-1} \sum_{j=i+1}^{n} \left(a^T (\tilde{x}_i - \tilde{x}_j) - \psi_{ij} \right)^2 \tag{11}$$

and substituing $\tilde{x}_i - \tilde{x}_j$ by $\tilde{x}_{ij}$ and considering the signs θ_{ij} one finally gets

$$E = \sum_{i=1}^{n-1} \sum_{j=i+1}^{n} \left(\theta_{ij} a^T \tilde{x}_{ij} - \psi_{ij} \right)^2. \tag{12}$$

Again, stress minimizing signs, in form of $\theta_{ij} \in \{1, -1\}$, can be iteratively determined by means of a greedy algorithm (see [2]).

2.3 Binning

The computational complexity of angle based mappings would be fairly high when intending to find the global minimum of E since all possible sign configurations should be checked. Of course, this would be unacceptable. In this regard, the use of polar coordinates for the target space and preserving the length of each feature vector allows the application of binning techniques.

The length perseveration already guarantees a roughly correct placement of the feature vectors in the lower dimensional space. This property enables to reduce the complexity of the algorithm based on the idea that it is chiefly important to map similar feature vectors in the original space X close to each other in the target space, whereas pairs of feature vectors with a large distance should also be mapped far away from each other. However, for vectors with a large distance, it is not important to match the original distance exactly, but it is sufficient to make sure that they will not be mapped close to each other. When the lengths of two vectors differ significantly, a certain distance between the projected vectors is already guaranteed, even if the angle between both does not match at all. Using this property, it is not necessary to consider the angles between all vectors. For those vectors having a significant difference in length, the angle can be neglected.

Consequently, bins containing subsets of data objects can be defined over the vector lengths. Feature vectors of similar length are represented by the same bin. Sorting the data according to the vector lengths permits to easily implement the binning concept. Then, in order to define the bins, the sorted dataset only has to be iterated until the bin criterion has been violated first. The bin criterion can be controlled by a binning function. In [1, 2], a generalization is discussed that introduces weighting functions with the objective to weight angle differences and to control the binning procedure. Introducing weights in MDS$_{polar}$ leads to

$$E = \sum_{k=2}^{n} \sum_{i=1}^{k-1} w_{ik} \left(\varphi_i - \varphi_k - \theta_{ik} \psi_{ik} \right)^2 \tag{13}$$

and in POLARMAP to

$$E = \sum_{i=1}^{n-1} \sum_{j=i+1}^{n} w_{ij} \left(\theta_{ij} a^T \tilde{x}_{ij} - \psi_{ij} \right)^2 . \tag{14}$$

When simply minimzing the relative error, $w_{ij} = 1/\psi_{ij}^2$ can be chosen. In respects of binning, an appropriate weighting function is used to control weights aiming to get a preferably low number of non-zero weights, which will guarantee computational efficiency.

3 Preprocessing for Angle Based Mappings

As discussed in the literature [1, 2], one preprocessing step is very important. Since angles ψ_{ij} of pairs of objects (x_i, x_j) in the original space are defined to be positive (or $0 \leq \psi_{ij} \leq \pi$ respectively), it cannot be guaranteed to approximate these angles on the plane properly, even for 2D datasets. This problem can be solved easily by translating all feature vectors into the first quadrant. More generally, for a high-dimensional dataset a translation can be applied that makes all components of data vectors non-negative. For this, the largest negative value of each component occurring in the dataset must be determined. These can be used as positive values of the corresponding components of the translation vector. In the following we discuss some new approaches tp preprocess the data in such a way that the mapping quality will be improved.

3.1 Increasing Vector Length Variability by Geometrical Transformations

As mentioned earlier, a roughly correct placement of the feature vectors in the target space can be achieved taking the vector lengths into account. According to this, we assume that mappings can be improved when the initial data is characterized by a great variability of vector lengths. Then, the starting stress should be considerably lower and either, or both, the number of iterations until convergence and the final layout quality should be improved.

Having this concept in mind, we propose to augment the vector length variability of the dataset by means of geometrical transformations such as reflections on axes and subsequent translation into the first quadrant. The terminal translation into the first quadrant, i.e. making all components of data vectors non-negative, is important as discussed above. Note, these transformations do not change any inter-data properties. Since MDS_{polar} and POLARMAP allow the transformation of new unseen data, all geometrical transformations must be stored in order to process new data accordingly.

A simple measure, measuring the vector lengths variability v can be

$$v = \frac{\sigma_l}{\bar{l}} \tag{15}$$

where σ_l is the standard deviation (i.e. the variation) of the vector lengths and $\bar{l}$ is the mean vector length of the dataset. Only considering vector lengths variation would be misleading sometimes. The quotient is suggestive because it describes the weighting of variation with the mean vector lengths. Of course, the number of possible combinations of consecutive geometrical transformations increases with the number of variables of the data. Thus, when mapping datasets with many variables, only a sample of all transformation combinations should be considered with regard to computational costs. From the list of all gathered v, the dataset with the greatest quotient v would be the choice to be mapped.

3.2   Increasing Vector Length Variability by Principal Axis Transformation

Principal axis transformation is a technique used to arrange a multi-dimensional dataset along its principal axes regarding their variances. As a result, a new dataset will be created whose inter-data properties have not changed but whose new variables comprise partial components of all original variables (i.e. the principal components). The first new component comprises the highest variance of the data. All remaining components will be ordered, decreasing with its respective variance.

This first step guarantees a fairly high variation in the vector lengths. However, since a translation into the first quadrand is mandatory, the vector lengths variation can be augmented by means of a rotation about 45° with respect to all axes except the x-axis (or generally the first axis).

Advantageous to the previous approach is the one-time transformation that provides an efficient arrangement of the data ensuring high vector lengths variations. The transformation of new data, as well as backward transformation is easily possible, when storing eigenvectors and translation vectors from the axis transformation and geometrical translation.

4   A 3D-Extension to Angle Based Mappings

Angle based mappings, as discussed above, are strictly limited to 2D so far. However, it is obvious that a third dimension for the mapping could lower the transformation stress

1: Given a dataset $X = \{x_1, x_2, \ldots, x_n\} \subset \mathbb{R}^p$

2: Compute $[X', \Phi] = \text{ANGLEBASEDMAPPING}(X, \text{BINSIZE})$

3: Randomly initialize $H = \{h_1, h_2, \ldots, h_n\} \subset \mathbb{R}$

4: Compute d_{ij}^x, $\quad i, j = 1, \ldots, n$

5: Define learning rate α

6: Define threshold $\tilde{E}$

7: **repeat**

8: $\quad$ Compute d_{ij}^y, $\quad i, j = 1, \ldots, n$

9: $\quad$ Compute $\partial E / \partial h_k$, $\quad k = 1, \ldots, n$

10: $\quad$ Update $h_k = h_k - \alpha \frac{\partial E}{\partial h_k}$, $\quad k = 1, \ldots, n$

11: **until** $\sum_{k=1}^{n} \frac{\partial E}{\partial h_k} < \tilde{E}$

12: Output projected data $Y = \{y_1, y_2, \ldots, y_n\} \subset \mathbb{R}^3$

Algorithm 1. 3D-Extension to angle based mappings

and up the information gain. For this reason, we propose in this section an extension that opens a third dimension on the basis of angle based mappings. As for conventional, i.e. distance based, multi-dimensional scaling, we propose to minimize a distance based stress function:

$$E = \sum_{k=1}^{n} \sum_{i=k+1}^{n} (d_{ik}^y - d_{ik}^x)^2 \tag{16}$$

with d_{ij}^x for the pairwise distances in the original space $d_{ij}^x = \|x_i - x_j\|$ and d_{ij}^y, the pairwise distances in the 3D target space $d_{ij}^y = \|y_i - y_j\|$. Then, vectors in the target space have the following form

$$y = \begin{pmatrix} l \cdot \cos \varphi \\ l \cdot \sin \varphi \\ h \end{pmatrix}$$

with h as the parameter zu optimize. Accordingly, distance d_{ik}^y of two vectors in the target space is

$$d_{ik}^y = \sqrt{(l_i \cos \varphi_i - l_k \cos \varphi_k)^2 + (l_i \sin \varphi_i - l_k \sin \varphi_k)^2 + (h_i - h_k)^2}. \tag{17}$$

Stress function (16) can be easily minimized applying a gradient descent technique. For this purpose we need the partial derivatives of E for h_k, the parameter we are looking for.

As a first we derive equation (17) partially for h_k we get

$$\frac{\partial d_{ik}^y}{\partial h_k} = \frac{1}{2}\Big((l_i \cos \varphi_i - l_k \cos \varphi_k)^2 + (l_i \sin \varphi_i - l_k \sin \varphi_k)^2 + (h_i - h_k)\Big)^{-\frac{1}{2}} \cdot 2(h_i - h_k) \cdot (-1)$$

simplifying to

$$\frac{\partial d_{ik}^y}{\partial h_k} = \frac{1}{\sqrt{(r_i \cos \varphi_i - l_k \cos \varphi_k)^2 + (l_i \sin \varphi_i - l_k \sin \varphi_k)^2 + (h_i - h_k)}} \cdot (h_i - h_k)$$

$$= -\frac{1}{d_{ik}^y} \cdot (h_i - h_k)$$

$$= -\frac{h_i - h_k}{d_{ik}^y}.$$

Finally, in order to minimize the stress function (16) we take the partial derivatives for h_k obtaining

$$\frac{\partial E}{\partial h_k} = -2 \sum_{i \neq k} (d_{ik}^y - d_{ik}^x) \frac{h_i - h_k}{d_{ik}^y}. \tag{18}$$

Considering a learning rate α we get the following update equation

$$h_k = h_k - \alpha \frac{\partial E}{\partial h_k}. \tag{19}$$

Algorithm 1 describes the general iterative procedure schematically. In order to preserve simplicity in this scheme, the use of bins is not considered. Of course, it is very efficient to use the same bins as already used by the angle based mapping since gradient calculations can then be limited to a small sample of the entire data yielding slightly higher stress values only.

5 Experiments

In this section we discuss some experimental results on various benchmark datasets: the Iris data, the Wine data and a synthetic dataset.

5.1 Preprocessing for Angle Based Mappings – Experimental Results

Figure 1(a) shows a simple 2-dimensional synthetic dataset that ideally shows some characteristics of the proposed preprocessing steps. The dataset contains one hundred data points that scatter around the point of origin with a radius of approximately ten length units. That means that the vector lengths are roughly identical and the data is primarily differentiated via the angles. Results for the proposed geometrical transformations and the principal axis transformation are shown in figure 2 for various bin sizes used for the angle based mapping[1]. The figure shows graphs for four different stress measures: (a) Sammon stress [8] on a POLARMAP transformation using absolute angles, (b) Sammon stress using weighted angles, (c) absolute POLARMAP stress and (d) weighted POLARMAP stress. From these graphs it can be seen that data representations having low vector length variations yield considerably smaller stress values, except for the Sammon stress for absolute angle optimization. The impact of the bin size, which is fairly high for low vector length variations, is negligible when increasing the vector length variations. The results for the geometrical transformation and the principle axis transformation (PAT) differ slightly. In the graphs these curves overlap almost completely.

Figures 3 and 4 show the results on the Iris dataset and the Wine dataset. In the majority of cases, increasing bin sizes improve the layout quality, which is not surprising. Regarding the proposed preprocessing steps, no definite picture can be gained. Sometimes the expected improvements can be observed, sometimes not. For high vector lengths variability based mappings it can be observed that an increase of the bin size has only little impcat on the layout quality, when a certain level is reached (see figure 4(a), 4(b) and 4(c)). This confirms that the vector lengths based bining strategy leads to reasonable results. Mostly, PAT based transformations lay between low and high vector length variability based tranformations and yield the most stable good quality results.

5.2   3D-Extension to Angle Based Mappings – Experimental Results

Figures 1(b) and 1(c) show experimental results of the proposed 3D-extension for angle based mappings on two well known benchmark datasets. The Iris dataset contains three classes of fifty instances each, where each class refers to a type of iris plant [9]. The Wine dataset results from a chemical analysis of wines grown in the same region in Italy but derived from three different cultivars. The analysis determined the quantities of thirteen constituents found in each of the three types of wines (which form the class attribute). In the figures, each class is represented be a respective symbol (class 1: □, class 2: ◇, class 3: ○). Both mappings are obtained using POLARMAP and the 3D-extension. Basis for the Iris mapping is a weighted POLARMAP transformation using a bin size of 20. As basis for the Wine mapping, a weighted POLARMAP transformation is used with a bin size of 40. Figures 3(b) and 4(b) show that these mappings have low stress values and should be suitable basis for the extension. The bin sizes from the basis mapping are kept. The Iris mapping clearly benefits from the 3D-extension. While class 1 can be distinguished easily on the plane already, the remaining two classes are stretched over the third dimension which helps to separate them. For the Wine data only little improvement can be denoted. Admittedly, class 1 and class 2 are hardly distinguishable also in higher dimensional spaces.

---

[1] All examples given in this paper are obtained using POLARMAP. Note, that similar results will be obtained using MDS_{polar}.

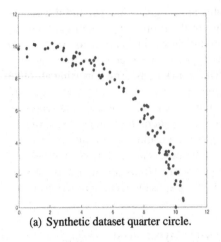

(a) Synthetic dataset quarter circle.

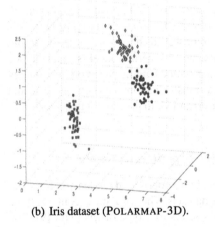

(b) Iris dataset (POLARMAP-3D).

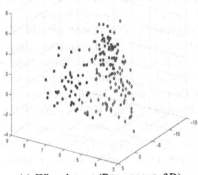

(c) Wine dataset (POLARMAP-3D).

Fig. 1.

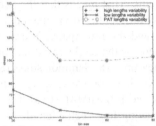

(a) Sammon stress on angle based mappings using absolute angles

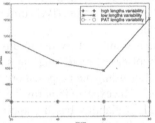

(b) Sammon stress on angle based mappings using weighted angles

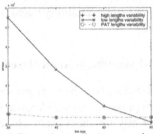

(c) Stress (according to equation 12) on angle based mappings using absolute angles

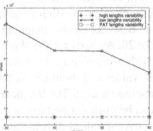

(d) Stress (according to equation 14) on angle based mappings using weighted angles

Fig. 2. Experimental results for the synthetic dataset

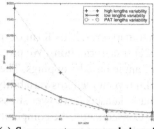

(a) Sammon stress on angle based mappings using absolute angles

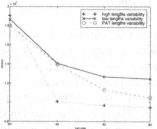

(a) Sammon stress on angle based mappings using absolute angles

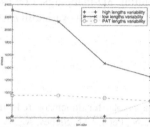

(b) Sammon stress on angle based mappings using weighted angles

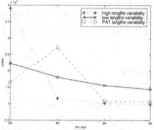

(b) Sammon stress on angle based mappings using weighted angles

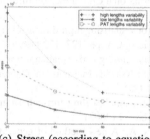

(c) Stress (according to equation 12) on angle based mappings using absolute angles

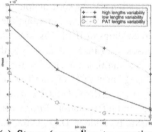

(c) Stress (according to equation 12) on angle based mappings using absolute angles

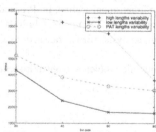

(d) Stress (according to equation 14) on angle based mappings using weighted angles

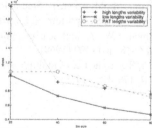

(d) Stress (according to equation 14) on angle based mappings using weighted angles

Fig. 3. Experimental results for the Iris dataset

Fig. 4. Experimental results for the Wine dataset

6 Conclusion

In this paper we considered the subject of angle based mappings. This form of multi-dimensional scaling allows efficient computations of 2D-transformations. We proposed two new techniques that improve the layout quality of angle based mappings. The first addresses the preprocessing of the raw data, such that high vector lengths variability can be gained. We could show by means of some benchmark datasets that lower stress values will be obtained and smaller bin sizes can be used. Consequently, the computational complexity can be slightly decreased. The second consists of a 3D-extension to angle based mapping techniques. Therewith, the earlier 2D-limitation can be compensated and more insight can be gained by means of the resulting 3D-mappings. Preprocessing methods that transform the raw data such that the vector lengths variability will be maximized will be subject of future research.

References

[1] Rehm, F., Klawonn, F., Kruse, R.: Mds$_{polar}$ - a new approach for dimension reduction to visualize high dimensional data. In: Famili, A.F., Kok, J.N., Pena, J.M., Siebes, A., Feelders, A. (eds.) IDA 2005. LNCS, vol. 3646, pp. 316–327. Springer, Heidelberg (2005)

[2] Rehm, F., Klawonn, F., Kruse, R.: Polarmap - a new approach to visualisation of high dimensional data. In: IEEE Proceedings of the Tenth International Conference on Information Visualisation (IV 2006), London, pp. 731–740 (2006)

[3] Chalmers, M.: A linear iteration time layout algorithm for visualising high-dimensional data. In: Proceedings of IEEE Visualization 1996, San Francisco, CA, pp. 127–132 (1996)

[4] Faloutsos, C., Lin, K.: A fast algorithm for indexing, data-mining and visualization of traditional and multimedia datasets. In: Proceedings of ACM SIGMOD International Conference on Management of Data, San Jose, CA, pp. 163–174 (1995)

[5] Morrison, A., Ross, G., Chalmers, M.: Fast multidimensional scaling through sampling, springs and interpolation. Information Visualization 2, 68–77 (2003)

[6] Pekalska, E., Ridder, D.D., Duin, R.P.W., Kraaijveld, M.A.: A new method of generalizing sammon mapping with application to algorithm speed-up. In: Boasson, M., Kaandorp, J.A., Tonino, J.F.M., Vosselman, M.G. (eds.) Proceedings of the 5th Annual Conference of the Advanced School for Computing and Imaging (ASCI 1999), pp. 221–228 (1999)

[7] Williams, M., Munzner, T.: Steerable, progressive multidimensional scaling. In: Proceedings the 10th IEEE Symposium on Information Visualization, Austin, TX, pp. 57–64 (2004)

[8] Sammon, J.W.: A nonlinear mapping for data structure analysis. IEEE Transactions Computer C-18, 401–409 (1969)

[9] Fisher, R.A.: The use of multiple measurements in taxonomic problems. Annual Eugenics 7, Part II, 179–188 (1936)

Mining Natural Language Programming Directives with Class-Oriented Bayesian Networks

Manolis Maragoudakis[1], Nikolaos Cosmas[2], and Aristogiannis Garbis[2]

[1] Artificial Intelligence Laboratory, University of the Aegean
83200 Samos, Greece
mmarag@aegean.gr
[2] Network Technologies Laboratory, Technical Education Institute of Messolonghi
30200, Messolonghi, Greece
{ncosmas,agarbis}@teimes.gr

Abstract. Learning a programming language is a painstaking process, as it requires knowledge of its syntax, apart from knowing the basic process of representing logical sequences to programming stages. This fact deteriorates the coding process and expels most users from programming. Particularly for novice users or persons with vision problems, learning of how to program and tracing the syntax errors could be improved dramatically by using the most natural of all interfaces, i.e. natural language. Towards this orientation, we suggest a wider framework for allowing programming using natural language. The framework can be easily extended to support different object-oriented programming languages such as C, C++, Visual Basic or Java. Our suggested model is named "Language Oriented Basic" and it concerns an intelligent interface that supports code creation, modification and control in Visual Basic. Users can use simple-structured Greek sentences in natural language and the system can output the corresponding syntactic tree. When users declare end of input, the system transforms the syntactic trees to source code. Throughout the whole interaction process, users can check the under-development code in order to verify its correspondence to their expectations. Due to the fact that using natural language can cause a great degree of ambiguity, Bayesian networks and learning from examples have been utilized as an attempt to reason on the most probable programming representation, given a natural language input sentence. In order to enhance the classifier, we propose a novel variation of Bayesian networks that favor the classification process. Experimental results have depicted precision and recall measures in a range of 73% and 70% respectively.

1 Introduction

Since the early 1980s, researchers have pointed out the significance of natural language as a means of instructing commands in a programming language. The term "Natural Language Programming" has been proposed ([2],[14],[17]) to represent the process where humans interact with machines in their own language. The ability to program in natural language instead of traditional programming languages would enable people to use familiar constructs in expressing their requests, thus making

C. Tang et al. (Eds.): ADMA 2008, LNAI 5139, pp. 15–26, 2008.

machines accessible to a wider user group. Automatic speech recognition and synthesis devices could eventually smooth the communication even further.

On the other side, scientists like [4],[15] and [18] have argued that the semantic and syntactic hypothesis space for such a task is too large to be handled by current technology. Users are able to use a plethora of natural language expressions instead of providing input in a strict syntactic manner like most programming languages define. This voluminous and very detailed set could deteriorate the parsing phase, leading to significant time delays. Moreover, this vagueness and ambiguity may result in poor translations of what users actually meant by the machine. A third argument asserts that no one would use a natural language programming system, even if one existed, because it would be too verbose. Why should one be willing to input long and wordy descriptions of a desired computation when there exist simple, easy to learn, and concise notations for doing the same thing?

Reasonable as these arguments may seem, the present work will attempt to show that some of them can be effectively handled using careful system design and the strength of an artificial intelligence discipline, called machine learning. Machine Learning describes the process of making machines able to automatically infer about the world. We propose a system called "Language-Oriented Basic" that can cope with simple Visual Basic programming commands, written in natural language. The system is based on learning from examples, in a sense that domain knowledge about the programming language is being encoded to it through past experience. By past experience we mean user input in natural language that has been annotated in order to form the training set for the machine learner. The collection of such data was carried out using the Wizard of Oz methodology, in which users were supposed to interact with a machine, instructing it using sentences in Modern Greek, only that a domain expert was behind the machine throughout the whole experiment. Upon completion of the annotation phase, Bayesian networks were utilized in order to infer on the most probable programming interpretation, given the input of the user. The whole architecture, as well as the linguistic tools that were used, shall be discussed in the next section.

1.1 Background

The first attempts in natural language programming were rather ambitious, targeting the generation of complete computer programs that would compile and run. As an example, the "NLC" prototype [1] aimed at creating a natural language interface for processing data stored in arrays and matrices, with the ability of handling low level operations such as the transformation of numbers into type declarations. This trend was not followed and thus, more recently, researchers have attempted to re-look at the problem of natural language programming, but with more realistic anticipations, and with a different, much larger pool of resources (e.g. broad spectrum commonsense knowledge, the Web) and a suite of significantly advanced publicly available natural language processing tools. Pane & Myers [12] conducted a series of studies with non-programming fifth grade users, and identified some of the programming models implied by the users' natural language descriptions. In a similar way, Lieberman & Liu [9] have conducted a feasibility study and showed how a partial understanding of a text, coupled with a dialogue with the user, can help non-expert users make their intentions more precise when designing a computer program. Their study resulted in a system called METAFOR [10], able to translate natural language statements into class descriptions with the associated objects and methods. A similar area that received a fair bit of attention in recent years is the construction of natural language interfaces to databases, which allows users to query structured data using natural language questions. For instance, the system described in [7], implements rules for mapping natural to "formal" languages using syntactic and semantic parsing of the input text.

This paper is structured as follows: Section 2 discusses the architecture of the proposed system describing the linguistic aspects of the approach. In Section 3, we refer to the Machine Learning algorithms that formed the basis of our inferring module, while Section 4 discusses the experimental results, followed by the concluding remarks.

2 The Language-Oriented Basic System

The system is comprised of three basic phases; a) a natural language processing subsystem, which takes a Greek sentence and uses Machine Learning methods to estimate the most probable interpretation to programming code (e.g. loops, arrays, control structures, etc) b) a module for transforming syntactic trees to source code and c) a module for managing the intercourse (e.g. if the user writes add, it may imply the addition operation of the inclusion of a new variable). Fig. 1 illustrates the interconnection of the system modules, as regards to the interaction process. Initially, the input is provided in text form, using Modern Greek, describing a programming directive. The natural language processing system is activated to retrieve any parts of the sentence triggering the programming elements such as arrays, variables, control structures, etc. By using intelligent techniques, the most probable element is identified, which is coded in the form of a tree. If the structure of the tree is complete, meaning that all nodes have the expected values (e.g. in a *for* loop, the initial count, the condition and the step have been identified) the source code module is transcribing the tree to code. The code is visible to the user for any corrections and can be saved to a file. If the tree is missing some parts, the interaction module asks the user for supplementary information.

2.1 Implementation

The association to programming directives of an input query could be considered as the process of searching for the optimal (most probable) programming commands through the space of candidate similar commands for a specific language, provided the lexical and syntactic items that define the meaning of the query. In our approach, a stochastic model for modeling programming code disambiguation is defined over a search space $H*T$, where H denotes the set of possible lexical contexts that could be identified within an input query $\{h_1,...,h_k\}$ or "*input variables*" and T denotes the set of the allowable programming commands $\{t_1,...,t_n\}$. Using Bayes' rule, the probability of the optimal interpretation T_{opt} equals to:

$$T_{opt} = \underset{T\in\{t_1...t_n\}}{\operatorname{argmax}} p(T\,|\,H) = \underset{T\in\{t_1...t_n\}}{\operatorname{argmax}} \frac{p(H\,|\,T)p(T)}{p(H)} = \underset{T\in\{t_1...t_n\}}{\operatorname{argmax}} p(H\,|\,T)p(T) \qquad (1)$$

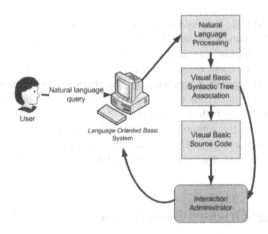

Fig. 1. Course of information when parsing the user input by the Language Oriented Basic system

The objective is to estimate the terms of the above equation for a given input vector of lexical items ($\{h_1,...,h_k\}$). As an example, consider the following input sentence:
"Declare an integer with value 0."
The system should first recognize the items of the input that define the meaning (*Declare, integer, value*) and estimate the probability the programming directive *"Variables"* have over the other directives (e.g. *Arrays, Loop, Functions*, etc). If this probability outclasses the other, then we can assume that the system has correctly recognized that this sentence implies the declaration of a variable. In other words, as section 3 explains, classification is needed in order to infer on the most probable programming command.

In order to obtain a pool of input examples, we ask 20 different users with varying experience in programming to supply 25 sentences, covering notions such as variable declaration, operands, loops, control structures with one condition (simple if then-else) and arrays. The set of training examples was annotated with morphology information, phrase chunking and simple SVO tags.

2.2 Linguistic Tools

As regards to the morphological analyzer, the problem is generally not deterministic and many approaches have been proposed to deal with it. In our implementation we have used a straightforward approach that is language independent, requires no model of the language or any other type of pre-programmed linguistic information and uses a single data structure. The structure is a specially structured lexicon that contains the lemmas, the inflected forms of the words and their grammatical features stored in a Directed Acyclic Word Graph (DAWG). The structure has certain similarities to a lexical transducer: it incorporates surface and lexical forms as well as the appropriate morphological information. It differs in the way these forms and information are stored. The analyzer is able to identify 10,000 words per second on a modest PC.

The phrase boundary detector, or chunker, is based on very limited linguistic resources, i.e. a small keyword lexicon containing some 450 keywords (articles, pronouns, auxiliary verbs, adverbs, prepositions etc.) and a suffix lexicon of 300 of the most common word suffixes in MG. In a first stage the boundaries of non-embedded, intra-sentential noun (NP), prepositional (PP), verb (VP) and adverbial phrases (ADP) are detected via multi-pass parsing. Smaller phrases are formed in the first passes, while later passes form more complex structures. In a second stage the head-word of every noun phrase is identified and the phrase inherits its grammatical properties. Upon completion of the afore-mentioned phase, a shallow syntactic parser is involved, in order to extract the tuples of SVO (subject, verb, direct and indirect object) of each main and secondary clause. This parser is a rule based one, where the rules were introduced by a linguist with experience in medical terminology.

3 Bayesian Classifiers

Classification is known to be a fundamental concept in the fields of data mining and pattern recognition. It requires the construction of a function that assigns a target or class label to a given example, described by a set of attributes. This function is referred to as a "classifier". There are numerous machine learning algorithms such as neural networks, decision trees, rules and graphical models that attempt to induce a classifier, given a set of annotated, pre-classified instances. The ability of that classifier to generalize over the training data, i.e. to perform well on new, unseen examples, is of great importance for any domain, including natural language programming.

While Bayesian graphical models were known for being a powerful mechanism for knowledge representation and reasoning under conditions of uncertainty, is was only after the introduction of the so-called Naïve Bayesian classifier ([5],[8]) that they were regarded as classifiers, with a prediction performance similar to state-of-the-art classifiers. The Naïve Bayesian classifier performs inference by applying Bayes rule to compute the posterior probability of a class C, given a particular vector of input variables A_i. It then outputs the class whose posterior probability is the highest. Regarding its computational cost, inference in Naïve Bayes is feasible, due to two assumptions, yet often unrealistic for real world applications:

- All the attributes A_i are conditionally independent of each other, given the classification variable.
- All other attributes are directly dependent on the class variable.

Despite the fact that Naïve Bayes performs well, it is obviously counterintuitive to ignore the correlation of the variables in some domains. Bayesian networks [13] provide a comprehensive means for effective representation of independence assumptions. They are capable of effectively coping with the non-realistic naïve Bayes restriction, since they allow stating conditional independence assumptions that apply to all or to subsets of the variables. A Bayesian network is consisted of a qualitative and quantitative portion, namely its structure and its conditional probability distributions respectively. Given a set of attributes $A=\{A_1,...,A_k\}$, where each variable A_i could take values from a finite set, a Bayesian network describes the probability distribution over this set of variables. We use capital letters as X,Y to denote variables and lower case as x,y to denote values taken by these variables. Formally, a Bayesian network is an annotated Directed Acyclic Graph (DAG) that encodes a joint probability distribution.

We denote a network B as a pair $B=<S,P>$ where S is a DAG whose nodes correspond to the attributes of A. P refers to the set of probability distributions that quantifies the network. S embeds the following conditional independence assumption:

Each variable A_i is independent of its non-descendants given its parent nodes. P includes information about the probability distribution of a value a_i of variable A_i, given the values of its immediate predecessors in the graph, which are also called "parents". This probability distribution is stored in a table, which is called conditional probability table. The unique joint probability distribution over A that a network B describes can be computed using:

$$p_B(A_1,...,A_n) = \prod_{i=1}^{n} p(A_i \mid parents(A_i))$$
(2)

3.1 Learning Bayesian Networks from Data

There are actually two known methodologies for determining the structure of a Bayesian network. The former is manually, by a human domain expert who should provide the interconnection of the variables. The latter is to having the structure determined automatically by learning from a set of training instances. Regarding the learning of the conditional probability table of a network, the same principle applies. The parameters of the table could either be provided manually by an expert or estimated automatically through a learning procedure. The task of handcrafting the parameters is a laborious one. Besides, in some applications it is simply infeasible for a human expert to know a priori both the structure and the conditional probability distributions.

The Bayesian learning process demonstrates an asymptotic correctness in terms of producing a learned network that is a close approximation of the probability distribution of a domain (assuming that the training instances are generated independently from a fixed distribution). However, in practice there are cases where the learning process returns a network with a relative good probability over the data, yet with a poor classification performance. In order to portray the reason for the discrepancy between good predictive accuracy and good Bayesian learning score, recall the Bayesian or MDL (Minimal Description Length) score [16], which provides a metric for determining the most probable network structure over a given training set. The MDL score of a network B given a training dataset D is given by:

$$MDL(B \mid D) = \frac{\log n}{2}|B| - LL(B \mid D)$$
(3)

where $|B|$ is the number of parameters in the network and n the number of features in the instances. In the above subtraction the first term represents the length of describing the network B in terms of bit while the second term is the log likelihood of B given D. Regarding a classification task, the log likelihood function is described by:

$$LL(B \mid D) = \sum_{i=1}^{n} \log p_B(C \mid A_1,...,A_n) + \sum_{i=1}^{n} \log p_B(A_1,...,A_n)$$
(4)

The first term in the above sum estimates how well the network B approximates the probability of a class given the attributes. This is actually the most classification-related among the two. The second term expresses the ability of B to reflect the joint distribution of the attributes. Unfortunately, the second term governs the first one since the number of possible attribute combinations grows exponentially in their number n. Thus, the log of the probability $p_B(A_1,...,A_n)$ will grow large [3].

It is more than obvious that we need a network structure that will accurately reflect the distribution of the attributes of a domain. Additionally, it will also perform well when it comes to classification. Some alternative network structures such as Tree-Augmented Naïve Bayes (TAN), and Bayesian Network Augmented Naïve Bayes (BAN) [6] consider that all attributes are affected by the class node. Perhaps this appears to be reasonable and sound, however when classifying, one might only want to take the really important attributes into account. The Bayesian theory suggests that only the nodes which are in the Markov blanket of the class node actually affect the class. This is not the case in the structures mentioned above, where their topology implies that all the attributes play a role in classification. In other words, no *feature selection* is performed.

Therefore, we propose a novel algorithm for learning Bayesian networks from data with a classification-oriented structure. This new type of network is called *Class-Oriented Bayesian Belief Network* or '*COr-BBN*'. We argue that a COr-BBN is suitable for classification since it retains the probability distribution of the domain and it also performs a feature selection for the given class. Unlike the unsupervised approach of the BBN learning technique, a COr-BBN knows the class prior to learning its structure and forces a potential arc from an attribute to the class to be reversed. By this approach, the class is always the cause of an attribute, thus when it comes to predict probability $p(C \mid A_1,...,A_n)$, by Bayes' rule it is transformed into

$$p(C \mid A_1,...,A_n) = \frac{p(A_1,...,A_n \mid C)p(C)}{p(A_1,...,A_n)}$$, where the term $p(A_1,...,A_n \mid C)$ can easily

be inferred according to the conditional probability table stored in the network. By imposing restrictions as regards to the direction of arcs, we can actually learn the optimal set of attributes that belong to the Markov Blanket of class C in computational time of $O(2^{n^2}/2)$. Recall that learning an undirected Bayesian network from data is an NP-hard problem [11].

The algorithmic analysis of the COr-BBN learning procedure is described below:

```
Given a dataset X, containing a set of attributes
A₁,…,Aₙ and a class C:
1. Compute the mutual information
```

$$I(A_i;C) = \sum_{a,c} p(a,c)\log\frac{p(a,c)}{p(a)p(c)}$$ between each attribute and

```
   the class C.
2. Set an edge constraint bias for arcs directing from
   each attribute to the class.
```

3. Using the MDL score, find the most probable network structure. Annotate the weight of each edge from X to Y found by $I(X;Y)$.
4. Build a maximum weighted Bayesian network and estimate the conditional probability table using the *Expectation-Maximization* (EM) algorithm.

Theorem 1. Given a dataset D of N instances, containing a set of n attributes $A_1,...,A_n$ and a class C, the COr-BBN learning procedure builds a network in time complexity of $O(2^{n^2}/2)$ and with maximum log likelihood.

Proof. The log-likelihood can be reformulated as follows [6]:

$$LL(B \mid D) = N \sum I(X_i; PAR_{x_i})$$ (5)

where X_i symbolizes any of the attributes or the class and PARXi is the set of parent nodes of X_i. Thus, if we maximize the first term of the above equation, we also maximize the log likelihood. Concerning the COr-BBN model, the class has no parents while the other attributes may have it as one. Thus, we have $I(C; PAR_C) = 0$ and $I(A_i; PAR_{A_i}) = I(A_i; PAR_{A_i}, C)$ if A_i has parent nodes other than C or $I(A_i; PAR_{A_i}) = I(A_i; C)$ if A_i has no other parents other than the class. So, we need to maximize the term $\sum I(A_i; PAR_{A_i}, C) + \sum I(A_i; C)$. By using the chain law ($I(X;Y,Z) = I(X;Z) + I(X;Y \mid Z)$), we can rewrite it as:

$$\sum I(A_i; C) + \sum I(A_i; PAR_{A_i} \mid C)$$ (6)

Note that the first term is independent of the parents of A_i. Therefore, it suffices to maximize the second term. Note also that the arc restriction that the COr-BBN imposes is guaranteed to maximize this term, and thus it maximizes the log likelihood. The complexity for the first step is $O(n^2N)$ and the complexity of the third step $O(2^{n^2}/2)$ due to the fact that we apply directional restrictions, posed in the second step. Since usually N>>n, we get the stated complexity, which refers to the case where during the search process, all the candidate pairs that invoke an arc from an attribute to the class are not considered.

4   Experimental Results

In order to evaluate the proposed methodology, we applied the 10-fold cross validation approach to the 500 instances data. The 90% of them was used for training and the remaining 10% as test. The process was repeated 10 times using different training and test sets. As for performance metrics, we chose precision and recall, borrowed from the information extraction domain. Accuracy in some domains, such as the one at hand, is not actually a good metric due to the fact that a classifier may reach high accuracy by simply always predicting the negative class. Furthermore, we also consider the F-measure metric. A set of well-known machine learning techniques have constituted the benchmark to which our results have been compared against the Bayesian networks approach. These algorithms were: C4.5, Naïve Bayes and ID3. Table 1 tabulates the performance of the system.

Table 1. Performance of the Language-Oriented Basic system

	Naïve Bayes	COR-BBN	C4.5	ID3
Precision	62,87	73,11	65,06	68,71
Recall	59,69	70,23	60,47	64,58
F-measure	61,28	71,67	62,765	66,64

The results can also be tabulated in Figure 2. As it can be seen, the Bayesian networks approach outperforms all the other algorithms by a varying factor of 5% to 11%. This supports our initial claim the Bayesian networks can effective encode the dependency assumptions of the input variables. On the contrast, the naïve Bayesian method is performing worse, due to the unrealistic assumption on the variable independency. Furthermore, the accuracy of the recognition system appears to be in acceptable levels, especially if we consider the classification process takes place in a large hypothesis space.

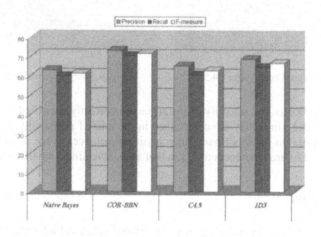

Fig. 2. Performance of the Language-Oriented system

Furthermore, in order to illustrate the difference in classification performance when incorporating the four classification methodologies, we provide the margin curves of the two Bayesian classifiers (Figures 3 to 6). The margin curve prints the cumulative frequency of the difference of the actual class probability and the highest probability predicted for the other classes (So, for a single class, if it is predicted to be positive with probability p, the margin is $p-(1-p)=2p-1$). Negative values denote classification errors, meaning that the dominant class is not the correct one.

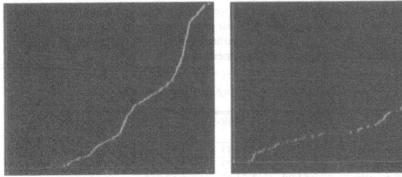

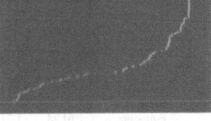

Fig. 3. Margin Curve using Naïve Bayes   **Fig. 4.** Margin Curve using COR-BBN

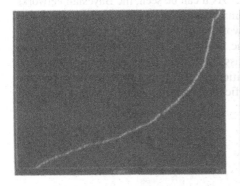

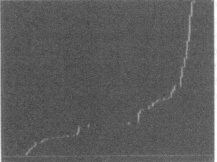

Fig. 5. Margin Curve using C4.5   **Fig. 6.** Margin Curve using ID3

As Figure 4 depicts, the majority of instances are correctly classified by the Bayesian network model, since they are centralized in the area of probability one (the right part of the graph). On the other hand, the classified instances of the other algorithms (Figures 3, 5 and 6) are not concentrated in that area, revealing a significant deviation.

5 Conclusions

Our objective in this study was to gain some refined empirical information about the nature of programming using natural language, to bring to bear on all these issues of increasing the usability and availability of computer language interfaces. Despite the fact that it was only a first attempt and keeping in mind that many essential linguistic tools such as semantic parsers and plan recognizers are not available for many languages, including Modern Greek, we established a data mining approach that is based on learning from past examples. Our major obstacles were style, semantics and world knowledge, however, some of this information could be identified within training examples and the learner was able to identify them in unseen instances, via the use of a well-formed mathematical framework, i.e. Bayesian networks. In order to enhance their classification performance, a novel variation as regards to the learning strategy was introduced. The complexity of this method lies within reasonable frames. Experimental data portrayed satisfactory results, a fact that does not necessarily point to the full adoption of natural language in programming but to the use of some natural language features in order to improve the structure of a program. As for example, such features could be used in very simple everyday routines like highly standardized office tasks (e.g. managements of data structures or spreadsheets) or financial and accounting tasks such as sums, averages and regression. Summing up, we are of the belief that the present study illustrates the great difficulties researchers face when attempting to implement an unconstrained natural language programming interface. Nonetheless, important initial steps have been proposed which can be followed to improve the notion of naturalness in computer systems.

Acknowledgements

The authors would like to express their thanks to some anonymous reviewers. This work is part of a research project, funded by the Greek government and the European Union (PYTHAGORAS II-Enhancement of Research Groups in Greek Universities).

References

1. Ballard, B., Bierman, A.: Programming in natural language: NLC as a prototype. In: Proceedings of the 1979 Annual Conference of ACM/CSC-ER (1979)
2. Balzer, R.M.: A Global View Of Automatic Programming. In: Proc. 3rd Joint Conference On Artificial Intelligence, pp. 494–499 (August 1993)
3. Cooper, J., Herskovits, E.: A Bayesian method for the induction of probabilistic networks from data. Machine Learning 9, 309–347 (1992)
4. Dijkstra, E.W.: On The Foolishness Of Natural Language Programming. unpublished report (1978)
5. Duda, R., Hart, P.: Pattern Classification and Scene Analysis. John Wiley & Sons, New York (1973)
6. Friedman, N., Geiger, D., Goldszmidt, M.: Bayesian network classifiers. Machine Learning 29, 131–163 (1997)
7. Kate, R., Wong, Y., Mooney, R.: Learning to transform natural to formal languages. In: Proceedings of the Twentieth National Conference on Artificial Intelligence (AAAI 2005), Pittsburgh (2005)
8. Langley, P., Iba, W., Thompson, K.: An analysis of Bayesian classifiers. In: Proceedings, Tenth National Conference on Artificial Intelligence, pp. 223–228. AAAI, Menlo Park (1992)
9. Lieberman, H., Liu, H.: Feasibility studies for programming in natural language. Kluwer Academic Publishers, Dordrecht (2005)
10. Liu, H., Lieberman, H.: Metafor: Visualizing stories as code. In: ACM Conference on Intelligent User Interfaces (2005)
11. Mitchell, T.: Machine Learning. Mc Graw-Hill, New York (1997)
12. Pane, J., Ratanamahatana, C., Meyers, B.: Studying the language and structure in non-programmers' solutions to programming problems. International Journal of Human Computer Studies 54(2) (2001)
13. Pearl, J.: Probabilistic Reasoning in Intelligent Systems: Networks of Plausible Inference. Morgan Kaufmann, San Mateo (1988)
14. Petrick, S.R.: On Natural Language Based Computer Systems. IBM J. Res. Develop., 314–325 (July 1976)

15. Simmons, R.F.: Personal Communication at TINLAP-2 Conference, Univ. of Illinois (July 1978)
16. Suzuki, J.: A construction of Bayesian networks from databases on a MDL scheme. In: Proceedings of the Ninth Conference on Uncertainty in Artificial Intelligence, San Francisco, CA, pp. 266–273 (1993)
17. Woods, W.A.: A Personal View Of Natural Language Understanding. In: Natural Language Interfaces, SIGART, Newsletter, pp. 17–20 (1977)
18. Voutilainen, A., Heikkila, J., Antitil, A.: Constraint grammar of English. Publication 21, Department of General Linguistics, University of Helsinki, Finland (1992)

Boosting over Groups and Its Application to Acronym-Expansion Extraction

Weijian Ni, Yalou Huang, Dong Li, and Yang Wang

College of Information Technical Science, Nankai University
No. 94 Weijin Road, Tianjin, China
niweijian@gmail.com,
huangyl@nankai.edu.cn,
{ldnet,wangyang022}@hotmail.com

Abstract. In many real-world classification applications, instances are generated from different 'groups'. Take webpage classification as an example, the webpages for training and testing can be naturally grouped by network domains, which often vary a lot from one to another in domain size or webpage template. The differences between 'groups' would result that the distribution of instances from different 'groups' also vary. Thus, it is not so reasonable to equally treat the instances as the independent elements during training and testing as in conventional classification algorithms. This paper addresses the classification problem where all the instances can be naturally grouped. Specifically, we give a formulation to this kind of problem and propose a simple but effective boosting approach, which is called AdaBoost.Group. The problem is demonstrated by the task of recognizing acronyms and their expansions from text, where all the instances are grouped by sentences. The experimental results show that our approach is more appropriate to this kind of problems than conventional classification approaches.

Keywords: Boosting, Acronym Extraction, Classification.

1 Introduction

One of the most basic assumptions of classification is that all the instances are independently and identically distributed. Based on the assumption, instances are often equally treated as independent elements during training and testing. However, in many real-world applications, the instances are generated from differently distributed groups, and our target is to obtain the labels of instances from new groups. Thus, it is not so reasonable to consider instance as the independent element during training and testing in these applications.

One typical example of these applications is acronym-expansion extraction. The target of the task is to recognize acronyms and their expansions from text, e.g., given a sentence 'Peer to peer, referred to as P2P, is a type of ad-hoc computer network.', we aim to recognize the acronym 'P2P' and its expansion 'Peer to peer'. Because of the popularity of acronym in Romanic language, automatic recognizing acronyms and the corresponding expansions is very helpful

C. Tang et al. (Eds.): ADMA 2008, LNAI 5139, pp. 27–38, 2008.

to further processing or understanding of the text. Supervised learning has been proved to be a novel approach for its high accuracy and robustness [1][2]. In the approach, pairs of token sequences within a sentence are firstly generated as possible acronym-expansion pairs, such as the pairs like ⟨P2P, Peer to peer⟩ and ⟨P2P, computer networks⟩ in the above sentence. Then each pair is characterized by a feature vector which is regarded as an instance. Using these instances with manual labels as training set, classification algorithm such as SVM or Boosting is employed to train a model to recognize genuine acronym-expansion pair against other candidates. In the problem, the possible pairs, i.e., instances, are grouped by sentences which often vary a lot in syntax or length.

Compared with conventional classification applications, acronym-expansion extraction has its own uniqueness. During the training stage, $O(n^3)$ pairs will be generate from a sentence with n tokens. The model can be easily biased by these long sentences which tend to generate much more pairs than the shorter ones. Since the genuine pair against other candidates within a same sentence imply a kind of pattern matched between acronym and expansion which should be considered equally, it is more reasonable to consider the sentence (group), rather than the pair (instance), as the independent element. During the inference stage, given a new sentence, users are often interested in whether it contains acronym and expansion, and of which pair is the genuine acronym-expansion pair. This implies that the model should be applied sentence-by-sentence, rather than pair-by-pair. So it is more practical to consider each sentence (group) as the independent element. Moreover, as the inference is conducted at group level, the model should be trained to minimize generalization error over group space, yet the conventional classification algorithms aim to train models to minimize the generalization error over instance space. This also indicates that the sentence (group) should be considered as the independent element in the application.

This kind of applications are common in real world, such as spam email filtering where emails are grouped by mailboxes, webpage classification where webpages are grouped by network domains. However, there seems few approach that can be applied to the problem directly. In this paper, we give a formulation to the problem and propose a boosting approach which is called AdaBoost.Group. In our approach, group of instances is considered as the independent element during training and testing, and the objective of training is to minimize a loss function w.r.t. group level training error. We give discrete and real versions of the proposed approach, in each of which the classification loss on groups is measured by either binary value in $\{0, 1\}$ or real value in $[0, 1]$. As the conventional AdaBoost, it can be verified that upper bounds hold for the group level training error and generalization error of both versions of AdaBoost.Group.

2   Related Work

2.1   Automatic Acronym-Expansion Extraction

The research on automatic acronym-expansion extraction is mainly focused on recognizing the genuine acronym-expansion pair from a given sentence. The

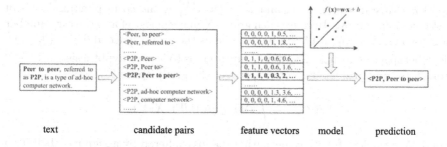

Fig. 1. Illustration of machine learning based acronym-expansion extraction approach

approaches roughly fall into two categories: pattern based approaches and machine learning based approaches. In pattern based approaches [3][4][5][6][7], a number of patterns are designed to evaluate how the acronym matches its expansion. Since the patterns are strong constrains on acronym and expansion, it is a hard task to design and tune these complex patterns to guarantee both precision and recall of the extraction results. Recently, machine learning has shown its effectivity to acronym-expansion extraction [1][2]. In these approaches, weak constraints can be encoded as the features of possible acronym-expansion pair, and machine learning algorithm such as SVM or Boosting is employed to learn a model to recognize the genuine pair against other candidates. The process of machine learning based approach is illustrated in Fig.1.

2.2   Boosting

Boosting is one of most popular classification algorithms for its effectivity and simplicity. The basic idea of boosting is to obtain an accurate hypothesis by combining many less accurate 'weak' hypotheses. Freund et al. [8] proposed the first well-known boosting algorithm AdaBoost in which the weighting scheme of 'weak' hypotheses is adaptive to their performance. Later, Schapire et al. [9] proposed an improved AdaBoost algorithm in which the hypotheses can give confidences to their predictions. Boosting also has been extended to other learning problems, such as regression [10], ranking [11][12], and etc. Although its simplicity, Boosting has soundness theoretical explanations. For example, Boosting can be viewed as a process of minimizing a type of exponential loss function w.r.t. the training error through forward stage-wise modeling procedure [13][14]. The algorithm proposed in this paper follows the framework of AdaBoost.

3   Proposed Approach - Boosting over Groups

3.1   Problem Formulations

Let $\mathcal{X}$ denotes the instance space and $\mathcal{Y} = \{+1, -1\}$ the labels. We are given a set of training groups $S = \{(X_i, Y_i)\}_{i=1}^{n}$, where $X_i = \{\boldsymbol{x}_{ij}\}_{j=1}^{n(i)}$ is the ith group made up of $n(i)$ instances $\boldsymbol{x}_{ij} \in \mathcal{X}$, and $Y_i = \{y_{ij}\}_{j=1}^{n(i)}$ is the corresponding labels of instances in group X_i. Because each group X may consist of an arbitrary number of instances, $\tilde{\mathcal{X}} = \bigcup_{k=1}^{\infty} \mathcal{X}^k$ can be denoted as the group space and $\tilde{\mathcal{Y}} = \bigcup_{k=1}^{\infty} \mathcal{Y}^k$ the label space of groups. Therefore, our target is to learn a hypothesis $f : \tilde{\mathcal{X}} \mapsto \tilde{\mathcal{Y}}$ from S to minimize the expected loss over the group space:

$$R^{\Delta}(f) = \int \Delta(Y, f(X)) d\Pr(X, Y) \tag{1}$$

where Δ is the loss function measuring the loss suffered by assigning label $f(X)$ to group X whose actual label is Y. One of the most straight forward way to define the loss function is $\Delta = \mathbb{1}_{[Y \neq f(X)]}$, i.e., we give 0/1 loss according to the correctness of the prediction. We can also give real valued loss to $f(X)$ according to its confidence. The usage of 0/1 loss and real valued loss bring about the discrete and real versions of our approach, respectively.

If all the groups can be assumed i.i.d. according to $\Pr(X, Y)$, then (1) can be estimated by the empirical loss on S:

$$\tilde{R}^{\Delta}(f) = \frac{1}{n} \sum_{i=1}^{n} \Delta(Y_i, f(X_i))$$

Since the hypothesis is applied to new groups, rather than new individual instances, the conventional performance measures such as *Accuracy*, *Precision*, *Recall*, F_β-score are no longer applicable. Therefore, we define the following measures to evaluate the 'goodness' of hypothesis for this kind of problems. Group level accuracy is defined as:

$$GAcc = \frac{\left| \{(X_i, Y_i) | Y_i = f(X_i), (X_i, Y_i) \in S\} \right|}{|S|}$$

The conventional measure of *Precision* and *Recall* can be adjusted to the problem, i.e., the group level precision and recall are defined as:

$$GPre = \frac{\left| \{(X_i, Y_i) | (Y_i = f(X_i)) \bigwedge (\exists j, y_{ij} = +1, j = 1 \ldots n(i)), (X_i, Y_i) \in S\} \right|}{\left| \{(X_i, Y_i) | \exists j, y_{ij} = +1, j = 1 \ldots n(i), (X_i, Y_i) \in S\} \right|}$$

$$GRec = \frac{\left| \{(X_i, Y_i) | (Y_i = f(X_i)) \bigwedge (\exists j, f(\boldsymbol{x}_{ij}) = +1, j = 1 \ldots n(i)), (X_i, Y_i) \in S\} \right|}{\left| \{(X_i, Y_i) | \exists j, y_{ij} = +1, j = 1 \ldots n(i), (X_i, Y_i) \in S\} \right|}$$

Then the group level F_β-score is defined based on *GPre* and *GRec*:

$$GF_\beta = \frac{(1 + \beta) \cdot GPre \cdot GRec}{\beta \cdot GPre + GRec}$$

Group level measures of *Precision*, *Recall* and F_β-score are especially useful to the applications where there only scarce positive instances that scatter among

Input: training set $S = \{(X_i, Y_i)\}_{i=1}^n$, number of iterations T.
Initialize: weights of each group $w_1^i = 1$.
For $t = 1, \ldots, T$

- Set the weight distribution $\mathbf{p}_t$ of groups in S: $p_t^i = \frac{w_t^i}{\sum_{i=1}^n w_t^i}$
- Train weak hypothesis $h_t : \widetilde{\mathcal{X}} \mapsto \widetilde{\mathcal{Y}}$ on S with distribution $\mathbf{p}_t$
- Calculate the weighted training error of h_t:

$$\varepsilon_t = \sum_{i=1}^n p_t^i \mathbb{1}_{[Y_i \neq f(X_i)]}$$

- Choose $\beta_t = \frac{\varepsilon_t}{1 - \varepsilon_t}$
- Update the weights

$$w_{t+1}^i = w_t^i \beta_t^{1 - \mathbb{1}_{[Y_i \neq f(X_i)]}}$$

Output: the final hypothesis

$$f_T(X) = \max_{Y \in \widetilde{\mathcal{Y}}} \sum_{t=1}^T (\log \frac{1}{\beta_t}) \mathbb{1}_{[h_t(X) = Y]}$$

Fig. 2. Discrete Version of the AdaBoost.Group Algorithm

only small number of groups. As in acronym extraction, only small number of sentences contain genuine acronym-expansion pairs and the acronyms appear once in most of them. It is reasonable to make use of these group level performance measures to evaluate how our model can recognize the sentences containing acronym and expansion and of which possible pair is the genuine pair.

3.2 Discrete Version

Based on the formulation of the problem, we propose a boosting approach following the framework of AdaBoost, referred to as AdaBoost.Group. Given a set of training groups $S = \{(X_i, Y_i)\}_{i=1}^n$, our approach outputs a hypothesis f in form of combination of T weak hypothesis h_t. The details are shown in Fig.2.

AdaBoost.Group maintains a distribution of weights w_t^i for each group i in training set and gives equal weights to them initially. At each round t, a weak hypothesis h_t is learned using the training set with current weight distribution $\mathbf{p}_t$, and its group level training error ε_t is calculated, which will reflect the importance of h_t in the final hypothesis. The weight of each group is adjusted at each round on the basis of the predictions of h_t, particularly, the weights of the misclassified groups are increased by a factor of β_t, and the correctly classified groups' remain unchanged. After the T rounds, AdaBoost.Group outputs a hypothesis f through weighted majority vote of the T 'weak' hypotheses.

Because the loss suffered by h_t on each group is measured by $\mathbb{1}_{[Y \neq h_t(X)]}$ which takes values in $\{0, 1\}$, we refer to the algorithm in Fig.2 as discrete version of AdaBoost.Group (AdaBoost.Group^{disc}).

Although AdaBoost.Group^{disc} follows the framework of AdaBoost, there are considerable differences between them. First, the weighting scheme are conducted on groups rather than on instances as in AdaBoost; Second, the 'goodness' of weak hypotheses is evaluated on group level rather than on instance level as in AdaBoost; Third, the prediction of hypothesis takes values in vector space rather than in discrete label space as in AdaBoost.

It is desirable that AdaBoost.Group^{disc} shares the theoretical soundness with AdaBoost. The following theorems give the theoretical justification of the convergency of AdaBoost.Group^{disc}. Specifically, Theorem 1 and 2 give upper bounds of training error and generalization error, respectively.

Theorem 1. *Using the notations in Fig.2, the following bound holds for the training error ε of the final hypothesis f_T:*

$$\varepsilon \leq 2^T \prod_{t=1}^{T} \sqrt{\varepsilon_t(1-\varepsilon_t)}$$

Theorem 2. *Using the notations in Fig.2 and let d be the VC-dimension of the weak hypothesis space, the following bound holds for the generalization error $\widetilde{\varepsilon}$ of the final hypothesis f:*

$$\widetilde{\varepsilon} \leq \varepsilon + O(\sqrt{\frac{Td}{n}})$$

We omit the proofs of the two theorems because they can be easily derived from the conclusions in [8][15].

3.3   Real Version

In the discrete version of AdaBoost.Group, all the inaccurate predictions on each group are given loss '1'. However, the confidence of different predictions are often not the same. For example, given a group X whose label $Y = (-1, +1, -1, -1)$ and two predictions $h_1(X) = (+1, +1, -1, -1)$ and $h_2(X) = (+1, -1, +1, -1)$, it is obvious that h_2 suffers more than h_1 on the group. In order to evaluate the confidence of predictions on groups, we design the following measure :

Definition 1 (Prediction Confidence). *The confidence of a prediction of hypothesis h on group X_i is the normalized inner product of the label vector and the prediction vector. That is:*

$$\gamma^i(h) = \frac{1}{n(i)}\langle Y_i, h(X_i)\rangle$$

It is easy to see that the following properties hold for *prediction confidence*:

1. $\gamma^i(h) \in [-1, 1]$;
2. $\gamma^i(\alpha \cdot h + \beta \cdot g) = \alpha \cdot \gamma^i(h) + \beta \cdot \gamma^i(g)$.

Then we propose the real version of AdaBoost.Group (AdaBoost.Group^{real}), which is shown in Fig.3. At each round, the *prediction confidence* γ_t^i

Input: training set $S = \{(X_i, Y_i)\}_{i=1}^n$, number of iterations T.
Initialize: the distribution of weights of each group $p_1^i = \frac{1}{n}$.
For $t = 1, \ldots, T$

- Train weak hypothesis $h_t : \widetilde{\mathcal{X}} \mapsto \widetilde{\mathcal{Y}}$ on S with distribution $\mathbf{p}_t$
- Calculate the classification confidence of h_t on the whole training set:

$$\gamma_t = \sum_{i=1}^n p_t^i \gamma^i(h_t)$$

- Choose $\alpha_t = \frac{1}{2} \ln \frac{1+\gamma_t}{1-\gamma_t}$
- Update the weights

$$p_{t+1}^i = \frac{1}{Z_t} p_t^i \exp\left(-\alpha_t \gamma^i(h_t)\right)$$

where Z_t is the normalization factor.

Output: the final hypothesis

$$f_T(X) = \sum_{t=1}^T \alpha_t h_t(X)$$

Fig. 3. Real Version of the AdaBoost.Group Algorithm

are used to calculate the weights updating factor for X_i. The final hypothesis in AdaBoost.Group^{real} takes the form of weighted linear combination of all the weak hypotheses, not just the weighted majority vote of weak hypotheses as in the discrete version.

The same as AdaBoost, it can be verified that AdaBoost.Group^{real} attempts to minimize a exponential loss w.r.t. the *classification confidence* on each group during its iterations:

$$\min_{f \in \mathcal{F}} \sum_{i=1}^n \exp\left(-\gamma^i(f)\right) \tag{2}$$

Because we make use of the linear combination of weak hypotheses as the final hypothesis, the minimization of (2) turns out to be:

$$\min_{h \in \mathcal{H}, \alpha_t \in \mathbb{R}^+} \sum_{i=1}^n \exp\left(-\gamma^i(f_{t-1} + \alpha_t h_t)\right)$$

$$= \sum_{i=1}^n \exp\left(-\gamma^i(f_{t-1}) - \alpha_t \gamma^i(h_t)\right) \tag{3}$$

The coefficient α_t of weak hypothesis h_t can be easily derived by minimizing (3) through forward stage-wise modeling procedure in [13]. Note that the upper bounds in Theorem 1 and 2 also hold for the real version of AdaBoost.Group.

3.4 Design of Weak Hypothesis

Theorem 1 indicates that, the errors suffered by weak hypotheses are required to be less than $1/2$ to guarantee the convergency of AdaBoost.Group. In AdaBoost, it means that the weak hypotheses only need to perform better than random guessing. However, the requirement is much stronger in our algorithm because the predictions of weak hypotheses are vectors. The weak hypotheses should be carefully designed to meet the requirement.

In this paper, we make use of the conventional AdaBoost with 30 rounds as the weak hypothesis. The choice is based on several considerations: First, AdaBoost performs well on instance level classification problems and the performance is also desirable when evaluated on group level. Second, AdaBoost can be adapted to weighted training set easily. Last, AdaBoost is efficient and easy to implement, which are desirable properties for weak hypothesis.

4   Experimental Results

In this section, we applied the AdaBoost.Group algorithm to the problem of acronym-expansion extraction. We also experimentally investigated the reason of our approaches outperforming baselines.

4.1   Settings

We made use of the UCI collection '*NSF Research Awards Abstracts 1990-2003*' [16] as the data set. It consists of 129,000 abstracts describing NSF awards for basic research. Acronyms often appear in the these abstracts. We random selected 1000 abstracts and segment each of them by natural sentences, then each appearance of acronyms and corresponding expansions are manually labeled. Finally, there are 495 genuine acronym-expansion pairs appear in 1546 sentences.

As for features, we extracted 106 binary or real valued features for each possible acronym-expansion pair. For example, the feature may be a test that whether the acronym candidate consists of letters in lower case, or whether the acronym candidate is made up of the first letters of each word of expansion candidate. The details of the features are shown in Tabel 1.

The state-of-the-art classification algorithms SVM and AdaBoost were selected as two baselines. The cost-sensitive version of AdaBoost (AdaBoost. CostSen) which gives different weights to possible pairs according to the length of sentences they belong to, was also selected as a baseline. Besides, a pattern based approach similar to [3] was another baseline, referred to as PatternMatch.

Table 1. Features for acronym-expansion extraction

Category	Number	Description
I	15	extracted from acronym candidates
II	28	extracted from expansion candidates
III	45	extracted from the pattern matched between acronym and expansion candidates
IV	18	extracted from the context

For our approaches, the parameter T was set to 100 experimentally. The results with the best performance in terms of $GAcc$ during the 100 rounds were reported as the final results. The parameters T for AdaBoost and AdaBoost.CostSen were selected in the same way. Decision tree with two leaves was used to train weak hypotheses for both of them.

4.2   Results

We randomly split the data set into four parts with equal number of groups and conduct 4-fold cross validations. The results reported in the section are the averages over the 4 trials.

Table 2 presents the performance of our approaches and baselines evaluated by the group level measures. We can see that the machine learning based approach are more effective than the pattern based approach for the problem of acronym-expansion extraction. Among these machine learning based approaches, AdaBoost.Group^{real} and AdaBoost.Group^{disc} outperform others in all the group level measures, which indicates that our approaches have the potential to improve the group level performance. Besides, we can note that the cost sensitive version of AdaBoost performs better than AdaBoost and SVM, which give an evidence that the cost sensitive approach can partially avoid the bias caused by large groups. However, the improvements are not so significant as that of our approaches. We also conduct significance test (t-test) on the improvements of our approaches to baselines and found that all the improvements are statistically significant (p-value ≤ 0.05).

Table 2. Results evaluated on group level performance measure

Methods	$GAcc$	$GPre$	$GRec$	$GF1$
AdaBoost.Group^{real}	**0.9412**	**0.8480**	**0.8208**	**0.8340**
AdaBoost.Group^{disc}	0.9398	0.8453	0.8157	0.8301
AdaBoost.CostSen	0.9356	0.8277	0.7901	0.8083
AdaBoost	0.9321	0.8235	0.7810	0.8015
SVM	0.9307	0.8162	0.7826	0.7985
PatternMatch	0.9011	0.7742	0.7597	0.7619

Table 3 presents the performance of the approaches evaluated by the instance level measures, i.e., the conventional measures. We can see that the machine learning based approaches outperform the pattern based approach again and our approaches perform as well as other machine learning based approaches in terms of instance level measure. It is not supervising because our approaches aims to optimize the loss defined on group level. The possible pairs generated from long sentences might be misclassified more easily since all the sentences were given equal weights.

Table 3. Results evaluated on instance level performance measure

Methods	Acc	Pre	Rec	F1
AdaBoost.Group^{real}	0.9995	0.8588	**0.8913**	0.8705
AdaBoost.Group^{disc}	0.9995	0.8601	0.8902	0.8703
AdaBoost.CostSen	0.9996	0.8626	0.8844	0.8724
AdaBoost	**0.9996**	**0.8798**	0.8749	**0.8768**
SVM	0.9992	0.8482	0.8957	0.8701
PatternMatch	0.9953	0.8011	0.8547	0.8320

4.3 Discussions

In this section, we experimentally investigated the reason of AdaBoost.Group outperforming the baselines.

In order to draw more insights into the problem of acronym-expansion extraction, we first make statistics on the data set used in our experiment. Fig.4 shows the distribution of sentences w.r.t. their length. We can see that most sentences contain medium numbers of tokens, but there are also a few of sentences which have the potential to generate large amount of possible pairs.

Then we made statistics on the performance of our approaches and baselines on the sentences with different length. As in Fig.4, we clustered all the sentences into 7 sets according to their length and examine the average performance of the approaches on each set, which is shown in Fig.5. The horizontal and vertical axes represent different sets of groups and the average performance on each set in terms of *GAcc*, respectively. We can see that the baselines perform better on long sentences than on the shorter ones, which indicates that the model can be easily biased by the minority of long sentences. While our approach performs well on most of the sentences, rather than on the few long sentences. Thus, our approach can be focused on the majority of groups, which has the potential to achieve better group level performance.

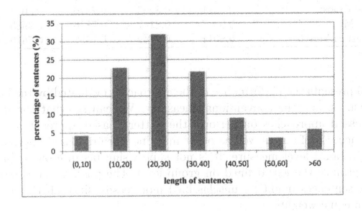

Fig. 4. Distributions of sentences w.r.t. the length

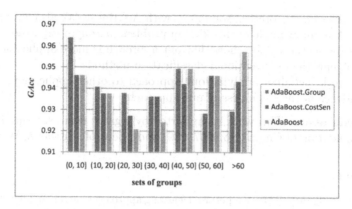

Fig. 5. Group level accuracies on different sets of sentences

At last, we investigated the convergency of our approaches. We drew the group level training curve of the two version of AdaBoost.Group in Fig.6. We can see that, although not very smooth, the group level training error of both versions are decreased continuously during training and converged finally. Moreover, AdaBoost.Group^{real} could converge to a bit lower bound that AdaBoost. Group^{disc}, which gives an experimental evidence that the *classification confidence* defined in Sect. 3.3 is helpful to guide the training process.

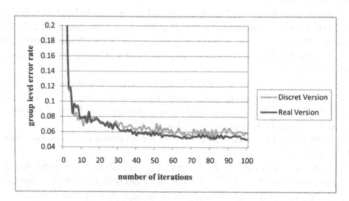

Fig. 6. Error rate curves of AdaBoost.Group on training set

5   Conclusion and Future Work

In this paper, we have addressed a new kind of classification problem where instances can be naturally grouped. The kind of problem has its own uniqueness and is widely existed in real-world applications. However, few approach can be applied to these problems directly. We have formulated the learning target and evaluation measure of the problem, and proposed an effective boosting approach. Our approach is an extension of the conventional AdaBoost algorithm and shares the same theoretical soundness with AdaBoost. We also have applied our approach to an example of this kind of problem, acronym-expansion extraction. The experiential results show that our approach is more applicable to the kind of problems than conventional classification methods.

Further work including applying our approach to other applications to give further evidence of the usefulness of our approach.

Acknowledgments. This work is supported by a grant from National Natural Science Foundation of China (No.60673009) and Microsoft Research Asia Fund.

References

1. Naueau, D., Turney, P.D.: A supervised learning approach to acronym identification. In: Proceedings of the 18th Canadian Conference on Aritifical Intelligence (2005)
2. Xu, J., Huang, Y.L.: A Machine Learning Approach to Recognizing Acronym and Their Expansions. In: Proceedings of the 4th International Conference on Machine Learning and Cybernetics, pp. 2313–2319 (2005)
3. Taghva, K., Gilbreth, J.: Recognizing Acronym and their Definitions. International Journal on Document Analysis and Recognition 1, 191–198 (1999)
4. Larkey, L.S., Ogilvie, P., Price, M.A., Tamilio, B.: Acrophile: An Automatic Acronym Extractor and Server. In: Proceedings of the 15th ACM Conference on Digital Libraries, pp. 205–214 (2000)
5. Park, Y., Byrd, R.J.: Hybrid Text Mining for Finding Abbreviations and Their Definitions. In: Proceedings of the 2001 Conference on Empirical Methods in Natural Language Processing (2001)
6. Yu, H., Hripcsak, G., Friedman, C.: Mapping abbreviations to full forms in biomedical articales. Journal of the American Medical Informatics Association 9, 262–272 (2002)
7. Schwartz, A., Hearst, M.: A simple algorithm for identifying abbreviation definitions in biomedical text. In: Proceedings of the Pacific Symposium on Biocomputing (2003)
8. Freund, Y., Schapire, R.E.: A Decision-Theoretic Generalization of Online Learning and an Application to Boosting. Journal of Computer Sciences 55, 119–139 (1997)
9. Schapire, R.E., Singer, Y.: Improved Boosting Algorithms Using Confidence-rated Predictions. Machine Learning 37, 297–336 (1999)
10. Duffy, N., Helmbold, D.: Boosting Methods for Regression. Machine Learning 47, 153–200 (2002)
11. Freund, Y., Iyer, R., Schapire, R.E., Singer, Y.: An Efficient Boosting Algorithm for Combining Preferences. Singer, Y.: An Efficient Boosting Algorithm for Combining Preferences. Journal of Machine Learning Research 4, 933–969 (2003)
12. Xu, J., Li, H.: AdaRank: A Boosting Algrithm for Information Retrieval. In: The proceedings of the 30th annual international ACM SIGIR conference on research and development in information retrieval, pp. 391–398 (2007)
13. Hastie, T., Tibshirani, R., Friedman, J.: The Elements of Statistical Learning - Data Mining, Inference, and Prediction. Springer, Heidelberg (2001)
14. Friedman, J., Hasite, T., Tibshirani, R.: Additive Logistic Regression: A Statistical View of Boosting. The Annals of Statistics 28, 337–407 (2000)
15. Schapire, R.E.: A Brief Introduction to Boosting. In: The proceedings of the 16th International Joint conference on Artifical Intelligence, pp. 1401–1406 (1999)
16. Hettich, S., Bay, S.D.: The UCI KDD Archieve. University of California, Department of Information and Computer Science, Irvine, http://kdd.ics.uci.edu

A Genetic-Based Feature Construction Method for Data Summarisation

Rayner Alfred

School of Engineering and Information Technology,
Universiti Malaysia Sabah,
Locked Bag 2073, 88999, Kota Kinabalu, Sabah, Malaysia
ralfred@ums.edu.my

Abstract. The importance of input representation has been recognised already in machine learning. This paper discusses the application of genetic-based feature construction methods to generate input data for the data summarisation method called Dynamic Aggregation of Relational Attributes ($DARA$). Here, feature construction methods are applied in order to improve the descriptive accuracy of the $DARA$ algorithm. The $DARA$ algorithm is designed to summarise data stored in the non-target tables by clustering them into groups, where multiple records stored in non-target tables correspond to a single record stored in a target table. This paper addresses the question whether or not the descriptive accuracy of the $DARA$ algorithm benefits from the feature construction process. This involves solving the problem of constructing a relevant set of features for the $DARA$ algorithm by using a genetic-based algorithm. This work also evaluates several scoring measures used as fitness functions to find the best set of constructed features.

Keywords: Feature Construction, Data Summarisation, Genetic Algorithm, Clustering.

1 Introduction

Learning is an important aspect of research in Artificial Intelligence (AI). Many of the existing learning approaches consider the learning algorithm as a passive process that makes use of the information presented to it. This paper studies the application of feature construction to improve the descriptive accuracy of a data summarisation algorithm, which is called Dynamic Aggregation of Relational Attributes ($DARA$) [1]. The $DARA$ algorithm summarises data stored in non-target tables that have many-to-one relationships with data stored in the target table. Feature construction methods are mostly related to classification problems where the data are stored in target table. In this case, the predictive accuracy can often be significantly improved by constructing new features which are more relevant for predicting the class of an object. On the other hand, feature construction also has been used in descriptive induction algorithms, particularly those algorithms that are based on inductive logic programming

C. Tang et al. (Eds.): ADMA 2008, LNAI 5139, pp. 39–50, 2008.

(e.g., Warmr [2] and *Relational Subgroup Discovery (RSD)* [3]), in order to discover patterns described in the form of individual rules. The *DARA* algorithm is designed to summarise data stored in the non-target tables by clustering them into groups, where multiple records exist in non-target tables that correspond to a single record stored in the target table. In this case, the performance of the *DARA* algorithm is evaluated based on the descriptive accuracy of the algorithm. Here, feature construction can also be applied in order to improve the descriptive accuracy of the *DARA* algorithm. This paper addresses the question whether or not the descriptive accuracy of the *DARA* algorithm benefits from the feature construction process. This involves solving the problem of constructing a relevant set of features for the *DARA* algorithm. These features are then used to generate patterns that represent objects, stored in the non-target table, in the *TF-IDF* weighted frequency matrix in order to cluster these objects.

Section 2 will introduce the framework of our data summarisation approach, *DARA* [1]. The data summarisation method employs the *TF-IDF* weighted frequency matrix (vector space model [4])to represent the relational data model, where the representation of data stored in multiple tables will be analysed and it will be transformed into data representation in a vector space model. Then, section 3 describes the process of feature construction and introduces genetic-based (i.e., evolutionary) feature construction algorithm that uses a non-algebraic form to represent an individual solution to construct features. This genetic-based feature construction algorithm constructs features to produce patterns that characterise each unique object stored in the non-target table. Section 4 describes the experimental design and evaluates several scoring measures used as fitness functions to find the best set of constructed features. The performance accuracy of the *J*48 classifier for the classification tasks using these summarised data will be presented and finally, this paper is concluded in section 5.

2   Dynamic Aggregation of Relational Attributes (*DARA*)

In order to classify records stored in the target table that have one-to-many relations with records stored in non-target tables, the *DARA* algorithm transforms the representation of data stored in the non-target tables into an $(n \times p)$ matrix in order to cluster these records (see Figure 1), where n is the number of records to be clustered and p is the number of patterns considered for clustering. As a result, the records stored in the non-target tables are summarised by clustering them into groups that share similar charateristics. Clustering is considered as one of the descriptive tasks that seeks to identify natural groupings in the data based on the patterns given. Developing techniques to automatically discover such groupings is an important part of knowledge discovery and data mining research.

In Figure 1, the target relation has a one-to-many relationship with the non-target relation. The non-target table is then converted into bags of patterns associated with records stored in the target table. In order to generate these

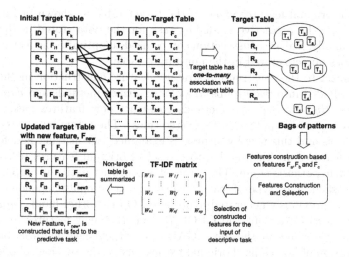

Fig. 1. Feature transformation process for data stored in multiple tables with one-to-many relations into a vector space data representation

patterns to represent objects in the $TF\text{-}IDF$ weighted frequency matrix, one can enrich the objects representation by constructing new features from the original features given in the non-target relation. The new features are constructed by combining attributes obtained from the given attributes in the non-target table randomly. For instance, given a non-target table with attributes (F_a, F_b, F_c), all possible constructed features are F_a, F_b, F_c, F_aF_b, F_bF_c, F_aF_c and $F_aF_bF_c$. These newly constructed features will be used to produce patterns or instances to represent records stored in the non-target table, in the $(n \times p)$ $TF\text{-}IDF$ weighted frequency matrix. After the records stored in the non-target relation are clustered, a new column, F_{new}, is added to the set of original features in the target table. This new column contains the cluster identification number for all records stored in the non-target table. In this way, we aim to map data stored in the non-target table to the records stored in the target table.

3   Feature Construction in Machine Learning

3.1   Feature Construction

The problem of *feature construction* can be defined as the task of constructing new features, based on some functional expressions that use the values of original features, that describe the hypothesis at least as well as the original set. The application of feature construction for the purpose of summarising data stored in the non-target tables has several benefits. First, by generating relevant patterns describing each object stored in the non-target table, the descriptive accuracy of the data summarisation can be improved. Next, when the summarised data are appended to the target table (e.g., the newly constructed feature, F_{new}, is added to the set of original features given in the target table as shown in Figure 1), it can facilitate the predictive modelling task for the data stored in the target table. And finally, feature construction can be used to optimise the feature space that describes objects stored in the non-target table.

With respect to the construction strategy, feature construction methods can be roughly divided into two groups: *Hypothesis-driven* methods and *data-driven* methods [5]. *Hypothesis-driven* methods construct new features based on the previously-generated hypothesis (discovered rules). They start by constructing a new hypothesis and this new hypothesis is examined to construct new features. These new features are then added to the set of original features to construct another new hypothesis again. This process is repeated until the stopping condition is satisfied. This type of feature construction is highly dependent on the quality of the previously generated hypotheses. On the other hand, *data-driven* methods, such as GALA [6] and GPCI [7], construct new features by directly detecting relationships in the data. GALA constructs new features based on the combination of booleanised original features using the two logical operators, AND and OR. GPCI is inspired by GALA, in which GPCI used an evolutionary algorithm to construct features. One of the disadvantages of GALA and GPCI is that the booleanisation of features can lead to a significant loss of relevant information [8].

There are essentially two approaches to constructing features in relation to data mining. The first method is as a separate, independent pre-processing stage, in which the new attributes are constructed before the classification algorithm is applied to build the model [9]. In other words, the quality of a candidate new feature is evaluated by directly accessing the data, without running any inductive learning algorithm. In this approach, the features constructed can be fed to different kinds of inductive learning methods. This method is also known as the Filter approach.

The second method is an integration of construction and induction, in which new features are constructed within the induction process. This method is also referred to as *interleaving* [10,11] or the wrapper approach. The quality of a candidate new feature is evaluated by executing the inductive learning algorithm used to extract knowledge from the data, so that in principle the constructed features' usefulness tends to be limited to that inductive learning algorithm. In this work, the filtering approach that uses the *data-driven* strategy is applied to construct features for the descriptive task, since the wrapper approaches are computationally more expensive than the filtering approaches.

3.2   Feature Scoring

The scoring of the newly constructed feature can be performed using some of the measures used in machine learning, such as information gain (Equation 1), to assign a score to the constructed feature. For instance, the $ID3$ decision-tree [12] induction algorithm applies information gain to evaluate features. The information gain of a new feature F, denoted *InfoGain(F)*, represents the difference of the class entropy in data set before the usage of feature F, denoted

$Ent(C)$, and after the usage of feature F for splitting the data set into subsets, denoted $Ent(C|F)$, as shown in Equation 1.

$$InfoGain(F) = Ent(C) - Ent(C|F) \tag{1}$$

where

$$Ent(C) = -\sum_{j=1}^{n} Pr\,(C_j) \cdot log_2 Pr\,(C_j) \tag{2}$$

$$Ent(C|F) = -\sum_{i=1}^{m} Pr(F_i) \cdot (-\sum_{j=1}^{n} Pr(C|F_i) \cdot log_2 Pr(C_j|F_i)) \tag{3}$$

where $Pr(C_j)$ is the estimated probability of observing the jth class, n is the number of classes, $Pr(F_i)$ is the estimated probability of observing the ith value of feature F, m is the number of values of the feature F, and $Pr(C_j|F_i)$ is the probability of observing the jth class conditional on having observed the ith value of the feature F. Information Gain Ratio (IGR) is sometimes used when considering attributes with a large number of distinct values. The Information Gain Ratio of a feature, denoted by $IGR(F)$, is computed by dividing the Information Gain, $InfoGain(F)$ shown in Equation 1, by the amount of information of the feature F, denoted $Ent(F)$,

$$IGR(F) = \frac{InfoGain(F)}{Ent(F)} \tag{4}$$

$$Ent(F) = -\sum_{i=1}^{m} Pr(F_i) \cdot log_2 Pr(F_i)) \tag{5}$$

and $Pr(F_i)$ is the estimated probability of observing the ith value of the feature F and m is the number of values of the feature F.

3.3   Feature Construction for Data Summarisation

In the $DARA$ algorithm, the patterns produced to represent objects in the TF-IDF weighted frequency matrix are based on simple algorithms. These patterns are produced based on the number of attributes combined that can be categorised into three categories. These categories include 1) a set of patterns produced from an individual attribute using an algorithm called P_{Single} 2) a set of patterns produced from the combination of all attributes by using an algorithm called P_{All} 3) a set of patterns produced from variable length attributes that are selected and combined randomly from the given attributes.

For example, given a set of attributes $\{F_1, F_2, F_3, F_4, F_5\}$, one could have $(F_1, F_2, F_3, F_4, F_5)$ as the constructed features by using the P_{Single} algorithm. In contrast, with the same example, one will only have a single feature $(F_1 F_2 F_3 F_4 F_5)$ produced by using the P_{All} algorithm. As a result, data stored across multiple tables with high cardinality attributes can be represented as

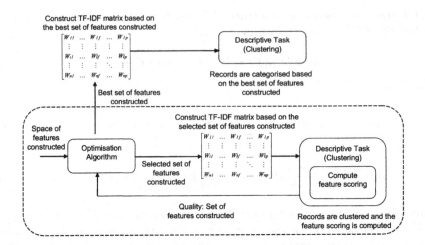

Fig. 2. Illustration of the Filtering approach to feature construction

bags of patterns produced using these constructed features. An object can also be represented by patterns produced on the basis of randomly constructed features (e.g., (F_1F_5, F_2F_4, F_3)), where features are combined based on some pre-computed feature scoring measures.

This work studies a filtering approach to feature construction for the purpose of data summarisation using the $DARA$ algorithm (see Figure 2). A set of constructed features is used to produce patterns for each unique record stored in the non-target table. As a result, these patterns can be used to represent objects stored in the non-target table in the form of a vector space. The vectors of patterns are then used to construct the TF-IDF weighted frequency matrix. Then, the clustering technique can be applied to categorise these objects. Next, the quality of each set of the constructed features is measured. This process is repeated for the other sets of constructed features. The set of constructed features that produces the highest measure of quality is maintained to produce the final clustering result.

3.4   Genetic-Based Approach to Feature Construction for Data Summarisation

Feature construction methods that are based on greedy search usually suffer from the local optima problem. When the constructed feature is complex due to the interaction among attributes, the search space for constructing new features has more variation. An exhaustive search may be feasible, if the number of attributes is not too large. In general, the problem is known to be NP-hard [14] and the search becomes quickly computationally intractable. As a result, the feature construction method requires a heuristic search strategy such as Genetic Algorithms to be able to avoid the local optima and find the global optima solutions [15,16].

Genetic Algorithms (GA) are a kind of multidirectional parallel search, and viable alternative to the intracable exhaustive search and complicated search space [13]. For this reason, we also use a GA-based algorithm to construct features for the data summarisation task, here. This section describes a GA-based feature construction algorithm that generates patterns for the purpose of summarising data stored in the non-target tables. With the summarised data obtained from the related data stored in the the non-target tables, the $DARA$ algorithm may facilitate the classification task performed on the data stored in the target table.

Individual Representation. There are two alternative representations of features: algebraic and non-algebraic [16]. In algebraic form, the features are shown by means of some algebraic operators such as arithmetic or Boolean operators. Most genetic-based feature construction methods like GCI [9], GPCI [7] and Gabret [17] apply the algebraic form of representation using a parse tree [18]. GPCI uses a fix set of operators, AND and NOT, applicable to all Boolean domains. The use of operators makes the method applicable to a wider range of problems. In contrast, GCI [9] and Gabret [17] apply domain-specific operators to reduce complexity. In addition to the issue of defining operators, an algebraic form of representation can produce an unlimited search space since any feature can appear in infinitely many forms [16]. Therefore, a feature construction method based on an algebraic form needs a restriction to limit the growth of constructed functions.

Features can also be represented in a non-algebraic form, in which the representation uses no operators. For example, in this work, given a set of attributes $\{X_1, X_2, X_3, X_4, X_5\}$, an algebraic feature like $((X_1 \wedge X_2) \vee (X_3 \wedge X_4 \wedge X_5))$ can be represented in a non-algebraic form as $\langle X_1 X_2 X_3 X_4 X_5, 2 \rangle$, where the digit, "2", refers to the number of attributes combined to generate the first constructed feature.

The non-algebraic representation of features has several advantages over the algebraic representation [16]. These include the simplicity of the non-algebraic form to represent each individual in the process of constructing features, since there are no operator required. Next, when using a genetic-based algorithm to find the best set of features constructed, traversal of the search space of a non-algebraic is much easier.

A genetic-based feature construction method can be designed to construct a list of newly constructed features. For instance, during the population initialisation, each chromosome is initialised with the following format, $\langle X, A, B \rangle$, where X represents a list of the attribute's indices, A represents the number of attributes combined, and B represents the point of crossover. Thus, given a chromosome $\langle 1234567, 3, 4 \rangle$, where the list 1234567 represents the sequence of seven attributes, the digit "3" represents the number of attributes combined and the digit "4" represents the point of crossover, the possible constructed features are $(F_1 F_3 F_4)$, $(F_6 F_7 F_5)$ and (F_2), with the assumption that the attributes are selected randomly from attribute F_1 through attribute F_7 to form the new features. The crossover process simply copies the sequence (string of attributes),

(1234567), and rearranges it so that its tail, (567), is moved to the front to form the new sequence (5671234). The mutation process simply changes the number of attributes combined, A, and the point of crossover in the string, B. The rest of the feature representations can be obtained by mutating A, and B, and these values should be less than or equal to the number of atttibutes considered in the problem. As a result, this form of representation results in more variation after performing genetic operators and can provide more useful features.

Fitness Function. Information Gain (Equation 1) is often used as a fitness function to evaluate the quality of the constructed features in order to improve the predictive accuracy of a supervised learner [19,8]. In contrast, if the objective of the feature construction is to improve the descriptive accuracy of an unsupervised clustering technique, one may use the Davies-Bouldin Index (DBI) [20], as the fitness function. However, if the objective of the feature construction is to improve the descriptive accuracy of a semi-supervised clustering technique, the total cluster entropy (Equation 6) can be used as the fitness function to evaluate how well the newly constructed feature clusters the objects.

In our approach to summarising data in a multi-relational database, in order to improve the predictive accuracy of a classification task, the fitness function for the GA-based feature construction algorithm can be defined in several ways. In these experiments, we examine the case of semi-supervised learning to improve the predictive accuracy of a classification task. As a result, we will perform experiments that evaluate four types of feature-scoring measures (fitness functions) including the Information Gain (Equation 1), Total Cluster Entropy (Equation 6), Information Gain coupled with Cluster Entropy (Equation 8), Davies-Bouldin Index [20]

The information gain (Equation 1) of a feature F represents the difference of the class entropy in data set before the usage of feature F and after the usage of feature F for splitting the data set into subsets. This information gain measure is generally used for classification tasks. On the other hand, if the objective of the data modelling task is to separate objects from different classes (like different protein families, types of wood, or species of dogs), the cluster's diversity, for the kth cluster, refers to the number of classes within the kth cluster. If this value is large for any cluster, there are many classes within this cluster and there is a large diversity. In this genetic approach to feature construction for the proposed data summarisation technique, the fitness function can also be defined as the diversity of the clusters produced. In other words, the fitness of each individual non-algebraic form of constructed features depends on the diversity of each cluster produced.

In these experiments, in order to cluster a given set of categorised records into K clusters, the fitness function for a given set of constructed features is defined as the total clusters entropy, $H(K)$, of all clusters produced (Equation 6). This is also known as the Shannon-Weiner diversity [21,22],

$$H(K) = \frac{\sum_{k=1}^{K} n_k \cdot H_k}{N} \qquad (6)$$

where n_k is the number of objects in kth cluster, N is the total number of objects, H_k is the entropy of the kth cluster, which is defined in Equation 7, where S is the number of classes, P_{sk}, is the probability that an object randomly chosen from the kth cluster belongs to the sth class. The smaller the value of the fitness function using the total cluster entropy (CE), the better is the quality of clusters produced.

$$H_k = -\sum_{s=1}^{S} P_{sk} \cdot log_2(P_{sk}) \tag{7}$$

Next, we will also study the effect of combining the *Information Gain* (Equation 1) and *Total Cluster Entropy* (Equation 6) measures, denoted as $CE - IG(F, K)$, as the fitness function in our genetic algorithm, as shown in Equation 8, where K is the number of clusters and F is the constructed feature.

$$CE - IG(F, K) = InfoGain(F) + \frac{\sum_{k=1}^{K} n_k \cdot H_k}{N} \tag{8}$$

Finally, we are also interested in evaluating the effectiveness of feature construction based on the quality of the cluster's structure, which is measured using the Davies-Bouldin Index (DBI) [20], to improve the predictive accuracy of a classification task.

4   Experiments and Results

In these experiments we observe the influence of the constructed features for the $DARA$ algorithm on the final result of the classification task. Referring to Figures 1, the constructed features are used to generate patterns representing the characteristics of records stored in the non-target tables. These characteristics are then summarised and the results appended as a new attribute into the target table. The classification task is then carried out as before. The Mutagenesis databases ($B1$, $B2$, $B3$) [23] and Hepatitis databases ($H1$, $H2$, $H3$) from PKDD 2005 are chosen for these experiments.

The genetic-based feature construction algorithm used in these experiments applies different types of fitness functions to construct the set of new features. These fitness functions include the Information Gain (IG) (Equation 1), Total Cluster Entropy (CE) (Equation 6), the combined measures of Information Gain and Total Cluster Entropy $(CE-IG)$ (Equation 8) and, finally, the Davies-Bouldin Index (DBI) [20]. For each experiment, the evaluation is repeated ten times independently with ten different numbers of clusters, k, ranging from 3 to 21. The $J48$ classifier (as implemented in WEKA [24]) is used to evaluate the quality of the constructed features based on the predictive accuracy of the classification task. Hence, in these experiments we compare the predictive accuracy of the decision trees produced by the $J48$ for the data when using P_{Single} and P_{All} methods. The performance accuracy is computed using the 10-fold cross-validation procedure.

Table 1. Predictive accuracy results based on leave-one-out cross validation using J48 (C4.5) Classifier

Datasets	P_{Single}	P_{All}	CE	CE-IG	IG	DBI
B1	80.9 ± 1.4	80.0 ± 2.0	**81.8 ± 1.3**	81.3 ± 0.7	81.3 ± 0.7	78.6 ± 2.9
B2	81.1 ± 1.4	79.2 ± 3.0	**82.4 ± 1.5**	80.3 ± 2.1	80.2 ± 2.3	78.8 ± 1.3
B3	78.8 ± 3.3	79.2 ± 5.7	**85.3 ± 3.9**	84.4 ± 3.9	75.5 ± 4.7	78.9 ± 4.6
H1	70.3 ± 1.6	72.3 ± 1.7	75.1 ± 2.5	**75.2 ± 2.4**	74.9 ± 2.5	74.0 ± 2.0
H2	71.8 ± 2.9	74.7 ± 1.3	**77.1 ± 3.3**	76.9 ± 3.0	76.3 ± 3.8	76.1 ± 2.1
H3	72.3 ± 3.0	74.8 ± 1.3	**77.1 ± 3.3**	76.4 ± 3.8	76.5 ± 3.9	76.3 ± 2.6

The results for the mutagenesis ($B1$, $B2$, $B3$) and hepatitis ($H1$, $H2$, $H3$) datasets are reported in Table 1. Table 1 shows the average performance accuracy of the $J48$ classifier (for all values of k), using a 10-fold cross-validation procedure. The predictive accuracy results of the $J48$ classifier are higher when the genetic-based feature construction algorithms are used compared to the predictive accuracy results for the data with features constructed by using the P_{Single} and P_{All} methods.

Among the different types of genetic-based feature construction algorithms studied in this work, the CE genetic-based feature construction algorithm produces the highest average predictive accuracy. The improvement of using the CE genetic-based feature construction algorithm is due to the fact that the CE genetic-based feature construction algorithm constructs features that develop a better organisation of the objects in the clusters, which contributes to the improvement of the predictive accuracy of the classfication tasks. That is, objects which are truly related remain closer in the same cluster.

In our results, it is shown that the final predictive accuracy for the data with constructed features using the IG genetic-based feature construction algorithm is not as good as the final predictive accuracy obtained for the data with constructed features using the CE genetic-based feature construction algorithm. The IG genetic-based feature construction algorithm constructs features based on the class information and this method assumes that each row in the non-target table represents a single instance. However, data stored in the non-target tables in relational databases have a set of rows representing a single instance. As a result, this has effects on the descriptive accuracy of the proposed data summarisation technique, $DARA$, when using the IG genetic-based feature construction algorithm to construct features. When we have unbalanced distribution of individual records stored in the non-target table, the IG measurement will be affected. In Figure 2, the data summarisation process is performed to summarise data stored in the non-target table before the actual classification task is performed. As a result, the final predictive accuracy obtained is directly affected by the quality of the summarised data.

5   Conclusions

In this paper, we have proposed a genetic-based feature construction algorithm that constructs a set of features to generate patterns that can be used to represent records stored in the non-target tables. The genetic-based feature construction method makes use of four predefined fitness functions studied in these experiments. We evaluated the quality of the newly constructed features by comparing the predictive accuracy of the $J48$ classifier obtained from the data with patterns generated using these newly constructed features with the predictive accuracy of the $J48$ classifier obtained from the data with patterns generated using the original attributes. This paper has described how feature construction can be used in the data summarisation process to get better descriptive accuracy, and indirectly improve the predictive accuracy of a classification task. In particular, we have investigated the use of Information Gain (IG), Cluster Entropy (CE), Davies-Bouldin Index (DBI) and a combination of Information Gain and Cluster Entropy ($CE - IG$) as the fitness functions used in the genetic-based feature construction algorithm to construct new features.

It is shown in the experimental results that the quality of summarised data is directly influenced by the methods used to create patterns that represent records in the $(n \times p)$ TF-IDF weighted frequency matrix. The results of the evaluation of the genetic-based feature construction algorithm show that the data summarisation results can be improved by constructing features by using the cluster entropy (CE) genetic-based feature construction algorithm. The results of the evaluation of the genetic-based feature construction algorithm show that the data summarisation results can be improved by constructing features by using the cluster entropy genetic-based feature construction algorithm. Finally, by improving the descriptive accuracy of the data summarisation approach, the predictive accuracy of a classfication problem can also be improved, provided that the summarised data is fed to the classification task.

References

1. Alfred, R., Kazakov, D.: Data Summarisation Approach to Relational Domain Learning Based on Frequent Pattern to Support the Development of Decision Making. In: 2nd ADMA International Conference, pp. 889–898 (2006)
2. Blockeel, H., Dehaspe, L.: Tilde and Warmr User Manual (1999), http://www.cs.kuleuvan.ac.be/~ml/PS/TWuser.ps.gz
3. Lavrač, N., Flach, P.A.: An extended transformation approach to Inductive Logic Programming. ACM Trans. Comput. Log. 2(4), 458–494 (2001)
4. Salton, G., Wong, A., Yang, C.S.: A Vector Space Model for Automatic Indexing. Commun. ACM 18(11), 613–620 (1975)
5. Pagallo, G., Haussler, D.: Boolean Feature Discovery in Empirical Learning. Machine Learning 5, 71–99 (1990)
6. Hu, Y.J., Kibler, D.F.: Generation of Attributes for Learning Algorithms. In: AAAI/IAAI, vol. 1, pp. 806–811 (1996)
7. Hu, Y.J.: A genetic programming approach to constructive induction. In: Proc. of the Third Annual Genetic Programming Conference, pp. 146–157. Morgan Kauffman, Madison (1998)
8. Otero, F.E.B., Silva, M.S., Freitas, A.A., Nievola, J.C.: Genetic Programming for Attribute Construction in Data Mining. In: Ryan, C., Soule, T., Keijzer, M., Tsang, E.P.K., Poli, R., Costa, E. (eds.) EuroGP 2003. LNCS, vol. 2610, pp. 384–393. Springer, Heidelberg (2003)

9. Bensusan, H., Kuscu, I.: Constructive Induction using Genetic Programming. In: ICML 1996, Evolutionary computing and Machine Learning Workshop (1996)
10. Zheng, Z.: Constructing X-of-N Attributes for Decision Tree Learning. Machine Learning 40(1), 35–75 (2000)
11. Zheng, Z.: Effects of Different Types of New Attribute on Constructive Induction. In: ICTAI, pp. 254–257 (1996)
12. Quinlan, R.J.: Decision-Tree. In: C4.5: Programs for Machine Learning. Morgan Kaufmann Series in Machine Learning (1993)
13. Holland, J.: Adaptation in Natural and Artificial Systems. University of Michigan Press (1975)
14. Amaldi, E., Kann, V.: On the Approximability of Minimising Nonzero Variables or Unsatisfied Relations in Linear Systems. Theory Computer Science 209(1-2), 237–260 (1998)
15. Freitas, A.A.: Understanding the Crucial Role of Attribute Interaction in Data Mining. Artif. Intell. Rev. 16(3), 177–199 (2001)
16. Shafti, L.S., Pérez, E.: Genetic Approach to Constructive Induction Based on Non-algebraic Feature Representation. In: R. Berthold, M., Lenz, H.-J., Bradley, E., Kruse, R., Borgelt, C. (eds.) IDA 2003. LNCS, vol. 2810, pp. 599–610. Springer, Heidelberg (2003)
17. Vafaie, H., DeJong, K.: Feature Space Transformation Using Genetic Algorithms. IEEE Intelligent Systems 13(2), 57–65 (1998)
18. Koza, J.R.: Genetic Programming: On the programming of computers by means of natural selection. Statistics and Computing 4(2) (1994)
19. Krawiec, K.: Genetic Programming-based Construction of Features for Machine Learning and Knowledge Discovery Tasks. Genetic Programming and Evolvable Machines 3, 329–343 (2002)
20. Davies, D.L., Bouldin, D.W.: A Cluster Separation Measure. IEEE Trans. Pattern Analysis and Machine Intelligence 1, 224–227 (1979)
21. Shannon, C.E.: A mathematical theory of communication. Bell system technical journal 27 (1948)
22. Wiener, N.: Cybernetics: Or Control and Communication in Animal and the Machine. MIT Press, Cambridge (2000)
23. Srinivasan, A., Muggleton, S., Sternberg, M.J.E., King, R.D.: Theories for Mutagenicity: A Study in First-Order and Feature-Based Induction. Artif. Intell. 85(1-2), 277–299 (1996)
24. Witten, I.H., Frank, E.: Data Mining: Practical Machine Learning Tools and Techniques with Java Implementations. Morgan Kaufmann, San Francisco (1999)

Suicidal Risk Evaluation Using a Similarity-Based Classifier

S. Chattopadhyay[1], P. Ray[1], H.S. Chen[2], M.B. Lee[3] and H.C. Chiang[3]

[1] Asia-Pacific ubiquitous Healthcare Research Center (APuHC),
School of Information Systems, Technology and Management,
Australian School of Business, Chiang
University of New South Wales (UNSW), 2052 Sydney, Australia
subhagata@unsw.edu.de, p.ray@unsw.edu.au
[2] Asia-Pacific ubiquitous Healthcare Research Center (APuHC)
[3] Taiwan Suicide Prevention Center (TSPC)
National Taiwan University, Taipei 10617, Taiwan
chenhs@ntu.edu.tw, mingbeen@ntu.edu.tw, d92845004@ntu.edu.tw

Abstract. Suicide remains one of the leading causes of death in the world and it is showing an increasing trend. Suicide is preventable by early screening of the risks. But the risk assessment is a complex task due to involvement of multiple predictors, which are highly subjective in nature and varies from one case to another. Moreover, none of the available suicide intent scales (SIS) are found to be sufficient to evaluate the risk patterns in a group of patients. Given this scenario, the present paper applies similarity-based pattern-matching technique for mining suicidal risks in vulnerable groups of patients. At first, medical data of groups of suicidal patients have been collected and modeled according to Pierce's Suicide Intent Scale (PSIS) and then engineered using a JAVA-based pattern-matching tool that performs as an intelligent classifier. Results show that addition of more factors, for example, age and sex of the patients brings more clarity to identify the suicidal risk patterns.

Keywords: Suicidality; Pierce's Suicidal Intent Scale (SIS), Suicide risk assessment, Similarity-based approach, JAVA platform.

1 Introduction

The term 'suicidality' means suicidal thoughts, intents or plans, actions and committing suicide [1]. It's a complex issue involving the orchestrated effects of several socio-biological parameters and environmental constructs [1]. The present scenario is quite gloomy as the incidence of suicide is showing an increasing trend irrespective of age and sex [2]. Environmental issues such as social loss, dejections, unemployment etc. put strong challenges to one's life and to overcome these one should be able to cope. Any event that demands coping may be termed as stressful life events. People usually cope with such stresses at a variable extent. But in some people, especially those who have psychiatric illness, such coping mechanism is often absent and interestingly, they are some times found to be hypersensitive in nature even to a minimal

C. Tang et al. (Eds.): ADMA 2008, LNAI 5139, pp. 51–61, 2008.

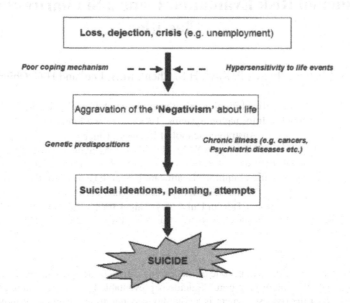

Fig. 1. Roles of environment and neurobiological factors behind suicide

amount of stress that is normally adapted by others. As a result there are aggravations of the negative thoughts about the life. They become cynic and often loose the meaning of living their lives further. Suicidal tendencies and in turn suicide emerge from this negativism, often remains unrecognised and then one day, it occurs suddenly (refer to Figure 1).

Thus suicidality is a challenging multi-disciplinary research area. The most critical challenge of suicidality is that its occurrence is absolutely unpredictable and in almost all occasions, it is abrupt and sudden. Therefore, early screening of risks could be useful to prevent its occurrence.

To address these issues in various domains of internal medicine, application of data mining and knowledge engineering techniques are gaining popularities as these are often useful for achieving the speedy solutions for a health problem e.g. psychiatric illnesses that often kills years of precious time [3]. Unfortunately due to involved complexities and subjectivity with psychiatry, the number of available literature does not score much. To engineer knowledge from a set of complex and subjective medical data of suicidal patients, the present paper is an attempt to screen suicidal risks with the help of a JAVA-based classifier.

The contribution of this paper may be three-fold. Firstly, it describes the methodology to simplify the subjectivity issues of complex medical data using data mining-based techniques and fit with Pierce's Suicide Intent Scale (PSIS). Secondly, using a similarity-based approach an intelligent classifier is developed on JAVA platform that can evaluate the suicidal risk pattern. This could be a significant contribution in neuropsychiatry and medical informatics. Finally, this analysis itself should give valuable insights that might be helpful for supporting medical doctors and psychologists to screen the degree of prospective vulnerability of suicide in future patients.

The present work is organized as follows. **Section 2** describes the background and motivations for the study. **Section 3** discusses the methodology that includes data collection, data modeling (based on PSIS), and development of the intelligent classifier. The performance of the developed classifier has been validated in **Section 4**. Finally in **Section 5** conclusions have been drawn, limitations of this work are explained and the possible extensions are discussed.

2 Background and Motivations

Suicidality has been one of the most challenging research fields because of its multi-faceted nature and socio-economic importance. It does cause loss of lives and resources, but preventable if screened and treated. Literature survey using Cochrane, MedLine, MedScape, Psycinfo and PubMed databases show that most of the studies on suicidality have focussed on a) meta-analysis of demographic scenario, b) neuro-biological basis, c) psychiatric predispositions, and d) questionnaire-based suicide intent scales (SIS) designs. Detail descriptions of all the studies are beyond the scope of this paper; however, some of the works, relevant to demonstrate the importance of suicidality as a research topic are discussed as follows.

Global studies on suicidality show that socially dejected, widowed or unemployed middle-aged males commit suicide more than females who attempts more [1]. Apart from adult populations, there are also evidences that the tendency of suicide is increasing among teenagers as well as in children [2]. Chronic illnesses, such as mental diseases [1], cancers [3], HIV [4], chronic pain disorders (e.g. rheumatoid arthritis [5]) contribute behind the onset of suicidality. Suicidality is also very common in those who are drug or alcohol abusers [6]. Thus, study (especially screening) of suicidality is of global interest.

Screening of vulnerability based on one's neurobiological status could be a useful guide for risk assessment. Studies have found a strong connection between suicide and serotonin deficiency in the brain [7], governed by serotonin transporter gene. More recently, attempts have been made to find a stable biomarker to study suicidality. A relationship between the lower ratios of homovanillic acid (HVA)-to-5-hydroxyindoleacetic acid (5-HIAA) is found to be correlating in the cerebrospinal fluid of suicide attempters who suffer from depressions [8] [9]. Such finding poses a strong presumption that suicidality is perhaps biologically pre-determined.

For early screening and assessment of suicidal risks, Suicide intent scales (SIS) or Intent Score Scales (ISS) remain the only way by which one can predict the vulnerability starting from suicidal ideations to committing suicide. Unfortunately there are only a few scales, available to measure the suicide risks. The Beck's suicide intent scale [10] is one of the most widely used SIS. In 1977 and 1981, respectively Pierce developed [11] and validated [12] a modified version of the Beck scale, called Pierce's Suicide Intent Scale (PSIS) that is used in this paper. Nurse's Global Assessment of Suicide Risk (NGASR) [13] is a recently developed scale that is especially useful for the novice scorers. Detail description of all these rating scales is beyond scope of the present paper. Generally speaking, SIS render a useful guidance, especially prevents complacency and over confidence but these are still very much manual and often the scorings are biased. For example, it may so happen that for similar cases, same person may score differently during different occasions for a particular patient. To address these issues, computerized intelligent systems may be useful.

This paper proposes that applications of various data mining approaches and intelligent computing could be interesting research areas, but due to involved complexities with the psychiatric data, the number of studies does not score much. However, to address it particularly, Chattopadhyay (2007) and Chatttopadhyay et al. (2007) have developed tools to identify suicidal risks in psychiatric patients using statistical modelling techniques [14] further extended to the development of an SVM-based controller [15]. This paper aims to develop a similarity-based classifier and test its performance (capacity to measure suicidal risks) with a set of known patients with varying degree of suicidal risks.

3 Methodology

This paper proposes to develop a similarity-based classifier that is able to grade the risk of suicidality in a group of patients. The steps are as follows,

Step 1: Data Collection

Retrospective information of a group of anonymous patients (n=50) with history of suicidal attempts and committed suicides are collected from the hospital records. It is important to mention here that proper ethical measures have been taken to conduct the data collection process. The data thus collected are structured according to PSIS-based rating tool, which is discussed as follows.

Table 1. Modified PSIS (a new factor 'M' is appended)

Circumstance scoring	Self reporting scoring	Medical scoring
A. Isolation	G. Lethality of the act	K. Predictable outcome
B. Time of act	H. Stated intent	L. Probability of death with or without treatment
C. Precautions against rescue	I. Premeditated act	M. Past history of suicide attempts
D. Activity gaining help	J. Reaction to act	
E. Final act in anticipation		
F. Writing a clear suicide note		

Originally PSIS is composed of the 12 factors under three broad scoring constructs (refer to Table 1), these are
- Circumstance Risk Scoring,
- Medical Risk Scoring, and
- Self-reporting risk scoring.

As studies have shown that suicidal risks are higher in patients with histories of past attempts [9], one more factor have been added in PSIS, i.e. 'past history of suicide attempts' (refer to factor 'M' in Table 1) under Medical Risk Scoring to make our study a more realistic one. The medical data are collected based on certain inclusion and exclusion criteria as follows,

Inclusion criteria

- Male and female adults,
- History of one or more suicide attempts,
- Predisposed with chronic illnesses (e.g. psychiatric co-morbidity, cancers etc.), and
- Patients having warning symptoms (e.g. IS PATH WARM **I** – Ideation, **S** - Substance abuse, **P** – Purposelessness, **A** – Anxiety, **T** – Trapped, **H** – Hopelessness, **W** – Withdrawal, **A** – Anger, **R** – Recklessness, and **M** – Mood changes [16]) prior to the suicidal act.

Exclusion criteria

- Eunuchs
- Children and adolescents, and
- Violent suicide without any warning sign.

The data thus collected are highly heterogeneous due to multiple entries in the hospital record as well as secondary in nature as the doctors and nurses collect these. Hence the data mandates pre-processing before the actual analysis is done.

Step 2: Data Pre-processing

Data pre-processing is an important step to prepare the data for classification and prediction study [17]. In this study following steps have been taken. This refers to cleaning of noise (errors), redundancies, and missing values. Noise is eliminated incorporating the expertise of psychiatrists and psychologists case-by-case. Missing values are filled up with the most common value of the corresponding attributes. Redundancies are removed as well. Some of the attributes in the data may be redundant. Correlation analysis has been done to identify which two data within an attribute are statistically similar. For example, a group of similar patients may be regarded as a particular group of patients, represented by a single patient than all patients. In this study the data has further been transformed by generalizing it to higher-level concepts, which are particularly useful for all the continuous-valued attributes. In this study, for example, each factor as well as their corresponding risks is weighted as 'low', 'medium' or 'high'. Intensive incorporation of domain knowledge remains pivotal to such transformation. Based on PSIS and the knowledge of domain experts the following parameters have been considered to structure the whole data,

- Independent variables (factors) - thirteen factors (A to M) into consideration for each patient. Each factor has 'low', 'medium' or 'high' contribution denoted by values 0, 1, or 2 according to their contribution or level of involvement,
- Dependent variables (responses) - Four risk levels (values from 1 to 4). Risk levels 1-4 express 'suicidal plans or thoughts', 'single suicidal attempts', 'multiple suicidal attempts' and 'committed suicide', respectively. In this study we have considered first three risk levels because at these stages, if properly screened, suicide is still preventable.

- Age of the patients (four levels; level 1 to 4 are represented by <40, >80, between 60 and 80, and 40-60 years), and
- Sex of the patients where 0 and 1 indicates female and male, respectively.

Thus an example of a patient within the matrix may be as follows

FACTORS				RESPONSE
A B...M AGE SEX				RISK

0	2	1	2	0		3

The rule thus may be created as follows

IF A is 0 AND B is 2 AND ... AGE is 2 AND SEX is 0 THEN RISK is 3.

Step 3: Development of Similarity-Based Classifier

Similarity measure is a known technique to identify look-alike classes in a case based or rule based reasoning system with some probability value of how much similarity. To accomplish it, distance measure is a way with a condition that more is the distance less is the similarity and vice versa. The challenge in this paper is to apply these techniques to a complex medical data set having multiple parameters. This is described as follows.

Let us consider N data points in M dimensional $[T]$ hyperspace, where each data point X_i ($i = 1, 2, 3, 4,..., N$) is represented by a set of M values (i.e., $X_{i1}, X_{i2},....X_{iM}$). The Euclidean distances (D) between two data points, 'i' and 'j' are calculated as follows,

$$D_{ij} = \sqrt{\sum_{k=1}^{M} (X_{ik} - X_{jk})^2} \tag{1}$$

There is a maximum of $N \times N$ distances values among N data points and out of which $^N C_2$ distances belong to D_{ij} (where $i<j$) and D_{ji} each. Moreover, there are N diagonal values, which are equal to zero (where $i=j$). Similarity (S) between any two points (i.e., i and j) may be determined like the following,

$$S_{ij} = D_{ij}^{-1} \tag{2}$$

It means more is the distance less is the similarity and vice versa.

In this study, the data matrix is generated with the collected patient data (i.e. training set, N=40) that is fed to a classifier that adopts a similarity-based approach, described above. The working principle of the classifier is to calculate the distances of two patient records (i and j) or between a patient and a class of records. Cumulating the absolute distance (δ) of all factors does this. For example,

FACTOR:	A	B	C	D	E	F	G	H	I	J	K	L	M	RISK
PT A:	1	2	0	1	1	0	2	0	1	0	2	2	1	3
PT B:	1	2	1	0	0	0	1	1	2	0	2	0	1	2
...														
PT 'n'	1	0	1	0	0	0	1	1	2	0	2	0	2	1
ABS.δ :	0	0	1	1	1	0	1	1	1	0	0	2	0	
SUM: 8														

Here, PT A and PT B represent patient A and B respectively. ABS δ is the deviation with absolute value and SUM denotes the total distance. In this example, the distance between these two cases is 8 (where as, the minimum is 0; the maximum is 13 x 2 = 26) and we know that less is the distance more is the similarity. Finally, the risk is estimated based on the closeness of the attributes, i.e. least cumulative distance. Additional feature of the developed classifier is that every new case dealt by it is appended with the training data letting it to be more robust, matured and more intelligent. The performance of this classifier has been validated on some test cases (N=10) as follows.

4 Validation of the Performance

Experiment has been carried out to test the performance of the developed classifier in two modules – module 1 (only with the PSIS-based factors without age and sex) and module 2 (PSIS-based factors plus age and sex of the patients). The objective of this experiment is to note whether additional factors might influence the overall performance of the classifier.

Module 1. *Analysis without taking sex and age into consideration*

First, search has been made to find the closest case in the past (i.e., the patient that is closest to the new patient). This is achieved by calculating the distances between this patient and all other patients (attribute-by-attribute).

Second, input data are separated and constructed into four classes with regard to the corresponding risk levels. This was supposed to give us some insight into the structure of the classes. Virtual class centre (i.e., a virtual patient whose record is closest to all other records), the mean, and the standard deviation (STD. DEV) for each factor have been calculated. Let us see this example,

FACTOR:	A	B	C	D	E	F	G	H	I	J	K	L	M
PT 1:	1	2	0	1	1	0	2	0	1	0	2	2	1
PT 2:	1	2	1	0	0	0	1	1	2	0	2	0	1
PT 3:	0	0	1	1	1	0	1	1	1	0	0	2	0

MEAN OF FACTOR 'A':   (1+1+0)/3 = 0.66
STD DEV. FACTOR 'A': SQRT (((1+1+0) - 4/9)/3) = 0.72

Third, the distances are measured between a patient and each of the four classes to find the class closest to this patient. For this, the overall distance (i.e., the cumulated distances between this patient and all patients of a particular class), the relative distance (i.e., the overall distance divided by the number patients in the class which results in the average distance), and the normalized distance (i.e., the relative distance transferred to a 0.0 to 1.0 spectrum) are calculated for the better understanding of the similarities. For example, let the following three patients be of the class "risk level 2"

FACTOR:	A	B	C	D	E	F	G	H	I	J	K	L	M
PT 1:	1	2	0	1	1	0	2	0	1	0	2	2	1
PT 2:	1	2	1	0	0	0	1	1	2	0	2	0	1
PT 3:	0	0	1	1	1	0	1	1	1	0	0	2	0
NEW PT 1:	1	0	0	2	1	0	1	1	2	0	0	1	1

ABS. DIST: 1 4 2 4 1 0 1 1 2 0 4 3 1
SUM: 24
REL. DIST. = ABS. DIST. / NO. OF ROWS = 24 / 3 = 8.00
NORM. DIST. =   REL. DIST. / MAX. DISTANCE   = 8 / 26 = 0.31
NEW PT 2: 0 2 1 1 0 0 1 1 1 0 2 2 1
ABS. DIST. 2 2 1 1 2 0 1 1 1 0 2 2 1
SUM: 16
REL. DIST. = 16 / 3 = 5.33
NORM. DIST. =   16 / 3x26 = 0.21

In the case, new patient no. 2 (NEW PT2) is closer to the given "risk level 2" class than new patient no. 1.

Fourth, probability of a patient being of risk level 1, 2, or 3, respectively (level 4 cases were disregarded for these patients have committed suicide and cannot be taken into account) has been estimated. To this end, it is found that all cases (independent of their risk level) within a certain distance (starting from 10 and decreased in single steps to 1). Based on the derived cases, the number of cases that were risk levels 1, 2, or 3 is counted and thus the probability can be calculated. For example, let us assume that for given patient record there were 8 cases within a given distance of 5. Let us further assume that of these 8 cases three had the risk level 1, four belong to the risk level 2 and one was at the risk level 3. Based on the aforementioned assumptions of the similarity of a patient's risk level to the other is coherent with the distance between those two. It may be said that this patient is with a probability of 3/8 (=37.5%) of the risk level 1, 4/8 (=50%) of risk level 2, and 1/8 (=12.5%) of risk level 3, respectively.

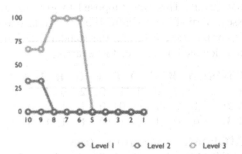

Fig. 2. (a)

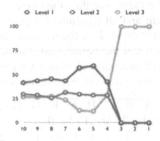

Fig. 2. (b)

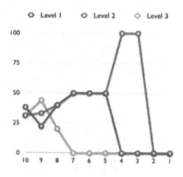

Fig. 2. (c)

Therefore the final diagnosis of the risk level for the given patient becomes 'risk level 2' or moderate risk. Refer to figure 2 (a) new patient values (all factors are set '0'), (b) new patient values (all factors are set '1'), and (c) new patient values (all factors are set '2'). The 'x' and 'y' axis in this figure denote the number of new patients and the probability of risk.

Module 2: *Analysis after considering age and sex into analysis*

First, six classes, each with regard to another attribute (male, female, age group 1, age group 2, age group 3, and age group 4) are constructed. Similar as done above, the virtual class centre (i.e., a virtual patient whose record is closest to all other records) is then calculated along with the means, and the standard deviations for each factor.

Second, in the same manner, the distances between a patient and each of the six classes are measured to find the class closest to this patient (which in an ideal world would be the two classes that correspond to the patient's age and sex). For this, the overall distance (i.e., the cumulated distances between this patient and all patients of a particular class) has been calculated along with the relative distance (i.e., the overall distance divided by the number patients in the class which results in the average distance), and the normalized distance [0.0,1.0].

Third, the probability of a patient being of risk level 1, 2, or 3, respectively needs to be estimated. To this end, all cases (independent of their risk level, but dependent on the patient's age and sex) within a certain distance (starting from 10 and decreased in single steps to 1) can be found. Based on the found-cases, then, counts of the number of cases that were with the risk levels 1, 2, or 3 including the probability values corresponding to the risk levels can be determined as shown in figure 3 (a) and (b), respectively.

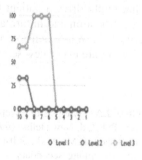

Fig. 3. (a)

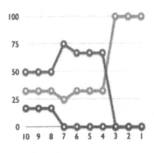

Fig. 3. (b)

In figure 3 (a) and (b) age group 1 and sex (both males and females) of the patients were considered. Similarly studies have been done with different other age groups, but age group 1 is found to be most at risk especially in male patients.

5   Conclusions and Future Scopes

From the above study the following conclusions may be drawn

- The classifier is able to evaluate the risk levels with certain probabilities. As the real-world scenario behind suicidality is extremely complex, it is not possible to make assumptions with absolute accuracy. However, with time and maturity, we hope that the accuracy can be improved. Moreover, certain more patterns may be captured with other different cases.
- It is also possible that the given model must be adjusted by, for example, weighting each factor according to the opinion and experience of psychologists. Defining the weights accurately behind individual case is a time taking process and impossible to some extent. Therefore, the proposed classifier may be used at least to get the clue towards to risk-level of an individual case at this stage of research, and
- The suicidal behaviour of each patient is so highly unique and special that is not really possible to evaluate a patient just based on historical data. But such a database could be very useful to fetch the hidden rules (refer to the example in page 7).

The world is so complex and intricate that it is probably never really possible to take all factors into consideration that might drive a patient to commit suicide. But this study can be proliferated with identification and in turn addition of more factors (predictors) within the classifier. Another useful extension of this tool can be that a rule base system can be constructed to capture every new scenario it comes across.

References

1. Kaplan, H.I., Saddock, B.J., Greb, J.A.: Synopsis of Psychiatry, Behavioural Sciences and Clinical Psychiatry. B.I. Waverly Pvt. Ltd, New Delhi (1994)
2. Fleming, T.M., Merry, S.N., Robinson, E.M., et al.: Self-reported suicide attempts and associated risk and protective factors among secondary school students in New Zealand. Aust. NZ J. of Psych. 41(3), 213–221 (2007)

3. Camidge, D.R., Stockton, D.L., Frame, S., et al.: Hospital admissions and deaths relating to deliberate self-harm and accidents within 5 years of a cancer diagnosis: a national study in Scotland, UK. Br. J. Cancer 96(5), 752–757 (2007)
4. Lacombe, K., Pacanowski, J.: HIV infection and comorbidities. Rev. Prat. 6(9), 995–1004 (2006)
5. Timonen, M., Viilo, K., Hakko, H., et al.: Suicides in persons suffering from rheumatoid arthritis. Rheumatology (Oxford) 42(2), 287–291 (2003)
6. Li, Y.M.: Deliberate self-harm and relationship to alcohol use at an emergency department in eastern Taiwan. Kaohsiung J. of Med. Sc. 23(5), 247–253 (2007)
7. Marcinko, D., Pivac, N., Martinac, M., et al.: Platelet serotonin and serum cholesterol concentrations in suicidal and non-suicidal male patients with a first episode of psychosis. Psych. Res. 150(1), 105–108 (2007)
8. Jokinen, J., Nordström, A.L., Nordström, P.: The relationship between CSF HVA/5-HIAA ratio and suicide intent in suicide attempters. Arch. Sui. Res. 11(2), 187–192 (2007)
9. Kisely, S., Smith, M., Lawrence, D., et al.: Mortality in individuals who have had psychiatric treatment: Population-based study in Nova Scotia. Br. J. of Psych. 187, 552–558 (2005)
10. Beck, A.T., Schuyler, D., Herman, J.: Development of Suicidal Intent Scales. In: Beck, A.T., Resnick, H., Lettieri, D. (eds.) The Prediction of Suicide (1974)
11. Pierce, D.W.: Suicidal Intent in Self-injuries. Br. J. of Psych. 130, 377–385 (1977)
12. Pierce, D.W.: The predictive validation of a suicide intent scale: a five year follow-up. Br. J. Psych. 139, 391–396 (1981)
13. Cutcliffe, J.R., Barker, P.: The Nurses' Global Assessment of Suicide Risk (NGASR): developing a tool for clinical practice. J. of Psych. Ment. Health Nurs. 11(4), 393–400 (2004)
14. Chattopadhyay, S.: A Study on Suicidal Risk Analysis. In: Proc. IEEE Healthcom2007 – 9th International conference on e-health Networking, Applications & Services, Taiwan Taipei. IEEE Press, Los Alamitos (2007)
15. Chattopadhyay, S., Ray, P., Lee, M.B., et al.: Towards the Design of an e-Health System for Suicide Prevention. In: Proc. 10th IASTED Conference on Artificial Intelligence and Soft Computing, Palma de Mallorca, Spain. ACTA Press (2007)
16. American Association of Suicidology [WWW page] (last accessed 03/3/08), http://www.suicidology.org/displaycommon.cfm?an=2
17. Han, J., Kamber, M.: Data Mining concepts and techniques. Morgan Kauffman, San Francisco (2006)
18. Yao, J., Dash, M., Tan, S.T., Liu, H.: Entropy-based fuzzy clustering and fuzzy modeling. Fuzzy Sets Syst. 113, 381–388 (2000)

Gene Selection for Cancer Classification Using DCA

Hoai An Le Thi*, Van Vinh Nguyen, and Samir Ouchani

Laboratory of Theoretical and Applied Computer Science (LITA)
UFR MIM, University of Paul Verlaine - Metz Ile du Saulcy, 57045 Metz, France
lethi@univ-mezt.fr

Abstract. Gene selection is a very important problem in microarray data analysis and has critical implications for the discovery of genes related to serious diseases. In this paper the problem of gene selection for cancer classification is considered. We develop a combined SVMs - feature selection approach based on the Smoothly Clipped Absolute Deviation penalty, minimizing directly the classifier performance. To solve our optimization problems, we apply the DCA (Difference of Convex functions Algorithms) which is a general framework for non-convex continuous optimization. This leads to a successive linear programming algorithm with finite convergence. Preliminary computational experiments on different real data demonstrate that our methods accomplish the desired goal: suppression of a large number of features with a small error of classification.

Keyword: Gene selection, Feature selection, Cancer classification, SVMs, nonconvex optimization, DC programming, DCA.

1 Introduction

Microarray data are used to understand and monitor genes expression in many areas of biomedical research. Microarrays are constantly delivering large amounts of data about the inner life of a cell. One of challenges today is to evaluate these gigantic data streams and extract useful information. Therefore robust and accurate gene selection methods are required to identify differentially expressed class of genes across low sample size. This task is also called feature selection, a commonly addressed problem in machine learning, where one has class-labeled data and wants to figure out which features best discriminate among the classes. If the genes are the features describing the cell, the problem is to select the features that have the biggest impact on describing the results and to drop the features with little or no effect.

The feature selection aims at picking out some original features to facilitate data collection, reducing storage space and classification time, and also defying the curse of dimensionality to improve prediction performance. Several methods

---

* Corresponding author.

C. Tang et al. (Eds.): ADMA 2008, LNAI 5139, pp. 62–72, 2008.

have been proposed in the literature for these aims, some methods put more emphasis on one aspect than another. In this work, focusing on gene selection for cancer classification we propose an embedded method by directly optimizing a two-part objective function with a goodness-of-fit term and a penalty for a large number of variables. The embedded methods are preferable to achieve good sparsity and accuracy because they proceed simultaneously classification and variable selection. However they usually lead to a nonconvex optimization problem that is hard to solve exactly. In the last years some efficient embedded methods based on Support Vector Machine (SVMs) have been proposed. They are distinguished from others in the use of the penalty functions ([1] - [7]).

Our Contribution: the starting point of our work is the approach of Zhang et al. ([7]) who have considered the linear SVMs model with a non-convex penalty called Smoothly Clipped Absolute Deviation (SCAD penalty). The SCAD penalty function has been proposed by Fan, J. and Li, R ([2]) in the context of regression and variable selection. In [2] computational experiments on a family of penalty functions indicated that the penalized likelihood with the SCAD penalty function gives the best performance in selecting significant variables without creating excessive biases. Zhang el al ([7]) have considered the so called SCAD SVM model where the optimization problem consists of two parts: the data fit is represented by the hinge loss function, and the regularization is defined as the SCAD penalty. This is a very hard nonsmooth nonconvex problem. Using a local quadratic approximation Zhang et al ([7]) have proposed an iterative algorithm to solve the SCAD SVM in which only a series of linear equation systems need to be solved. Our main contribution is to approximate the SCAD penalty by a DC (Difference of Convex functions) function and then develop an efficient algorithm based on DC programming and DCA (DC Algorithm) for solving the resulting optimization problem. DCA is a robust approach for nonconvex continuous optimisation ([8,9,10]). Preliminary computational experiments indicate that the proposed method is promising and more efficient than the standard L_1- SVM algorithm.

The paper is organized as follows. In the next section we present the SCAD SVM model developed in [7] and our new formulation for SCAD SVM. The algorithm to solve the resulting problem is presented in Section 3 while the numerical results are reported in Section 4.

2   Models

To construct an SVM, we consider the training set $\{(x_i, y_i)\}_{i=1}^{n}$ where $x_i \in \mathbb{R}^d$ is the input vector, and $y_i \in \{+1, -1\}$ indicates its class label; the classification problem is to learn a discrimination rule $c : \mathbb{R}^d \to \{+1, -1\}$ which permits us to assign a class label to any new subject observed in the future. For microarray gene expression data, x_i represents the expression levels of d genes of the ith sample tissue and y_i is "normal" or "not"; often we have $d >> n$.

2.1 The SCAD SVM

The SCAD penalty proposed by Fan and Li [2] has been expressed as follow, for $t \in \mathbb{R}$:

$$p_\lambda(|t|) = \begin{cases} \lambda|t| & \text{if} \quad |t| \le \lambda, \\ -\frac{|t|^2 - 2\alpha\lambda|t| + \lambda^2}{2(\alpha-1)} & \text{if} \quad \lambda < |t| \le \alpha\lambda, \\ \frac{(\alpha+1)\lambda^2}{2} & \text{if} \quad |t| > \alpha\lambda, \end{cases} \tag{1}$$

where $\alpha > 2$ and $\lambda > 0$ are two tuning parameters. The function in (1) is a quadratic spline function with two knots at λ and $\alpha\lambda$. It is singular at the origin, and do not have continuous second order derivatives. The Figure 1 shows the SCAD penalty function with $\alpha = 3$ and $\lambda = 0.4$.

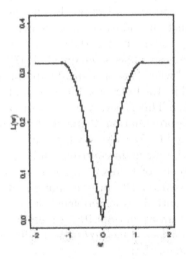

Fig. 1. The SCAD penalty function

For achieving the gene selection to classification of tissues, Zhang et al [7] proposed the following formulation called SCAD SVM (they focused on linear SVMs, i.e. the classifier is defined by the hyperplane $w^T x + b$)

$$\min_{b,w} \quad (1/n) \sum_{i=1}^{n} [1 - y_i(b + \langle w, x_i \rangle)]_+ + \sum_{j=1}^{d} p_\lambda(|w_j|). \tag{2}$$

The objective function in (2) consists of the hinge loss part and the SCAD penalty on w. The parameter λ balances the trade-off between data fitting and model parsimony. If λ is too small, the procedure tends to overfit the training data and gives a classifier with a little sparsity; If λ is too large, the produced classifier can be very sparse but have a poor discriminating power.

2.2 The SCAD SVM DC

In this work we attempt to use DC programming and DCA which is a robust approach for non-convex continuous optimisation ([8,9,10]) to solve the SCAD SVM problem. For this purpose, we express the SCAD penalty function by an appropriate way such that the resulting problem can be formulated in term of a DC program.

To eliminate the absolute symbol in the objective function of (14) we define the function f_λ which coincides with p_λ for all $t \geq 0$, namely:

$$f_\lambda(t) := \begin{cases} \lambda t & \text{if} \quad 0 \leq t \leq \lambda, \\ -\frac{t^2 - 2\alpha\lambda t + \lambda^2}{2(\alpha-1)} & \text{if} \quad \lambda < t \leq \alpha\lambda, \\ \frac{(\alpha+1)\lambda^2}{2} & \text{if} \quad t > \alpha\lambda, \\ f_\lambda(-t) & \text{if} \quad t < 0. \end{cases} \quad (3)$$

Our new model called SCAD SVM DC takes then the form:

$$\text{(SCAD SVM DC)} \quad \begin{aligned} \min \quad & F(\xi, w, b) := (1/n) \sum_{i=1}^{n} \xi_i + \sum_{j=1}^{d} f_\lambda(w_j) \\ \text{s.t.:} \quad & y_i(b + \langle w, x_i \rangle) \geq 1 - \xi_i \quad (i = 1, \ldots, n) \\ & \xi_i \geq 0 \quad (i = 1, \ldots, n), \end{aligned} \quad (4)$$

where the nonnegative slack variables $\xi_i, i = 1, \ldots n$ represent the error of the linear classifier. We will show in the next section that SCAD SVM DC is a DC program for which DCA can be successfully applied.

3 DCA for Solving SCAD SVM DC Problem

First, let us describe some notations and background materials that will be used in the next. For a convex function θ defined on $\mathbb{R}^p$ and $x_0 \in \text{dom } \theta := \{x \in \mathbb{R}^p : \theta(x_0) < +\infty\}$, $\partial\theta(x_0)$ denotes the subdifferential of θ at x_0 that is

$$\partial\theta(x_0) := \{y \in \mathbb{R}^p : \theta(x) \geq \theta(x_0) + \langle x - x_0, y \rangle, \forall x \in \mathbb{R}^p\}.$$

The subdifferential $\partial\theta(x_0)$ is a closed convex set in $\mathbb{R}^n$. It generalizes the derivative in the sense that θ is differentiable at x_0 if and only if $\theta(x_0)$ is reduced to a singleton which is exactly $\{\theta'(x_0)\}$. A convex function θ is called *convex polyhedral* if it is the maximum of a finite family of affine functions, i.e.

$$\theta(x) = \max\{\langle a_i, x \rangle + b : i = 1, \ldots p\}, a_i \in \mathbb{R}^p.$$

A point x^* is called *critical point* of the function $G - H$ if:

$$\partial H(x^*) \cap \partial G(x^*) \neq \emptyset. \quad (5)$$

DC programming and DCA which have been introduced by Pham Dinh Tao in 1985 and extensively developed by Le Thi Hoai An and Pham Dinh Tao since 1994 (see e.g. [8,9,10]) constitute the backbone of smooth/nonsmooth nonconvex programming and global optimization.

A general DC program takes the form:

$$\inf\{F(x) := (Gx) - H(x) : x \in \mathbb{R}^p\} \quad (P_{dc})$$

where G and H are lower semicontinuous proper convex functions on $\mathbb{R}^p$. Such a function F is called DC function, and $G - H$, DC decomposition of F while G and H are DC components of F. The convex constraint $x \in C$ can be incorporated in the objective function of (P_{dc}) by using the indicator function on C denoted χ_C which is defined by $\chi_C(x) = 0$ if $x \in C$; $+\infty$ otherwise.

The idea of DCA is simple: each iteration of DCA approximates the concave part $-H$ by its affine majorization (that corresponds to taking $y^k \in \partial H(x^k)$) and minimizes the resulting convex function.

Generic DCA Scheme:

Initialization. Let $x^0 \in \mathbb{R}^p$ be a best guest, $0 \leftarrow k$.
Repeat
    Calculate $y^k \in \partial H(x^k)$
    Calculate $x^{k+1} \in \arg\min\{G(x) - H(x^k) - \langle x - x^k, y^k \rangle : x \in \mathbb{R}^p\} \quad (P_k)$
    $k + 1 \leftarrow k$
Until. convergence of x^k.

Convergence properties of DCA and its theoretical basis can be found in [8,9,10], for instant it is important to mention that:

- DCA is a descent method (the sequences $\{G(x^k) - H(x^k)\}$ is decreasing) *without linesearch*;
- If the optimal value of problem (P_{dc}) is finite and the infinite sequence $\{x^k\}$ is bounded then every limit point x^* of $\{x^k\}$ is a critical point of $G - H$.
- DCA has a *linear convergence* for general DC programs.
- DCA has a finite convergence for polyhedral DC programs ((P_{dc}) is called polyhedral DC program if either G or H is polyhedral convex).

The construction of DCA involves DC components G and H but not the function F itself. Hence, for a DC program, each DC decomposition corresponds to a different version of DCA. Since a DC function F has an infinite number of DC decompositions which have crucial impacts on the qualities (speed of convergence, robustness, efficiency, globality of computed solutions,...) of DCA, the search of a "good" DC decomposition is important from algorithmic point of views. How to develop an efficient algorithm based on the generic DCA scheme for a practical problem is thus a judicious question to be studied, the answer depending on the specific structure of the problem being considered. In the current paper, we propose a DCA that has interesting convergence properties: our algorithm converges to a critical point after a many finitely iterations and its consists of solving a linear program at each iteration.

We note that the convex concave procedure (CCCP) for constructing discrete time dynamical systems studied in [11] is nothing else a special case of DCA. Whereas the approach by Yuille and Rangarajan ([11]) assumes differentiable objective functions, DCA handles both smooth and nonsmooth nonconvexe optimization. In the last five years DCA has been successfully applied in several works in Machine Learning for SVM-based Feature Selection [3], for improving boosting algorithms [12], for implementing - learning [13,14], for Transductive SVMs [15] and for clustering [16,17], ect.

3.1 A DC Decomposition of the SCAD SVM DC Objective Function

First, let us show a DC decomposition of $f_\lambda(t)$. Let g and h be the functions given by:

$$g(t) = \begin{cases} \lambda t & \text{if } t \geq 0, \\ -\lambda t & \text{if } t < 0, \end{cases} \tag{6}$$

and:

$$h(t) = \begin{cases} 0 & \text{if } 0 \leq t \leq \lambda, \\ \frac{1}{2(\alpha-1)}(t-\lambda)^2 & \text{if } \lambda < t \leq \lambda\alpha, \\ \lambda t - \frac{(\alpha+1)\lambda^2}{2} & \text{if } t > \lambda\alpha, \\ h(-t) & \text{if } t < 0. \end{cases} \tag{7}$$

Clearly that g and h are convex functions and:

$$f_\lambda(t) = g(t) - h(t).$$

Consider now the functions G and H defined by:

$$G(\xi, w, b) := (1/n) \sum_{i=1}^{n} \xi_i + \sum_{j=1}^{d} g(w_j); \quad H(\xi, b, w) = \sum_{j=1}^{d} h(w_j) \tag{8}$$

which are obviously convex. Then we have the following DC decomposition of the SCAD SVM DC objective function:

$$F(\xi, w, b) := G(\xi, w, b) - H(\xi, w, b).$$

Since the function G (reps. H) depends only on ξ and w (resp. w), in the sequence without ambiguity we use $G(\xi, w)$ (resp. $H(w)$) instead of $G(\xi, w, b)$ (resp. $H(\xi, w, b)$). By the very definition of g, say: $g(t) = \max(\lambda t, -\lambda t)$, it is convex polyhedral and so is G. Finally, the SCAD SVM DC problem can be written as the next DC polyhedral problem:

$$\begin{aligned} \min \quad & G(\xi, w) - H(w) \\ \text{s.t.:} \quad & y_i(b + \langle w, x_i \rangle) \geq 1 - \xi_i \quad (i = 1, \dots, n) \\ & \xi_i \geq 0 \quad (i = 1, \dots, n). \end{aligned} \tag{9}$$

In the standard form of a DC program (9) is expressed as

$$\min \left\{ \chi_K(\xi, w, b) + G(\xi, w) - H(w) : \xi, w, b) \in K \right\}, \tag{10}$$

where:

$$K := \left\{ (\xi, w, b) \in \mathbb{R}^{n+d+1} : y_i(b + \langle w, x_i \rangle) \geq 1 - \xi_i, \xi_i \geq 0 \quad (i = 1, \ldots, n) \right\}. \tag{11}$$

3.2   DCA Applied to the DC Program (9)

According to the generic DCA scheme given above, apply DCA on the last problem (10) amounts to computing a subgradient v^k of $H(w^k)$ and then solving the next convex program (at each iteration k)

$$\min \left\{ G(\xi, w) - \langle v^k, w \rangle : (\xi, w, b) \in K \right\}. \tag{12}$$

Clearly that v can be chosen as

$$v_j = \begin{cases} 0 & \text{if} & -\lambda \leq w_j \leq \lambda \\ (\alpha - 1)^{-1}(w_j - \lambda) & \text{if} & \lambda < w_j \leq \alpha\lambda \\ (\alpha - 1)^{-1}(w_j + \lambda) & \text{if} & -\alpha\lambda < w_j \leq -\lambda & , j = 1, \ldots d, \\ \lambda & \text{if} & w_j > \alpha\lambda \\ -\lambda & \text{if} & w_j < -\alpha\lambda \end{cases} \tag{13}$$

and the convex problem (12) is equivalent to:

$$\begin{aligned} \min \quad & (1/n) \sum_{i=1}^{n} \xi_i + \sum_{j=1}^{d} \eta_j - \langle v^k, w \rangle \\ \text{s.t.:} \quad & (\xi, w, b) \in K \\ & g(w_j) \leq \eta_j \quad (j = 1, \ldots, d) \end{aligned}$$

that is in fact a linear program:

$$\begin{aligned} \min \quad & (1/n) \sum_{i=1}^{n} \xi_i + \sum_{j=1}^{d} \eta_j - \langle v^k, w \rangle \\ & (\xi, w, b) \in K \\ \text{s.t.:} \quad & \lambda w_j \leq \eta_j \quad (j = 1, \ldots, d) \\ & -\lambda w_j \leq \eta_j \quad (j = 1, \ldots, d). \end{aligned} \tag{14}$$

Finally the DCA applied to (9) can be described as follows:

3.3   Algorithm DCA

Step 0. Choose $u^0 = (\xi^0, , w^0, b^0) \in \mathbb{R}^n \times \mathbb{R} \times \mathbb{R}^d$; $k = 0$. Let τ be a tolerance sufficiently small, set $k = 0$.

Step 1. Compute $v^k \in \partial H(w^k)$ via (13).
Step 2. Compute $u^{k+1} := (\xi^k, w^k, b^k)$ by solving the linear program (14).
Step 3. If

$$\left\| \xi^{k+1} - \xi^k \right\| + \left\| w^{k+1} - w^k \right\| + \left| b^{k+1} - b^k \right| \leq \tau \left(1 + \left\| \xi^k \right\| + \left\| w^k \right\| + \left| b^k \right| \right)$$

then STOP
Otherwise, set $k = k + 1$ and go to Step 1.

Theorem 1. *(Convergence properties of Algorithm **DCA**)*

*(i) **DCA** generates a sequence $\{(y^k, z^k, w^k, \gamma^k)\}$ such that the sequence $\{F(\xi^k, w^k, b^k)\}$ is monotonously decreasing.*

(ii) The sequence $\{((\xi^k, w^k, b^k))\}$ converges to (ξ^*, w^*, b^*) after a finite number of iterations.

(iii) The point (ξ^*, w^*, b^*) is a critical point of the SCAD SVM DC objective function.

Proof: (i) and (iii) are direct consequent of the convergence properties of general DC programs while (ii) is a convergence property of a DC polyhedral program.

4 Computational Experiments

In this section, we compare our approach DCA with L_1-SVM downloaded from http://svm.sourceforge.net/docs/3.00/api/ on different real datasets concerning gene selection for cancer classification.

4.1 Data Sets

Different public microarray gene expression datasets are used for the both *training* and *testing* phases: Breast cancer from van't Veer et al. [18] , Leukemia from Golub et al. [19], Prostate from Dinesh [20], Arcene is a benchmark from [21]. Here, we present a brief description of each one of them:

- *Breast Cancer data*: this dataset is described and used in van't Veer et al. [18]. It can be downloaded from:http://www.rii.com/publications/2002/vantveer.html and corresponds to the selection of 24481 genes to refer 78 patient in training set, 34 of which are labeled as "relapse", and the rest as "non-relapse". Correspondingly, there are 12 relapse and 7 non-relapse samples in the testing data set.
- *Leukemia data*: the Leukemia dataset represents gene expression patterns of 7129 probes from 6817 human genes. The training dataset consists of 38 bone marrow samples (27 ALL and 11 AML), versus 20 ALL and 14 AML for testing dataset. It's used by Golub et al. [19] and we can download it from http://www.broad.mit.edu.

- *Prostate data*: in this dataset used by Dinesh [20], the expression profiles 12600 genes. The training set contains 52 prostate tumor samples and 50 non-tumor (labeled as "Normal") prostate samples which can be downloaded from http://www-genome.wi.mit.edu/mpr/prostate. The testing set of 8 patients having relapsed and 13 patients having remained relapse free can be founded in http://carrier.gnf.org/welsh/prostate.
- *Arcene data*: this is among the benchmarks datasets of feature selection which can be downloaded from http://www.nipsfsc.ecs.soton.ac.uk/. The task of Arcene is to distinguish cancer versus normal patterns from mass spectrometric data. The number of features is 10000.

4.2   Parameters

The following parameters are used during running DCA for all datasets:

- *The parameter α, λ*: we choose $\alpha = 3.4$ as suggested by Fan and Li [2], and $\lambda = 0.4$.
- *The initial points* : the components of w, and b are randomly chosen between -5, and $+5$.

4.3   Numerical Results

We are implemented both of the approaches in the environment V.S C++ *v6.0* and performed the experiments on an Intel Weon Processor 3.00GHz with 2.00 MBytes of RAM. In the table 1 we show the number of selected genes by DCA and L_1 SVM while in the table 2 we compare the errors of cancer classification of both methods on the *training* sets and the *test* sets. We also indicate in Table 2 the CPU time in seconds of the two algorithms.

Table 1. The number of selected genes

Data Set Name	Number of genes	L_1 SVM selected genes	DCA selected genes
Breast Cancer	24481	24045 (98%)	19 (0.078%)
Leukemia	7129	7103 (99.6%)	10 (0.1%)
Prostate	12600	12423 (98.6%)	34 (0.27%)
Arcene	10000	9943 (99.4%)	34 (0.34%)

We observe from the computational results that

- DCA applied to the SCAD SVM DC problem suppressed more than 99% of genes while the standard L_1 SVM deletes only less than 2%.
- On the same dataset the classification error of DCA is always smaller than that of L_1 SVM, except for the training set of Breast Cancer data.
- DCA is faster than L_1 SVM, except for the Breast Cancer data.

Table 2. The error of cancer classification on training sets and test sets and CPU time of the two algorithms

Dataset	Training error		Testing error		CPU time	
	DCA	L_1 SVM	DCA	L_1 SVM	DCA	L_1 SVM
BreastCancer	0.06	0	0.26	0.36	107.96	15.78
Leukemia	0	0.36	0	0.36	4.34	15.93
Prostate	0.12	0.47	0.26	0.32	46.93	58.90
Arcene	0.05	0.56	0.44	0.56	9.73	193.75

Conclusion. We have proposed in this paper a continuous nonconvex optimization approach based on DC programming and DCA for the SCAD SVM model. Using a suitable DC decomposition we get a successive linear programming algorithm that converges after a finite number of iterations to a critical point of the SCAD SVM DC objective function. Preliminary computational concerning gene selection for cancer classification shows that the proposed algorithm is promising and better than the standard L_1 SVM method. Our approach can be used for the common feature selection - classification problem in machine learning. We will extended the computational experiments on other kinds of data.

References

1. Bredley, P.S., Mangasarian, O.L.: Feature Selection via concave minimization and support vector machines. In: Proceeding of International Conference on Machina Learning ICML 2008 (2008)
2. Fan, J., Li, R.: Variable selection via nonconcave penalized likelihood and its Oracle Properties. J. Am. Stat. Assoc. 96, 1348–1360 (2001)
3. Neumann, J., Schnörr, C., Steidl, G.: SVM-based Feature Selection by Direct Objective Minimisation, Pattern Recognition. In: Proc. of 26th DAGM Symposium, pp. 212–219 (2004)
4. Liu, Y., Zheng, Y.F.: FS_SFS: Anovel feature selection method for support vector machines. Pattern recognition (2005), doi:10.1016/j.patcog.2005.10.006
5. Jaeger, J., Sengupta, R., Ruzzo, W.L.: Improved Gene Selection for Classification of Microarrays Pacific Symposium on Biocomputing, vol. 8, pp. 53–64 (2003)
6. Liua, Y., Zhang, H.H., Parkc, C., Ahnc, J.: Support vector machines with adaptive L_q penalty. Computational Statistic and Data Analysis 51, 6380–6394 (2007)
7. Zhang, H.H., Ahn, J., Lin, X., Park, C.: Gene selection using support vector machines with non-convex penalty, vol. 22(1), pp. 88–95 (2006), doi:10.1093/bioinformatics/bti736
8. Le Thi, H.A., Pham Dinh, T.: The DC (difference of convex functions) programming and DCA revisited with DC models of real world nonconvex optimization problem. Ann. Oper. Res. 133, 23–46 (2005)
9. Pham Dinh, T., Le Thi, H.A.: Convex analysis approach to DC programming: Theory, Algorithms and Applications. Acta Mathematica Vietnamica, dedicated to Professor Hoang Tuy on the occasion of his 70th birthday 22, 289–355 (1997)
10. Pham Dinh, T., Le Thi, H.A.: DC optimization algorithms for solving the trust region subproblem. SIAM J. Optimization, 476–505 (1998)

11. Yuille, A.L., Rangarajan, A.: The Convex Concave Procedure (CCCP), Advances in Neural Information Processing System 14. MIT Press, Cambridge (2002)
12. Krause, N., Singer, Y.: Leveraging the margin more carefully. In: International Conference on Machine Learning ICML (2004)
13. Liu, Y., Shen, X., Doss, H.: Multicategory ψ-Learning and Support Vector Machine: Computational Tools. Journal of Computational and Graphical Statistics 14, 219–236 (2005)
14. Liu, Y., Shen, X.: Multicategoryψ -Learning. Journal of the American Statistical Association 101, 500–509 (2006)
15. Ronan, C., Fabian, S., Jason, W., Léon, B.: Trading Convexity for Scalability. In: International Conference on Machine Learning ICML (2006)
16. Le Thi, H. A., Belghiti, T., Tao, P.D.: A new efficient algorithm based on DC programming and DCA for Clustering. Journal of Global Optimization 37, 593–608 (2007)
17. Le Thi, H.A., Le Hoai, M., Tao, P.D.: Optimization based DC programming and DCA for Hierarchical Clustering. European Journal of Operational Research (2006)
18. Van't Veer, L., et al.: Gene expression profiling predicts clinical outcome of breast cancer. Nature 415, 530–536 (2002)
19. Golub, T.R., Slonim, D.K., Tamayo, P., Huard, C., Gaasenbeek, M., Mesirov, J.P., Coller, H., Loh, M.L., Downing, J.R., Caligiuri, M.A., Bloomfield, C.D., Lander, E.S.: Molecular Classifcation of Cancer: Class Discovery and Class Prediction by Gene Expression Monitoring. Science 286, 531–537 (1999)
20. Singh, D., Febbo, P.G., Ross, K., Jackson, D.G., Manola, J., Ladd, C., Tamayo, P., Renshaw, A.A., D'Amico, A.V., Richie, J.P., Lander, E.S., Loda, M., Kantoff, P.W., Golub, T.R., Sellers, W.R.: Gene expression correlates of clinical prostate cancer behavior Copyright © 2002 Cell Press. Cancer Cell 1, 203–209 (2002)
21. http://www.nipsfsc.ecs.soton.ac.uk/

FARS: A Multi-relational Feature and Relation Selection Approach for Efficient Classification

Bo Hu[1], Hongyan Liu[2], Jun He[1], and Xiaoyong Du[1]

[1] Key Labs of Data Engineering and Knowledge Engineering, MOE, China
Information School, Renmin University of China, Beijing, 100872, China
{erichu2006, hejun, duyong}@ruc.edu.cn
[2] School of Economics and Management, Tsinghua University, Beijing, 100084, China
hyliu@tsinghua.edu.cn

Abstract. Feature selection is an essential data processing step to remove the irrelevant and redundant attributes for shorter learning time, better accuracy and better comprehensibility. A number of algorithms have been proposed in both data mining and machine learning area. These algorithms are usually used in single table environment, where data are stored in one relational table or one flat file. They are not suitable for multi-relational environment, where data are stored in multiple tables joined each other by semantic relationships. To solve this problem, in this paper we propose a novel approach called *FARS* to do both feature and relation selection for efficient multi-relational classification. By this approach, we not only extend traditional feature selection method to selects relevant features from multi-relations, but also develop a new method to reconstruct the multi-relational database schema and get rid of irrelevant tables to further improve classification performance. Results of experiments conducted on several real databases show that *FARS* can effectively choose a small set of relevant features, enhancing the classification efficiency significantly and improving prediction accuracy.

1 Introduction

It is easy and convenient to collect data through Internet, and data accumulates in an unprecedented speed. We analyze this collected data for data mining, such as classification, clustering etc. With the increasing number of dimensionalities, most machine learning and data mining techniques will meet a big problem: curse of dimensionality. They may be ineffective for high-dimensional dataset: the prediction accuracy will degrade and the processing time will be longer. How to solve the problem? Since 1970s scientists have found that feature selection is an effective method to solve the problem. It is frequently used as a preprocessing step for machine learning. It is a process of choosing a subset of attributes according to a certain evaluation criterion, and has shown effective in removing irrelevant and redundant attributes. In addition, the data is not collected only for data mining, but also more comprehensive for users when there are only relevant and useful attributes left. Also downsizing the data is helpful for efficient storage and retrieval.

C. Tang et al. (Eds.): ADMA 2008, LNAI 5139, pp. 73–86, 2008.

There are many approaches [1-16] for single table feature selection. They can be divided into two categories of model: *Filter* and *Wrapper*. In the filter model, feature selection is performed as a preprocessing step to induction, and it relies on general characteristic of the training data to select some features without involving any learning algorithms. Some well-known algorithms are *Focus* [1], *Relief* [2], *CFS* [12, 13], and *FCBF* [16]. While in the wrapper model, it requires one predetermined learning algorithm in feature selection and uses its performance to evaluate and determine which feature to select. As for each new subset of features, the wrapper model needs to learn a hypothesis (or a classifier). It tends to give superior performance as it finds features better suited to the predetermined learning algorithm, but it also tends to be more computationally expensive. When the number of features becomes very large, the filter model is usually a better choice due to its computational efficiency.

Due to the advantages of the filter feature selection methods, a large number of algorithms have been proposed. But, none of them is suitable for the multi-relational database. As we all know, relational database is the most popular format for structured data, and is thus one of the richest sources of knowledge in the world. Since data usually exist in multi-relations of database instead of one single table or one flat file, it is urgent to propose an approach for multi-relational feature selection. By comparing many single table feature selection algorithms, in this paper, we use Correlation-based Feature Selection method (*CFS*) that shows good performance. Then we extend this method into multi-relational database. By this way, the total number of features can be reduced. But the number of relations does not change a lot. So the efficiency improvement is limited. This motivates us to do relation selection.

There are several challenges in this work: How can we apply single table feature selection method to multi-relational database? How can we traverse the database schema so that classifier be built and use efficiently? How can we determine the degree of a table's relevance to class label? How can we prune tables according to their relevance?

In this paper, we try to address the challenges discussed above. Our contributions are as follows:

1 We update *CFS* method to deal with multi-relational feature selection. With this method, features in different tables can be processed directly, and no transformation is needed.
2 In order to further enhance the learning performance, we propose an approach to compute the relevance of a table to the class label attribute and reconstruct the database schema. By this way, we change the original relationship graph between tables into a linear linked list of tables. We also give a method to do efficient joining between tables for this database schema.
3 Based on these approaches mentioned above, we design and implement an algorithm called *FARS* (Feature And Relation Selection). Experimental results indicate that it adapts well for multi-relational classifier such as *CrossMine* [18] and *Graph-NB* [20]. Experiments were conducted on three real datasets. Both *CrossMine* and *Graph-NB* shows that the learning time can be largely reduced and the accuracy can be improved by this approach. This attributes to the construction of simpler relationship structure based on effective selection of important features and tables.

The rest of the paper is organized as follows. In the second section, we review related work. In the third section, we introduce the multi-table feature selection approach, including traverse method, non-target table feature selection and reconstruction of the multi-table structure. The fourth section describes our algorithm. Finally, the experimental study of this algorithm with different multi-table classification algorithms is given in section five and conclusion is in the last section.

2 Related Work

In filter model, a lot of statistic and information theoretical methods have been used on feature evaluation. We divide the existing filter algorithms into three categories according to the feature evaluation methods, and choose several representative algorithms from each category: 1. the well-known filter algorithm *RELIEF* and *FOCUS*. *RELIEF* is first proposed by Kira and Rendell in 1992, it finds near-miss and near-hit and calculates the correlated value between feature and class, then set a threshold. Any features that greater than this threshold will be selected. In 1994, Kononenko [5] extended the *RELIEF* algorithm and made it applicable for different types of data. Another classic algorithm of filter is *FOCUS*, it is proposed by Almullim and Dietterich in 1991. It assumes that there is a bias of min-feature in each dataset, and it searches over the entire feature space to find out the minimum feature subset that is corresponding to the min-feature bias. The disadvantage is that its entire space searching is expensive. 2. Evaluated by information gain, Clardie [3] proposed an algorithm which combines the decision tree feature selection and nearest neighbor algorithm in 1993; Hall proposed correlation-based feature selection (*CFS*) in 1999 and 2000 [12, 13]; Liu proposed *FCBF* [16] that combines selecting optimal subset and feature relevance weight method. 3. Selecting features by cross-entropy, the algorithm that proposed by Koller Sahami [9] in 1996 searches for Markov Blanket. If the left set of attributes could replace the feature items in Markov Blanket, then remove it.

We compared the algorithms that mentioned in the previous paragraph, and chose *CFS* that is with good performances to apply on the multi-relational database.

We also worked with multi-relational classification algorithms. *CrossMine* is an algorithm that has high efficiency in multi-relational classification. It uses the method of tuple ID propagation to join tables virtually. By avoiding the cost of physical joins, *CrossMine* achieves better performance than several other multi-relational algorithms. Another multi-relational algorithm *Graph-NB* is a multi-relational Naïve Bayes classifier which uses semantic relationship graph to describe different relationships between tables, and use a straight-forward way to exclude some tables from the classifier.

3 Multi-relational Feature and Relaiton Selection

In multi-relational classification, there is a table that includes class label attribute. We call this table "*target table*" and this class attribute "*target attribute*". The join chains of other tables are linked with the target table through primary keys and foreign keys directly or indirectly. In the following parts, we will discuss how to express the correlation between table and class, the method of traversing the table space, and the method of reconstructing the database schema.

3.1 Correlation Measurement between Table and Class

In this section, we discuss how to evaluate the goodness of tables for classification. In single table feature selection, a feature is good if it is relevant to the class concept but is not redundant to any other relevant features. We adopt this concept in multi-relational feature selection too, that is to say, a table is good if it is relevant to the class concept but not redundant to any other relevant tables. Considering different tables represent different aspects of database information, we assume that the redundancy between relevant tables is so low that can be ignored. In this sense, our key point can be focused on finding relevant tables based on multi-relational feature selection.

First let's discuss how to calculate the correlation between two attributes or two variables. We can use the method of getting information gain that based on information-theoretical concept of *entropy*, a measure of the uncertainty of a random variable.

If X and Y are discrete random variables (nominal), equation 1 gives the entropy of a variable X:

$$H(X) = -\sum_i P(x_i) \log_2 (P(x_i))$$

(1)

Where $P(x_i)$ is the prior probabilities for all values of X. Equation 2 gives the entropy of X after observing values of another variable Y:

$$H(X \mid Y) = -\sum_j P(y_j) \sum_i P(x_i \mid y_j) \log_2 (P(x_i \mid y_j))$$

(2)

The amount by which the entropy of X decreases after observing values of another variable Y reflects additional information about X provided by Y and is called *information gain* (Quinlan, 1993) , which is defined in Equation 3:

$$InformationGain(X \mid Y) = H(X) - H(X \mid Y)$$

(3)

Information gain is regarded a measure to evaluate relevance between two variables. Unfortunately, information gain is biased in favor of features with more values. Therefore, we choose *symmetrical uncertainty* (*SU*) (Press et al., 1988), defined as follows in Equation 4:

$$SU(X,Y) = 2 \left[\frac{InformationGain(X \mid Y)}{H(X) + H(Y)} \right]$$

(4)

It corrects the bias of features with more values that made by information gain, and standardizes the value into [0, 1]. We've explained how to calculate the correlation between two attributes, next let's discuss how to calculate the correlation between table and class, since the table is a set of attributes, we calculate attributes set's correlation with class, according to the following Equation 5.

$$TSU = \frac{n\overline{SU}_{cf}}{\sqrt{n + n(n-1)\overline{SU}_{ff}}}$$ (5)

In Equation 5, variable n is the number of features, $\overline{SU}_{cf}$ is the average SU value between features and class, and $\overline{SU}_{ff}$ is the average SU value of feature-feature intercorrelation. Equation 5 is Pearson's correlation, where all variables have been standardized. Similarly, this equation can be used to describe the correlation between table and class: TSU is the SU value between table and class.

3.2 Non-target Table

When calculating the SU value of feature and class, it is easy to work with the target table, but not with other tables, because there's no class attribute in non-target tables, then how can we work with them? Fig.1 shows an example database. Arrows go from primary-keys to corresponding foreign-keys. Tables 1 and 2 are two example tables named Researcher and University respectively of this database, among which Researcher is the target table. Attribute *status* in Researcher is the target attribute.

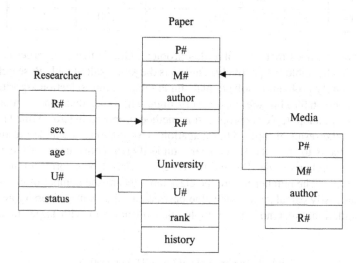

Fig. 1. An example of multi-relational database

Table 1. Researcher

R#	sex	age	U#	status
r1	F	48	u1	Y
r2	M	51	u2	N
r3	M	62	u3	Y
r4	F	36	u1	N

Table 2. University

U#	rank	history
u1	2	≥100
u2	2	≥100
u3	1	< 100
u4	2	< 100
u5	1	< 100

Table 3. The join of Researcher and University

Researcher ⋈ University						
R#	sex	age	U#	rank	history	status
r1	F	48	u1	2	≥100	Y
r2	M	51	u2	2	≥100	N
r3	M	62	u3	1	< 100	Y
r4	F	36	u1	2	≥100	N

There are two methods that can solve this problem. One is that join target table Researcher with other tables respectively. Table 3 is the join result of table Researcher and University. Surely problem is solved, and single table feature selection algorithm can be used in every table, but the cost is very high. The other that can overcome this shortcoming, we adopt tuple ID propagation method proposed in CrossMine [18].

Table 4 is the result of tuple ID propagation. Two columns are added to the table University. One is to store the Researcher's tuple ID (for convenience, R# can be regarded as Researcher's tuple ID), and the other are class labels corresponding to the target table tuple. The number before the class label means the number of class labels. Thus we can easily calculate the SU value between attributes in University and class. During calculation, we ignore those tuples that do not join with target table since

Table 4. The example of tuple ID propagation

University				
U#	rank	history	IDs	class labeles
u1	2	≥100	1,4	1Y,1N
u2	2	≥100	2	1N
u3	1	< 100	3	1Y
u4	2	< 100		

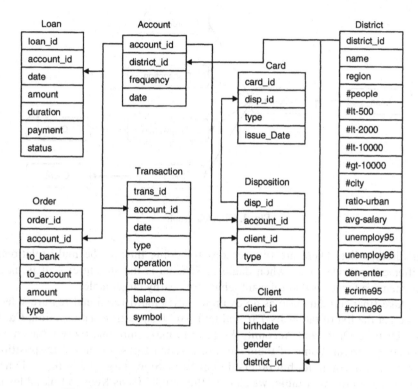

Fig. 2. The example of financial database from PKDD CUP 99

there's no impact on class, and sometimes calculate one tuple twice or more (first tuple in table 4) since this tuple has been linked with two tuples of the target table.

3.3 Width-First Traverse Whole Database

In the last section, we know that we have to propagate target table tuple ID to non-target tables in order to select every table's relevant features. Now we discuss the traverse approach. There are primary keys and foreign keys in every table, tables are joined together through these keys or other attributes as long as they links two tables. Fig.2 shows a financial database from PKDD CUP 99. The ER diagram of this database is an undirected graph. When we traverse the whole database from the target table, there may be unnecessary repeat work with the same table. In order to avoid this problem, we convert the undirected graph to directed graph. Fig.3 is a directed graph based on our approach.

3.4 Database Schema Reconstruction

After finish of feature selection in every table, we sort the tables by their relevance to class label, and convert the ER diagram of database which is anundirected graph into

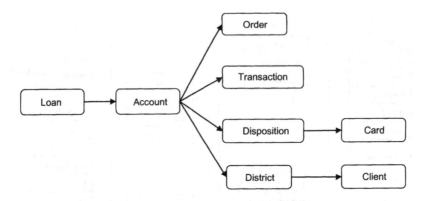

Fig. 3. Directed graph

linear directed list. There are two reasons for doing this: 1, the multi-relational classifier can process faster when database schema is list structure; 2, it is more comprehensive for users that relevant tables are nearby target table.

We take financial database as an example: after multi-relational feature selection, we get the list of tables by *TSU* value: Loan, Disposition, Transaction, Card, Client, District, Order and Account. We have to make sure that these tables have Keys between them. Some of them can use original Keys: Loan and Disposition both have key account_id, but others do not have. Since target table tuple ID has been propagated to every table, we can use these tuple ID as Keys to link tables in the list.

4   Algorithm

Based on the methodology presented above, we develop an algorithm called *FARS* in this selection. As in the following Fig. 4, given a multi-relational database, *tt* represents target table, *G* is the ER diagram of dataset, Q_w is a queue of waiting tables, and the output includes the reconstructed database schema, and a list of tables with relevant features left.

From line 1 to line 3, this algorithm initializes Q_w, L_t and L_f to NULL, sets threshold (default value = 0) and puts *tt* into Q_w. From line 4 to line 13, algorithm will repeat major steps on every table in the waiting queue until the queue is empty. In line 5, 6, and 7, algorithm reads the table that Q_w pops. If the table has been handled before, it continues next loop. Otherwise, it selects *CurrentTable* features (line8), adds *CurrentTable* into L_t if *CurrentTable*'s *TSU* is above the threshold, and propagates *tt*'s tuple id to its near neighbor tables and puts them into waiting table list (line11, 12). In line 14 and 15, to achieve the reconstruction of database schema, we sort tables by their *TSU* value and generate a new schema G_o in the end.

Algorithm *FARS*

Input
   mintst   threshold of *TSU*
   tt   a training target table
   G   dataset's ER diagram
   Q_w a queue of waiting tables

Output
   G_o an optimized dataset ER diagram
   L_t a list of selected tables
   L_f a list of selected features

Major steps
```
1  begin
2       Init: Qw, Lt and Lf
3       add tt into Qw
4       do begin
5            CurrentTable = Qw.pop ()
6            if (CurrentTable is in Lt)
7              continue
8            TSU(CurrentTable)
9               if (CurrentTable.TSU >= mintst)
10              add CurrentTable into Lt
11           T = GetLinkedTable (G, Lt, CurrentTable)
12           propagate TID to T and add add T into Qw
13      end until (Qw == NULL)
14      sort tables and reconstruct schema
15      generate Go
16 end
```

Fig. 4. Major steps of algorithm *FARS*

5 Experiment Study

The objective of this section is to evaluate our proposed algorithm in terms of the effectiveness of the selection of features and tables.

We conducted experiments on three real databases. The effectiveness of the selection results is further verified by comparing the performance of classifiers that has been working with and without our approach. The comparison includes run time and accuracy. Classifiers that we choose are *CrossMine* [18] and *Graph-NB* [20]. Our approach demonstrates its efficiency and effectiveness in dealing with high dimensional data for classification.

All experiments were performed on an HP NX6325 laptop with AMD Turion 1.6Ghz CPU and 1024MB RAM, running windows XP Professional. All runtimes for algorithm *Graph-NB* include both computation time and I/O time, and runtimes for *CrossMine* only include computation time. In each database, ten-fold experiments are used. In addition, we discretized the continuous attributes into 10 intervals for each attribute in every database.

The first database is the financial database used in PKDD CUP 1999. Its schema is shown in Fig. 1. We adopt the same way as [18] did to modify it. There are 8 tables and 36 attributes in this database. The second database is a mutagenesis database, which is a frequently used ILP benchmark. These two databases are often used in multi-relational classification experiments. The third database is a real database from educational area [21].

Fig.5 shows the effectiveness of the dimension reduction achieved by *FARS*. It compares the original number of features without feature selection (*Full Features* in the Fig. 5) and the number of features after feature selection (*Selected Features* in Fig. 5) on three datasets. From Fig. 5, we can see the pruning effectiveness of *FARS* is significantly.

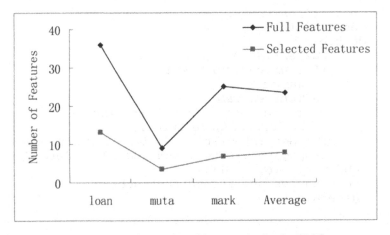

Fig. 5. The effectiveness of feature selection by *FARS*

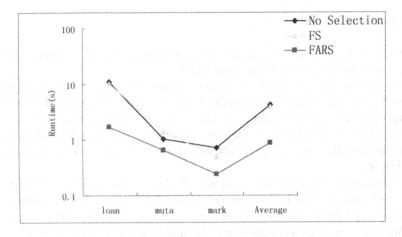

Fig. 6. Running Time of *CrossMine* on three datasets

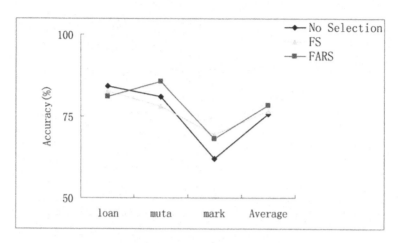

Fig. 7. Accuracy of *CrossMine* on three datasets

The experiment results of two classifiers' performance are given in figures from Fig 6 to Fig 9.

We compare three kinds of experimental results on these datasets: running classifier without feature or table selection (*No Selection*), running classifier after feature selection (*FS*) and running classifier after feature and relation selection (*FARS*). The runtime in the following figures is in logarithmic (10) scale.

Fig. 6 and Fig. 7 show the results of *CrossMine*.

Fig. 6 indicates that *FARS*'s feature and relation selection method is more effective than both *No Selection* and *FS* (only doing feature selection) for efficiency improving. Fig. 7 tell us that the accuracy after doing both feature and relation selection is slightly better than only doing feature selection or without doing feature or relation selection on the average. Fig. 8 and Fig. 9 show the results of *Graph-NB*.

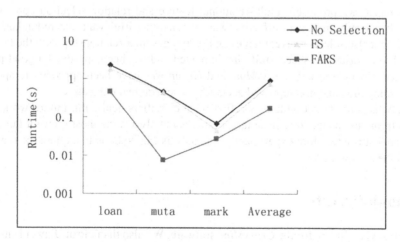

Fig. 8. Running Time of *Graph-NB* on three datasets

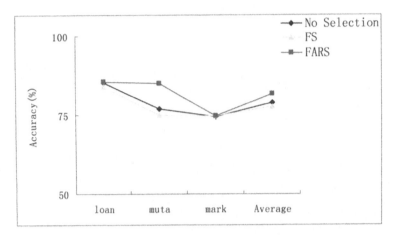

Fig. 9. Accuracy of *Graph-NB* on three datasets

Fig. 8 and 9 almost tell the same story as Fig. 6 and 7. Therefore, from these figures we can conclude that, in general, (1) *FARS* improves the accuracy of both *CrossMine* and *Graph-NB*; (2) *FARS* decreases the runtime of both *CrossMine* and *Graph-NB*; (3) *FARS* have better performance than doing feature selection without relation selection. From individual accuracy values, we also observe that for most of the data sets, *FARS* can maintain or even increase the accuracy. (4) The dimension reduction is significantly, which leads to the improvement of the classifiers' enhanced efficiency. In sum, the approach proposed in this paper is an effective feature and relation selection method for improving classification performance.

6 Conclusion and Future Work

In this paper, we propose a multi-relational feature and relation selection approach, *FARS*. It not only makes an effective way of removing irrelevant and redundant attributes, but also selects relevant tables and rearranges their relationship with the target table. The algorithm is successfully implemented and has been approved a good performance. Two classifiers, *CrossMine* and *Grahp-NB*, have been approved to spend less learning time and get improved accuracy on several real databases.

FARS fixes the target table as the first table classifiers deal with. Future work includes trying to change this, since target table is not always the most relevant table to class label attribute. More experiments and analysis can be done to explain the reason behind these approaches.

Acknowledgments

We thank Xiaoxin Yin for the *CrossMine* software. We also thank Prof. Jiawei Han for his helpful comments on this work. This work was supported in part by the National

Natural Science Foundation of China under Grant No. 70471006, 70621061, 60496325 and 60573092; the 985 Project of Renmin University under Grant No. 21357232.

References

1. Almuallim, H., Dietterich, T.G.: Learning with Many Irrelevant Features. In: Proceedings of the Ninth National Conference on Artificial Intelligence (AAAI-91), Anaheim, California, July 1991, vol. 2, pp. 547–552. AAAI Press, Menlo Park (1991)
2. Kira, K., Rendell, L.: The Feature Selection Problem: Traditional Methods and A New Algorithm. In: Proceedings of the Tenth National Conference on Artificial Intelligence, pp. 129–134. AAAI Press/The MIT Press, Menlo Park (1992)
3. Cardie, C.: Using Decision Trees to Improve Case–based Learning. In: Proceedings of the Tenth International Conference on Machine Learning, pp. 25–32. Morgan Kaufmann Publishers, Inc., San Francisco (1993)
4. Langley, P.: Selection of Relevant Features in Machine Learning. In: Proceedings of the AAAI Fall Symposium on Relevance. AAAI Press, New Orleans (1994)
5. Kononenko, I.: Estimating attributes: Analysis and Extension of RELIEF. In: Proceedings of the European Conference on Machine Learning, Catania, Italy, pp. 171–182. Springer, Berlin (1994)
6. Caruana, R., Freitag, D.: Greedy attribute selection. In: Proceedings of the Eleventh International Conference on Machine Learning, pp. 180–189. Morgan Kaufmann, San Francisco (1994)
7. John, G., Kohavi, R., Pfleger, K.: Irrelevant Features and the Subset Selection Problem. In: Proceedings of the Eleventh International Conference on Machine Learning, pp. 121–129. Morgan Kaufmann, San Francisco (1994)
8. Aha, D., Bankert, R.: A Comparative Evaluation of Sequential Feature Selection Algorithms. In: Fisher, D., Lenz, H. (eds.) Proceedings of the Fifth International Workshop on Artificial Intelligence and Statistics, Ft. Lauderdale, FL, pp. 1–7 (1995)
9. Koller, D., Sahami, M.: Toward Optimal Feature Selection. In: Proceedings of the Thirteenth International Conference on Machine Learning (1996)
10. Kohavi, R., John, G.: Wrappers for Feature Subset Selection. Artificial Intelligence, 273–324 (1997)
11. Blum, A., Langley, P.: Selection of Relevant Features and Examples in Machine Learning. Artificial Intelligence, 245–271 (1997)
12. Hall, M.: Correlation Based Feature Selection for Machine Learning. Doctoral dissertation, University of Waikato, Dept. of Computer Science (1999)
13. Hall, M.: Correlation-based Feature Selection for Discrete and Numeric class Machine Learning. In: Proceedings of the Seventeenth International Conference on Machine Learning, pp. 359–366 (2000)
14. Boz, O.: Feature Subsets Selection by Using Sorted Feature Relevance. In: Proc. Intl. Conf. on Machine Learning and Applications (June 2002)
15. Liu, H., Motoda, H., Yu, L.: Feature Selection with Selective Sampling. In: Proceedings of the Nineteenth International Conference on Machine Learning, pp. 395–402 (2002b)
16. Yu, L., Liu, H.: Feature Selection for High-Dimensional Data: A Fast Correlation Based Filter Solution. In: 12th Int. Conf. on Machine Learning (ICML) (2003)
17. Quinlan, J.: C4.5: Programs for Machine Learning. Morgan Kaufmann, San Francisco (1993)

18. Yin, X., Han, J., Yang, J., Yu, P.S.: CrossMine: Efficient Classification across Multiple Database Relations. In: Proc. 2004 Int. Conf. on Data Engineering (ICDE 2004), Boston, MA (March 2004)
19. Yin, X.: CrossMine software, http://www-sal.cs.uiuc.edu/~hanj/pubs/software.htm
20. Liu, H., Yin, X., Han, J.: An Efficient Multi-relational Naïve Bayesian Classifier Based on Semantic Relationship Graph. In: Proc. ACM-SIGKDD MRDM Workshop (2005)
21. Wang, R., Liu, H., Fang, M.: Research for the Relation between Learning Behaviors and Results. In: ICITM (2007)

Enhancing Text Categorization Using Sentence Semantics

Shady Shehata, Fakhri Karray, and Mohamed Kamel

Pattern Analysis and Machine Intelligence (PAMI) Research Group
University of Waterloo
Waterloo, Ontario, Canada N2L 3G1
{shady,karray,mkamel}@pami.uwaterloo.ca

Abstract. Most of text categorization techniques are based on word and/or phrase analysis of the text. Statistical analysis of a term frequency captures the importance of the term within a document only. However, two terms can have the same frequency in their documents, but one term contributes more to the meaning of its sentences than the other term. Thus, the underlying model should indicate terms that capture the semantics of text. In this case, the model can capture terms that present the concepts of the sentence, which leads to discover the topic of the document.

A new concept-based model that analyzes terms on the sentence and document levels rather than the traditional analysis of document only is introduced. The concept-based model can effectively discriminate between non-important terms with respect to sentence semantics and terms which hold the concepts that represent the sentence meaning.

A set of experiments using the proposed concept-based model on different datasets in text categorization is conducted. The experiments demonstrate the comparison between traditional weighting and the concept-based weighting enhances the quality of categorization quality of sets of documents substantially.

Keywords: Data mining, text categorization, concept-based model.

1 Introduction

Text mining attempts to discover new, previously unknown information by applying techniques from natural language processing and data mining. Categorization, one of the traditional text mining techniques, is supervised learning paradigm where categorization methods try to assign a document to one or more categories, based on the document content. Classifiers are trained from examples to conduct the category assignment automatically. To facilitate effective and efficient learning, each category is treated as a binary classification problem. The issue here is whether or not a document should be assigned to a particular category or not.

Most of current document categorization methods are based on the vector space model (VSM) [1,14,15], which is a widely used data representation.

C. Tang et al. (Eds.): ADMA 2008, LNAI 5139, pp. 87–98, 2008.

The VSM represents each document as a feature vector of the terms (words or phrases) in the document. Each feature vector contains term weights (usually term-frequencies) of the terms in the document. The similarity between documents is measured by one of several similarity measures that are based on such a feature vector. Examples include the cosine measure and the Jaccard measure.

Usually, in text categorization techniques, the frequency of a term (word of phrase) is computed to explore the importance of the term in the document. However, two terms can have the same frequency in a document, but one term contributes more to the meaning of its sentences than the other term. Thus, some terms provide the key concepts in a sentence, and indicate what a sentence is about. It is important to note that extracting the relations between verbs and their arguments in the same sentence has the potential for analyzing terms within a sentence. The information about who is doing what to whom clarifies the contribution of each term in a sentence to the meaning of the main topic of that sentence.

In this paper, a novel concept-based model is proposed. In the proposed model, each sentence is labeled by a semantic role labeler that determines the terms which contribute to the sentence semantics associated with their semantic roles in a sentence. Each term that has a semantic role in the sentence, is called concept. Concepts can be either a word or phrase and it is totally dependent on the semantic structure of the sentence. The concept-based model analyzes each term within a sentence and a document using the concept-based statistical analysis that analyzes each term on the sentence and the document levels. After each sentence is labeled by a semantic role labeler, each term is statistically weighted based on its contribution to the meaning of the sentence. This weight discriminates between non-important and important terms with respect to the sentence semantics.

The explanations of the important termimilogies, which are used in this paper, are listed as follows:

- *Verb-argument structure*: (e.g John hits the ball). "hits" is the verb. "John" and "the ball" are the arguments of the verb "hits",
- *Label*: A label is assigned to an argument. e.g: "John" has subject (or Agent) label. "the ball" has object (or theme) label,
- *Term*: is either an argument or a verb. Term is also either a word or a phrase (which is a sequence of words),
- *Concept*: in the new proposed model, concept is a labeled term.

The rest of this paper is organized as follows. Section 2 presents the thematic roles background. Section 3 introduces the concept-based model. The experimental results are presented in section 4. The last section summarizes and suggests future work.

2   Thematic Roles

Generally, the semantic structure of a sentence can be characterized by a form of verb argument structure. This underlying structure allows the creation of a composite meaning representation from the meanings of the individual concepts in a sentence. The verb argument structure permits a link between the arguments in the surface structures of the input text and their associated semantic roles.

Consider the following example: *My daughter wants a doll.* This example has the following syntactic argument frames: (Noun Phrase (NP) wants NP). In this case, some facts could be driven for the particular verb "wants" (1) There are two arguments to this verb (2) Both arguments are NPs (3) The first argument "my daughter" is pre-verbal and plays the role of the subject (4) the second argument "a doll" is a post-verbal and plays the role of the direct object. The study of the roles associated with verbs is referred to a thematic role or case role analysis [8]. Thematic roles, first proposed by Gruber and Fillmore [4], are sets of categories that provide a shallow semantic language to characterize the verb arguments.

Recently, there have been many attempts to label thematic roles in a sentence automatically. Gildea and Jurafsky [6] were the first to apply a statistical learning technique to the FrameNet database. They presented a discriminative model for determining the most probable role for a constituent, given the frame, predicator, and other features. These probabilities, trained on the FrameNet database, depend on the verb, the head words of the constituents, the voice of the verb (active, passive), the syntactic category (S, NP, VP, PP, and so on) and the grammatical function (subject and object) of the constituent to be labeled. The authors tested their model on a pre-release version of the FrameNet I corpus with approximately 50,000 sentences and 67 frame types. Gildea and Jurafsky's model was trained by first using Collins' parser [2], and then deriving its features from the parsing, the original sentence, and the correct FrameNet annotation of that sentence.

A machine learning algorithm for shallow semantic parsing was proposed in [11][12][13]. It is an extension of the work in [6]. Their algorithm is based on using Support Vector Machines (SVM) which results in improved performance over that of earlier classifiers by [6]. Shallow semantic parsing is formulated as a multi-class categorization problem. SVMs are used to identify the arguments of a given verb in a sentence and classify them by the semantic roles that they play such as AGENT, THEME, GOAL.

3   Concept-Based Model

This work is an extension of the work in [16] which enhances text clustering quality. In this paper, a new concept-based model that generates concept vectors is used to enhance the text categorization quality.

A raw text document is the input to the proposed model. Each document has well defined sentence boundaries. Each sentence in the document is labeled automatically based on the PropBank notations [9]. After running the semantic role labeler[9], each sentence in the document might have one or more labeled verb argument structures. The number of generated labeled verb argument structures is entirely dependent on the amount of information in the sentence. The sentence that has many labeled verb argument structures includes many verbs associated with their arguments. The labeled verb argument structures, the output of the role labeling task, are captured and analyzed by the concept-based model on the sentence and document levels.

In this model, both the verb and the argument are considered as *terms*. One term can be an argument to more than one verb in the same sentence. This means that this term can have more than one semantic role in the same sentence. In such cases, this term plays important semantic roles that contribute to the meaning of the sentence. In the concept-based model, a labeled term either word or phrase is considered as *concept*.

The proposed concept-based model consists of concept-based statistical analysis. The aim of the concept-based analysis is to weight each term on the sentence and the document levels rather than the traditional analysis of document only.

The proposed model assigns new weight to each concept in a sentence. The newly proposed $weight_{stat}$ is computed by the concept-based statistical analysis.

3.1   Concept-Based Statistical Analysis

The objective of this task is to achieve a concept-based statistical analysis (word or phrase) on the sentence and document levels rather than a single-term analysis in the document set only.

To analyze each concept at the sentence-level, a concept-based frequency measure, called the conceptual term frequency (ctf) is utilized. The ctf is the number of occurrences of concept c in verb argument structures of sentence s. The concept c, which frequently appears in different verb argument structures of the same sentence s, has the principal role of contributing to the meaning of s.

To analyze each concept at the document-level, the term frequency tf, the number of occurrences of a concept (word or phrase) c in the original document, is calculated.

The concept-based weighting is one of the main factors that captures the importance of a concept in a sentence and a document. Thus, the concepts which have highest weights are captured and extracted.

The following is the concept-based weighting $weight_{stat}$ which is used to discriminate between non-important terms with respect to sentence semantics and terms which hold the concepts that present the meaning of the sentence.

$$weight_{stat_i} = tfweight_i + ctfweight_i \qquad (1)$$

In calculating the value of $weight_{stat_i}$ in equation (1), the $tfweight_i$ value presents the weight of concept i in document d at the document-level and the $ctfweight_i$ value presents the weight of the concept i in the document d at the sentence-level based on the contribution of concept i to the semantics of the sentences in d. The sum between the two values of $tfweight_i$ and $ctfweight_i$ presents an accurate measure of the contribution of each concept to the meaning of the sentences and to the topics mentioned in a document.

In equation (2), the tf_{ij} value is normalized by the length of the document vector of the term frequency tf_{ij} in the document d, where $j = 1, 2, ..., cn$

$$tfweight_i = \frac{tf_{ij}}{\sqrt{\sum_{j=1}^{cn} (tf_{ij})^2}}, \qquad (2)$$

where cn is the total number of the concepts which has a term frequency value in the document d.

In equation (3), the ctf_{ij} value is normalized by the length of the document vector of the conceptual term frequency ctf_{ij} in the document d where $j = 1, 2, ..., cn$

$$ctfweight_i = \frac{ctf_{ij}}{\sqrt{\sum_{j=1}^{cn} (ctf_{ij})^2}}, \qquad (3)$$

where cn is the total number of concepts which has a conceptual term frequency value in the document d.

Concept-Based Statistical Analysis Algorithm

---

1. d is a new Document
2. L is an empty List (L is a top concept list)
3. **for** each labeled sentence s in d **do**
4. c_i is a new concept in s
5.   **for** each concept c_i in s **do**
6.   compute tf_i of c_i in d
7.   compute ctf_i of c_i in s in d
8.   compute $weight_{stat_i}$ of concept c_i
9.   add concept c_i to L
10.   **end for**
11. **end for**
12. sort L descendingly based on $max(weight_{stat})$
13. output the $max(weight_{stat})$ from list L

The concept-based statistical analysis algorithm describes the process of calculating the tf and the ctf of concepts in the documents. The procedure begins with processing a new document (at line 1) which has well defined sentence boundaries. Each sentence is semantically labeled according to [9].

For each labeled sentence (in the for loop at line 3), concepts of the verb argument structures which represent the sentence semantics are weighted by the $weight_{stat}$ according to the values of the tf and the ctf (at lines 6, 7, and 8). The concepts list L is sorted descendingly based on the $weight_{comb}$ values. The maximum weighted concepts are chosen as top concepts from the concepts list L. (at line 13)

The concept-based statistical analysis is capable of extracting the top concepts in a document (d) in $O(m)$ time, where m is the number of concepts.

3.2   Example of the Concept-Based Model

Consider the following sentence:

*We have **noted** how some electronic techniques, **developed** for the defense effort, have eventually been **used** in commerce and industry.*

In this sentence, the semantic role labeler identifies three target words (verbs), marked by bold, which are the verbs that represent the semantic structure of the meaning of the sentence. These verbs are *noted*, *developed*, and *used*. Each one of these verbs has its own arguments as follows:

- [ARG0 We] [TARGET **noted**] [ARG1 how some electronic techniques developed for the defense effort have eventually been used in commerce and industry]
- We have noted how [ARG1 some electronic techniques] [TARGET **developed**] [ARGM-PNC for the defense effort] have eventually been used in commerce and industry
- We have noted how [ARG1 some electronic techniques developed for the defense effort] have [ARGM-TMP eventually] been [TARGET **used**] [ARGM-LOC in commerce and industry]

Arguments labels[1] are numbered Arg0, Arg1, Arg2, and so on depending on the valency of the verb in sentence. The meaning of each argument label is defined relative to each verb in a lexicon of Frames Files [9].

Despite this generality, Arg0 is very consistently assigned an Agent-type meaning, while Arg1 has a Patient or Theme meaning almost as consistently [9]. Thus, this sentence consists of the following three verb argument structures:

1. First verb argument structure:
   - [ARG0 We]
   - [TARGET noted]
   - [ARG1 how some electronic techniques developed for the defense effort have eventually been used in commerce and industry]
2. Second verb argument structure:
   - [ARG1 some electronic techniques]
   - [TARGET developed]
   - [ARGM-PNC for the defense effort]

---

[1] Each set of argument labels and their definitions is called a frameset and provides a unique identifier for the verb sense. Because the meaning of each argument number is defined on a per-verb basis, there is no straightforward mapping of meaning between arguments with the same number. For example, arg2 for verb *send* is the recipient, while for verb *comb* it is the thing searched for and for verb *fill* it is the substance filling some container [9].

3. Third verb argument structure:
   - [ARG1 some electronic techniques developed for the defense effort]
   - [ARGM-TMP eventually]
   - [TARGET used]
   - [ARGM-LOC in commerce and industry]

Table 1. Example of Concept-based Statistical Analysis

Number	Concepts	CTF
(1)	noted	1
(2)	electronic techniques developed defense effort eventually commerce industry	1
(3)	electronic techniques	3
(4)	developed	3
(5)	defense effort	3
(6)	electronic techniques developed defense effort	2
(7)	used	2
(8)	commerce industry	2
	Individual Concepts	**CTF**
(9)	electronic	3
(10)	techniques	3
(11)	defense	3
(12)	effort	3
(13)	used	2
(14)	commerce	2
(15)	industry	2

After each sentence is labeled by a semantic role labeler, a cleaning step is performed to remove stop-words that have no significance, and to stem the words using the popular Porter Stemmer algorithm [10]. The terms generated after this step are called *concepts*. In this example, stop words are removed and concepts are shown without stemming for better readability as follows:

1. Concepts in the first verb argument structure:
   - noted
   - electronic techniques developed defense effort eventually commerce industry

2. Concepts in the second verb argument structure:
   - electronic techniques
   - developed
   - defense effort
3. Concepts in the third verb argument structure:
   - electronic techniques developed defense effort
   - used
   - commerce industry

It is imperative to note that these concepts are extracted from the same sentence. Thus, the concepts mentioned in this example sentence are:

- noted
- electronic techniques developed defense effort eventually commerce industry
- electronic techniques
- developed
- defense effort
- electronic techniques developed defense effort
- used
- commerce industry

The traditional analysis methods assign same weight for the words that appear in the same sentence. However, the concept-based statistical analysis discriminates among terms that represent the concepts of the sentence. This discrimination is entirely based on the semantic analysis of the sentence. In this example, some concepts have higher conceptual term frequency ctf than others as shown in Table 1. In such cases, these concepts (with high ctf) contribute to the meaning of the sentence more than concepts (with low ctf).

As shown in Table 1, the concept-based statistical analysis computes the ctf measure for:

1. The concepts which are extracted from the verb argument structures of the sentence, which are in Table 1 from row (1) to row (8).
2. The concepts which are overlapped with other concepts in the sentence. These concepts are in Table 1 from row (3) to row (8),
3. The individual concepts in the sentence, which are in Table 1 from row (9) to row (15).

In this example, the topic of the sentence is about the *electronic techniques*. These concepts have the highest ctf value with 3. In addition, the concept *noted* which has the lowest ctf, has no significant effect on the topic of the sentence.

4   Experimental Results

To test the effectiveness of using the concepts extracted by the proposed concept-based model as an accurate measure to weight terms in the document, an extensive set of experiments for a large scale evaluation of the proposed model in document categorization is conducted.

The experimental setup consisted of four datasets. The first data set contains 23,115 ACM abstract articles collected from the ACM digital library. The ACM articles are classified according to the ACM computing classification system into five main categories: general literature, hardware, computer systems organization, software, and data. The second data set has 12,902 documents from the Reuters 21578 dataset. There are 9,603 documents in the training set, 3,299 documents in the test set, and 8,676 documents are unused. Out of the 5 category sets, the topic category set contains 135 categories, but only 90 categories have at least one document in the training set. These 90 categories were used in the experiment. The third dataset consisted of 361 samples from the Brown corpus [5]. Each sample has 2000+ words. The Brown corpus main categories used in the experiment were: press: reportage, press: reviews, religion, skills and hobbies, popular lore, belles-lettres, learned, fiction: science, fiction: romance, and humor. The fourth dataset consists of 20,000 messages collected from 20 Usenet newsgroups.

In the datasets, the text directly is analyzed, rather than, using metadata associated with the text documents. This clearly demonstrates the effect of using concepts on the text categorization process.

For each dataset, stop words are removed from the concepts that are extracted by the proposed model. The extracted concepts are stemmed using the Porter stemmer algorithm [10]. Concepts are used to build standard normalized feature vectors using the standard vector space model for document representation.

The concept-based weights which are calculated by the concept-based model are used to compute a document-concept matrix between documents and concepts. Four standard document categorization techniques are chosen for testing the effect of the concepts on categorization quality: (1) Support Vector Machine (SVM), (2)Rocchio, (3) Naive Bayesian (NB), and (4) k-Nearest Neighbor (k-NN). These techniques are used as binary classifiers in which they recognize documents from one specific topic against all other topics. This setup was repeated for every topic.

For the single-term weighting, the popular TF-IDF [3] (Term Frequency/ Inverse Document Frequency) term weighting is adopted. The TF-IDF weighting is chosen due to its wide use in the document categorization literature.

In order to evaluate the quality of the text categorization, three widely used evaluation measures in document categorization and retrieval literatures are computed with 5-fold cross validation for each classifier. These measures are the Macro-averaged performance F1 measure (the harmonic mean of precision and recall), the Micro-averaged performance F1 measure, and the error rate.

Recall that in binary classification (relevant/not relevant), the following quantities are considered:

- p^+ = the number of relevant documents, classified as relevant.
- p^- = the number of relevant documents, classified as not relevant.
- n^- = the number of not relevant documents, classified as not relevant.
- n^+ = the number of not relevant documents, classified as relevant.

Table 2. Text Classification Improvement using Concept-based Model ($weight_{stat}$)

DataSet		Single-Term			Concept-based			Improvement
		Micro Avg(F1)	Macro Avg(F1)	Avg Error	Micro Avg(F1)	Macro Avg(F1)	Avg Error	
Reuters	SVM	0.9023	0.7421	0.0871	0.9254	0.8521	0.0523	+ 2.56%, +14.82%, -39.95%
	NB	0.8132	0.6127	0.2754	0.8963	0.7843	0.0674	+10.21%, +27.97%, -72.62%
	Rocchio	0.8543	0.6513	0.1632	0.9052	0.8062	0.0625	+ 5.95%, +23.78%, -61.7%
	kNN	0.8736	0.6865	0.1074	0.9174	0.8153	0.0541	+ 5.01%, +18.76%, -49.62%
ACM	SVM	0.6851	0.4973	0.1782	0.7621	0.6854	0.1264	+11.23%, +37.82%, -87.36%
	NB	0.6134	0.4135	0.4215	0.7063	0.6213	0.2064	+15.14%, +37.87%, -79.36%
	Rocchio	0.6327	0.4826	0.2733	0.7248	0.6457	0.1537	+14.55%, +33.79%, -43.76%
	kNN	0.6543	0.4952	0.2103	0.7415	0.6821	0.1325	+13.32%, +37.74%, -36.99%
Brown	SVM	0.8537	0.6143	0.1134	0.9037	0.8054	0.0637	+ 5.85%, +31.10%, -43.82%
	NB	0.7864	0.5071	0.3257	0.8461	0.7613	0.0891	+ 7.95%, +50.12%, -72.64%
	Rocchio	0.8067	0.5728	0.2413	0.8837	0.7824	0.0765	+ 9.54%, +36.59%, -68.29%
	kNN	0.8291	0.5934	0.1256	0.8965	0.7965	0.0652	+ 8.12%, +34.22%, -48.08%
Newsgroups	SVM	0.7951	0.5923	0.1325	0.8723	0.7835	0.0534	+ 9.7%, +32.28%, -59.69%
	NB	0.7023	0.4975	0.3621	0.8134	0.7253	0.0721	+15.81%, +45.78%, -80.08%
	Rocchio	0.7124	0.5346	0.2571	0.8503	0.7481	0.0683	+19.35%, +39.93%, -73.43%
	kNN	0.7341	0.5581	0.1423	0.8647	0.7524	0.0542	+17.79%, +34.81%, -56.44%

Obviously, the total number of documents N is equal to:

$$N = p^+ + n^+ + p^- + n^- \qquad (4)$$

For the class of relevant documents:

$$Precision(P) = \frac{p^+}{p^+ + n^+} \qquad (5)$$

$$Recall(R) = \frac{p^+}{p^+ + p^-} \qquad (6)$$

The $F - measure_\alpha$ is defined as:

$$F_\alpha = \frac{(1 + \alpha) * P * R}{(\alpha * P) + R} \qquad (7)$$

The error rate is expressed by:

$$Error = \frac{n^+ + p^-}{N} \qquad (8)$$

Generally, the Macro-averaged measure is determined by first computing the performance measures per category and then averaging these to compute the global mean. The Micro-averaged measure which is determined by first comput-ing the totals p^+, p^-, n^+, and n^- for all categories and then use these totals to compute the performance measures. Micro-averaged gives equal weight to every document, while Macro-averaged gives equal weight to each category.

Basically, the intention is to maximize *Macro-averaged F1* and *Micro-averaged F1* and minimize the *error rate* measures to achieve high quality in text categorization.

The results listed in Table(2) show the improvement on the categorization quality obtained by the the concept-based statistical analysis. The popular SVM-light implementation [7] is used with parameter C = 1000 (tradeoff between training error and margin). A k of 25 is used in the kNN method as illustrated in Table(2). The parameters chosen for the different algorithms were the ones that produced best results.

The percentage of improvement ranges from +14.82% to +50.12% increase (higher is better) in the Macro-averaged F1 quality and from +2.56% to +19.35% increase (higher is better) in the Micro-averaged F1 quality, and -39.95% to -80.08% drop (lower is better) in the error rate as shown in Table(2).

Weighting based on the matching of concepts in each document, is showed to have a more significant effect on the quality of the text categorization due to the similarity's insensitivity to noisy terms that can lead to an incorrect similarity measure. The concepts are less sensitive to noise when it comes to calculating normalized feature vectors. This is due to the fact that these concepts are orig-inally extracted by the semantic role labeler and analyzed with respect to the sentence and document levels. Thus, the matching among these concepts is less likely to be found in non-relevant documents to a category. The results produced by the proposed concept-based model in text categorization have higher quality than those produced by traditional techniques.

5 Conclusions

This work bridges the gap between natural language processing and text catego-rization disciplines. A new concept-based model is proposed to improve the text categorization quality. By exploiting the semantic structure of the sentences in documents, a better text categorization result is achieved. The introduced model analyzes the semantic structure of each sentence to capture the sentence con-cepts using the conceptual term frequency *ctf* measure. This analysis captures the structure of the sentence semantics which represents the contribution of each concept to the meaning of the sentence. This leads to perform concept matching and weighting calculations in each document in a very robust and accurate way.

The concept-based analysis assigns weight to each concept in a document. The top concepts which have maximum weights are used to build standard normalized feature vectors using the standard vector space model (VSM) for the purpose of text categorization. The quality of the categorization results achieved by the proposed model surpasses that of traditional weighting approaches significantly.

There are a number of suggestions to extend this work. One direction is to link the presented work to web document categorization. Another future direction is to investigate the usage of such models on other corpora and its effect on document categorization results, compared to that of traditional methods.

References

1. Aas, K., Eikvil, L.: Text categorisation: A survey. technical report 941. Tech. rep., Norwegian Computing Center (June 1999)
2. Collins, M.: Head-driven statistical model for natural language parsing. Ph.D. thesis, University of Pennsylvania (1999)
3. Feldman, R., Dagan, I.: Knowledge discovery in textual databases (kdt). In: Proceedings of First International Conference on Knowledge Discovery and Data Mining, pp. 112–117 (1995)
4. Fillmore, C.: The case for case. Chapter in: Universals in Linguistic Theory. Holt, Rinehart and Winston, Inc., New York (1968)
5. Francis, W., Kucera, H.: Manual of information to accompany a standard corpus of present-day edited american english, for use with digital computers (1964)
6. Gildea, D., Jurafsky, D.: Automatic labeling of semantic roles. Computational Linguistics 28(3), 245–288 (2002)
7. Joachims, T.: Text categorization with support vector machines: learning with many relevant features. In: Nédellec, C., Rouveirol, C. (eds.) ECML 1998. LNCS, vol. 1398, pp. 137–142. Springer, Heidelberg (1998)
8. Jurafsky, D., Martin, J.H.: Speech and Language Processing. Prentice Hall Inc., Englewood Cliffs (2000)
9. Kingsbury, P., Palmer, M.: Propbank: the next level of treebank. In: Proceedings of Treebanks and Lexical Theories (2003)
10. Porter, M.F.: An algorithm for suffix stripping. Program 14(3), 130–137 (1980)
11. Pradhan, S., Hacioglu, K., Krugler, V., Ward, W., Martin, J.H., Jurafsky, D.: Support vector learning for semantic argument classification. Machine Learning 60(1-3), 11–39 (2005)
12. Pradhan, S., Hacioglu, K., Ward, W., Martin, J.H., Jurafsky, D.: Semantic role parsing: Adding semantic structure to unstructured text. In: Proceedings of the 3th IEEE International Conference on Data Mining (ICDM), pp. 629–632 (2003)
13. Pradhan, S., Ward, W., Hacioglu, K., Martin, J., Jurafsky, D.: Shallow semantic parsing using support vector machines. In: Proceedings of the Human Language Technology/North American Association for Computational Linguistics (HLT/NAACL) (2004)
14. Salton, G., McGill, M.J.: Introduction to Modern Information Retrieval. McGraw-Hill, New York (1983)
15. Salton, G., Wong, A., Yang, C.S.: A vector space model for automatic indexing. Communications of the ACM 18(11), 112–117 (1975)
16. Shehata, S., Karray, F., Kamel, M.S.: Enhancing text clustering using concept-based mining model. In: IEEE International Conference on Data Mining (ICDM), pp. 1043–1048 (2006b)

Mining Evolving Web Sessions and Clustering Dynamic Web Documents for Similarity-Aware Web Content Management

Jitian Xiao

School of Computer and Information Science, Edith Cowan University,
2 Bradford Street, Mount Lawley, WA 6050, Australia
j.xiao@ecu.edu.au

Abstract. Similarity discovery has become one of the most important research streams in web usage mining community in the recent years. The knowledge obtained from the exercise can be used for many applications such as predicting user's preference, optimizing web cache organization and improving the quality of web document pre-fetching. This paper presents an approach of mining evolving web sessions to cluster web users and establish similarities among web documents, which are then applied to a Similarity-aware Web content Management system, facilitating offline building of the similarity-ware web caches and online updating of sub-caches and cache content similarity profiles. An agent-based web document pre-fetching mechanism is also developed to support the similarity-aware caching to further reduce the bandwidth consumption and network traffic latency, therefore to improve the web access performance.

Keywords: Web usage mining, web caching, similarity discovery, web document pre-fetching.

1 Introduction

Similarity discovery has become one of the most important research streams in web usage mining community in the recent years. One example of this research stream is discovering similarities between web users, and another is establishing similarities among web documents. The former is to discover clusters of users that exhibit similar information needs, e.g., users that access similar pages. By analyzing the characteristics of the clusters, web users can be understood better and thus can be provided with more suitable and customized services [1]. And the latter is to cluster dynamic web documents under certain similarity measures [2]. By grouping web documents of similar themes, it is possible to make better recommendation to users who are viewing particular topic/s of web documents, thus to provide better services to the web users. The knowledge obtained from these exercises can also be used for many other applications such as predicting user's preference [3], optimizing web cache organization [4] and improving the quality of web document pre-fetching [5, 6, 7].

Most previous research efforts in web usage mining have worked with assumption that the web usage data is static [3]. However, the dynamic aspects of the web access

C. Tang et al. (Eds.): ADMA 2008, LNAI 5139, pp. 99–110, 2008.

patterns, as a result of user interaction with the web, have more potential impact on mining effectiveness and predicting web users' access preference. This is because web access patterns on the web site are dynamic due not only to the dynamics of web content and structure but also to changes in the user's interests and their navigation patterns. Thus it is desirable to study and discover web usage patterns at a higher level, where such dynamic tendencies and temporal events can be distinguished. We focus on both static and dynamic web usage mining in this work in order to facilitate web caching organization and improve web pre-fetching performance in our Similarity-aware Web Content Management (SaWCM) system [4].

In this paper we present approaches to perform web usage and web content mining to facilitate similarity-aware web content caching and document pre-fetching between the caching proxy and web browsers/users. A means of similarity based web content management is described to improve the relative performance of pre-fetching techniques based upon user similarities and document similarities detected. Web document caching in the context of this study will be based upon similarity detection. Document similarities will be sought from previously and newly cached documents by employing several concurrently applied, but differing, algorithms to detect equivalences of broad-content or keywords and links contained within pages under scrutiny. Similarities between web documents, having been detected, will then be ranked for candidature to be fetched in anticipation of a user's intentions. Following the ranking exercise, content settings may be realized for sub-caches and pre-fetching may then proceed.

The rest of the paper is organized as follows. Section 2 defines the similarity measures. Section 3 presents the offline web mining approach to build initial web user clusters and sub-cache content similarity profiles (CSP). In Section 4, we first review the similarity-based web cache architecture [8], and then outline the online approach to dynamically update the similarity-aware web caches and CSP. The similarity-aware web document pre-fetching strategy is also presented in this section. Section 5 concludes the paper.

2 Similarities Measures Used in This Work

In our previous work, two types of similarity measures were defined for web usage mining, one for measuring similarities among web users [2] and the other for measuring similarities among web documents [4]. The similarity measures of web users are used to clustering web users, while the similarity measures of the web documents are used to establishing links between web documents that share similar themes in their contents. Both of these similarity measures (and related mining approaches proposed) were based on the data collected in a certain period of time.

However, web usage data is *evolutionary* in nature. The information needs of users may vary over time. Consequently, pages accessed by users in different time periods may be different as well. Responding to this change, the web contents cached in a particular (sub-)caches may change dramatically over time. Such evolutionary nature of the web usage data poses challenges to web usage mining: How to maintain the web user clustering results and discover new web user clusters, and how to update similarity-aware web caching contents to reflect evolutionary nature of web usage data. To deal with this change, we now describe briefly the new similarity measures to be used in this work to ease the mining result updating.

2.1 Measuring Similarities among Web Users

There are quite a few methods for clustering web users proposed in the literature [1, 3, 7, 8, 9, 10]. In general, web user clustering consists of two phases, i.e., *data preparation* and *cluster discovery* (probably followed by another phase, *cluster analysis*, depending on application scenarios). In the first phase, *web sessions*[1] of users are extracted from the web server log by using some user identification and session identification techniques [11]. Most existing web user clustering methods cluster users based on the snapshots of their web sessions. However, this type of web user clustering methods does not capture the dynamic nature of the web usage data. As the information needs of users may vary over time, pages accessed by users in different time periods may change as well. For example, Fig. 1 shows the historical web sessions of users u_1, u_2 and u_3 at time periods p_1, p_2 and p_3, respectively, with a specific time granularity (e.g. *day, week, month* etc). It can be observed that pages visited by web users at different time periods are different. This can be attributed to various factors, such as users' variation of their information needs and changes to the content of the web site etc [1].

In the second phase, clustering techniques are applied to generate clusters of users. Based on the web sessions shown in Fig. 1 (a) (i.e., in time period p_1), existing web user clustering methods which use commonly accessed web pages as the clustering feature, such as the work in [2], will group the three users together as their web sessions share common pages. However, for web sessions shown in time periods p_2 and p_3, different clustering methods may results in different user cluster/s.

Among those recent web user clustering methods, the one reported by Chen et al. [1] is able to cluster web users based on the evolutions of their historical web sessions. They defined the similarity between web users using the *Frequently Changed Subtree Pattern (FCSP)*, which is a set of subtrees, in a *page hierarchy*[2], whose structures frequently change together in a sequence of historical web sessions. With FCSP, the sequences of historical web sessions of web users are represented as sequences of page hierarchies, where a page that will disappear in the next web session and a page that newly occurs in current session are distinguished. The changes to the structure of a page hierarchy, e.g. the insertions and deletions of pages, reflect the variation of user's information needs. Based on the similarity measure defined, their

---

[1] A *web session*, which is an episode of interaction between a web user and the web server, consists of pages visited by a user in the episode [1]. For example, a request extracted from the server log:

      foo.cs.ntu.edu – [21/Feb/2008:10:22:02 – 0800]

      "GET / www.ecu.edu.au/library/students.html HTTP/1.0" 200 3027

means a user at *foo.cs.ntu.edu* accessed the page www.ecu.edu.au/library/students.html at 10:22:02 on February 21, 2008. For simplicity, the web session contains only the page visited, e.g., "www.ecu.edu.au/library/students.html", which is further simplified to "a/b/c", as shown in Fig 1. All other information is omitted.

[2] According to [1], pages accessed in a web session are organized into a hierarchical structure, called a *page hierarchy*, based on the URLs of the pages.

algorithm, called *COWES,* clusters web users in three steps. First, for a given set of web users, it mines the history of their web sessions to extract interesting patterns that capture the characteristics of their usage data evolution. Then, the similarity between web users is computed based on their common interesting patterns. And finally, the desired clusters are generated by a partitioning clustering technique.

p_1		p_2		p_3	
UID	sessions	UID	sessions	UID	sessions
u_1	< a/b/e, a/c/i, a/d/m >	u_1	< a/b/f, a/b/g, a/c/i/q, a/d/m >	u_1	< a/b/e, a/b/f, a/c/i/q, a/d/m >
u_2	< a/b/e, a/c/i, a/d/m >	u_2	< a/b/e, a/c/h, a/c/i, a/d/m, a/d/k >	u_2	< a/b/e, a/c/h, a/c/j, a/d/l, a/d/m >
u_3	< a/b/e, a/c/i, a/d/m >	u_3	< a/b/e, a/c/h, a/c/j, a/d/l >	u_3	< a/b/e, a/c/h, a/c/i, a/d/k >
	(a)		(b)		(c)

Fig. 1. Historical Web sessions of users u_1, u_2, and u_3

We combine our work as reported in [7] with the method proposed by Chen et al. [1]. In particular, we adopt the similarity measures defined in [1].We implemented the algorithm and embedded it into an agent, *i.e., Access Pattern Agent,* (see Section 4.3 for details) in this work.

2.2 Measuring Similarities among Web Contents

In this sub-section, we define similarity measures of web documents for effective web document caching and pre-fetching. To pre-fetch documents that are of similar topic to the document a user is currently viewing, we need to derive the similarity of contents of web documents, ignoring any structural elements, e.g. HTML formatting. For efficacy of on-line pre-fetching, we propose different levels of similarity measures to capture levels of similarity between web documents.

The similarities among web documents are computed based on a document model similar to that of [12], wherein structured web documents are represented as unordered labeled trees. We consider containment rather than order of appearance of words within a document. Our model differs from that of Flesca's in two ways: first, we don't consider the HTML formatting elements and, second, we consider a document's structure to be based on sectional elements, e.g. *Abstract* and *subsections,* while their work specifies texts in terms of pairs of start and end tags, e.g., <table> ... </table>, <ul. ... </ul>.

In the resultant tree, each non-leaf node corresponds to a subsection of the document (e.g. characterizing the title of the subsection), except that the root-node might also contain a set of *keywords*, a list of *authors*, a string for *title*, or/and a set of words comprising the *abstract*. Each leaf node corresponds to the text of that (sub)section. Notably, such a structure allows us to determine sectional similarities between particular elements such as titles; between the various contents, and, implicitly, between the structures of compared documents. In brief, a document tree is an unordered tree wherein each node is characterized by an associated set of type-value pairs. Given a document tree T, of root r, with a node n_r we may represent a sub-tree of T rooted at nr as $T(n_r)$. We define a set of functions, each characterizing some element, on the document tree: *keyword(r)*, *title(r)*, *authors(r)*, *abstract(r)* and *text(r)*. For a document tree rooted at r, *keyword(r)* = {$s \mid s$ is a keyword contained in the keyword section of r}. The *title(r)*, *authors(r)* and *abstract(r)* can be defined similarly. If $n_1, n_2, \ldots, n_k$ are child nodes of r, then

$$
text(r)= \begin{cases} title(r) \cup \cup_{i=1}^{k} \{s \mid s \in text(n_i)\} & \text{if } r \text{ is a non-leaf node, with children} \\ & n_1, \ldots, n_k \\ \{s \mid s \text{ is a word in } leaf(T(r))\} & \text{if } r \text{ is a leaf node of } T \end{cases}
$$

Essentially *text(r)* is a set of words contained in the various strings associated with nodes of the (sub-)tree rooted at r. *text(r)* is defined recursively.

The similarity computation algorithm works on this tree structure by exploiting the information contained in individual nodes and the whole tree. Observe that each node keeps track of its level in the tree, its content and the content of its child nodes.

When a user finds a web page that is on-topic, she or he may desire to view other documents of similar topic (this is one of the main driven points for similarity-aware pre-fetching). There are different parameters which determine the similarity of two documents: some are related according to their content and others by their in and out hyperlinks. In this section we consider only document content.

We combine the TFIDF [13] and DCS [14] models to forming our new document similarity measures in this work. Levels of document similarity measures are defined by making use of the text extracted from elements of document (sub-)trees. To compute the similarities efficiently, the measures must be normalized, allowing the comparison of pairs of documents and the selection of different levels of elements/components.

Given two document trees T_1 and T_2, and two nodes $r_1 \in T_1$ and $r_2 \in T_2$, we define an intersection function, which is based on Broder's resemblance function [15], to assess the similarity between the document components represented by r_1 and r_2,

$$
intersect(w(r_1), w(r_2)) = \frac{\mid w(r_1) \cap w(r_2) \mid}{\mid w(r_1) \cup w(r_2) \mid} \tag{1}
$$

where $w(r)$ is a set of strings associated with nodes of the (sub-)tree rooted at r. The function $intersect(w(r_1), w(r_2))$ returns the percentage of the number of common words divided by the number of all words that appear in both $w(r_1)$ and $w(r_2)$. Clearly, *intersect(w(r_1),w(r_2))* ≤ 1, while equality exists when $w(r_1) = w(r_2)$.

For two trees rooted at r_1 and r_2, their similarities of keywords, titles and abstracts, respectively, may be defined by the formulae (2) through (4):

$$
SIM_{KB}(r_1, r_2) = intersect(keyword(r_1), keyword(r_2)) \tag{2}
$$

$$
SIM_{TB}(r_1, r_2) = intersect(title(r_1), title(r_2)) \tag{3}
$$

$$
SIM_{AB}(r_1, r_2) = intersect(abstract(r_1), abstract(r_2)) \tag{4}
$$

while the content-based similarity is defined as

$$SIM_{CB}(r_1, r_2) = intersect(w(r_1), w(r_2)) \tag{5}$$

where $w(r_i) = text(r_i) \cup keywords(r_i) \cup abstract(r_i)$, $i = 1, 2$.

Generally, the higher a word occurrence in a document, the closer that word relates to the theme of the document and this may be used to measure similarity between documents. To take the significance level of words into account, let $weight_r(s)$ be the number of occurrence of the word s in document represented by r, then the intersect function defined in (1) can be re-defined as

$$intersect_{wt}(w(r_1), w(r_2)) = \frac{\sum_{s \in w(r_1) \cap w(r_2)} \min\{weight_{r_1}(s), weight_{r_2}(s)\}}{\frac{1}{2}\sum_{s \in w(r_1) \cup w(r_2)} |weight_{r_1}(s) + weight_{r_2}(s)|} \tag{6}$$

Formula (6) is similar to the definition of TFIDF weight of documents, but it is used to calculating the similarity between two documents rather than evaluating how important a word is to a document. Based on this function, the *weighted* similarity measures $SIM_{KB}()$, $SIM_{TB}()$, $SIM_{AB}()$ and $SIM_{CB}()$ can all be re-defined by replacing *intersect*() in (2) to (5) with *intersect*$_{wt}$() defined in (6). The weighted similarity measures will be used only when the frequency of word occurrences is considered important to the content of the documents.

3   Data Pre-processing – An Offline Phase

The pre-processing phase in this work consists of two separate tasks: One is to cluster web users and the other is to compute the similarities among cached documents collected in a specific time period. The first task, like many other web usage mining process, is performed in the following steps to achieve its goal:

- *collection of web data* such as activities/click streams recorded in web server log;
- *preprocessing the web data* such as filtering crawlers requests, requests to graphics, and identifying unique sessions;
- *analysis of web data* to discover interesting web usage patterns; and
- *interpretation/evaluation* of the discovered usage patterns thus to cluster web users into clusters.

Note that the above data pre-process phase is performed once before the subcaches and similarity profile, etc., are created, and subsequently applied once a while when the SaWCM needs to update its profiles on a regular time interval. Due to space limitation, the detailed algorithm of clustering web users are omitted here (interested readers are referred to [1] and our previous work in [2, 4].

The second data pre-processing task, i.e., computing the similarities among cached documents, is combined to the initial task of building caching architecture and similarity profile of the SaWCM, which will be detailed in Section 4. Before this is done, to calculate similarities among documents, a *text filter* was developed to extract meaningful words from related sections of a document, and count them per section. The detailed description of the text filter can be found in [4].

4 The Similarity-Based Web Cache Scheme

The basic idea of web-caching is to reduce network traffic load and reduce retrieval latency by holding recent requested documents at the proxy caches so that they do not have to be fully retrieved upon identical request. In this section, we describe a similarity-based multi-cache web content management scheme and on-line algorithm to capture and maintain an opposite similarity profile of documents requested through a caching proxy.

4.1 Caching Architecture

SaWCM is a similarity-based multi-cache web caching architecture (see Fig. 2). It has four major components: *central router, similarity profiles, Cache Similarity Knowledge Base, sub-caches,* and *document allocator.* Of these, the central router is pivotal in controlling and coordinating other components.

To configure the multi-cache web caching architecture, based on particular caching similarity level, we first cluster documents in cache based on combination of the similarity measures (2), (3) and (4) introduced before (i.e., by taking a similarity measure SIM(r_1, r_2) = intersect (w(r_1) , w(r_2)) where w(r_i) = title(r_i) $\cup$ keywords(r_i) $\cup$ abstract (r_i), i = 1, 2), and determine the number, N, of themes of the documents. For the initial cache content clustering purpose, we examined a number web content classification approaches (e.g., decision trees, k-nearest neighbor classifiers, neural networks and support vector machine (SVM) [16] and finally adopted SVM classification algorithm (with slightly modification on it) for this purpose. SVM classification algorithm is more suitable than others to this work because it can work with short summary descriptions of web pages (such as title, keywords and/or a small number of starting words of the document body), and it has been shown to be both very fast and effective for text classification problems [16].

For each theme (or cluster), a number of *stems* relating to it were chosen (e.g., by looking at all stems produced by the text filter when similarity profile vectors were computed). Then the cache is divided into N+1 sub-caches. Each of the first N sub-caches stores documents of one particular theme, and the last sub-cache stores other documents not belonging to any of the N themes. In this way, we ensure that similarities among documents in any sub-cache are relatively higher, while relegating those among documents across sub-caches.

The *similarity profile* (SP) comprises N two-dimensional arrays Ai(*, *), i=1, 2, ..., N, of which each corresponds to one of the first N sub-caches. For each document j in sub-cache *i*, SP counts the number of occurrences of the stems that relate to the theme of the sub-cache, storing the numbers in vector Ai(j,*). This information is useful when performing similarity-aware pre-fetching from the sub-cache to a client. For each theme, we limit the number of stems to be a specific number (e.g., 128).

The *Cache Similarity Knowledge Base* (CSKB) consists of a set of rules designed for classification of web contents. Semantics information can be used here to direct the cache. Based on these rules, more advanced caching management can be implemented. For example, the rule

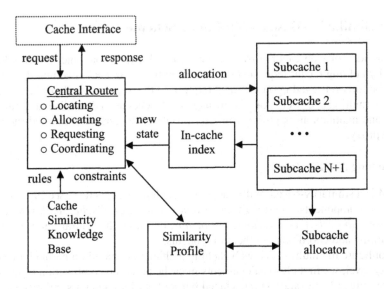

Fig. 2. The similarity-based web cache scheme

*R1: allocate(X, y):- url(X, U), match(U, *.au), content(X, y(football)).*

directs a document in sub-cache y if it is about football and comes from Australia. The number of sub-cache y is determined by the theme most closely related stem "football".

The CSKB not only directs similarity information in its rules but it may also impose various restrictions on sub-caches. For example, it is essential that dynamic documents, too large documents, or documents that are prohibited from caching will not be accepted in any sub-cache. These conditions can be combined into CSKB rules. As an example, the following rule R2 restricts that only those football related documents whose size is less than 2 megabytes could be cached.

R2: allocate(X, y):- content(X, y(football)), size(X, <2M).

A *sub-cache* is an independent cache that has its own cache space, contents and replacement policy. Since documents in a same sub-cache are usually of similar theme, simpler replacement policies, such as LRU, LFU and FIFO, may be applied.

The *sub-cache allocator* assesses comprehensively a candidate set of evictions selected by sub-caches, with possible results of: re-caching, eviction or probation. Of these, re-caching and eviction are instantaneous, while a probation document will be held by the allocator in its own space pending a final decision. A document to be re-cached will be cached at once in a certain sub-cache. An eviction document will be purged immediately.

The *central router* in Fig. 2 mediates between cooperating sub-caches. Although a document may be cached "conceptually" in several sub-caches in terms of sub-cache document allocator evaluation, only one actual copy will be maintained.

4.2 Online Updating of Cache Content and Similarity Profile

A request for a document d invokes the similarity-aware caching algorithm as follows: an instance of d is sought in an in-cache index; if d is already cached (i.e., cache hit) and still fresh its containing sub-cache is noted whereupon d will be returned to the requesting client. If the instance of d is not fresh, then re-cache from an origin server, updating related parameters such as SP vectors. For a cache miss, a request for d will be forwarded to the origin server and a resultant downloaded document d_{new} is returned to the client. Based on the content of d_{new}, a SP vector will be calculated to determine a sub-cache c_d in which d_{new} is to be cached. If there is insufficient space for d_{new}, the sub cache c_d makes room according to its eviction (e.g. LRU, LFU) and/or space sharing policies. The document allocator of c_d will then assess and purge any eviction candidates.

4.3 Agent-Based Similarity-Aware Document Pre-fetching

We now briefly describe the web document pre-fetching between caching proxies and browsing clients. If the proxy can predict those cached documents a user might access next, the idle periods of network links may be used to push (or to have the browser/client pull) them to the user while the user is viewing the web document. Since the proxy only initiates pre-fetches for documents in its caches, there is no extra internet traffic increase.

We employ both proxy-side and client-side agents that exchange messages using a predefined protocol for performing similarity detection, document prediction, network traffic monitoring and proxy-client coordination intentions during the process where they negotiate to reach the most probable solution. We are concerned with coordinating intelligent behavior among these agents, i.e. how they coordinate their knowledge, goals and plans jointly to take action or to solve problems.

In the similarity-aware web document pre-fetching process, three activities are crucial and are the focuses in this section, including (1) identifying similarities between documents in the proxy cache and the document a user is viewing; (2) predicting documents that a client is most likely to access next; and (3) monitoring idle network periods to pre-fetch the documents. The first activity is similar to the similarity detection in caching new document (see Section 3 and 4.2). The third activity involves traffic handling and resource utilization, and is, thus, beyond the scope of this chapter. Therefore, we focus on the second activity. In this architecture, agents and other software components are described as follows:

The *Client Agent (CA)* plays the role of a client. It delivers a pre-fetching request to the *Coordination Agent* (CoA). Upon receipt of an initial pre-fetching plan (i.e., a list of candidate documents to be pre-fetched) from the CoA, it modifies the plan by removing the candidates that were hit by its local cache, and then returns the modified plan to the CoA for final pre-fetching. The CoA is responsible for receiving the pre-fetching requests from clients, and coordinates among the *similarity detection agent*

(SDA), *access pattern matching agent* (PMA), *pre-fetching agent* (PFA) and *network traffic monitoring agent* (TMA) for document pre-fetching. The SDA determines a set of documents whose similarity with the given document surpasses the given similarity threshold. These documents will be referenced when similarity-aware PFA performs document prediction. The PMA matches a number of other users whose past access patterns with the given user's is greater than or equal to a certain threshold. These access patterns will also be referenced when the PFA performs document prediction. The PFA is responsible for predicting a set of cached documents as candidates of an initial pre-fetching plan (see Section 4.2). The TMA is responsible for monitoring the network traffic between the proxy and a given client. Once a suitable idle period is identified, the agent sends (if a proxy-side agent) a candidate document of the pre-fetch plan from the proxy cache to the client within the idle period. This monitoring-identifying-sending process continues until all candidate documents were sent, or the pre-fetching time limit is reached. The *Conversation Manager (CM)* coordinates the activities of agents in the documents pre-fetching circle. It is responsible for receiving events from an agent, and informing other agents of messages. For example, each agent routes all its outgoing messages through the CM, and all its incoming messages are received via the CM as well.

We propose two agent-based prediction algorithms to guide similarity-aware pre-fetching from proxy caches to clients. The first one is a pure similarity-based pre-fetching predictor which considers only those documents whose similarities with the document in viewing surpass a certain threshold. The second algorithm (i.e., similarity-aware pre-fetching) combines the *prediction by partial matching (PPM)* method [6] and the pure similarity-based pre-fetching strategies. These algorithms are the main functionalities and behavior of PFAs.

The similarity-based pre-fetching agent predicts the next k documents in the proxy cache based on document similarities. With the support of the similarity-aware web cache architecture, the similarity-based document pre-fetching predictor works based on a very simple rule. Suppose a client is viewing a document, say d (at this time, a copy of d must be cached in a certain sub-cache, say c_i, or being held by the allocator). When a pre-fetching request is received, the CoA invokes an SDA which computes the similarities between d and those documents in sub-cache c_i by referencing the similarity information in i_{th} SP. No documents in other sub-caches are considered because of their low similarities with d. Then the predictor simply chooses k documents whose similarities with d are among the top k highest ones. These k documents, together with those cached pages to which hyperlinks exist from d, will form an initial pre-fetching plan and be returned to CoA for possible pre-fetching.

Palpanas adopted the PPM [6] to predict the next l requests based on the past m accesses of a user, limiting candidates by an access probability threshold t. The performance metrics of the algorithm depend on the (m, l, t) configurations [5]. The algorithm uses patterns observed from all users' references to predict a particular user's behavior. Referencing too many contexts makes the prediction inaccurate, inefficient and unwieldy. Our previous work [7] extended the PPM algorithm by referencing only those access patterns from a small group of other users exhibiting high similarities in their past access patterns to predict a current user's next accesses. The number of times the algorithm can make prediction is reduced because of the smaller sample size, but the hit ratio of the pre-fetching increases because more related access patterns are referenced. We call the method *pattern-similarity based PPM* (or *psPPM*).

The similarity-aware pre-fetching algorithm is formed by modifying *psPPM*, i.e., by replacing the access threshold t with s, where s is the similarity threshold between the document to be pre-fetched and the document the client is viewing.

Suppose a user u is viewing a document d. When a pre-fetching request is received, the CoA invokes a PMA to assess and identify a set of r users' access patterns of relatively high similarities with u (sorted in descending order). For $l>1$, not only the immediate next request, but the next few requests after a URL are also considered for potential pre-fetching. For example, if $l = 2$, the PFA predicts both the immediate next and its successor for the user. If $m > 1$, more contexts of the r users' past accesses are referenced for the purpose of improving the accuracy of the prediction.

The PFA maintains a data structure that tracks the sequence of URLs for every user. For prediction, the past reference, the past two references, and up to the past m references are matched against the collection of succession to the users' past access patterns to produce a list of URLs for the next l steps. If a longer match sequence can be found from the other r users' patterns, the next URL to the longest match is also taken as a potential document to be accessed next by the user. The outcome of each prediction is a list of candidate documents, ordered by their similarities with d. For those candidate documents with the same similarity value, the URL matched with longer prefix is put first in the list.

5 Conclusions

In order to make best use of large scale web caches, it is important to develop suitable content management strategies, because semantics information related to a document are important indicators to its usage. This paper described an approach of mining evolving web sessions to cluster web users and establish similarities among web documents. The knowledge obtained from the mining exercise is then used to facilitating offline building of the similarity-aware web cache and online updating of sub-caches and cache content similarity profiles. Upon reviewing the underlying web-caching architecture of SaWCM, we developed similarity-based and similarity-aware predictors, respectively, for web document pre-fetching between proxy caches and browsing clients. It builds on regular web caching and tries to predict the next set of documents that will be requested, and guide the pre-fetching accordingly. This greatly speeds up access to those documents, and improves the users' experience.

References

1. Chen, L., Bhowmick, S.S., Li, J.: COWES: Clustering Web Users Based on Historical Web Sessions. In: Li Lee, M., Tan, K.-L., Wuwongse, V. (eds.) DASFAA 2006. LNCS, vol. 3882, pp. 541–556. Springer, Heidelberg (2006)
2. Xiao, J., Zhang, Y.: Clustering of web users using session-based similarity measures. In: Proc. of ICCNMC 2001 (2001)
3. Nasraoui, O., Soliman, M., Saka, E., Badia, A., Germain, R.: A Web usage mining Framework for mining Evolving user profiles in Dynamic Web sites. IEEE Transaction on Knowledge and Data Engineering 20(2) (2008)

4. Xiao, J., Wang, J.: A Similarity-Aware Multiagent-Based Web Content Management Scheme. In: Yeung, D.S., Liu, Z.-Q., Wang, X.-Z., Yan, H. (eds.) ICMLC 2005. LNCS (LNAI), vol. 3930, pp. 305–314. Springer, Heidelberg (2006)
5. Fan, L., Cao, P., Lin, W., Jacobson, Q.: Web Prefetching between Low-Bandwidth Client and Proxies: Potential and Performance. In: SIGMETRICS 1999 (1999)
6. Palpanas, T.: Web Prefetching using Partial Matching Prediction, Technical report CSRG-376, University of Toronto (1998)
7. Xiao, J.: Agent-based Similarity-aware Web Document Pre-fetching. In: Proc. of the CIMCA/IAWTIC 2005, pp. 928–933 (2005)
8. Wang, W., Zaiane, O.R.: Clustering web sessions by sequence alignment. In: Proc. of DEXA (2002)
9. Fu, Y., Sandhu, K., Shih, M.: A generalization-based approach to clustering of web usage sessions. In: Masand, B., Spiliopoulou, M. (eds.) WebKDD 1999. LNCS (LNAI), vol. 1836, pp. 21–38. Springer, Heidelberg (2000)
10. Wen, J.R., Nie, J.Y., Zhang, H.J.: Querying Clustering Using User Logs. ACM Transactions on Information Systems 20(1), 59–81 (2002)
11. Popescul, A., Flake, G., Lawrence, S., Ungar, L.H., Gile, C.L.: Clustering and Identifying Temporal Trends in Document Database. In: Proceedings of the IEEE advances in Digital Libraries, Washington (2000)
12. Flesca, S., Masciari, E.: Efficient and Effective Web Change Detection. In: Data & Knowledge Engineering. Elsevier, Amsterdam (2003)
13. Salton, G., Yang, C.: On the specification of term values in automatic indexing. Journal of Documentation 29, 351–372 (1973)
14. Barfourosh, A.A., Nezhad, H.R.M., Anderson, M.L., Perlis, D.: Information Retrieval on the World Wide Web and Active Logic: A Survey and Problem Definition, Technical report UMIACS-TR-2001-69, DRUM: Digital Repository at the University of Maryland (2002)
15. Broder, A.Z.: On the Resemblance and Containment of Documents. In: Proceedings of Compression and Complexity of SEQUENCES 1997, Salerno, Italy, pp. 21–29 (1997)
16. Fox, E.: Extending the Boolean and Vector Space Models on Information Retrieval with P-Norm Queries and Multiple Concepts Types. Cornell University Dissertation (1983)

Data Quality in Privacy Preservation for Associative Classification

Nattapon Harnsamut[1], Juggapong Natwichai[1], Xingzhi Sun[2], and Xue Li[3]

[1] Computer Engineering Department, Faculty of Engineering
Chiang Mai University, Chiang Mai, Thailand
harnsamut@gmail.com, juggapong@eng.cmu.ac.th
[2] IBM Research Laboratory
Beijing, China
sunxingz@cn.ibm.com
[3] School of Information Technology and Electrical Engineering
The University of Queensland, Brisbane, Australia
xueli@itee.uq.edu.au

Abstract. Privacy preserving has become an essential process for any data mining task. In general, data transformation is needed to ensure privacy preservation. Once the privacy is preserved, data quality issue must be addressed, i.e. the impact on data quality should be minimized. In this paper, k-Anonymization is considered as the transformation approach for preserving data privacy. In such a context, we discuss the metrics of the data quality in terms of classification, which is one of the most important tasks in data mining. Since different type of classification may use different approach to deliver knowledge, data quality metric for the classification task should be tailored to a certain type of classification. Specifically, we propose a frequency-based data quality metric to represent the data quality of the transformed dataset in the situation that associative classification is to be processed. Subsequently, we validate our proposed metric with experiments. The experiment results have shown that our proposed metric can effectively reflect the data quality for the associative classification problem.

1 Introduction

When data are to be release to another business collaborator for data mining purpose, the privacy issue must be addressed. Typically all identifiers such as ID or name must be removed. Unfortunately, there could be another dataset which can "link" to the released data. The link can be establish by common attributes between the two datasets. For example, consider the datasets in Table 1. Suppose that the dataset in Table 1a) is released from a hospital to be used to build a classifier by a data analysis company. By considering this dataset alone could misjudge that the privacy of the individuals which contain in this dataset has been already preserved due to the removal of the identifiers. However, suppose that there is another dataset which is released publicly for voting purpose as shown in Table 1b). If an adversary wants to find private information about a

C. Tang et al. (Eds.): ADMA 2008, LNAI 5139, pp. 111–122, 2008.

man named "Somchai" who lives in an area with postal code "50200", and his age is approximately 50 years-old. The adversary can link two datasets together by using postal code and age attributes, subsequently, his medical condition will be disclosed.

Table 1. Linkable datasets and its 2-Anonymity

Postal code	Age	Sex	Disease
50211	1-25	Female	Fever
50211	1-25	Female	Fever
50202	26-50	Male	Flu
50202	26-50	Male	Flu
50200	26-50	Male	Cancer

a)

Name	Postal code	Age	Sex
Manee	50211	19	Female
Wanthong	50211	24	Female
Tawan	50202	32	Male
Sutee	50202	41	Male
Somchai	50200	50	Male

b)

Postal code	Age	Sex	Disease
5021*	1-25	Female	Fever
5021*	1-25	Female	Fever
5020*	26-50	Male	Flu
5020*	26-50	Male	Flu
5020*	26-50	Male	Cancer

c)

k-Anonymity [1] is a well-known privacy model for datasets, in which a dataset is said to satisfy the anonymity, if for every tuple in the dataset, there are another k-1 tuples which are in-distinguishable from the tuple for all "linkable" attributes. If a dataset does not satisfy the standard, we can transform such the dataset by generalize it until the standard is reached. For example, from the dataset in Table 1a) we can generalized it into a 2-Anonymity dataset by changing the last digit of the postal code as shown in Table 1c). However, data quality issue in the transformation processes must be addressed, i.e. the transformed datasets should have enough quality to be used by the designate data processing which is decided at the first place. As in our example, the transformed dataset should be able to served the classification purpose.

Generally, the metrics proposed to determine the data quality can be categorized into two classes[2]: general data quality and data-mining-algorithm dependence data quality. The examples of well-known general data quality metrics are precision metric (*Prec*) in [3], k-minimal generalization in [4], or general loss metric in [2].

For data-mining-algorithm dependence data quality, there are several metrics proposed, particularly, classification data quality metrics [2,5]. Generally, this type of metrics measures whether a transformed dataset can be used to build a classification model accurately. However, there are many different approaches for classification, e.g., gain-ratio based classification, associative classification, or probability-based classification. In fact, these classification approaches are very different in terms of both concept and methodology. Therefore, a classification data quality metric should be tailored to a particular classification approach.

In this paper, we propose a new classification data quality metric for an important classification approach, associative classification [6,7]. The associative classification works on support and confidence scheme as association rules [8], but having a designate attribute as class label. Based on the new proposed metrics, we formalize the problem of data transformation by k-Anonymization. After defining the problem, we conduct experiments to illustrate the applicability of the metric. For the investigation purpose, we implement an exhaustive search algorithm which transforms datasets, and meanwhile optimizes data quality. In the experiments, various characteristics of the problem are investigated to validate the new proposed metric.

The organization of this paper is as follows. Related work is reviewed in the next section. Section 3 presents the basic definitions used in this paper. Subsequently, we give the problem definition which includes our proposed data quality metric in Section 4. Our metric is validated by experiments in Section 5. Finally, we presents the conclusion and future work in Section 6.

2   Related Work

k-Anonymity is a well-known privacy model which was firstly proposed in [1]. There has been a lot of work applied the k-Anonymity because its simplicity and meaningful of the transformed data. The examples of such the proposed works are presented in [3,5,9,10,11,12,13]. As data quality of the transformed datasets is concerned, transformation problem is not trivial. In [9], the authors have proved that achieving an optimal anonymization, i.e. satisfying k while having minimal impact on data quality, is an NP-hard problem.

In order to transform data to satisfy k-Anonymity, there are a few techniques have been proposed. Such the techniques can be categorized into generalization techniques [14], suppression techniques [9], and generalization with suppression techniques [10]. While our work focuses on the first technique.

For classification data quality metric, there have been a few proposed metrics. In [9], the authors suggested that data transformation weakens the ability to classify data into classes. Therefore, a tuple will have less data quality and subject to the penalty, if it is transformed and its class label is not the majority class in the equivalence-quasi-identifer values. In [5], tuples are grouped together to determine classification data quality by using information loss created by the transformation processes. In this work the information loss is based on gain-ratio.

There have been a few privacy models built based on the k-Anonymity model such as ℓ-diversity [12] or (α,k)-Anonymity model [13] in which our new proposed metric can be included in the models as an additional metric, or it can replace the generic classification metric when associative classification is to be used.

3   Basic Definitions

In this section, the basic definitions of the problem are presented as follows.

Definition 1 (Dataset). *Let a dataset D be a collection of tuples, $D = \{d^1, d^2, \ldots, d^n\}$ and $I = (1, ..., n)$ be a set of identifiers for elements of D. Tuples in a table is not necessary to be unique.*

The dataset D is defined on a schema $\mathbf{A} = \{A_1, A_2, \ldots, A_k\}$, and $J = (1, \ldots, k)$ be a set of identifiers for elements of $\mathbf{A}$.

For each $j \in J$, attribute domain of A_j is denoted as $dom(A_j)$. For each $i \in I$, $d^i(\mathbf{A}) = (d^i(A_1), d^i(A_2), \ldots, d^i(A_k))$, denoted as $(d^i_1, d^i_2, \ldots, d^i_k)$.

Let C be a set of class labels, such that $C = \{c_1, c_2, \ldots, c_o\}$, and $M = \{1, \ldots, o\}$ be a set of identifiers for elements of C. For each $m \in M$, c_m is a class label.

The label is just an identifier of a class. A class which is labelled as c_m defines a subset of tuples which is described by data assigned to the class. The class label of a tuple d^i is denoted as $d^i.Class$. The classification problem is to establish a mapping from D to C.

Definition 2 (Associative Classification). A literal p is a pair, consisting of an attribute A_j and a value v in $dom(A_j)$. A tuple d^i will **satisfy** the literal $p(A_j, v)$ iff $d_j^i = v$.

Given a dataset D, and a set of class labels C, let R be a set of classification rules, such that $R = \{r_1, r_2, \ldots, r_q\}$, and $L = \{1, \ldots, q\}$ be a set of identifiers for elements of R.

For all $l \in L$, $r_l : \bigwedge p \to c_m$, where p is the literal, and c_m is a class label. The left hand side (LHS) of the rule r_l is the conjunction of the literals, denoted as $r_l.LHS$. The right hand side (RHS) is a class label of the rule r_l, denoted as $r_l.RHS$.

A tuple d^i **satisfies** the classification rule r_l iff it satisfies all literals in $r_l.LHS$, and has a class label c_m as $r_l.RHS$.

A tuple d^i which satisfies the classification rule r_l is called **supporting tuple** of r_l. The **support** of the rule r_l, denoted as $Sup(r_l)$, is the ratio between the number of supporting tuples of r_l and the total number of tuples. The **confidence** of rule r_l, denoted as $Conf(r_l)$, is the ratio between $Sup(r_l)$ and the total number of tuples which satisfy all literals in LHS of r_l.

Generally, the set of attributes of a dataset which can "link" to another dataset is called "quasi-identifier". The linkage process is also called "re-identifying" as it can identify the de-identified data. A quasi-identifier attribute is not necessary to be a sensitive attribute, i.e. it can be disclosed but may be used to re-identify individuals.

Definition 3 (Quasi-Identifier). A quasi-identifier of the dataset D, written Q_D, is the minimal subset of the attributes **A** that can re-identify the tuples in D by using given external data.

Definition 4 (k-Anonymity). A dataset D with a schema **A** and a quasi-identifier Q_D satisfies k-Anonymity iff for each tuple $d^i \in D$, there exist at least $k - 1$ other tuples $d^{i^1}, d^{i^2}, \ldots, d^{i^{k-1}} \in D$ such that $d_j^i = d_j^{i^1} = d_j^{i^2} = \ldots = d_j^{i^{k-1}}, \forall A_j \in Q_D$.

Definition 5 (Generalization). Let a domain $dom^*(A_j) = \{P_1, P_2, \ldots\}$ be a generalization of a domain $dom(A_j)$ of an attribute A_j where $\bigcup P_{jt} = dom(A_j)$ and $P_{jt} \bigcap P_{jt'} = \emptyset$, for $jt \neq jt'$. For a value v in $dom(A_j)$, its generalized value Pjt in a generalized domain $dom^*(A_j)$ is denoted as $\phi_{dom^*(A_j)}(v)$.

Let $\prec_G$ be a partial order on domains, $dom(A_j) \prec_G dom^*(A_j)$ iff $dom^*(A_j)$ is a generalization of $dom(A_j)$.

For a set of attributes $\mathbf{A'}, \mathbf{A'} \subseteq \mathbf{A}$, *let* $dom^*(\mathbf{A'})$ *be a generalization of a domain* $dom(\mathbf{A'})$. *A dataset D can be generalized to* D^* *by replacing the values of* $d^i(\mathbf{A'})$ *with a generalized value* $\phi_{dom^*(\mathbf{A'})}(d^i(\mathbf{A'}))$ *to get a new tuple* d^{i*}. *The tuple* d^{i*} *is defined as a generalization of the tuple* d^i.

For an attribute, the set of generalization domains on it forms a hierarchy deriving from the priori knowledge of the given data, or domain partitioning. From the dataset in Table 1, we can apply the hierarchies shown in Figure 1a), 1b), and 1c).

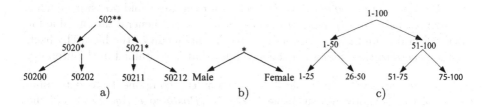

Fig. 1. Postal Code, Sex, and Age Hierarchies

Definition 6 (k-Anonymization). k-*Anonymization is the transformation from D to* D^* *where* D^* *is the generalization of D and* D^* *satisfies the* k-*Anonymity property.*

4   Problem Definition

After giving the basic definitions, we formalize the problem of privacy preserving for associative classification focusing on defining the new metric for data quality of the transformed dataset.

Problem 1. Given a dataset D with a set of class label C, a quasi-identifier Q_D, a k value, and a minimal support threshold *minsup* for associative classification, find D^* by anonymization such that 1) D^* satisfies k-Anonymity property, and 2) the impact on data quality (defined below) is minimized.

1. First, we define a general impact on data quality metric C_{GM} as the one originally proposed in [13]:

$$C_{GM} = \frac{\sum_{j \in J} \frac{h_j}{Full\ Generalization_j}}{|Q_D|} \tag{1}$$

In the formula, for an attribute $A_j \in Q_D$, h_j is the height of the generalized value of A_j in D^*, and h_j starts from zero when there is no generalization. *Full Generalization$_j$* is the height of the hierarchy from the generalization domain of attribute A_j.

2. As the transformed dataset is intended to be used to build associative classifiers, we define the frequency-based classification impact C_{FCM} as follows:

$$C_{FCM} = \frac{\sum_{fp \in FP}[\frac{hp_{fp}}{Full\ Generalization_{fp}} \times Sup(fp)]}{\sum_{fp \in FP} Sup(fp)} \tag{2}$$

In the formula, fp is a frequency-pair of (p, c_m) such that 1) p is a literal on the attribute in the quasi-identifier Q_D, 2) c_m is a class label, and 3) the support of rule $p \to c_m$ in D is no less than $minsup$. Note that we use $Sup(fp)$ to denote the number of supporting tuples for the rule $Sup(p \to c_m)$. FP is denoted as the set of all fp from D for the threshold $minsup$. Given a frequent pair $fp = (p, c_m)$, hp_{fp} is the height of the generalization value for the literal p, and $Full\ Generalization_{fp}$ is the height of the hierarchy from the generalization domain of the attribute that is contained in the literal p.

For the sake of clarity, in Table 2, we present the components to determine C_{FCM} of the 2-Anonymity in Table 1 (Q_D is $\{Postalcode, Age, Sex\}$ and the hierarchies are shown in Figure 1). Given a minimum support as 0.2, we can see that all frequency-pairs are listed in the left-most column. After using Equation 2, the C_{FCM} can be calculated. In this case, the value is 0.33.

Table 2. An example of C_{FCM} calculation

Pair	$Sup(fp)$	$\frac{hp_{fp}}{Full\ Generalization_{fp}}$
(50211, Fever)	2	$\frac{1}{2}$
(1-25, Fever)	2	0
(Female, Fever)	2	0
(50202, Flu)	2	$\frac{1}{2}$
(26-50, Flu)	2	0
(Male, Flu)	2	0

According to formula (2), the value domain of the frequency-based metric is [0,1], in which the larger the value is, the greater impact on the result dataset. Also, we can see that the frequency-based metric will penalty any transformation which degrades pairs (p, c_m) with the support no less than $minsup$. The intuition is: because such frequency-pairs will be used to derive the associative classification rules, reducing the penalty on the frequency-pairs will preserve the characteristics of the classifier. When comparing the generalizations of two different attributes, for a single level of generalization, the attribute with higher hierarchy levels will cause less penalty since it introduces relatively less generalized values. Additionally, any transformation that affects the frequent pairs with higher support will be punished more than the transformation that affects the ones with less support.

Intuitively, the first metric can put a global constraint on the generalization of all values, while the second metric can take care of the values relevant for associative classification. As the datasets are intended for associative classification building, therefore, the C_{FCM} will be optimized firstly. If there are more

```
Input:
D: a dataset
Q_D: a quasi-identifier
minsup: a minimal support threshold
k: a condition for k-Anonymity
dom*(Q_D): a generalization on Q_D
Output:
D'_FCM: the output dataset, which satisfies the k-Anonymity property,
        and the frequency-based classification impact on data quality is minimal
Method:
 1 Initialize MIN_GM and MIN_FCM as 0;
 2 Determine the set GD*, whose elements are all possible generalized dataset D*
 3    based on dom*(Q_D) for each attribute in Q_D;
 4 for all generalized D* ∈ GD*
 5    if D* satisfies k-Anonymity
 6       Determine C_FCM and C_GM of D*
 7       if C_FCM < MIN_FCM or (C_FCM = MIN_FCM and C_GM < MIN_GM)
 8          D'_FCM = D*;
 9          MIN_FCM = C_FCM;
10          MIN_GM = C_GM;
11       end if
12    end if
13 end for
```

Fig. 2. An exhaustive search algorithm

than one generalization which provide optimal solution in term of C_{FCM}, the one with the least general impact C_{GM} will be selected as the final solution.

5 Experimental Validation

In this section, we present the experiments to validate whether the proposed frequency based metric can well reflect the data quality for associative classification. Firstly, we present an exhaustive search algorithm which transforms the given datasets to meet k-Anonymity standard and guarantees optimal data quality. Then, we give the experiment setting for our validation. At the end, we present the experiment results with discussions. Note that the results reported in this section are five-time-average results.

5.1 Algorithm

Figure 2 shows the pseudo code of the exhaustive algorithm. This generates the set of all possible generalization D^* by using the hierarchies created from generalization domains for the attributes in quasi-identifiers Q_D. After the generation, we determine whether a generalized dataset satisfies the pre-specified k-Anonymity. For each k-Anonymity dataset, the general metric C_{GM} and frequency-based metric C_{FCM} are determined. The transformed dataset with minimum impact is selected as the output of the algorithm.

It is apparent that exhaustive algorithm explores very large search space and is not practical for large datasets. However, since our focus in this paper is to demonstrate the effectiveness of the proposed metric, we apply this algorithm to find the optimal solution. We are aware that some heuristics could be used to find the near-optimal result efficiently.

5.2 Setting

We evaluate our proposed work by using "adult" and "crx" datasets from UCI repository [15]. Both datasets are pre-processed by removing the tuples with unknown values, and discretizing continuous attributes. Subsequently, the adult dataset has 8 attributes available for quasi-identifier selection, and consists of 45,222 tuples. The crx dataset has 9 attributes for quasi-identifier, and consists of 671 tuples. In Table 3, we show the detail of quasi-identifier attributes, including attribute names, the number of distinct values, generalization method, and the height of the hierarchy.

Table 3. Quasi-Identifiers of Adult and Crx Datasets

Adult			
Attribute	Distinct Values	Generalization	Height
Age	42	5-,10,20-year ranges	4
Sex	2	Suppression	1
Race	3	Suppression	1
Martial Status	6	Taxonomy Tree	2
Education	13	Taxonomy Tree	4
Native Country	41	Taxonomy Tree	3
Work Class	6	Taxonomy Tree	2
Occupation	12	Taxonomy Tree	3
Crx			
A1, A9, A10, and A12	2	Suppression	1
A4	3	Taxonomy Tree	2
A5	3	Suppression	1
A6	14	Taxonomy Tree	3
A7	9	Taxonomy Tree	3
A13	3	Suppression	1

The experiments are conducted on a 3.00 GHz Intel Pentium D PC with 3 gigabytes main memory running Microsoft Window Vista. The exhaustive algorithm is implemented by using JDK 5.0 based on Weka Data Mining Software.

5.3 Results

We investigate two aspects of the transformed datasets in the experiments. Firstly, because the transformed datasets are intended for associative classification, we investigate whether the transformed dataset (with the least C_{FCM}) preserves the data quality for associative classification. Specifically, we derive the classification model from the result dataset, and compute its classification correction rate (CCR) as proposed in [5]. Given a testing dataset, the CCR is computed by classifying each tuple into the predicted class label from the model, subsequently, comparing the predicted class label with the actual class label, finally determining the ratio between the number of the correct prediction and the total number of the tuples. The higher CCR value means the classification model can be used to classify the target data better. Secondly, the effect of the

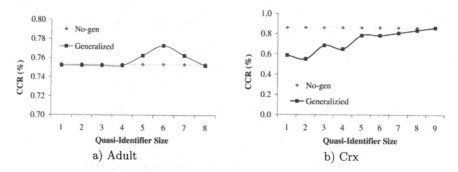

Fig. 3. Effect of the size of QI to classification correction rate

size of quasi-identifier, and the k value on the proposed data quality metric is investigated. In all experiments, the *minsup* are set as 10 % and 30 % and *minconf* as 10 % and 50% for the adult and crx datasets respectively.

Classification Correction Rate. In these experiments, we apply the algorithm to find a transformed dataset that satisfies the k-Anonymity on a specific quasi-identifier and has the minimum value of the metric. Then, we build the set of associative classification rules from the transformed dataset to classify the testing datasets as explained in [6]. The classification correction rate (CCR) of the generalized data will be compared with the "No-gen" dataset, which is the original dataset without transformation.

The effect of the quasi-identifier size to the CCR is reported in Figure 3. In these experiments, k is fixed at 4. From Figure 3a), the result shows that the size of quasi-identifier does not have a significance effect on the CCR from the adult dataset. As the CCR from the "No-gen" dataset is not high at the first place, the generalization could not make the result worse significantly. However, from Figure 3b), the CCR from the crx dataset rises when the size of quasi-identifier increases. This is because, with the large size of quasi-identifer, the algorithm has more candidates to select when discovering the optimal solution. Therefore, the optimal dataset, which tends to preserve the frequency-pairs for building the classification rules later, will have a better data quality. In general, this result suggests that choosing the large size of quasi-identifer is appropriate in our problem. It can not only block dataset linkage from linkable attributes, but also yield a better classification correction rate.

In Figure 4, the effect of the k value to the CCR is presented. The size of quasi-identifier is set at maximum value (i.e., 8 and 9 for dataset adult and crx respectively) in these experiments. From Figure 4a), we can see that CCR from the adult dataset remains constant with the change of k value. The reason is: because this dataset has a very poor CCR at the first place, the generalization causes it to derive only associative classification rules with one class label from the majority classes of the dataset. Meanwhile, we can see that for the crx dataset, the CCR is decreased with the increase of the value k. However, it can be seen that the CCR starts to decrease after the k value is increased at 75. This

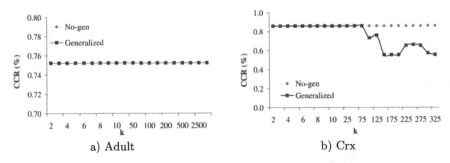

Fig. 4. Effect of the k value to classification correction rate

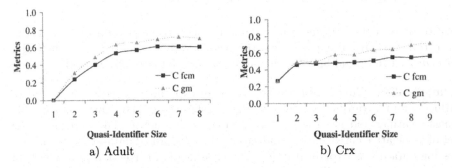

Fig. 5. Effect of the size of QI to frequency-based data quality

means that there is a specific "falling-point" of the CCR when k is increasing. Such the point could allow the practitioners to set the suitable k value by which the possible privacy threat level is acceptable, while the very high CCR could be obtained.

To summarize, we can see that the generalized datasets with optimal data quality metric C_{FCM} can derive the sets of associative classification rules with high CCR. This shows that our proposed metric works effectively for the defined problem. In the next section, we will further investigate the characteristics of the proposed metric.

Frequency-Based Classification Metric Characteristics. First, the effect of the size of quasi-identifier to the frequency-based metric is reported in Figure 5. In this experiment, the k value is fixed at 4 for both datasets.

Figure 5 shows the effect of the size of quasi-identifier on the frequency-based cost metric. Let consider the sparse dataset adult first. When the adult dataset is generalized, it is not hard to find the optimal solution with the least cost metric. As shown in Figure 5a), the dataset can even satisfy k-Anonymity when no generalization has taken place. For such the dataset, if the size of quasi-identifier is increased, the optimal value of C_{fcm} is also increased. For the very dense dataset as the crx dataset, it is often the case that k-Anonymity property does not hold at the first place. By the way, the optimal value of C_{fcm} increases when the size of quasi-identifier is increased.

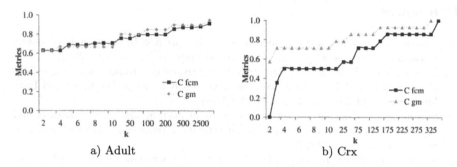

Fig. 6. Effect of the k value to frequency-based data quality

Secondly, the effect of the k value to the proposed data quality metric is reported in Figure 6. The number of attributes in quasi-identifier is fixed at maximum value of each dataset. From Figure 6, we can see that when the k value is increased, the cost metric also increases. For the dense dataset crx, the cost could be even 1.00 when the k value is set at 325. This means that all attributes that are related to frequency-pairs have been generalized to the highest level. However, this could be considered as an extreme case as the number of tuples in this dataset is small (671).

Also, in Figure 5 and 6, we report the general impact C_{GM} of the datasets which have optimal frequency-based metric. From the results, we can see that the curves for C_{GM} and C_{GM} have the same trend. Intuitively, with the increase of the size of Quasi-Identifer and the value k, more generalization is made to satisfy the k-Anonymity property. As a result, the impact on both metric will be increased.

6   Conclusion

In this paper, we address the problem of k-Anonymization under the circumstance that the transformed dataset are used to build associative classification models. The main contributions are twofold. Firstly, we have introduced a new data-mining-algorithm dependent data quality metric, called "frequency-based" metric. Secondly, we have conducted the experiments to validate the new metric, and the results have shown that the optimal transformed datasets are able to perform classification tasks effectively. Also, from the experiment results, we have shown that the larger size of quasi-identifier not only makes a generalized dataset harder to link, but also could help to improve the classification correction rate (CCR). Additionally, the results have shown that the CCR will remain as similar as the CCR from the original dataset at some period of k value. This observation could help to select a suitable k in practice. In our future work, we will focus on the efficiency of algorithms for this problem. Some heuristics will be applied to efficiently search the near-optimal solution. Also, we will target on investigating the problem where other privacy standards are applied.

References

1. Sweeney, L.: k-anonymity: a model for protecting privacy. International Journal on Uncertainty, Fuzziness and Knowledge-based Systems 10, 557–570 (2002)
2. Iyengar, V.S.: Transforming data to satisfy privacy constraints. In: Proceedings of the Eighth ACM International Conference on Knowledge Discovery and Data Mining, pp. 279–288. ACM, New York (2002)
3. Sweeney, L.: Achieving k-anonymity privacy protection using generalization and suppression. International Journal on Uncertainty, Fuzziness and Knowledge-based Systems 10, 571–588 (2002)
4. Samarati, P.: Protecting respondents' identities in microdata release. IEEE Transactions on Knowledge and Data Engineering 13, 1010–1027 (2001)
5. Fung, B.C.M., Wang, K., Yu, P.S.: Top-down specialization for information and privacy preservation. In: Proceedings of the IEEE International Conference on Data Engineering, pp. 205–216. IEEE Computer Society, Los Alamitos (2005)
6. Liu, B., Hsu, W., Ma, Y.: Integrating classification and association rule mining. In: Proceedings of the ACM International Conference on Knowledge Discovery and Data Mining, pp. 80–86. AAAI Press, Menlo Park (1998)
7. Li, W., Han, J., Pei, J.: Cmar: Accurate and efficient classification based on multiple class-association rules. In: Proceedings of the IEEE International Conference on Data Mining, Washington, DC, USA, pp. 369–376. IEEE Computer Society, Los Alamitos (2001)
8. Agrawal, R., Imielinski, T., Swami, A.: Mining association rules between sets of items in large databases. In: Proceedings of the ACM International Conference on Management of Data, pp. 207–216. ACM Press, New York (1993)
9. Meyerson, A., Williams, R.: On the complexity of optimal k-anonymity. In: Proceedings of the ACM Symposium on Principles of Database Systems, pp. 223–228. ACM, New York (2004)
10. Bayardo Jr., R.J., Agrawal, R.: Data privacy through optimal k-anonymization. In: Proceedings of the IEEE International Conference on Data Engineering, pp. 217–228. IEEE Computer Society, Los Alamitos (2005)
11. Truta, T.M., Campan, A.: K-anonymization incremental maintenance and optimization techniques. In: Proceedings of the Symposium on Applied Computing, pp. 380–387. ACM, New York (2007)
12. Machanavajjhala, A., Gehrke, J., Kifer, D., Venkitasubramaniam, M.: ℓ-diversity: Privacy beyond κ-anonymity. In: Proceedings of the International Conference on Data Engineering, Washington, DC, USA, p. 24. IEEE Computer Society, Los Alamitos (2006)
13. Wong, R.C.W., Li, J., Fu, A.W.C., Wang, K. (α, k)-anonymity: an enhanced k-anonymity model for privacy preserving data publishing. In: Proceedings of the ACM International Conference on Knowledge Discovery and Data Mining, pp. 754–759. ACM Press, New York (2006)
14. LeFevre, K., DeWitt, D.J., Ramakrishnan, R.: Incognito: efficient full-domain k-anonymity. In: Proceedings of the ACM International Conference on Management of Data, pp. 49–60. ACM Press, New York (2005)
15. Blake, C., Merz, C.: UCI repository of machine learning databases (1998)

Timeline Analysis of Web News Events[*]

Jiangtao Qiu[1,2], Chuan Li[1], Shaojie Qiao[1], Taiyong Li[1,2], and Jun Zhu[3]

[1] Computer School, Sichuan University, Chengdu, China 610065
[2] School of Economic Information Engineering, South Western University of Finance and Economics, Chengdu, China 610074
[3] National Center for Birth Defects Monitoring, Chengdu,China 610041

Abstract. With a large number of news available on the internet everyday, it is an interesting work to automatically organize news events by time order and dependencies between events. The work may help users to conveniently and quickly browse news event evolution. This paper defines an Event Timeline Analysis (ETA) task to meet the need. Compared with existing works, ETA presents event evolution in graph manner, and incrementally updates the process of events evolving so as to better fit feature of stream of news on the internet. In order to complete ETA task, this paper proposes an Event Evolving Graph (EEG) structure and building and tidying algorithm of EEG. Experiments demonstrate the utility and feasibility of the method.

Keywords: Web mining, Events Timeline Analysis, Event Evolution Graph.

1 Introduction

We may almost find out any interested news by surfing the internet today. But massive information on the internet also raises a problem that it is very difficult to navigate through a news topic. Perhaps search engine is helpful for the problem. However, it only provides a large number of Hyperlinks about the topic. Search Engine lacks ability to organize news event. If users want to know how news events evolve in a period, they have to depend on themselves. Therefore, if we may automatically organize news event about a topic by time order and dependency between events, and then present the result to users, it may help users to conveniently navigate through events evolution.

In this paper, we define a web news Event Timeline Analysis (ETA for short) task to meet the above need. Because web news occur every day in stream manner, ETA should incremental present the process of news events evolution. Fig.1 illustrates an example of events evolution about a topic.

Some works are similar with ETA, such as Topic Detection and Tracking, Comparative Text Mining, Temporal Text Mining and Event Treading. We will discuss these works in Section 2.

---

[*] This work was supported by NSFC Grant Number: 60773169, 11-th Five Years Key Programs for Sci. &Tech. Development of China under grant No. 2006BAI05A01 and Youth Grant of Computer School and Sichuan University. LI Chuan is the corresponding author.

C. Tang et al. (Eds.): ADMA 2008, LNAI 5139, pp. 123–134, 2008.

Parts of these works only present event evolution in a list view, for example TDT task. Such are too restrictive for user understanding news events evolution. We want to give a graph view that may present rich structure of events evolution. Parts of these works analyze events evolving based on the web pages collection. However, they will be inefficient in news stream. For example, TTM [2] need a background model that will be generated in text collection. Event Threading [3] derive events on text collection.

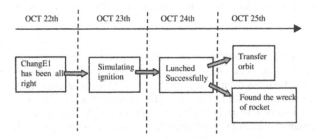

Fig. 1. An example of Events Evolution Graph

To analyzing news events evolution in news stream, it is important for ETA to have ability to incrementally present events evolution. This paper defines ETA task that may incrementally present events evolution about a topic along timeline. This paper also proposes EEG structure and building and tidying algorithm of EEG to complete ETA task.

The rest of this paper is organized as follows. Section 2 gives a brief introduction to related works. Section 3 formally describe ETA task. Section 4 introduces EEG building algorithm and tidying algorithm. Section 5 gives a thorough study on performance of new method. Section 6 summarizes our study.

2 Related Work

Zai study CTM (Comparative Text Mining) [1] problem to find out themes on multiple text collections. Zai proposes a probability mixed model. Theme is one of parameters of the model, then use EM algorithm and the text collection to estimate the parameters. So theme can be derived.

TTM (Temporal Text Mining) [2] task use model in [1] to find out theme and use K-L Divergence to calculate similarity between themes, then build theme evolution graph and analyze theme life-cycle. It partitioned documents to possibly overlapping subcollections with time intervals, then extract themes by probability mixed model. TTM needs a background model. It is built using text collection. Therefore, TTM is inefficient to incrementally update Theme Evolution Graph in news stream.

Event Threading [3] supposes that all texts about one topic have been derived before analyzing events. Then it employs text clustering method to get events on the text collection. Event (each cluster is one event) is presented in a series of story. Because Event Threading is based on text collection, it also cannot incremental present events evolution.

In TDT [10, 11], researchers have traditionally considered topics as flat clusters. However, in TDT-2003, a hierarchical structure of topic detection has been proposed and made useful attempts to adopt the new structure. However this structure still did not explicitly model any dependencies between events.

Kuo[6] used documents clustering to group documents of describing same event to one cluster. However, it cannot analyze dependency between events and event evolution along timeline. Some works [7, 8, 9] may detect new events but cannot present events evolution.

3 Problem Description

We considers a piece of news web page as a event.

Table 1. Symbol Table

Symbol	Description	symbol	Description	Symbol	Description
e	Event	c	Documents collection	O	Node
d	Document	t	Time stamp	l	Interval of levels
w	word	v	Vocabulary	s	Cluster

Definition 1 (Event). Let d be a piece of web page, event e be words probability distribution $\{P(w\,|\,d)\}_{w\in d}$ in d, naturally $\sum_{w\in d} P(w\,|\,d)=1$.

Definition 2 (Topic). In an event collection, we call the background of events as Topic.

Topic is a higher-level concept than event. For example, *Chang E1 was launched successfully* and *Chang E1 completed first orbital transfer successfully*, are two events. *Chang E1* is background of the two events, which is called Topic.

Definition 3 (Event Evolution Graph). EEG is a directed acyclic graph with the level structure:

1) Each node in EEG consists of four fields: *Child_List, Next, TC, e* where *Child_list* registers a list storing pointer that point to its children nodes, *Next* registers a pointer that point next node in same level, *TC* registers text classifier and *e* registers a event that the node represents.
2) Link between a node and its child node is called edge.
3) EEG contains an array of level. Each record in the array consists of two fields: *L* and *t* where *L* registers a pointer that point to first node in a level, *t* represent time stamp of the level whose granularity is day.

Fig.2 illustrates EEG. Node in same level have same time stamp. Same events are grouped to one cluster, and then build a node using the cluster. i.e., each node in EEG represents an event. Each edge represents dependency between two events. Edge only link nodes lied on different level.

Definition 4 (Events Timeline Analysis). For a web pages collection c with same time stamp t, we call the task that either build EEG or incrementally update EEG using c as news Event Timeline Analysis (ETA).

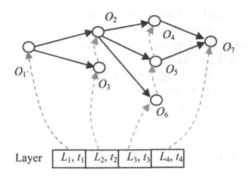

Fig. 2. Structure of EEG

4 Construction of EEG

Observation 1. Let A and B be two events. A is usually considered being associated to B if the following two conditions are met: 1) time stamp of B is older than that of A; 2) A and B have high similarity.

In fact, the construction of EEG is a process of finding out events and confirming dependencies between events. By Observation 1, we propose following steps to construct EEG.

1) Collect web pages about a topic, then put web pages into different sets $C=\{c_1,...,c_k\}$ by their time stamp where c_i has older time stamp than c_{i+1}.
2) Construct first level of EEG: get c_1, which has the oldest time stamp in C, then implement text clustering for c_1 according to topic. Detect noise clusters and delete them. Build nodes of first level by using the remained clusters.
3) Construct i+1th level using c_{i+1} (updating operation): use classifier in i-l+1 ~ i level in EEG to classify each web page in c_{i+1}, then each web page build a node in i+1 level. Use merging operation to merge nodes that have same parent nodes.
4) Implement tidying operation for EEG.

From the above steps, we can observe that key techniques of constructing EEG include: 1) web page clustering and noise cluster detection; 2) building text classifier; 3) building nodes of EEG and tidying EEG.

We use text clustering method OHC in [4] to group web pages by topic and use PRAC method in [5] to build classifiers. This paper focuses on constructing, updating and tidying of EEG.

4.1 Generating Nodes of EEG

EEG consists of multiple levels. We use different methods to generate first level and other levels. We think that each piece of web pages represents an event. Every day, there are a large number of news events being generated. When we focus on important events, it needs a technique to determine whether an event is important.

Observation 2. Compared with unimportant events, important events can have much more reports. The more news reports about an event are, the more import the event is.

Experiment 1 in Section 5.2 gives a statistics test for Observation 2. On building first level of EEG, we use clustering method to group web pages about same event to a cluster. Because one cluster represents one event, therefore, by Observation 2, the quantity of web pages in a cluster reflects importance of the event.

Definition 5 (Outlier Cluster). Let $S=\{s_1,.., s_n\}$ be a clustering solution, there are k_i data in cluster $s_i \in S$. If the number of data k_i in cluster s_i is obvious little than the number of data in others cluster, then cluster s_i is called as outlier cluster.

Outlier clusters means the corresponding events are unimportant. After detecting and deleting outlier clusters in a clustering solution. The remains clusters in the clustering solution all are important events. We will generate nodes of first level of EEG by using the remained clusters.

By Definition 5, there exists obvious difference on the number of web pages between important and unimportant events. Hence we use the number of web pages in a cluster as attribute and employ outlier detection method to detect outlier cluster in clustering solution, and then delete outlier clusters.

For each cluster, we will build a text classifier by using PARC approach [5]. Algorithm 1 represents detailed steps of building first level of EEG.

On building ith ($i>1$)level (updating EEG), it is necessary to confirm association between each new web page (each piece of web page is considered as a event) and events of other levels. We use classifier in each node to determine whether there are associations between new web page and old event. For every piece of web page in new level, it needs to be classified by classifiers in nodes of i-l~i-1 level. If a web page d is recognized by a classifier in node o, then we will generate a new cluster, and o is called parent node of the cluster. If d is not recognized by any classifier, it will be regarded as noise and will be deleted. After n piece of web pages ($d_1,.., d_n$) are explored, k ($k<=n$) clusters ($s_1,.., s_k$) will be generated. Each cluster s_k contains parent node set PO_k. For two cluster s_h and s_j, if $PO_h=PO_j$, then we call s_h and s_j are equivalent cluster. After merging all equivalent clusters, we will get m ($m<=k$) clusters at last. For each cluster, we build node of new level, then EEG is updated. Algorithm 1 shows updating process of EEG.

Algorithm 1. Construction of EEG

Input: web pages collection c
Output: EEG
Steps:
Procedure buildEEG(c) // building first level of EEG
1 $cs \leftarrow$ OHC (c);   // get clustering solution using OHC algorithm
2 DelNoise (cs);
3 eeg=new EEG(); buildLevel(eeg);
4 **For** each cluster $s \in cs$ **DO**
5   BuildNode (s, eeg);

Procedure updateEEG (c) //building ith (i>1) level of EEG
7 **For** each document d in c **DO**

---

8   build a cluster s_j and put it into set cs;
9   **For each** node o in i-l ~ i-1 levels **DO**
10   **If** $(o.TC(d)=true)$ **Then**
11   put o into parent node set of s_j PO_j;
12   MergeCluster (cs); //merge equivalent clusters
13   buildLevel (eeg);
14   **For** each cluster s in cs **DO**
15   BuildNode (s, eeg);

Procedure BuildNode (s, eeg) // building nodes
18    $e \leftarrow$ getEvent(s); $tc \leftarrow$ PARC(s);
19   insertEEG (new Node(e, tc));
20   **For** each node po in PO of s
21   update child-list of po; //updating children nodes of parent node

Function buildLevel in step 3 and 13 update level array and *next* pointer of node in new level. When events of a topic evolve, for some hot topic, it is possible that there are many events happening every day. So l may be set to 1. For some topics are not so hot, l may be set to lager than 1 so that EEG may keep continuity.

Function GetEvent in step 20 derived events from clusters. By definition 1, event is represented by a unigram language model. On deriving event from cluster (web pages collection), all web pages in the cluster will be regarded as train sample and event is regarded as parameter. By using following model, we can derive event.

$$p(w \mid e) = \frac{\sum_{d \in s} c(w, d)}{\sum_{w' \in v} \sum_{d \in s} c(w', d)}$$

Where s is a cluster, v is all words in web pages collection, d is a piece of web page, $c(w, d)$ is the count of word w in d.

Function DelNoise in step 2 detect and delete outlier clusters.

4.2 Tidying of EEG

EEG derived from Algorithm 1 is probably very complicated. It needs to be tidied so as to reduce complexity when we are only concerned about main events in EEG. Twigs and equivalent nodes are direct reasons that result in complexity of EEG.

Definition 6 (Twig). Let n be the number of levels of EEG. If there exists paths from first level to n-l+1 th level, the path is called trunk. Those nodes not in trunks are called twigs.

We think that two events having $l+1$ day far on time stamp are almost impossible associated (parameter l is set by users). Events in leaf nodes from first level to n-l th level have little possibility to evolve to new events in n+1th level. So these leaf nodes are not considered as nodes in trunk.

Definition 7 (Equivalent node). Given two nodes in EEG, O_1 and O_2, their parent nodes set are $PO_1=\{O_i,.., O_j\}$ and $PO_2=\{O_{i'},..., O_{j'}\}$ and their children nodes set are $CO_1=\{O_k,..,O_n\}$ and $CO_2=\{O_{k'},...,O_{n'}\}$ respectively. If $PO_1=PO_2$ and $CO_1=CO_2$, we call O_1 and O_2 being Equivalent Node.

Deleting twigs and merging equivalent nodes in EEG may effectively reduce complexity of EEG. Fig.3 (a) illustrates EEG before being tidied where bold lines represent trunks. Parameter l is set to 2. Node O_3 is not in trunk, so it is twig. Node O_4 and O_5 have same parent node O_2 and same child node O_7, so they are equivalent node. After deleting twig and merging equivalent nodes, we get the tidied EEG shown in Fig.3 (b).

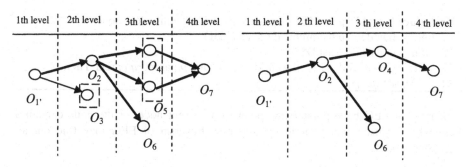

Fig. 3(a). EEG before tidying   **Fig. 3(b).** EEG after tidying

Tidying of EEG contains two operations, *twig pruning* and *nodes merging*. In operation of twigs pruning, it is firstly needed to find out twigs in EEG, and then delete twigs. In operation of node merging, we will merge equivalent nodes, and then build new classifier for new node.

Lemma 1. Let O_1 and O_2 be two nodes in EEG. O_3 is parent node of O_1. If $O_2 \notin O_3.Child\_List$, it is impossible that O_1 and O_2 are equivalent node.

Proof: if O_1 and O_2 are equivalent node, by definition 7, O_1 and O_2 should have equal parent nodes set. Because O_3 is parent node of O_1, so O_3 must be parent of O_2. Because of O_2 not in $O_3.$Child_List, so it can be conclude that O_1 and O_2 are not equivalent node.

By lemma 1, equivalent nodes only exist in child nodes of a node. Hence it only needs to explore equivalent nodes in child node of a node. Such will be more efficient than comparing a node with all other nodes.

We firstly breadth-first traverse EEG when tidying EEG, then find out equivalent nodes in child node of each node. Algorithm 2 give detailed description.

Algorithm 2. Tidying EEG

Input: EEG
Output: tidied EEG
1 set all nodes in EEG as twig node;
2 **For** each node o in first layer **DO**
3   DepthFirTraverse(st, o); // st is a aiding stack
5 delete all twig;
6 NodeMerge ();

Procedure DepthFirTraverse(st, node o) //depth-first traversal from node o
9 st.push(o);
10 **If** o is leaf in last l layer **Then**

```
11   set each o in st as non-twig node; // in trunk
12   Else If (o is null)
13   Return;
14   For each child of o DO
15   depthFirTraverse (st, child)
16   st.pop();
```

```
Procedure NodeMerge() // finding out and merging equivalent nodes
19   For each node v in hierarchical traversal DO
20     For p in v.Child_List DO
21       If ∃q in v.Child_List s.t. p.child=q.child and p.parent=q.parent Then
22         Merge (p, q);
```

If node in EEG have pointer that point to its parent node, or the node contain a field where register parent node set, one-pass traversal of EEG may find out all equivalent nodes.

5 Experiments

In this section, we will perform a thorough analysis of our method. All experiments were implemented in Java and conducted on an Intel P2.6G system with 512M of RAM.

5.1 Data Set

We collect web pages about tow topics from the internet. Dataset D1 contain 18 days web pages about *Chang E1 launching*. Dataset D2 contains 26 days web pages about *the south China tiger have been Seen in ShanXi*. Some information about data sets are shown in Table 2

Table 2. Data sets

Data set	Topic	Period (2007)	Number of pages
D1	Chang E1	10.24-11.11	1840
D2	South China Tiger	10.12-11.10	1585

5.2 Experiment 1

Experiment 1 gives a statistics test for Observation 2. Nodes in trunk should be important event and twigs are unimportant events. In order to test whether important events have much more reports than unimportant event, we build EEG on D1 and D2 respectively. And parameter l is correspondingly set to 1 and 2. Twigs in EEG have not been deleted. Then we count the number of web pages of every event.

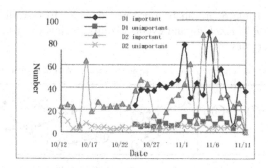

Fig. 4. Average reported number of important and unimportant event

Fig.5 illustrates the average number of web pages of important and unimportant events every day. We can directly observe that important events have more reports than unimportant events.

Furthermore, we use t test to determine whether a significant difference between the reported number of import and unimportant events exists.

Table 3. Parameters for t text

Dataset	Important events	Unimportant events
D1	$n_1=29$ $\bar{x}_1=42.2$ $s_1^2=308$	$n_2=115$ $\bar{x}_2=8.2$ $s_2^2=13.9$
D2	$n_1=29$ $\bar{x}_1=31.1$ $s_1^2=393$	$n_2=84$ $\bar{x}_2=5.4$ $s_2^2=6.1$

Regarding the reported number of important and unimportant events every day as two populations P_1 and P_2 respectively, we use t test to investigate difference between two population means. Alpha(α)level is 0.05. Table 3 shows parameters where n is size of sample, $\bar{x}$ is mean, s^2 is population variance.

Let u_1, u_2 be mean of two populations P_1, P_1 respectively. Null hypothesis is H_0: $u_1 - u_2 = 0$; alternative hypothesis is H_1: $u_1 - u_2 \neq 0$.

On two datasets, we derived the value of test statistics z=10.4 and z=6.9. Because alpha level is set to 0.05, the reject region is -1.96 <z< -1.96. We reject null hypothesis because 10.4 and 6.9 are far lager than 1.96. Therefore, we can conclude that there exists a statistically significant difference between the reported number of important and unimportant events.

5.3   Experiment 2

Experiment 2 constructs EEG on two datasets D1 and D2. We get an Event list for each EEG while each event was represented using title of a news web page in the event. Because the collected web pages are Chinese web pages, we keep events represented in Events List in Chinese.

The EEG of D1 and events list are shown in Fig.4 and Table 5. Parameter l is set to 1. The EEG in Fig.4 has been tidied and retains parts of twigs.

From Fig.4 and Table 5, it can be observed that the EEG well represent main events about *Chang E1 launching* and events evolution. New events about Chang E1 happened nearly every day.

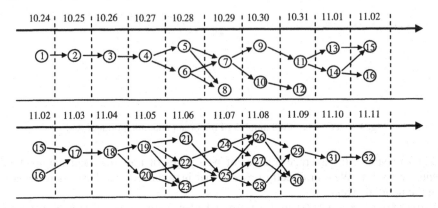

Fig. 5. EEG of dataset D1

Table 5. Events List

1	外电：承载中国人希望，嫦娥一号成功发射升空	17	嫦娥一号今离月还有3万公里 仍需飞行1天。嫦娥一号昨天实施首次轨道中途修正。
2	嫦娥一号卫星首次变轨成功	18	嫦娥一号直飞月球捕获点。胡锦涛家宝致电祝贺嫦娥一号卫星近月制动圆满成功
3	嫦娥一号卫星成功实施第二次变轨。嫦娥一号第一次变轨成功，推进系统工作正常。	19	胡锦涛温家宝致电祝贺嫦娥一号卫星近月制动圆满成功
4	月球探测卫星嫦娥一号运行正常各系统状态良好	20	嫦娥一号将实施首次近月制动 将成为月球卫星
5	嫦娥一号卫星10月29日将实施第二次近地点变轨。	21	胡锦涛温家宝贺嫦娥一号首次近月制动成功
6	嫦娥一号状态良好 深空测控网全面启动	22	嫦娥一号最快可于7日宣布"奔月"成功喜讯
7	北京时间29日18时01分 嫦娥一号第三次变轨成功。嫦娥一号卫星今起给地月照相	23	"嫦娥一号"今日11时左右进行第二次近月制动
8	嫦娥一号卫星第三次变轨成功 未来十天有四大看点	24	嫦娥一号卫星完成第三次近月制动
9	嫦娥一号有关数据将在一年后国际共享。嫦娥一号探月卫星成为我国飞行最远的航天器	25	国家航天局发言人宣布嫦娥一号卫星成功绕月
10	黄江川:嫦娥一号卫星紫外敏感器达国际先进水平	26	嫦娥一号开始环月工作 11月下旬传回图片语音。嫦娥一号11月下旬传回第一段语音
11	嫦娥一号卫星飞离地面高度11月1日将再创新高。已达远地点12万公里嫦娥一号今奔月。	27	嫦娥一号测控开展国际合作 卫星运行面临四风险
12	为什么说嫦娥一号发射环节取得圆满成功	28	专家称日凌现象可能干扰嫦娥一号通信
13	嫦娥一号卫星正式脱离地球怀抱 开始奔月旅程	29	图文:嫦娥一号探月卫星进入近月工作轨道
14	嫦娥一号预计11月5日11时25分进入月球捕获轨道	30	嫦娥一号升空 VIEWGOOD应用进入新领域
15	嫦娥一号卫星测控首次实现国际联网。嫦娥一号预计11月5日11时25分进入月球轨道	31	嫦娥一号全面体检 首次面对日凌考验
16	嫦娥一号首次轨道修正取消	32	嫦娥一号成功经受"日凌"挑战

EEG of D2 and its events list are shown in Fig.5. Parameter *l* is set to 2. The topic of the EEG is about *South China Tiger had been seen in ShanXi*. Fig.5 illustrates events evolution about the topic from Oct 12 to Nov 3.

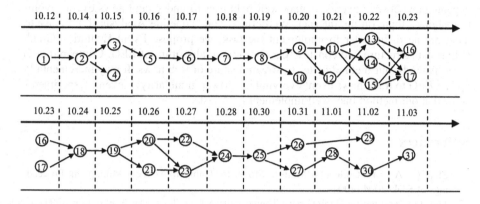

Fig. 6. EEG of dataset D2

Table 6. Events List

1	最新照片证实野生华南虎再现陕西巴山腹地	17	华南虎风波法律审视:拍虎英雄是否越法律禁区
2	重庆曾出现华南虎踪迹 林业局建百万亩保护区。野生华南虎再现"江湖"的惊喜与启示	18	陕西就华南虎一事上报国家林业局 尚未得到意见
3	最新照片证实野生华南虎在中国没有灭绝	19	华南虎"身世"仍是谜
4	我们能给华南虎多大的生存空间	20	国家林业局不会研究华南虎照片真假
5	华南虎发现地停止一切狩猎活动	21	陕西到底有没有华南虎
6	陕西华南虎重现地停止狩猎	22	争论华南虎照片真假已没有意义
7	拍摄华南虎者称照片绝对真实 拍照为获利	23	镇坪神州湾华南虎事件:"华南虎是篇大文章"
8	陕西镇坪经贸局长讲述华南虎照片出笼经过	24	陕西省公安扣押探查华南虎记者的调查
9	"拍虎英雄"欲卖华南虎胶片	25	陕西林业厅展示野外华南虎照片胶卷
10	拍照者称陕西镇坪华南虎起码有9只	26	陕西省林业厅昨日又公布2张野生华南虎照片
11	拍摄者称若华南虎照片作假可以去坐牢	27	中科院动物学家质疑陕西存在华南虎
12	中科院专家:华南虎照片造假	28	国际野生动物保护组织首次就华南虎事件表态
13	华南虎照片没拼接痕迹	29	华南虎研究者通过模拟实验证明虎照作假
14	华南虎拍摄者将赴京向国家林业局汇报	30	华南虎质疑中将上《科学》杂志
15	华南虎谜团追踪 记者进山探虎被扣查勘索	31	美国《科学》将登争议华南虎照片
16	中科院专家继续炮轰华南虎照片造假 吁司法介入		

6 Conclusions

The internet has become fourth media. Every day, a large number of web news occur in the internet in form of text stream. If news events can be organized by time and dependency between events, it may well help user to understand news events evolution about a topic on the internet. We define Event Timeline Analysis (ETA) task to meet the need. In order to implement the task, we propose Event Evolution Graph (EEG) data structure and constructing and tidying algorithm of EEG. Compared with other methods, our method better fit stream feature of web news. It may incrementally update EEG to track news event evolving in a lower granularity of event. Experiments show that our method may well implement ETA tasks.

References

1. Zhai, C.: A Cross-Collection Mixture Model for Comparative Text Mining. In: Proceedings of KDD 2004 (2004)
2. Mei, Q.: Discovering Evolutionary Theme Pattern from Text –An Exploration of Theme Text Mining. In: Proceedings of KDD 2005 (2005)
3. Event Threading within News Topics. In: Proceedings of CIKM 2004 (2004)
4. Qiu, J., Tang, C.: Topic-Oriented Semi-supervised Documents Clustering. In: Proceedings of SIGMOD 2007 Workshop IDAR (2007)
5. Qiu, J., et al.: A Novel Text Classification Approach based on Enhanced Association Rules. In: Alhajj, R., Gao, H., Li, X., Li, J., Zaïane, O.R. (eds.) ADMA 2007. LNCS (LNAI), vol. 4632, pp. 252–263. Springer, Heidelberg (2007)
6. Kuo, J.-J., Chen, H.-H.: Event Clustering on Streaming News Using Co-Reference Chains and Event Words. In: ACL 2004 Workshop (2004)
7. Ping-bo, W., Qun-xiu, C., Liang, M.: Research on Extraction and Integration of Developing Event Based on Analysis of Space-time Information. Journal of Chinese Information Processing 20(1) (January 2006)
8. Hua, Z., Tie-Jun, Z., Hao, Y., Shu, Z.: Dynamic evolvement-oriented topic detection research Chinese High Technology Letters, vol. 16(12) (December 2006)
9. Zi-Yan, J., Qing, H., Hai-Jun, Z., Jia-You, L., Zhong-Zhi, S.: A News Event Detection and Tracking Algorithm Based on Dynamic Evolution Model. Journal of Computer Research and Development 41(7) (July 2004)
10. Allan, J., Carbonell, J., Doddington, G., Yamron, J., Yang, Y.: Topic detection and tracking pilot study: Final report. In: Proceedings of the DARPA Broadcast News Transcription and Understanding Workshop, pp. 194–218 (1998)
11. Allan, J., Feng, A., Bolivar, A.: Flexible intrinsic evaluation of hierarchical clustering for TDT. In: Proc. Of the ACM Twelfth International Conference on Information and Knowledge Management, pp. 263–270 (2003)
12. Han, J., Kamber, M.: Data Mining Concepts and Techniques, 2nd edn. China Machine Press (2007)

Analysis of Alarm Sequences in a Chemical Plant

Savo Kordic[1], Peng Lam[1], Jitian Xiao[1], and Huaizhong Li[2]

[1] The School of Computer and Information Science, Edith Cowan University, Perth 6050, Western Australia
skordic@student.ecu.edu.au, {c.lam,j.xiao}@ecu.edu.au
[2] The School of Computer Science and Engineering, Wenzhou University Town, Zhejiang 325035, China
hli@wzu.edu.cn

Abstract. Oil and gas industries need secure and cost-effective alarm systems to meet safety requirements and to avoid problems that lead to plant shutdowns, production losses, accidents and associated lawsuit costs. Although most current distributed control systems (DCS) collect and archive alarm event logs, the extensive quantity and complexity of such data make identification of the problem a very labour-intensive and time-consuming task. This paper proposes a data mining approach that is designed to support alarm rationalization by discovering correlated sets of alarm tags. The proposed approach was initially evaluated using simulation data from a Vinyl Acetate model. Experimental results show that our novel approach, using an event segmentation and data filtering strategy based on a *cross-effect* test is significant because of its practicality. It has the potential to perform meaningful and efficient extraction of alarm patterns from a sequence of alarm events.

Keywords: Chemical plants, Data mining and Correlated alarms.

1 Introduction

Large and complex industrial processes such as chemical plants and petroleum refineries are regularly equipped with distributed control systems (DCS) which allow users to increase the number of alarms for the purpose of better monitoring process-variables. As such industrial processes increase in size, the volume of alarm information being presented to the operators also increases. Nimmo [1] pointed out that hazard and operability analyses (HAZOP) have added more alarms to control systems, and gave an example of a plant in which 14,000 DCS alarms were added from only 150 physical alarms. Not only may there be thousands of individual alarms, nuisance alarms could also distract the operator's attention from more important problems. One example of the consequences of too many inappropriate alarms being generated in an emergency situation was the incident at the Texaco Refinery, Milford Haven in 1994, where large amounts of alarm information overwhelmed the operators for a 5 hour duration, ending in a major explosion [2]. Clearly, because of over-alarming and a lack of configuration management practices there is a need for tools and techniques that can increase overall understanding of what is happening within alarm systems.

C. Tang et al. (Eds.): ADMA 2008, LNAI 5139, pp. 135–146, 2008.
© Springer-Verlag Berlin Heidelberg 2008

This paper proposes a strategy that investigates event relationships when there are no clear boundaries between consecutive time windows. When an alarm triggers other alarms, there is a "time lag" while the entire event sequence finishes. In an ideal situation, a group of associated alarms should all return well before any new activation of the alarms takes place within the group. But if the cause alarm returns and activates again before the first group of associated alarms returns, there is a cross-effect between two consecutive activations of an associated alarm group. In order to find alarm dependencies in such a situation we segment and filter events with respect to the entire alarm propagation area. The emphasis is not only on discovery of frequent patterns related to the time-interval when alarm tags are active, but also on generalization over time for determining which alarms are significant.

The main contribution of this paper is the demonstration of an event-based segmentation and filtering strategy which removes spurious data points in a chemical process sense, while preserving the richness of alarm information through reducing the number of unrelated time-interval windows. Once groups of correlated alarms are identified via a data mining process, they can be used to support alarm rationalization by minimizing false alarm rates, and eliminating alarm system bad actors.

The rest of this paper is organized as follows: Section 2 describes related work and Section 3 introduces necessary notations and definitions. Section 4 presents the segmentation method for more accurate and efficient extraction of alarm data. Section 5 covers generation of simulated alarms for the process and presents relevant results. Section 6 concludes this paper.

2 Related Work

A related research area is fault management in telecommunications networks where huge numbers of generated alarms could overwhelm the network operators. TASA [3] was an alarm system for extracting useful knowledge from network alarm databases in terms of "episodes", which were defined as partially ordered collections of events. Basically, because alarms are time-stamped sequences of events, the so-called *temporal windows* can be formed from alarms that fall inside *time-interval* boundaries. WINEPI [4] recognises episodes by "sliding a window" on the input sequence, and then calculates the frequency of an episode as the fraction of windows in which the episode occurs. One of the main difficulties when analysing event sequences in WINEPI was to specify the window *width* within which an episode must occur. If the user given fixed width of the window is too small then alarm information will be lost, or if it is too big, then "noise" can be added in the window's data. Srikant and Agrawal [5] used the term "sliding time windows" for a union of items from multiple transactions that can fit inside the maximum and minimum transaction times. Keogh et al. [6] describe a "growing" sliding window for *segmenting* time series, which works by anchoring the first left point of a potential segment, and then a subsequence is grown until it exceeds some error threshold. In contrast, MINEPI [7] does not rely on the *sliding window* strategy since it counts minimal occurrences of episodes (*mo*) with respect to user specified time bounds. As the number of recognized individual alarms will almost linearly depend on the bounds between the first and last event,

MINEPI needs the maximal window size for practical mining purposes, to reduce search space.

Approaches for improving alarm management in industrial processes such as nuclear power plants and petrochemical industries include the concept of alarm sanitation [8] for finding alarms that are badly tuned, and alarm cleanup [9] for removing nuisance alarms. However, while alarm cleanup and alarm sanitation use the signal processing technique for suggesting changes to existing alarm settings, in this paper we are interested in finding groups of co-occurring alarms from discrete alarm data.

The novel contribution of the proposed approach is in segmentation and extraction of all temporal patterns that are related to a particular tag of interest, and then in using the extracted patterns as the basis for discovery of local relationships by identifying primary and consequential alarms. Our event-based segmentation[1] not only dynamically determines time intervals for each alarm tag but also at the same time eliminates unrelated temporal windows with automatic and novel stopping criteria based on a *cross-effect-test*. There are two sets of temporal relationships that must be taken into account: 1) The **A-R window** is an activation event time interval. We did not limit the duration of this interval because the events in the activation windows are pruned in a chemical process sense if their return events do not appear in the associated verifying group. 2) The **R-A or R-w window** interval is the period of time for alarms to return. In essence, if the cause of the problem is eliminated then all subsequent alarm tags related to the problem should return after a short time. Since there can be causal action at a short temporal distance we use the **R-w window** to limit the duration of the return-activation time interval. It should be noted that the larger the return-activation time-interval, then the more likely it is that external factors could affect the relationship.

3 Preliminaries

3.1 Alarm and Alarm Sequences

We follow the basic concepts and definitions introduced by Manilla et al. [5] in defining alarm sequences.

Given a class of event types T, an *alarm* is a pair of terms (a, t) where $a \in T$ and t is the *occurrence time* represented as an integer. Additionally, in our research an alarm sequence is a collection of alarm types which includes alarm *activation* and alarm *return* knowledge. While activations are represented as positive integers, returns are represented as negative integers. An *alarm sequence s* is an ordered collection of alarms defined as $s = \{(a_1,t_1),(a_2, t_2),...,(a_n,t_n)\}$, for all $i=1,2,...n$, $a_i \in T$, and $t_{i+1} \geq t_i$ for all $i = 1,...,n - 1$.

Example 1. Now consider a simple example of such a sequence: $S = \{(1, 15), (2, 19), (-1, 21), (-2, 23)\}$. Notice that a pair of terms (*alarm tag* and *occurrence time*), have been recorded for each event that occurred in the time interval [15, 23]. For instance, the first member of the sequence $(1, 15)$ indicates that TAG 1 is activated at the

---

[1] The data segmentation takes place in an event based context.

occurrence time = 15, and the third element of the sequence (-1, 21), indicates that TAG 1 is returned at occurrence time equals 21.

Since we consider both activation and return knowledge, it is possible to perform an event-based segmentation with a clear contextual meaning. That is, we can segment the entire alarm sequence by using the activation instances of a target tag, where the activation event marks the beginning of a sliding widow and the return event of the target alarm indicates the end of a window. All alarm activation events in the mining window form the items in a new transaction. In a similar manner, the entire alarm sequence can also be segmented in relation to the return-activation boundary of a target alarm type. All alarm return events in the verifying window form the items in the verifying transaction which is associated with the activation transaction. For simplicity and without loss of generality, let us consider only two alarms, namely, Alarm A and Alarm B in a chemical process. If we think of A as the cause alarm, and B as the consequence alarm, then Alarm B must come on after Alarm A. If the activation of A causes the activation of B, then when Alarm A returns, the cause for Alarm B is eliminated. Therefore, it should be expected that Alarm B will return shortly after Alarm A returns.

3.2 Activation-Return (A-R) Window

Formally, let s be an event sequence. An activation-return (A-R) sliding window $W_{A\text{-}R}$ is another sequence of an entire event sequence s with respect to an event interval $W_{A\text{-}R}=(s, t_{act}, t_{ret})$. It consists of the alarm pairs (a, t) from sequence s, where $a \in T$ and $t_{ret} > t \geq t_{act}$. Note that in our research the time difference $t_{ret} - t_{act}$ is not given by the user; instead, it is determined dynamically with respect to the activation-return time interval within which events are observed.

3.3 Return-Activation (R-A) or Return-Time Width (R-w) Window

A verifying return-activation (R-A) sliding window $W_{R\text{-}A}$ is another sequence of an entire event sequence s with respect to an event interval $W_{R\text{-}A}=(s, t_{ret}, t_{act})$. It consists of the alarm pairs (a, t) from sequence s, where $a \in T$ and $t_{act} > t \geq t_{ret}$. In our research the time difference $t_{act} - t_{ret}$ is not only determined dynamically with respect to the return-activation time interval but also with respect to the user given maximal width w of the window. Thus the sliding window will be formed either if an alarm tag is re-activated or the window's width w is reached.

3.4 Transactional Windows and Data Filtering

During the shift of each sliding window a set of ordered unique events is automatically recognized and extracted from the corresponding (A-R), (R-A) or (R-w) sliding windows. It should be noted that we do not consider a number of events of the same type - so only the first occurrence of an event is recorded. As a result, the output of the event segmentation algorithm is a "transactional window" containing unique events ordered by the time of their occurrence.

Filtering is a simple pre-processing procedure for removing the *bad* data points in a chemical process sense since a *dependent* variable (consequent alarm) should return after the *independent* variable (cause alarm) is returned. Thus activation events in the (A-R) transactional windows are filtered if their return events do not appear in the associated verifying (R-A) or (R-w) (comparison) group. Formally we could write this criterion as:

$$Activations\ (A\text{-}R) \cap Returns\ (R\text{-}A,\ or\ R\text{-}w)$$

Therefore, the relationship can be described in terms of the intersection between activation events in the activation-return (A-R) transactional window and return events in the return-activation (R-A) or return-time (R-w) transactional window. If the total number of activations and returns of a specified alarm tag is n, then the whole alarm sequence can be transformed into n "*intersectional*" windows of ($A\text{-}R \cap R\text{-}A$, or $R\text{-}w$).

Example 2. Figure 1 shows graphically the alarm sequence $s = \{(1,2),(2,10),(3,20), (-1,30),(-3,40),(-2,50),(1,60)\}$. Note that sliding windows are created with respect to TAG 1 and the maximal width of return windows $w = 45$ seconds.

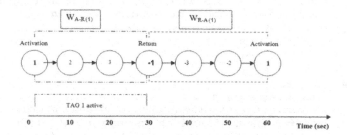

Fig. 1. Example of alarm sequence and two sliding windows with respect to TAG 1

As can be seen in figure 1, one resulting sliding window $W_{A\text{-}R\,(1)} = \{1, 2, 3\}$ is created based on the A-R event segmentation, and one resulting window $W_{R\text{-}A\,(1)} = \{|\text{-}1|,|\text{-}3|,|\text{-}2|\}$ is created based on the R-A event segmentation because the width of the R-A window interval [30, 60] < w. The intersection of sets $W_{A\text{-}R\,(1)} \cap W_{R\text{-}A\,(1)} = \{1, 2, 3\}$, since tags 1, 2 and 3 are in both sets.

4 Method

The first phase employs event-based segmentation and filtering that consider the temporal context and the causal process in an interval, and the second phase finds association rules from a list of time ordered transactions.

4.1 Temporal Windows

The preceding example showed that in our research two sets of temporal relations need to be taken into account. However, it is difficult to decide *how close is close enough* when giving the width of the (R-w) window as it depends on the size as well as the causal significance of the time intervals.

If the return-activation (R-A) window is very short then there cannot be observable relationships as other associated events will still be in an active state. Thus rather than constructing a sliding window for each activation and return event, we join together consecutive windows until the stopping criterion is met.

Suppose we are given a sequence s, an integer n representing the total number of activations of a specified alarm tag, and a return window width w. We form from s all windows $W_{R-A/R-w\,(1)}, W_{R-A/R-w\,(2)},..., W_{R-A/R-w\,(n)}$. Assume we have a duration win $(W_{R-A/R-w(i)})$ of every window where i = 1,2 ,..., n, and the user given minimum time span of the $W_{R-A/R-w}$ window is called *minw*. These time-interval durations can be used for more efficient segmentation of W_{A-R} and $W_{R-A/R-w}$ subsequences into corresponding activation and return transactional windows respectively, in the case of $win < minw$.

4.2 Algorithm

The pseudocode for the main algorithm is shown below.

```
Input: a sequence s, a time window w, a time span length
       minw, and a number of returns events n
Output: a set E of transactional windows
    initialise A = {∅}, R = {∅}, E = {∅}
             tA = {∅}, tR = {∅}
    union_flag = false
FOR i = 1 to n
        read sequence s
        //extract-recognize activations and returns
        tA ← subset of activation segment (W_A-R (i))
        tR ← subset of return segment (W_R-A/R-w (i), w)
    IF (W_R-A/R-w (i)) interval width < minw
        IF union_flag = true
                   E ← intersection (A ∩ R)
        ELSE
                   E ← intersection (tA ∩ tR)
                   A = {∅} R = {∅}
                     union_flag = false
        END IF
    ELSE
            A ← union (A, tA)
            R ← union (R, tR)
            union_flag = true
        END IF
    END FOR
Output E
```

The main idea of the algorithm is the following: during each shift of the window $W_{A-R\,(i)} + W_{R-A/R-w\,(i)}$, we recognize all unique activations and return events and place them into sets (tA and tR). If the width of the $W_{R-A/R-w\,(i)}$ window is greater than the time span threshold *minw*, then we can stop. If only one activation and return window is recognized (union_flag = false) then we store the intersection of two sets tA ∩ tR into a list of transactions E. Otherwise, we update both Activation transaction set A

and Return transaction set R with the corresponding activation and return events respectively. Next, the window is shifted to $W_{A-R\ (i+1)}$ and $W_{R-A/R-w\ (i+1)}$ and the event recognition continues until the *cross-effect-test* stopping criterion is met. If the stop criterion is met we then output the intersection of A and R into E.

4.3 Rule Discovery from Transactions

In this paper we are interested in finding local relationships from the list of transactions obtained in the data segmentation and filtering phase. We are favouring the idea that the closer together the cause and consequence alarms are in time, then the less chance there is that irrelevant factors will influence the association. A simple example of such a rule is: "if Alarm A occurred, then (B and C) will occur within transactional time T_E". We wrote the above rule as: A=> (B, C, T_E). The confidence of the *serial*[2] episodes A => (B, C, T_E) is the fraction of occurrences of A followed by, B and C

$$conf(A \Rightarrow B,C) = \frac{freq(A,B,C,T_E)}{freq(A)}$$

where *freq* $(A, B, C, T_E) = \{i \mid a_i = (A \wedge B \wedge C) \in T_{E(i)}\}$ *is the number of occurrences of B and C that occur after A* within interval of time T_E.

Calculating the confidences of target episodes is not difficult since the alarm sequence is segmented into sets of transactions associated with each specific alarm tag.

5 Simulated Alarms and Results

Due to the enormous complexity of a chemical plant, the proposed approach was initially evaluated using simulated data generated from a Matlab model of the Vinyl Acetate chemical process. Figure 2 illustrates the Vinyl Acetate process flowsheet showing locations of the simulated alarm monitors (AM) denoted in the figure as AM01 to AM27. Vinyl data consists of records of alarm logs which characterize the actual state of the plant at particular points in time, representing the status of 27 alarm monitors.

It is observed that setpoint changes and injection of disturbances will cause changes in plant measurements, while the measurement outputs of the model under normal operation conditions remain unchanged. So the differences between the disturbed and normal measurement outputs were used to generate discrete alarm data. For simplicity, it is assumed that a simulated alarm is activated if the following condition is satisfied:

$$Abs(\frac{(D_m - N_m)}{N_m}) \geq S_{am}$$

where D_m is the disturbed output magnitude, N_m is the normal output magnitude and S_{am} is the sensitivity of the simulated alarm monitor. Note that the simulated alarm will return to normal if the above condition is not satisfied. The signal detection sensitivity for all alarm monitors is set to be equal 0.0005.

---

[2] Note that the episode A=> (B, C) is a serial combination of an episode consisting of A, and a parallel episode consisting of B and C.

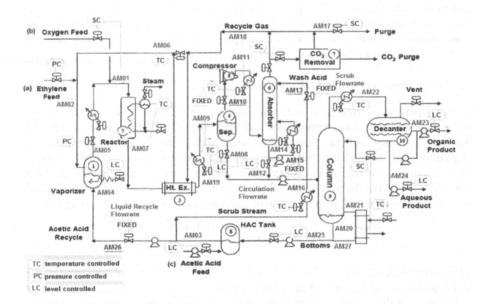

Fig. 2. Vinyl Acetate process flowsheet showing location of the simulated alarm monitors (modified from [10])

5.1 Simulated Data

To evaluate the proposed method three simulated data sets were generated with varying complexity and fault durations. *Simulation data 1* - disturbances of one type, loss of %O2 in the Reactor Inlet (associated with alarm monitor **AM01**), were injected into the Vinyl Acetate process to induce a response in measurement outputs. The fault was injected 10 times and each injected fault lasted for different durations. The measurement outputs were monitored and sampled at a frequency of 1 sample in one second. *Simulation data 2* - only one type of disturbance was introduced, namely the loss of the fresh HAc feed stream (associated with alarm monitor **AM03**), with various durations. The fault was injected 10 times and the measurement outputs were monitored and sampled at a frequency of 1 sample in five seconds. Finally, for *Simulation data 3* - frequency disturbances of one type, the loss of the fresh HAc feed stream (alarm monitor **AM03**) was introduced. The fault was injected 150 times, with various durations, and the measurement outputs were monitored and sampled at a frequency of 1 sample in 60 seconds.

5.2 Results and Discussion

In our experiments we focused primarily on the questions of how well the proposed method discovers patterns from the alarm sequences and how accurate the algorithm is. The *complexity* of the rule refers to the number of unique event types it contains, and another important aspect is the likehood that the approach yields accurate results.

From a practical viewpoint, our aim is to find only a concise set of frequent itemsets called maximal frequent itemsets [11] for comparison purposes. A modified FP-growth [12] algorithm has been implemented to output only maximal frequent itemsets (i.e. the smallest frequent itemsets) that are associated with each alarm tag of interest. For the first simulated data set, we wanted to discover all maximal itemsets, so we set minimum support equal to 1% frequency and then experimented with different confidence levels and window width w. Note that we only present selected results due to an obvious lack of space.

For the simulated data 1, the quality of findings with respect to the *complexity* of the rules achieved by the proposed method is compared to the results of a simple sliding window algorithm (in which the flow of data is not controlled by the cross-effect test) as shown in Table 1.

Table 1. Comparative results for Simulated Data Set 1 with respect to minimum confidence = 20% and 70%, and window width w = 1200 and 1500 seconds

TAG w=1200s	Simple Sliding min conf=20%	Proposed min conf=20%	Sliding min conf=70%	Proposed min conf=70%
1 %O2	1=>6 7 9 4 17 (20%)	1=>6 7 9 4 17 (20%)	1=>6 7 9 4 (70%)	1=>6 7 9 4 (70%)
2 Press	2=>5 (20%)	2=>5 7 14 23 (20%)	-	2=>5 (90%)
TAG w=1200s	Simple Sliding m. conf=20%	Proposed min conf=20%	Sliding min conf=70%	Proposed min conf=70%
...				
4 Vap-L	4=>7 9 (23%)	4=> 5 7 14 2 (20%)	-	4=>7 (80%)
...				
7 RCT-T	7=>12 (34%)	7=> 9 11 12 14 16 19 (20%)	-	7=>9 12 (90%)
...				
w=1500s	Simple Sliding m. conf=20%	Proposed min conf=20%	Sliding min conf=70%	Proposed min conf=70%
1 %O2	1=>6 7 9 4 14 17 19 (20%)	1=>6 7 9 4 14 17 19 (20%)	1=>6 7 9 4 (70%)	1=>6 7 9 4 (70%)
2 Press	2=>5 (20%)	2=>5 7 14 23 (20%)	-	2=>5 (90%)
...				
4 Vap-L	4=>7 19 (23%)	4=>7 9 17 19 (40%)	-	4=>7 9 (70%)
...				
7 RCT-T	7=>12 16 (31%)	7=>9 11 12 14 4 16 19 (20%)	-	7=>9 12 (90%)
...				

As can be seen in Table 1 the resulting set of associated alarm tags with respect to the proposed method has greater overall *complexity* of the rules. One possible interpretation will be that in a case of *repeating alarms* the link between activations and returns is broken, so a simple sliding window cannot always find associations between alarms. Figure 3 plots the total number of these two rule sets with respect windows width w= 1500 seconds and minimum confidence threshold between 1 and 100%.

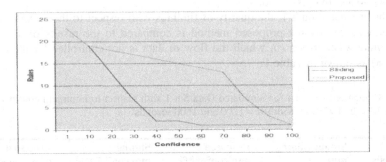

Fig. 3. Comparative results with respect to total number of rules

Rules associated with the proposed approach generally have a higher confidence value as a result of the smaller number of transactional windows which arises from the application of the event-based segmentation approach.

We also compared the proposed method with sliding windows to assess the validity or "trustworthiness" of the discovered pattern. This time we set minimum support equal to 10% to find more meaningful rules. The results in Table 2 associated with mining the second and third data set can be easily validated against the flowsheet.

Table 2. Comparative results for Simulated Fault data Set 2 and 3 with respect to minimum confidence = 20% and 70%, and window width w = 1200 seconds. Note that only in the third set there are no clear boundaries between consecutive transactions.

TAG w=1200s	Simple Sliding min conf=20%	Proposed min conf=20%	Sliding min conf=70%	Proposed min conf=70%
Simulated Fault **data Set 2** with clear boundaries				
fault	3=>16 23	3=>16 23	3=>16	3=>16
3 HAc-L	(20%)	(20%)	(100%)	(100%)
Simulated Fault **data Set 3** with no clear boundaries				
fault	3=> 16 25	3=>16 20 9	-	3=>16
3 HAc-L	(21%)	25 (29%)		(92%)

In terms of checking whether the group of associated alarms is correct, the results sets associated with TAG 3 (AM03) can be checked against the Vinyl Acetate process flowsheet in Figure 1. A careful examination of the process reveals that as AM13 is fixed the change to level monitors AM12, AM 23 and AM25 should be minimal and will require a longer period for any changes to be registered; as AM 15 is fixed, temperature change monitored by AM14 is not significantly affected by temperature change in AM16. Similarly, temperature change in AM16 is unlikely to cause significant change in the component percentages monitored by AM17 and AM18. Therefore, the real process will have the following significant alarm correlation when alarm TAG 3 is the cause alarm:

TAG 3, TAG 16

Obviously, if the causal process takes time and the user given period is too short, we could lose certain variables. However, TAG 16 being close to TAG 3 would return within a time frame = 1200 seconds.

6 Conclusions

In this paper we have presented and experimentally validated our methodology for meaningful and efficient extraction of alarm patterns from a sequence of alarm events, which is required in application domains such as chemical plant data. The discovery algorithm can quickly identify initial alarm groupings with different parameter settings and then the process engineer can use the identified alarm patterns to further examine the data. Future work will focus on extending the algorithm for mining multiple types of faults as well as alarm data from petrochemical industries.

References

1 Nimmo, I.: Distributed control systems: Rescue your plant from alarm overload. In: Chemical Processing (January 2005) (accessed February 8, 2008),
   http://www.chemicalprocessing.com
2 Health & Safety Executive: The explosion and fires at the Texaco Refinery, Milford Haven, July 24, 1994. Report published by the HSE C30 (1997)
3 Hatonen, K., Klemettinen, M., Mannila, H., Ronkainen, P., Toivonen, H.: Knowledge Discovery from Telecommunication Network Alarm Databases. In: 12th International Conference on Data Engineering (ICDE 1996), New Orleans, pp. 115–122 (1996)
4 Mannila, H., Toivonen, H., Verkamo, A.I.: Discovering frequent episodes in sequences. In: The First International Conference on Knowledge Discovery and Data Mining (KDD 1995), Montreal, pp. 210–215 (1995)
5 Srikant, R., Agrawal, R.: Mining Sequential Patterns: Generalizations and Performance Improvements. In: Apers, P.M.G., Bouzeghoub, M., Gardarin, G. (eds.) EDBT 1996. LNCS, vol. 1057, pp. 3–17. Springer, Heidelberg (1996)
6 Keogh, E., Chu, S., Hart, D., Pazzani, M.: An online algorithm for segmenting time series. In: ICDM 2001, IEEE International Conference on Data Mining, San Jose, pp. 289–296 (2001)
7 Mannila, H., Toivonen, H.: Discovering generalized episodes using minimal occurrences. In: The Second Int'l Conference on Knowledge Discovery and Data Mining (KDD 1996), Portland, pp. 146–151 (1996)
8 Larsson, J.E.: Simple Methods for Alarm Sanitation. In: Proc. of IFAC Symposium on Artificial Intelligence in Real-Time Control, AIRTC 2000, Budapest (2000)

9 Ahnlund, J., Bergquist, T., Spaanenburg, L.: Rule-Based Reduction of Alarm Signals in Industrial Control. Journal of Intelligent and Fuzzy Systems 10, 1–12 (2004)
10 Chen, R., Dave, K., McAvoy, T.J., Luyben, M.: A Nonlinear Dynamic Model of a Vinyl Acetate Process. Ind. Eng. Chem. Res. 42, 4478–4487 (2003)
11 Burdick, D., Calimlim, M., Gehrke, J.: MAFIA: A Maximal Frequent Itemset Algorithm for Transactional Databases. IEEE Transactions on Knowledge and Data Engineering 17(11), 1490–1504 (2005)
12 Han, J., Pei, J., Yin, Y.: Mining Frequent Patterns without Candidate Generation. In: Proc. of the 2000 ACM SIGMOD International Conference on Management of Data, pp. 1–12 (2000)

Speed Up SVM Algorithm for Massive Classification Tasks

Thanh-Nghi Do[1], Van-Hoa Nguyen[2], and François Poulet[3]

[1] College of Information Technology, Can Tho University, 1 Ly Tu Trong street,
Can Tho city, Vietnam
dtnghi@cit.ctu.edu.vn
[2] IRISA Symbiose, Campus de Beaulieu, 35042 Rennes Cedex, France
vhnguyen@irisa.fr
[3] IRISA Texmex, Campus de Beaulieu, 35042 Rennes Cedex, France
francois.poulet@irisa.fr

Abstract. We present a new parallel and incremental Support Vector Machine (SVM) algorithm for the classification of very large datasets on graphics processing units (GPUs). SVM and kernel related methods have shown to build accurate models but the learning task usually needs a quadratic program so that this task for large datasets requires large memory capacity and long time. We extend a recent Least Squares SVM (LS-SVM) proposed by Suykens and Vandewalle for building incremental and parallel algorithm. The new algorithm uses graphics processors to gain high performance at low cost. Numerical test results on UCI and Delve dataset repositories showed that our parallel incremental algorithm using GPUs is about 70 times faster than a CPU implementation and often significantly faster (over 1000 times) than state-of-the-art algorithms like LibSVM, SVM-perf and CB-SVM.

1 Introduction

Since Support Vector Machine (SVM) learning algorithms were first proposed by Vapnik [23], they have shown to build accurate models with practical relevance for classification, regression and novelty detection. Successful applications of SVMs have been reported for such varied fields as facial recognition, text categorization and bioinformatics [12]. In particular, SVMs using the idea of kernel substitution have been shown to build high quality models, and they have become increasingly popular classification tools.

In spite of the prominent properties of SVMs, current SVM algorithms cannot easily deal with very large datasets. A standard SVM algorithm requires solving a quadratic or linear program; so its computational cost is at least $O(m^2)$, where m is the number of training data points and the memory requirement of SVM frequently make it intractable. There is a need to scale up these learning algorithms for dealing with massive datasets. Efficient heuristic methods to improve SVM learning time divide the original quadratic program into series of small problems [2], [18]. Incremental learning methods [3], [6], [7], [11], [19], [21] improve memory performance for massive datasets by updating solutions in a growing training set without needing to load the entire dataset into memory at once. Parallel and distributed algorithms [7], [19]

C. Tang et al. (Eds.): ADMA 2008, LNAI 5139, pp. 147–157, 2008.

improve learning performance for large datasets by dividing the problem into components that are executed on large numbers of networked personal computers (PCs).
Active learning algorithms [22] choose interesting data point subsets (active sets) to
construct models, instead of using the whole dataset.

In this paper, we describe methods to build the incremental and parallel LS-SVM
algorithm for classifying very large datasets on GPUs, for example, an Nvidia Ge-
Force 8800 GTX graphics card. Most of our work is based on LS-SVM classifiers
proposed by Suykens and Vandewalle [20]. They replace standard SVM optimization
inequality constraints with equalities in least squares error; so the training task only
requires solving a system of linear equations instead of a quadratic program. This
makes training time very short. We have extended LS-SVM in two ways.

1. We developed an incremental algorithm for classifying massive datasets (at least
   billions data points).
2. Using a GPU (massively parallel computing architecture), we developed a parallel
   version of incremental LS-SVM algorithm to gain high performance at low cost.

Some performances in terms of learning time and accuracy are evaluated on datasets from the UCI Machine Learning repository [1] and Delve [5], including Forest
cover type, KDD cup 1999, Adult and Ringnorm datasets. The results showed that our
algorithm using GPU is about 65 times faster than a CPU implementation. An example of the effectiveness of our new algorithm is its performance on the 1999 KDD cup
dataset. It performed a binary classification of 5 million data points in a 41-
dimensional input space within 0.7 second on the Nvidia GeForce 8800 GTX graphics
card (compared with 55.67 seconds on a CPU, Intel core 2, 2.6 GHz, 2 GB RAM).
We also compared the performances of our algorithm with the highly efficient standard SVM algorithm LibSVM [4] and with two recent algorithms, SVM-perf [13] and
CB-SVM [25].

The remainder of this paper is organized as follows. Section 2 introduces LS-SVM
classifiers. Section 3 describes how to build the incremental learning algorithm with
the LS-SVM algorithm for classifying large datasets on CPUs. Section 4 presents a
parallel version of the incremental LS-SVM using GPUs. We present numerical test
results in section 5 before the conclusion and future work.

Some notations are used in this paper. All vectors are column vectors unless trans-
posed to row vector by a T superscript. The inner dot product of two vectors, x, y is
denoted by $x.y$. The 2-norm of the vector x is denoted by $\|x\|$. The matrix A[mxn] is m
data points in the n-dimensional real space R^n.

2   Least Squares Support Vector Machine

Consider the linear binary classification task depicted in figure 1, with m data points x_i
($i=1..m$) in the n-dimensional input space R^n. It is represented by the [mxn] matrix A,
having corresponding labels $y_i = \pm1$, denoted by the [mxm] diagonal matrix D of ±1
(where $D[i,i] = 1$ if x_i is in class +1 and $D[i,i] = -1$ if x_i is in class -1). For this problem, a
SVM algorithm tries to find the best separating plane, i.e. the one farthest from both
class +1 and class -1. Therefore, SVMs simultaneously maximize the distance between
two parallel supporting planes for each class and minimize the errors.

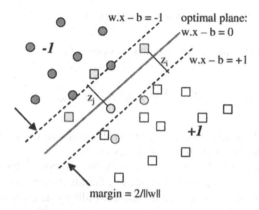

Fig. 1. Linear separation of the data points into two classes

For the linear binary classification task, classical SVMs pursue these goals with the quadratic program (1):

$$\min \Psi(w, b, z) = (1/2) \|w\|^2 + cz$$
$$\text{s.t.: } D(Aw - eb) + z \geq e \tag{1}$$

where the slack variable $z \geq 0$ and the constant $c > 0$ is used to tune errors and margin size.

The plane (w, b) is obtained by the solution of the quadratic program (1). Then, the classification function of a new data point x based on the plane is: predict(x) = sign($w.x - b$).

SVM can use some other classification functions, for example a polynomial function of degree d, a RBF (Radial Basis Function) or a sigmoid function. To change from a linear to non-linear classifier, one must only substitute a kernel evaluation in (1) instead of the original dot product.

Unfortunately, the computational cost requirements of the SVM solutions in (1) are at least $O(m^2)$, where m is the number of training data points, making classical SVM intractable for large datasets. The LS-SVM proposed by Suykens and Vandewalle has used equality instead of the inequality constraints in the optimization problem (2) with a least squares 2-norm error into the objective function Ψ as follows:

- minimizing the errors by $(c/2)\|z\|^2$
- using the equality constraints $D(Aw - eb) + z = e$

Thus substituting for z from the constraint in terms w and b into the objective function Ψ of the quadratic program (1), we get an unconstraint problem (2):

$$\min \Psi(w, b) = (1/2)\|w\|^2 + (c/2)\|e - D(Aw - eb)\|^2 \tag{2}$$

In the optimal solution of (2), the gradient with respect to w and b will be 0. This yields the linear equation system of $(n+1)$ variables $(w_1, w_2, \ldots, w_n, b)$ as follows:

$$\Psi'(w) = cA^T(Aw - eb - De) + w = 0 \tag{3}$$

$$\Psi'(b) = ce^T(-Aw + eb + De) = 0 \tag{4}$$

(3) and (4) are rewritten by the linear equation system (5):

$$[w_1 w_2 w_3 ... w_n b]^T = \left(\frac{1}{c}I^o + E^T E\right)^{-1} E^T De \tag{5}$$

where $E = [A \quad -e]$, I^o denotes the $(n+1)\times(n+1)$ diagonal matrix whose $(n+1)^{th}$ diagonal entry is zero and the other diagonal entries are 1.

The LS-SVM formulation (5) requires thus only the solution of linear equations of $(n+1)$ variables (w_1, w_2, ..., w_n, b) instead of the quadratic program (1). If the dimensional input space is small enough, even if there are millions data points, the LS-SVM algorithm is able to classify them in some minutes on a single PC.

The numerical test results have shown that this algorithm gives test accuracy compared to standard SVM like LibSVM but the LS-SVM is much faster than standard SVMs. An example of the effectiveness is given in [7] with the linear classification into two classes of one million data points in 20-dimensional input space in 13 seconds on a PC (3 GHz Pentium IV, 512 MB RAM).

3   Incremental Algorithm of LS-SVM

Although the LS-SVM algorithm is fast and efficient to classify large datasets, it needs to load the whole dataset in memory. With a large dataset e.g. one billion data points in 20 dimensional input space, LS-SVM requires 80 GB RAM. Any machine learning algorithm has difficulties to deal with the challenge of large datasets. Our investigation aims at scaling up the LS-SVM algorithm to mine very large datasets on PCs (Intel CPUs).

The incremental learning algorithms are a convenient way to handle very large datasets because they avoid loading the whole dataset in main memory: only subsets of the data are considered at any time and update the solution in growing training set.

Suppose we have a very large dataset decomposed into small blocks of rows Ai, Di. The incremental algorithm of the LS-SVM can simply incrementally compute the solution of the linear equation system (5). More simply, let us consider a large dataset split into two blocks of rows A_1, D_1 and A_2, D_2(6):

$$A = \begin{bmatrix} A_1 \\ A_2 \end{bmatrix}, D = \begin{bmatrix} D_1 & 0 \\ 0 & D_2 \end{bmatrix}, e = \begin{bmatrix} e_1 \\ e_2 \end{bmatrix}$$

$$E = [A \quad -e] = \begin{bmatrix} A_1 & -e_1 \\ A_2 & -e_2 \end{bmatrix} = \begin{bmatrix} E_1 \\ E_2 \end{bmatrix} \tag{6}$$

We illustrate how to incrementally compute the solution of the linear equation system (5) as follows:

$$E^T De = \begin{bmatrix} E_1 \\ E_2 \end{bmatrix}^T \begin{bmatrix} D_1 & 0 \\ 0 & D_2 \end{bmatrix} \begin{bmatrix} e_1 \\ e_2 \end{bmatrix} = \begin{bmatrix} E_1^T & E_2^T \end{bmatrix} \begin{bmatrix} D_1 & 0 \\ 0 & D_2 \end{bmatrix} \begin{bmatrix} e_1 \\ e_2 \end{bmatrix} \tag{7}$$

$$E^T De = E_1^T D_1 e_1 + E_2^T D_2 e_2$$

$$E^T E = \begin{bmatrix} E_1 \\ E_2 \end{bmatrix}^T \begin{bmatrix} E_1 \\ E_2 \end{bmatrix} = \begin{bmatrix} E_1^T & E_2^T \end{bmatrix} \begin{bmatrix} E_1 \\ E_2 \end{bmatrix} \tag{8}$$

$$E^T E = E_1^T E_1 + E_2^T E_2$$

$$[w_1 w_2 ... w_n b]^T = \left(\frac{1}{c} I^o + \sum_{i=1}^{2} E_i^T E_i \right)^{-1} \sum_{i=1}^{2} E_i^T D_i e_i \tag{9}$$

From the formulas (7), (8) and (9), we can deduce the formula (10) of the incremental LS-SVM algorithm with a very large dataset generally split into k small blocks of rows $A_1, D_1, ..., A_k, D_k$:

$$[w_1 w_2 ... w_n b]^T = \left(\frac{1}{c} I^o + \sum_{i=1}^{k} E_i^T E_i \right)^{-1} \sum_{i=1}^{k} E_i^T D_i e_i \tag{10}$$

Consequently, the incremental LS-SVM algorithm presented in table 1 can handle massive datasets on a PC. The accuracy of the incremental algorithm is exactly the same as the original one. If the dimension of the input space is small enough, even if there are billions data points, the incremental LS-SVM algorithm is able to classify them on a simple PC. The algorithm only needs to store a small $(n+1)x(n+1)$ matrix and two $(n+1)x1$ vectors in memory between two successive steps. The numerical test has shown the incremental LS-SVM algorithm can classify one billion data points in 20-dimensional input into two classes in 21 minutes and 10 seconds (except the time needed to read data from disk) on a PC (Pentium-IV 3 GHz, 512 MB RAM).

Table 1. Incremental LS-SVM algorithm

```
Input:
- training dataset represented by k blocks: A1, D1,
..., Ak, Dk
- constant c to tune errors and margin size
Training:
init: E E=0, d=E De=0
for i = 1 to k do
     load Ai and Di
     compute E E=E E+E E  and d=d+d  (d =E D e )
                      i  i            i  i  i  i
end for
solve the linear equation system (10)
get the optimal plane (w,b)=w , w , ..., w , b
                            1   2        n
Classify new datapoint x according to f(x)=sign(w.x-b)
```

4 Parallel Incremental LS-SVM Algorithm Using GPU

The incremental SVM algorithm described above is able to deal with very large datasets on a PC. However it only runs on one single processor. We have extended it to build a parallel version using a GPU (graphics processing unit).

During the last decade, GPUs described in [24] have developed as highly specialized processors for the acceleration of raster graphics. The GPU has several advantages over CPU architectures for highly parallel, compute intensive workloads, including higher memory bandwidth, significantly higher floating-point, and thousands of hardware thread contexts with hundreds of parallel compute pipelines executing programs in a single instruction multiple data (SIMD) mode. The GPU can be an alternative to CPU clusters in high performance computing environments. Recent GPUs have added programmability and been used for general-purpose computation, i.e. non-graphics computation, including physics simulation, signal processing, computational geometry, database management, computational biology or data mining.

NVIDIA has introduced a new GPU, the GeForce 8800 GTX and a C-language programming API called CUDA [16] (Compute Unified Device Architecture). A block diagram of the NVIDIA GeForce 8800 GTX architecture is made of 16 multiprocessors. Each multiprocessor has 8 streaming processors for a total of 128. Each group of 8 streaming processors shares one L1 data cache. A streaming processor contains a scalar ALU (Arithmetic Logic Unit) and can perform floating point operations. Instructions are executed in SIMD mode. The NVIDIA GeForce 8800 GTX has 768 MB of graphics memory, with a peak observed performance of 330 GFLOPS and 86 GB/s peak memory bandwidth. This specialized architecture can sufficiently meet the needs of many massively data-parallel computations. In addition, NVIDIA CUDA also provides a C-language API to program the GPU for general-purpose applications. In CUDA, the GPU is a device that can execute multiple concurrent threads. The CUDA software package includes a hardware driver, an

Table 2. Incremental LS-SVM algorithm

```
Input:
- training dataset represented by k blocks: A1, D1,
..., Ak, Dk
- constant c to tune errors and margin size
Training:
init: E E=0, d=E De=0 in GPU memory
for i = 1 to k do
     load Ai and Di into CPU memory
     copy Ai and Di to GPU memory
     use CUBLAS to perform matrix computations on GPU
     E E=E E+E  E  and d=d+d  (d =E D e )
             i   i             i   i   i i
end for
copy E E and E De in CPU memory
solve the linear equation system (10) in CPU
get the optimal plane (w,b)=w , w , ..., w , b
                            1   2        n
Classify new datapoint x according to f(x)=sign(w.x-b)
```

API, its runtime and higher-level mathematical libraries of common usage, an implementation of Basic Linear Algebra Subprograms (CUBLAS [17]). The CUBLAS library allows access to the computational resources of NVIDIA GPUs. The basic model by which applications use the CUBLAS library is to create matrix and vector objects in GPU memory space, fill them with data, call a sequence of CUBLAS functions and finally, upload the results from GPU memory space back to the host. Furthermore, the data transfer rate between GPU and CPU memory is about 2 GB/s.

Thus, we developed a parallel version of incremental LS-SVM algorithm based on GPUs to gain high performance at low cost. The parallel incremental implementation in table 2 using the CUBLAS library performs matrix computations on the GPU massively parallel computing architecture. It can be used on any CUDA/CUBLAS compatible GPU (today around 200 different ones, all from NVidia). Note that in CUDA/CUBLAS, the GPU can execute multiple concurrent threads. Therefore, parallel computations are done in an implicit way.

First, we split a large dataset A, D into small blocks of rows A_i, D_i. For each incremental step, a data block A_i, D_i is loaded into the CPU memory; a data transfer task copies A_i, D_i from CPU to GPU memory; and then GPU computes the sums of $E_i^T E_i$ and $d_i = E_i^T D_i e_i$ in a parallel way. Finally, the results $E_i^T E_i$ and $d_i = E_i^T D_i e_i$ are uploaded from GPU memory space back to the CPU memory to solve the linear equation system (9). The accuracy of the new algorithm is exactly the same as the original one.

5   Results

We prepared an experiment setup using a PC, Intel Core 2, 2.6 GHz, 2 GB RAM, Nvidia GeForce 8800 GTX graphics card with NVIDIA driver version 6.14.11.6201 and CUDA 1.1, running Linux Fedora Core 6. We implemented two versions (GPU and CPU code) of parallel and incremental LS-SVM algorithm in C/C++ using NVIDIA's CUDA, CUBLAS API and the high performance linear algebra package, Lapack++ [9]. The GPU implementation results are compared with the CPU results under Linux Fedora Core 6. We have only evaluated the computational time without the time needed to read data from disk and for the GPU implementation, the time for GPU/CPU data transfer is taken into account (so the only computational time is about 10 to 50% lower than the ones listed).

We focus on numerical tests with large datasets from the UCI repository, including Forest cover type, KDD Cup 1999 and Adult datasets (cf. table 3). We created two

Table 3. Dataset description

Dataset	# dimensions	Training set	Test set
Adult	110	32,561	16,281
Forest Cover Types	20	495,141	45,141
KDD Cup 1999	41	4,868,429	311,029
Ringnorm-1M	20	1,000,000	100,000
Ringnorm-10M	20	10,000,000	1,000,000

Table 4. Classification results

Dataset	Time (s)			Accuracy (%)
	GPU	CPU	ratio	
Adult	0.03	2.00	66.67	85.08
Forest Cover Types	0.10	10.00	100	76.41
KDD Cup 1999	0.70	55.67	79.53	91.96
Ringnorm-1M	0.07	3.33	47.57	75.07
Ringnorm-10M	0.61	31.67	51.92	76.68

other massive datasets by using the RingNorm software program with 20 dimensions, 2 classes and 1 and 10 million rows. Each class is created from a multivariate normal distribution. Class 1 has mean equal to zero and covariance 4 times the identity. Class 2 (considered as -1) has unit covariance with mean = 2/sqrt(20).

First, we have split the datasets into small blocks of rows. For the CPU implementation, we have varied the block size for each incremental step from one thousand data points to fully in main memory to compare the time needed to perform the classification task, the best results are obtained for small sizes using only the main memory (and not the secondary memory). Therefore we have finally split the datasets into small blocks of fifty thousand data points to reach good performances on our experiment setup.

The classification results obtained by GPU and CPU implementations of the incremental LS-SVM algorithm are presented in table 4. The GPU version is about 70 times faster than the CPU implementation.

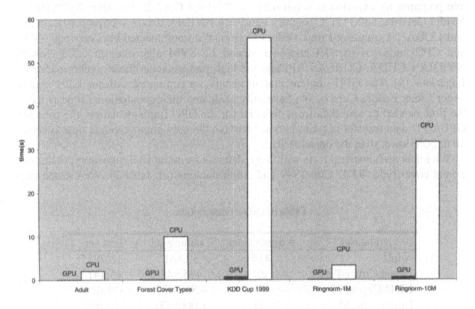

Fig. 2. GPU vs. CPU execution times

For the Forest cover type dataset, the standard LibSVM algorithm ran during 21 days without any result. However, recently-published results show that the SVM-perf algorithm performed this classification in 171 seconds on a 3.6 GHz Intel Xeon processor with 2 GB RAM. This means that our GPU implementation of incremental LS-SVM is probably about 1500 times faster than SVM-Perf.

The KDD Cup 1999 dataset consists of network data indicating either normal connections (negative class) or attacks (positive class). LibSVM ran out of memory. CB-SVM has classified the dataset with over 90 % accuracy in 4750 seconds on a Pentium 800 MHz with 1GB RAM, while our algorithm achieved over 91 % accuracy in only 0.7 second. It appears to be about 6000 times faster than CB-SVM.

The numerical test results showed the effectiveness of the new algorithm to deal with very large datasets on GPUs.

Furthermore, we have said our new algorithm is an incremental one, but it is also decremental and so it is particularly suitable for mining data stream. We add blocks of new data and remove blocks of old data, the model is then updated from the previous step. It is very easy to get any temporal window on the data stream and compute the corresponding model.

Domingos and Hulten [8] have listed the criteria a data mining system needs to meet in order to mine high-volume, open-ended data streams:

- it must require small constant time per record: our algorithm has a linear complexity with the number of data points,
- it must use only a fixed amount of main memory, irrespective of the total number of records it has seen: the amount of memory used is determined by the block size and is fixed,
- it must be able to build a model using at most one scan of the data: we only read and treat each data point once,
- it must make a usable model available at any point in time: we can compute the model at any time with the data points already read,
- ideally, it should produce a model that is equivalent (or nearly identical) to the one that would be obtained by the corresponding ordinary database mining algorithm, operating without the above constraints: the results obtained are exactly the same as the original sequential algorithm,
- when the data-generating phenomenon is changing over time (i.e., when concept drift is present), the model at any time should be up-to-date, but also include all information from the past that has not become outdated: our algorithm is incremental and decremental and can follow concept drift very easily and efficiently.

Our algorithm meets all the criteria to deal efficiently with very large datasets.

6 Conclusion and Future Work

We have presented a new parallel incremental LS-SVM algorithm being able to deal with very large datasets in classification tasks on GPUs. We have extended the recent LS-SVM algorithm proposed by Suyken and Vandewalle in two ways. We developed an incremental algorithm for classifying massive datasets. Our algorithm avoids loading the whole dataset in main memory: only subsets of the data are considered at any one time and updates the solution in growing training set. We developed a parallel version of incremental LS-SVM algorithm based on GPUs to get high performance at low cost.

We evaluated the performances in terms of learning time on very large datasets from the UCI repository and Delve. The results showed that our algorithm using GPU is about 70 times faster than a CPU implementation. We also compared the performances of our algorithm with the efficient standard SVM algorithm LibSVM and with two recent algorithms, SVM-perf and CB-SVM. Our GPU implementation of incremental LS-SVM is probably more than 1000 times faster than LibSVM, SVM-Perf and CB-SVM.

We also applied these ideas to build other efficient SVM algorithms proposed by Mangasarian and his colleagues: Newton SVM (NSVM [14]) and Lagrangian SVM (LSVM [15]) in the same way, because they have the same properties as LS-SVM. The new implementation based on these algorithms is interesting and useful for classification on very large datasets.

We have only used one GPU (versus one CPU) in our experiments and we have shown the computation time is already more than 1000 times faster than standard SVM algorithms like LibSVM, SVM-Perf and CB-SVM. The GPU parallel implementation is performed implicitly by the library, may be it can be improved. A first and obvious improvement is to use a set of GPUs. We have already shown [19] the computation time is divided by the number of computers (or CPU/GPU) used (if we do not take into account the time needed for the data transfer), if we use for example 10 GPUs, the computation time is divided by 10,000 compared to usual algorithms. This means a classification task needing previously one year can now be performed in only one hour (using 10 GPUs). This is a significant improvement of the machine learning algorithms to massive data-mining tasks and may pave the way for new challenging applications of data-mining.

Another forthcoming improvement will be to extend our methods to construct other SVM algorithms that can deal with non-linear classification tasks.

References

1. Asuncion, A., Newman, D.J.: UCI Repository of Machine Learning Databases, http://archive.ics.uci.edu/ml/
2. Boser, B., Guyon, I., Vapnik, V.: A Training Algorithm for Optimal Margin Classifiers. In: Proc. of 5th ACM Annual Workshop on Computational Learning Theory, Pittsburgh, Pennsylvania, pp. 144–152 (1992)
3. Cauwenberghs, G., Poggio, T.: Incremental and Decremental Support Vector Machine Learning. In: Advances in Neural Information Processing Systems, vol. 13, pp. 409–415. MIT Press, Cambridge (2001)
4. Chang, C.-C., Lin, C.-J.: LIBSVM – A Library for Support Vector Machines (2003), http://www.csie.ntu.edu.tw/~cjlin/libsvm/
5. Delve, Data for evaluating learning in valid experiments (1996), http://www.cs.toronto.edu/~delve
6. Do, T.-N., Fekete, J.-D.: Large Scale Classification with Support Vector Machine Algorithms. In: Proc. of ICMLA 2007, 6th International Conference on Machine Learning and Applications, pp. 7–12. IEEE Press, Ohio (2007)

7. Do, T.-N., Poulet, F.: Classifying one Billion Data with a New Distributed SVM Algorithm. In: Proc. of RIVF 2006, 4th IEEE International Conference on Computer Science, Research, Innovation and Vision for the Future, Ho Chi Minh, Vietnam, Vietnam, pp. 59–66 (2006)
8. Domingos, P., Hulten, G.: A General Framework for Mining Massive Data Streams. Journal of Computational and Graphical Statistics 12(4), 945–949 (2003)
9. Dongarra, J., Pozo, R., Walker, D.: LAPACK++: a design overview of object-oriented extensions for high performance linear algebra. In: Proc. of Supercomputing 1993, pp. 162–171. IEEE Press, Los Alamitos (1993)
10. Fayyad, U., Piatetsky-Shapiro, G., Uthurusamy, R.: Summary from the KDD-03 Panel – Data Mining: The Next 10 Years. In: SIGKDD Explorations, vol. 5(2), pp. 191–196 (2004)
11. Fung, G., Mangasarian, O.: Incremental Support Vector Machine Classification. In: Proc. of the 2nd SIAM Int. Conf. on Data Mining SDM 2002 Arlington, Virginia, USA (2002)
12. Guyon, I.: Web Page on SVM Applications (1999), http://www.clopinet.com/isabelle/Projects/SVM/app-list.html
13. Joachims, T.: Training Linear SVMs in Linear Time. In: Proc. of the ACM SIGKDD Intl Conf. on KDD, pp. 217–226 (2006)
14. Mangasarian, O.: A Finite Newton Method for Classification Problems. Data Mining Institute Technical Report 01-11, Computer Sciences Department, University of Wisconsin (2001)
15. Mangasarian, O., Musicant, D.: Lagrangian Support Vector Machines. Journal of Machine Learning Research 1, 161–177 (2001)
16. NVIDIA® CUDA^{TM}, CUDA Programming Guide 1.1 (2007)
17. NVIDIA® CUDA^{TM}, CUDA CUBLAS Library 1.1 (2007)
18. Platt, J.: Fast Training of Support Vector Machines Using Sequential Minimal Optimization. In: Schoelkopf, B., Burges, C., Smola, A. (eds.) Advances in Kernel Methods – Support Vector Learning, pp. 185–208 (1999)
19. Poulet, F., Do, T.-N.: Mining Very Large Datasets with Support Vector Machine Algorithms. In: Camp, O., Filipe, J., Hammoudi, S. (eds.) Enterprise Information Systems V, pp. 177–184. Kluwer Academic Publishers, Dordrecht (2004)
20. Suykens, J., Vandewalle, J.: Least Squares Support Vector Machines Classifiers. Neural Processing Letters 9(3), 293–300 (1999)
21. Syed, N., Liu, H., Sung, K.: Incremental Learning with Support Vector Machines. In: Proc. of the 6th ACM SIGKDD Int. Conf. on KDD 1999, San Diego, USA (1999)
22. Tong, S., Koller, D.: Support Vector Machine Active Learning with Applications to Text Classification. In: Proc. of ICML 2000, the 17th Int. Conf. on Machine Learning, Stanford, USA, pp. 999–1006 (2000)
23. Vapnik, V.: The Nature of Statistical Learning Theory. Springer, New York (1995)
24. Wasson: Nvidia's GeForce 8800 graphics processor, Technical report, PC Hardware Explored (2006)
25. Yu, H., Yang, J., Han, J.: Classifying Large Data Sets Using SVMs with Hierarchical Clusters. In: Proc. of the ACM SIGKDD Intl Conf. on KDD, pp. 306–315 (2003)

Mining Supplemental Frequent Patterns[*]

Yintian Liu[1,2], Yingming Liu[1], Tao Zeng[3], Kaikuo Xu[1], and Rong Tang[1]

[1] College of Mathematics, Sichuan University, Chengdu, China, 610065
[2] DB&KE Lab., Chengdu University of Information Technology, Chengdu, China, 610225
[3] Tianjin Normal University, Tianjin, China, 300074
liuyintian@gmail.com

Abstract. The process of resource distribution and load balance of a distributed P2P network can be described as the process of mining Supplement Frequent Patterns (SFPs) from query transaction database. With given minimum support (*min_sup*) and minimum share support (*min_share_sup*), each SFP includes a core frequent pattern (BFP) used to draw other frequent or sub-frequent items. A latter query returns a subset of a SFP as the result. To realize the SFPs mining, this paper proposes the structure of SFP-tree along with relative mining algorithms. The main contribution includes: (1) Describes the concept of Supplement Frequent Pattern; (2) Proposes the SFP-tree along with frequency-Ascending order header table FP-Tree (AFP-Tree) and Conditional Mix Pattern Tree (CMP-Tree); (3) Proposes the SFPs mining algorithms based on SFP-Tree; and (4) Conducts the performance experiment on both synthetic and real datasets. The result shows the effectiveness and efficiency of the SFPs mining algorithm based on SFP-Tree.

1 Introduction

Peer-to-peer systems have recently drawn a lot of attention in the social, academic, and commercial communities. The central strength of P2P system is sharing resources on different sites and distributing proper sites to provide file blocks for a resource query efficiently. For a single file resource in a P2P system, there are many sites owning the copy of this file. These sites respond to the query on this file. A P2P system contains so many sites owning large quantity of different resource copies that the task of ensuring the load balance of sites and the efficiency of resource share is difficult. To finish the task, this paper proposes a strategy to manage the sites resource and file resource efficiently. For a given file resource, we first find out the sites providing enough response for the queries on this file; the second step is to find out limited groups from these sites and each group provides enough response for the queries on this file; and the last step is to add proper sites to each group to reinforce the share power of each group. To answer a latter query, we select a group and return a subset of this group. The result of a query is a list of sites that can provide blocks of needed resource synchronously. Each site is a transaction item and each site list is a query

---

[*] This work is supported by the National Natural Science Foundation of China under Grant No. 60773169 and No. 60702075, Development Foundation of Chengdu University of Information Technology(KYTZ200811).

C. Tang et al. (Eds.): ADMA 2008, LNAI 5139, pp. 158–169, 2008.

transaction. For a query transaction database in a P2P system, the process of resource distribution and load balance can be described as the process of mining k-item pattern based on core frequent patterns under given minimum support threshold (min_sup) and minimum share support threshold ($min\_share\_sup < min\_sup$) with k. k is the number of sites which own a copy of a given file resource.

Any subset of a frequent pattern should be frequent too and the length of frequent pattern should be smaller than the maximum transaction length. Unlike the traditional frequent pattern, the k-item pattern X proposed in this paper has follow characters:

a) The value of k can be larger than the maximum transaction length and should be smaller than the copy number of a file resource existing in a system.

b) $Support(X) < min\_sup$, the support of X can be equal to 0 when k is bigger than the maximum transaction length.

c) There existis a subset $B \subset X$, $Support(B) > (min\_sup + min\_share\_sup)$.

d) $Support(B \cup a_i) > min\_share\_sup$, $(a_i \in (X\text{-}B))$.

In a word, this k-item pattern contains a core subset with big support count. And the number of each item appearing together with this core subset in many transactions may not arrive at min_sup. We define this k-item pattern as a Supplement Frequent Pattern (SFP) relative to Traditional Frequent Pattern. For a given file resource F and its relative k-item supplement frequent pattern P, a query on F returns a subset of P providing partitions of F synchronously. All the other sites not included in P no longer respond to later queries of F, and the copy of F are cancelled from these items when these sites stop providing file partitions service of F.

To ensure the optimality of the query result, there should exist a subset B of P. The subset B is a traditional frequent pattern standing for the most efficient sites set for a given file resource and the support of B should be high enough to ensure that it has the power to draw other sites into it.

The existing frequent mining algorithms can only mine frequent pattern shorter than maximum transaction length because the items in frequent pattern are required to appear together in transactions. We can not mine SFP through existing frequent pattern mining algorithms. Anymore with required minimum support min_sup, the length of maximum frequent pattern mining through existing mining methods is usually much shorter than k because of the sparseness of query transaction database in a P2P system.

To realize the SFPs mining, this paper proposes the structure of SFP-Tree along with its constructing algorithms and mining algorithm. The main contribution includes:

1. Constructs the Ascending frequent-item-header table FP-Tree (AFP-Tree) of transaction database;
2. Generates Conditional Mix Pattern Tree (CMP-Tree) recursively until the base pattern size is k-1;
3. For each k-1 item frequent base pattern, constructs its SFP-Tree;
4. Mines each SFP-Tree to construct all SFPs.

The rest of the paper is as follows: We present related work in Section 2 and present the problem description in Section 3. Section 4 presents the structure of AFP-Tree, CMP-Tree, and SFP-Tree. Section 5 presents the results of our performance study. We conclude our work in Section 6.

2 Related Work

Frequent pattern mining is a basic issue in data mining domain with deeply research and variant algorithms have been proposed to support different frequent pattern generation. Traditional frequent pattern mining methods include Classic Frequent Pattern Mining, Maximum Frequent Pattern Mining and Closed Frequent Pattern Mining. The classic algorithms include Apriori[1], Partition[2], Eclat[3], DHP[4], FP-grwoth[5] and relative extended algorithms[6-11]. Algorithms MFPs[16, 17] and CFPs[12-15] are the result of enhanced Classic Frequent Pattern with restriction conditions, and the relative algorithms are usually proposed from the algorithms of CFPs. The traditional frequent pattern has a basic property, i.e. any subset of a frequent itemset must be frequent too.

Supplement Frequent Pattern is an extension of traditional frequent pattern. The closest work to this paper is prefix-tree structure FP-tree (frequent-pattern tree) and corresponding mining method FP-growth. As a DFS algorithm, FP-growth method can avoid the costly generation of a large number of candidate sets. It uses a partitioning-based, divide-and-conquer method to decompose the mining task into a set of smaller tasks for mining confined patterns in conditional databases, which dramatically reduces the search space.

3 Problem Description

In this paper data partitioning and searching strategy of distributed P2P networks are based on the Query Transaction DataBase(QTDB). To mining Supplemental Frequent Patterns from QTDB, relative conceptions are proposed firstly.

Definition 1 (Full Transaction). Given a transaction database D with items set $A=\{I_1, I_2, ..., I_m\}$, for a transaction $t = \{I_i \mid I_i \in A\}$, we say $t' = \{I_i, \neg I_j \mid I_i \in t, I_j \in A$ and $I_j \notin t\}$, $\neg I_j$ is the negative item of positive item I_j in transaction t meaning item I_j not appearing in t, and t' is named the full transaction of t. The database composed by t' is Full Database D'.

The length of each full transaction is identical $|A|$, i.e. the total item number of D. SFPs mining is actually based on database D' so that it is factually impossible to

Table 1. Sample transaction database

TID	Items	Frequent Items	Full Frequent Items
1	b, h, i, o, p	h, p, o, b	h, p, o, b, l ⌐a, ⌐c, ⌐l, ⌐m
2	c, d, g, i, m	c, m	c, m, l ⌐a, ⌐b, ⌐h, ⌐l, ⌐o, ⌐p
3	a, b, l, m, o	l, a, o, m, b	l, a, o, m, b l ⌐c, ⌐h, ⌐p
4	b, h, m, o	h, o, m, b	h, o, m, b l ⌐a, ⌐c, ⌐l, ⌐p
5	b, c, k, h, p, s	h, p, c, b	h, p, c, b l ⌐a, ⌐l, ⌐m, ⌐o
6	a, c, e, l, m, n, p	l, p, a, c, m	l, p, a, c, m l ⌐b, ⌐h, ⌐o
7	a, b, c	a, c, b	a, c, b l ⌐h, ⌐l, ⌐m, ⌐o, ⌐p
8	b, c, h, j, m	h, c, m, b	h, c, m, b l ⌐a, ⌐l, ⌐o, ⌐p
9	a, b, k, m, o, s	a, o, m, b	a, o, m, b l ⌐c, ⌐h, ⌐l, ⌐p
10	a, c, e, l, n, o, p	l, p, a, o, c	l, p, a, o, c l ⌐b, ⌐h, ⌐m

realize SFPs mining using any existing frequent pattern mining algorithms within limited space complexity and time complexity. A sample query transaction database is shown in table 1.

Definition 2 (Base Frequent Pattern). The frequent pattern of database D are all composed of positive items. A frequent pattern with k positive items is called a k-item **Base Frequent Pattern**.

Definition 3 (Supplement Frequent Pattern). Let the frequent 1-itemsets of database D be F_l, given a base frequent pattern $B \subset F_l$, a positive itemsets $P \subset F_l$, an item a_i ($a_i \in F_l$), and two thresholds *mini_sup*, *mini_share_sup*, the item sets $F = B \cup P \cup \neg a_i$ having following conditions is a Supplement Frequent Pattern based on B:

1. support($B \cup P$) >= *mini_sup*
2. *mini_share_sup* <= support($B \cup P \cup a_i$) <= *mini_sup*
3. support($B \cup P \cup \neg a_i$) >= *mini_sup* (a_i not appears with all items in B in a same transaction, $\neg a_i$ named negative item of positive item a_i)
4. support(a_i) ≤ Support(a_j) ($a_j \in B \cup P$);

Items in set P are the positive supplement items and Item $\neg I_n$ is the negative supplemental item of SFP F base on BFP B, the number of both negative supplement items and positive supplement items in a SFP can be more than 1. The traditional frequent pattern is just the special case of SFP with zero negative item.

Condition 2 ensures item a_i and set B is an optimal combination to a given resource although the count they appearing together not reach minimum support count. Condition 3 ensures set B is powerful enough to draw a proper item into it to form a new itemset. Condition 4 ensures the load of the joined item is lighter than any item in B to ensure the load balance.

4   Mining of Supplemental Frequent Patterns

4.1   Construction of Ascending Frequent Pattern Tree (AFP-Tree)

Like FP-Tree used to mine frequent patterns quickly, we need construct a structure AFP-tree firstly to describe the whole transactions in QTDB. The construction principle of AFP-tree is similar to traditional FP-tree. The difference between these two tree structures is that AFP-tree produces a frequency-ascending header table. This modification decreases the share degree of node inevitably with more new nodes being created and inserted in AFP-tree. As a result the space complexity and time complexity of AFP-tree construction increase relatively for the operations on AFP-tree. The ascending order tree structure character of AFP-tree can ensure the conditions 3 and 4 of SFP.

By analysis the structure of FP-tree, we modify the generation of node link. In original FP-tree, each node of header table points to its relative item first occurrence in the tree. When a new node is created and inserted in FP-tree, it is add to the end of its node-link with the same item-name. Each time a new node is add to its node link, the corresponding node-link is entirely scanned a time to locate the end position of node-link. The time complexity of node-link generation is O(n). In this paper we change the insert strategy, i.e. each item in header table points to the lastest occurrence node of its node-link. Every time a new node is inserted into AFP-tree, it become the header of its node-link. The insert operation just need to find the node in header table with the same item-name and replace it as the front of their node-link. The time complexity of this strategy is O(1). This method can entirely avoid the trace of node-link with no change of the data structure of header table node, and decrease the time complexity of node insert.

Set the minimum support count be 3, figure 1 shows the AFP-tree of sample database shown in table 1. To the nodes with the same item-name, the node-link direction is reversed with first appearance node as the end of node-link and the laterest inserting node is registered in header table.

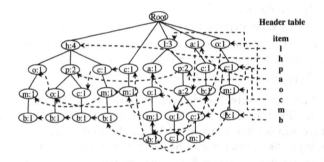

Fig. 1. AFP-Tree of sample database

4.2 Construction of Conditional Mix Pattern Tree (CMP-Tree)

Once the AFP-tree of transaction database is constructed, we can generate the Conditional Mix Pattern Tree recursively. Comparing with Conditional Frequent Pattern Tree, CMP-tree includes not only frequent items but also sub-frequent items. The sub-frequent items of a frequent suffix pattern is the prefix items with support smaller than *mini_sup* but.bigger than *mini_share_sup*.

Definition 4 (CMP-tree). The Conditional Mix Pattern Tree of a Base Frequent Pattern is a tree structure defined below.

1. It consists of a root node labeled as *"null"*, a set of item-prefix subtrees as the children of the root, and a mix-item-header table.
2. Nodes structure of CMP-tree is similar to the nodes of FP-tree.
3. The support-ascending order mix-item-header table consists of both frequent items and sub-frequent items.
4. Only frequent items of CMP-tree have their node-links used to generate CMP-tree and SFP-tree recursively.

Set the minimum share support count be 1, to the AFP-tree shown in figure 1, the conditional pattern base of frequent itemset {b} is {(ocm:1), (ac:1), (laom:1), (hcm:1), (hpc:1), (hpo:1), (hom:1)}. The count of items l, a, p are all smaller than minimum support count 3 but not smaller than minimum share support count 1. They are the sub-frequent items of frequent itemset {b} and should insert into {b}'s CMP-tree. Because no CMP-tree is generated for these items, we needn't generate the node links of these items and then decrease the space and time complexity of CMP-tree. We can say AFP-tree of database is the CMP-tree of pattern {*Null*} without sub-frequent items.

Figure 2 gives the CMP-trees of frequent pattern {b} and {m} respectively, and The algorithm of CMP-Tree construction is shown in table 2.

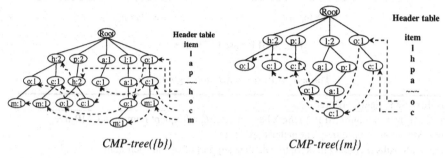

CMP-tree({b})   CMP-tree({m})

Fig. 2. CMP-tree construction

Table 2. Generation algorithm of CMP-tree

Procedure CMP_gen(CMP-tree$_\beta$, α_i)
Input: CMP-tree of base itemset β, a frequent item α_i in CMP-tree$_\beta$
Output: CMP-trees of base frequent patterns {$\beta \cup \alpha_i$}
1:    travel paths including node α_i to calculate support count of α_i and each item I_j on path
// Travel means to visit upwards from node α_i to root node
2:    **for each** item I_j **do**
3:        **if** support(I_j) >= *min_sup* **then**
4:            add frequent item I_j to mix 1-item set and add the count of frequent items by 1
5:        **else**
6:            **if** support(I_j) >= min_share_sup **then**
7:                add item I_j to mix 1-item set and add the count of sub-frequent items by 1
8:    generate support-ascending order header table of CMP-tree$_{(\beta \cup \alpha i)}$
9:    **for each** path beginning at α_i **do**
10:       select out frequent items and sub-frequent items
11:       index-ascending sort these items
12:       **for each** item **do**
13:           **if** item is a sub-frequent item **then**
14:               insert it into CMP-tree and add to its node-link
15:           **else**
16:               insert it into CMP-tree
17:   **return**

4.3 Construction of Supplement Frequent Pattern Tree (SFP-Tree)

SFP-tree is the conditional frequent pattern tree of CMP-tree including not only frequent positive items but also frequent negative items. To the CMP-Trees shown in figure 2, The SFP-Trees of BFP {b, m} and {m, c} are shown in figure 3. The algorithm of SFP-Tree generation is also given in table 3.

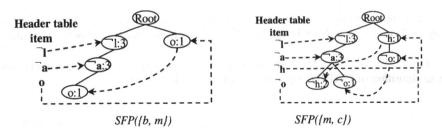

$SFP(\{b, m\})$ $SFP(\{m, c\})$

Fig. 3. BFP-based SFP-tree

Table 3. SFP-tree generation algorithm

Procedure SFP_gen(CMP-tree$_\beta$, α_i)
Input: CMP-tree of a num_BFP-1 length base itemset β, a frequent item α_i in CMP-tree$_\beta$ Output: SFP-trees of base frequent pattern $\{\beta \cup \alpha_i\}$ 1: travel all paths including node α_i to calculate support of α_i and each item I_j on path   2: **for each** item I_j **do**   3:   **if** support(I_j) >= *min_sup* **then**   4:   add I_j to frequent 1-item set   5:   **else**   6:   **if** support(I_j)>=min_share_sup and (support($\beta \cup \alpha_i$)–support(I_j))>=*min_sup* **then**   7:   add $\bar{}I_j$ to frequent 1-item set   8: generate support-descending order header table of SFP-tree$_{(\beta \cup \alpha_i)}$ 9: **for each** path beginning at α_i **do**   10:   select out frequent items and supply frequent negative items   11:   index-ascending sort these items and insert each item into SFP-tree   12: **return**

4.4 Generation of Supplement Frequent Patterns Based on SFP-Tree

The SFP-tree can be regard as a common Conditional FP-tree including both frequent
and sub-frequent items, by executing FP-growth method on SFP-tree we can generate
all SFPs of transaction database. For the SFP-tree shown in figure 3, the SFPs with
base freqeunt pattern $\beta=\{b, m\}$ is SFPs($\{b, m\}$) = $\{bmo, bm\bar{}a, bm\bar{}l, bm\bar{}a\bar{}l\}$, and
the SFPs with base frequent pattern $\beta=\{m, c\}$ is SFPs($\{m, c\}$) = $\{mc\bar{}o, mc\bar{}a, mc\bar{}h,$
$mc\bar{}l, mc\bar{}a\bar{}l\}$.

Theorem 1 (Completeness). SFP-tree based mining method generates the complete
set of SFPs in transaction database.

Proof. To guarantee the completeness of SFPs, we just need to ensure two factors.
The first factor is SFP-tree based mining algorithm can generate all base frequent
patterns, and the second factor is the SFP-tree of a BFP includes all relative frequent
items and sub-frequent items.

The FP-growth method based on FP-Tree can ensure the completeness of frequent
patterns because the FP-tree contains the complete information for frequent pattern
mining. AFP-tree and CMP-tree also contain can the complete information too, and all
frequent patterns including BFPs can be generated based on AFP-tree and CMP-tree.

To the second factor can be ensured by three points. The AFP-tree and CMP-tree are constructed with ascending frequent-item-header table; An sub-frequent item of an itemset must be the sub-frequent item of any subset of this itemset; The sub-frequent items are generate based on base frequent pattern, and the BFP and SFP-tree are generated with a growth method from lower nodes to upper nodes.   □

By integrating the techniques of AFP-tree, CMP-tree and SFP-tree, we can generate all the base frequent patterns and corresponding supplemental frequent patterns. The supplemental frequent pattern generation algorithm is shown in table 4.

Table 4. SFPs mining algorithm

Procedure *SFP-growth(AFP-tree, min_sup, min_share_sup, num_BFP)*

Input: AFP-tree, min_sup, min_share_sup, num_BFP
Output: complete supplemental frequent patterns
1: **for each** item α in headertable of AFP-tree **do**
2:      call **CMP_gen**(AFP-tree, α) until base itemset length equal to (num_BFP-1)
3:      **for each** CMP-tree with (num_BFP-1)-item base itemset β **do**
4:          **for each** item α_i in CMP-tree **do**
5:              call **SFP_gen**(CMP-tree$_\beta$, α_i)
6:              call **FP-growth**(SFP$_{\beta \cup \alpha i}$)
7: **return**

---

5 Performance Study

SFPs mining algorithm is used to find supplemental items of a base frequent pattern in sparse query transaction databases in P2P system. We test SFPs mining method on two sparse data sets. *T10I4D100K* is the synthetic dataset and *Bms-pos* is the real dataset. The *mini_share_sup* is set as half of *mini_sup* to all experiments.

5.1 Header Table Node-Link Generation Modification

AFP-tree and CMP-tree are support-ascending order header table tree structure, which decrease the share degree of nodes. For the node scan operation consumes large part

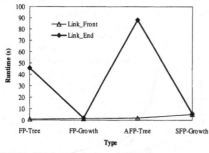
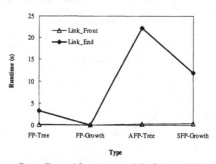

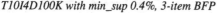

T10I4D100K with min_sup 0.4%, 3-item BFP   *Bms_Pos with min_sup 4%, 3-item BFP*

Fig. 4. Runtime performance results for different headertable link

of mining time, we modify the node-link generation method by placing new node on the front of node-link with the same item-name. Figure 4 shows the runtime of tree construction and patterns mining. The result reflects the time of node-link scan holds the majority mining time and the modification of node-link generation greatly improve the efficiency of tree construction.

5.2 Synthetic Data Set

Data set T10I4D100K is a sparse database containing 100,000 transactions with 1000 items and the average transaction length is 10. Figure 5 reflects the storage consumption and time consumption of different mining phase.

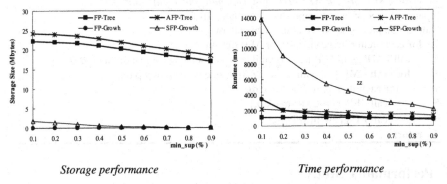

Storage performance   *Time performance*

Fig. 5. Performance results

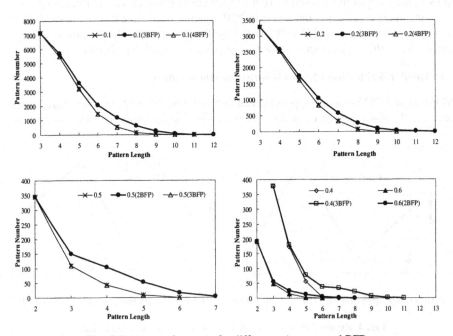

Fig. 6. Pattern performance for different *min_supp* and BFP

Comparing with traditional frequent pattern mining method based on FP-tree, the storage size of frequency-ascending order header table tree is a little bigger than frequency-descending order header table tree because the decrease of node share degree. The mining time of SFPs decreases along with the increase of *min_sup*. But according to figure 6 showing the effectness of SFPs on different minimum support and BFP length, we can find the most effective SFPs are generated within 6 seconds when *min_sup* is 0.4% and base frequent pattern length is 3.

5.3 Real Dataset

Data set BMS-POS is real dataset containing several years worth of point-of sale data from a large electronics retailer. It has 65,000 transactions with 1300 items and the maximum transaction size of this dataset is 164. Figure 7 presents the mining performance under different parameters. According to the result we can know under min_sup 3% no efficient SFPs can mined even though consuming much time. The mining efficiency is relative outstanding when *min_sup* is 4% and base frequent pattern size is 3.

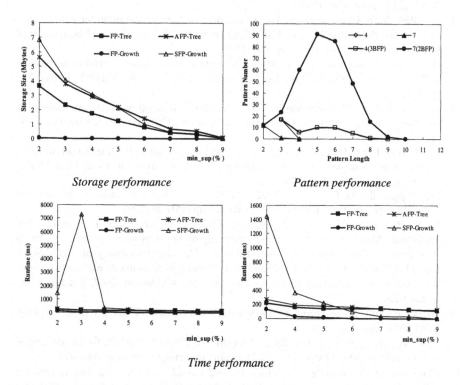

Storage performance

Pattern performance

Time performance

Fig. 7. Performance results

6 Conclusion

This paper proposes the conception of Supplemental Frequent Pattern. SFP phenomena exist in many applications such as the resource distribution and load balance of

P2P networks. To mine SFPs efficiently this paper presents a novel prefix-tree structure, Supplemental Frequent Pattern tree (SFP-tree), to store both frequent and subfrequent items of a base frequent pattern. We present the generation method of Base Frequent Pattern and its SFP-tree. SFPs can be efficiently generated by executing FP-growth algorithm on SFP-tree.

References

1. Agrawal, R. and Srikant, R. 1994. Fast algorithms for mining association rules. In Proc. 1994 Int. Conf. Very Large Data Bases (VLDB'94), Santiago, Chile, pp. 487–499.
2. Savasere, A., Omiecinski, E., and Navathe, S. 1995. An efficient algorithm for mining association rules in large databases. In Proc. 1995 Int. Conf. Very Large Data Bases (VLDB'95), Zurich, Switzerland, pp. 432–443.
3. M.J.Zaki,S.Parthasarathy,M.Ogihara,and W.Li.New algorithms for fast discovery of association rules.In Proc.of the 3rd Int'l Conf.on KDD and Data Mining(KDD'97), Newport-Beach,California,August 1997.
4. J. S. Park, M. S. Chen, and P. S. Yu. An effective hash-based algorithm for mining association rules. Proceedings of ACM SIGMOD International Conference on Management of Data, pages 175-186, San Jose, CA, May 1995.
5. Han, J., Pei, J., and Yin, Y. 2000. Mining frequent patterns without candidate generation. In Proc. 2000 ACMSIGMOD Int. Conf. Management of Data (SIGMOD'00), Dallas, TX, pp. 1–12.
6. Pei, J., Han, J., and Lakshmanan, L.V.S. 2001. Mining frequent itemsets with convertible constraints. In Proc. 2001 Int. Conf. Data Engineering (ICDE'01), Heidelberg, Germany, pp. 433–332.
7. Pei, J., Han, J., Lu, H., Nishio, S., Tang, S., and Yang, D. 2001. H-Mine: Hyper-structure mining of frequent patterns in large databases. In Proc. 2001 Int. Conf. Data Mining (ICDM'01), San Jose, CA, pp. 441–448.
8. Prefix(fpgrowth): G. Grahne and J. Zhu, "Efficiently Using. Prefix-trees in Mining Frequent Itemsets," In. Proc. IEEE ICDM'03 Workshop FIMI'03, 2003.
9. Pei, J., Han, J., Mortazavi-Asl, B., Pinto, H., Chen, Q., Dayal, U., and Hsu, M.-C. 2001. PrefixSpan: Mining sequential patterns efficiently by prefix-projected pattern growth. In Proc. 2001 Int. Conf. Data Engineering (ICDE'01), Heidelberg, Germany, pp. 215–224.
10. David Lo, Siau-Cheng Khoo, and Chao Liu: Efficient mining of iterative patterns for software specification discovery. In Proc. KDD 2007: 460-469 August, 2007, San Jose, California, USA.
11. Fosca Giannotti, Mirco Nanni, Fabio Pinelli, Dino Pedreschi: Trajectory pattern mining. KDD 2007: 330-339.
12. closeZaki, M.J. and Hsiao, C.J. 2002. CHARM: An efficient algorithm for closed itemset mining. In Proc. 2002 SIAM Int. Conf. Data Mining, Arlington, VA, pp. 457–473.
13. ClosePasquier, N., Bastide, Y., Taouil, R., and Lakhal, L. 1999. Discovering frequent closed itemsets for association rules. In Proc. 7th Int. Conf. Database Theory (ICDT'99), Jerusalem, Israel, pp. 398–416.
14. closePei, J., Han, J., and Mao, R. 2000. CLOSET: An efficient algorithm for mining frequent closed itemsets. In Proc. 2000 ACM-SIGMOD Int. Workshop Data Mining and Knowledge Discovery (DMKD'00), Dallas, TX, pp. 11–20.

15. N. Pasquier, Y. Bastide, R. Taouil, and L. Lakhal. Discovering frequent closed itemsets for association rules. In Proceeding of the 7th International Conference on Database Theory, pages 398-416, 1999.
16. maxJ. Roberto J. Bayardo. Efficiently mining long patterns from databases. In Proceedings of the 1998 ACM SIGMOD international conference on Management of data, pages 85-93, 1998.
17. maxLin DI, Kedem ZM. Pincer-Search: A new algorithm for discovering the maximum frequent set. In: Schek HJ, ed. Proceedings of the 6th European Conference on Extending Database Technology. Heidelberg: Springer-Verlag, 1998. 105~119.

A Distributed Privacy-Preserving Association Rules Mining Scheme Using Frequent-Pattern Tree

Chunhua Su* and Kouichi Sakurai**

Dept. of Computer Science and Communication Engineering,
Kyushu University, Japan
http://itslab.csce.kyushu-u.ac.jp
su@itslab.csce.kyushu-u.ac.jp

Abstract. Association rules mining is a frequently used technique which finds interesting association and correlation relationships among large set of data items which occur frequently together. Nowadays, data collection is ubiquitous in social and business areas. Many companies and organizations want to do the collaborative association rules mining to get the joint benefits. However, the sensitive information leakage is a problem we have to solve and privacy-preserving techniques are strongly needed. In this paper, we focus on the privacy issue of the association rules mining and propose a secure frequent-pattern tree (FP-tree) based scheme to preserve private information while doing the collaborative association rules mining. We show that our scheme is secure and collusion-resistant for n parties, which means that even if $n-1$ dishonest parties collude with a dishonest data miner in an attempt to learn the associations rules between honest respondents and their responses, they will be unable to success.

Keywords: association rules, privacy-preserving, cryptographic protocol.

1 Introduction

Association rules mining techniques are generally applied to databases of transactions where each transaction consists of a set of items. In such a framework the problem is to discover all associations and correlations among data items where the presence of one set of items in a transaction implies (with a certain degree of confidence) the presence of other items. Association rules are statements of the form $X_1, X_2, ..., X_n \Rightarrow Y$, meaning that if we find all of $X_1, X_2, ..., X_n$ in the transactions, then we have a good chance of finding Y. The probability of finding Y for us to accept this rule is called the confidence of the rule. We normally would search only for rules that had confidence above a certain

---

* Supported by the Research Fellowship of Japan Society for the Promotion of Science (JSPS) and Grant-in-Aid for Scientific Research of JSPS No. 2002041.
** Supported by Japan Society for the Promotion of Science, Grant-in-Aid for Scientific Research (B) No. 20300005.

C. Tang et al. (Eds.): ADMA 2008, LNAI 5139, pp. 170–181, 2008.

threshold. The problem is usually decomposed into two sub-problems. One is to find those itemsets whose occurrences exceed a predefined threshold in the database; those itemsets are called frequent or large itemsets. The second problem is to generate association rules from those large itemsets with the constraints of minimal confidence. Much data mining starts with the assumption that we only care about sets of items with high support, they appear together in many transactions. We then find association rules only involving a high-support set of items. That is to say that $X_1, X_2, ..., X_n \Rightarrow Y$ must appear in at least a certain percent of the transactions, called the support threshold. How to do the global support threshold counting with respecting clients' privacy is a major problem in privacy-preserving rules mining.

$support_{X \Rightarrow Y} = \frac{|T_{X \cup Y}|}{|DB|}$ means that the support is equal to the percentage of all transactions which contain both X and Y in the whole dataset. And then we can get that: $confident_{X \Rightarrow Y} = \frac{support_{X \Rightarrow Y}}{support_X}$

The problem of mining association rules is to find all rules whose support and confidence are higher than certain user specified minimum support and confidence.

Distributed mining can be applied to many applications which have their data sources located at different places. In this paper, we assume that there are n parties possess their private databases respectively. They want to get the common benefit for doing association rules analysis in the joint databases. For the privacy concerns, they need a private preserving system to execute the joint association rules mining. The concern is solely that values associated with an individual entity not being revealed.

1.1 Related Work

The research of privacy-preserving techniques for data mining began in Year 2000, R. Agrawal et al [2] proposed a reconstruction procedure which is possible to accurately estimate the distribution of original data values from the random noise perturbed data. However, Evfimievski et al[3] pointed out that the privacy breach will occur in R. Agrrawal's proposal and proposed a new randomization techniques to mine association rules from transactions consisting of categorical items where the data has been randomized to preserve privacy of individual transactions. The method presented in Kantarcioglu et al. [9] is the first cryptography-based solutions for private distributed association rules mining, it assumes three or more parties, and they jointly do the distributed Apriori algorithm with the data encrypted. In the recent research papers [5][13][15], some privacy-preserving association rules schemes are proposed. These papers are similar and developed a secure multi-party protocol based on homomorphic encryption.

1.2 Motivation and Our Contributions

The related works we mentioned above have three problems. The first one is low efficiency by using the Apriori algorithm. As we know, the Apriori algorithm

is not so efficient because of its candidates generation scan. The second one is
the accuracy problem in [3] in which there is a trade-off between the accuracy
and security. The third one is the security problem, the schemes proposed in
the related works are not collusion-resistant. We propose an improved scheme
to overcome these three problems.

- We apply frequent-pattern tree (FP-tree) structure proposed in [8] to execute the association rules mining and extend it to distributed association
  rules mining framework. We use FP-tree to compress a large database into
  a compact FP-tree structure to avoid costly database scans.
- We present a privacy-preserving protocol which can overcoming the accuracy
  problem causes randomization-based techniques and improve the efficiency
  compared to those cryptography-based scheme [5][13][15].
- Our privacy-preserving protocol provide a perfect security and collusion-
  resistant property. Our scheme uses the attribute-based encryption to create
  the global FP-tree for each party and then uses the homomorphic encryption
  to merger the FP-tree to get the final result of the global association rules.

2   Preliminaries

2.1   Problem Definition

We assume that there are n parties want to do cooperation on the joint databases
$DB_1 \cup DB_2 \cup ... \cup DB_n$ without revealing the private information of database.
And we assume the standard synchronous model of computation in which n
parties communicate by sending messages via point-to-point channels. There
are some distributed parties who want to get the global result from their data
transactions over the internet. Every party P_i has their private transaction T_i^1.
They all have serious concern about their privacy while they want to get the
accurate result to help their following decision. No Party should be able to
learn contents of a transaction of any other client. And we want to use some
cryptographic toolkits to construct a secure multi-party computation protocol
to perform this task. Let $I = \{a_1, a_2, ..., a_m\}$ be a set of items, and a transaction
database $DB = \langle T_1, T_2, ..., T_n \rangle$, where $T_i(i \in [1...n])$ is a transaction which
contains a set of items in I. The support (or occurrence frequency) of a pattern
A, where A is a set of items, is the number of transactions containing A in DB.
A pattern A is frequent if A's support is no less than a predefined minimum
support threshold $MinSupp$.

2.2   Cryptographic Primitives

Public Key Encryption with Homomorphic Property: In modern terms, a
public-key encryption scheme on a message space M consists of three algorithms
(K, E, D):

1. The key generation algorithm $K(1^k)$ outputs a random pair of private/public
   keys (sk, pk), relatively to a security parameter k.

2. The encryption algorithm $E_{pk}(m;r)$ outputs a ciphertext c corresponding to the plaintext $m \in M$, using random value r.
3. The decryption algorithm $D_{sk}(c)$ outputs the plaintext m associated to the ciphertext c. We will occasionally omit the random coins and write $E_{pk}(m)$ in place of $E_{pk}(m;r)$. Note that the decryption algorithm is deterministic.

In this paper we use Palliler encrytion as public key encryption. Paillier homomorphic encryption proposed by Pallier [11]. It is provably secure and one-way based on the Decisional Composite Residuosity Assumption and the Computational Composite Residuosity Assumption : If the public key is the modulus m and the base g, then the encryption of a message x is $E(x) = g^x r^m \mod m^2$. Then it has the homomorphic property $E(x_1) \cdot E(x_2) = (g^{x_1} r_1^m)(g^{x_2} r_2^m) = g^{x_1+x_2}(r_1 r_2)^m = E(x_1 + x_2 \mod m) \cdot$ and $+$ denote modular multiplication and addition, respectively.

Attributes-based Encryption (ABE) The ABE scheme is developed from Identity based encryption(IBE) which introduced by Shamir [12], is a variant of encryption which allows users to use any string as their public key (for example, an email address). This means that the sender can send messages knowing only the recipient's identity (or email address), thus eliminating the need for a separate infrastructure to distribute public keys. In their scheme, there is one authority giving out secret keys for all of the attributes. Each encryptor then specifies a list of attributes such that any user with at least d of those attributes will be able to decrypt. They show that the scheme they present is secure.

2.3 Security Definition and Adversary Model

This paper considers both semi-honest and malicious adversaries. For Semi-honest adversaries, every party are assumed to act according to their prescribed actions in the protocol. The security definition is straightforward, particularly as in our case where only one party learns an output. The definition ensures that the party does not get more or different information than the output of the function. This is formalized by considering an ideal implementation where a trusted third party (TTP) gets the inputs of the two parties and outputs the defined function. We require that in the real implementation of the protocol— that is, one without a TTP the client C does not learn different information than in the ideal implementation. We say that π privately computes a function f if there exist probabilistic, polynomial-time algorithms S_A and S_B such that:

$$\{(S_A(a, f_A(x)), f_B(x))\} \equiv \{(VIEW_A^\pi(x), OUPUT_B^\pi(x))\} \tag{1}$$

$$\{(f_A(x), S_B(b, f_B(x)))\} \equiv \{(OUPUT_A^\pi(x), VIEW_B^\pi(x))\} \tag{2}$$

where $\equiv$ denotes computational indistinguishability, which means that there is no probabilistic polynomial algorithm used by an adversary A can distinguish the probability distribution over two random string. It means that no matter how the adversary tries to derive the private information from the computation, what he can get only his inputs and the random values.

3   Secure Multi-party Protocol for Association Rules Mining Based on FP-tree

3.1   Problem in Apriori-Based Distributed Association Rules Mining

Most distributed association rules mining algorithms are adaptations of existing sequential (serial) algorithms. Generally speaking two strategies for distributing data for parallel computation can be identified:

1. Data distribution: The data is apportioned amongst the processes, typically by "horizontally" segmenting the dataset into sets of records. Each process then mines its allocated segment (exchanging information on-route as necessary).
2. Task distribution: Each process has access to the entire dataset but is responsible for some subset of the set of candidate itemsets.

The Apriori heuristic achieves good performance gained by (possibly significantly) reducing the size of candidate sets. However, in situations with a large number of frequent patterns, long patterns, or quite low minimum support thresholds, an Apriori-like algorithm may suffer from the following two nontrivial costs:

- It is costly to handle a huge number of candidate sets. For example, if there are 10^4 frequent 1-itemsets, the Apriori algorithm will need to generate more than 10^7 length-2 candidates and accumulate and test their occurrence frequencies. Moreover, to discover a frequent pattern of size 100, such as $\{a_1, ..., a_{100}\}$, it must generate $2^{100} - 2 \approx 10^{30}$ candidates in total. This is the inherent cost of candidate generation, no matter what implementation technique is applied.
- It is tedious to repeatedly scan the database and check a large set of candidates by pattern matching, which is especially true for mining long patterns.

3.2   The General Description of Our Proposal

our protocol construction is based on secure multi-party computation techniques. The history of the multi-party computation problem is extensive since it was introduced by Yao [14] and extended by Goldreich, Micali, and Wigderson [7]. Secure multi-party computation (MPC) protocols allow a set of n players to securely compute any agreed function on their private inputs, where the following properties must be satisfied: *privacy*, meaning that the corrupted players do not learn any information about the other players' inputs. and *correctness*, meaning that the protocol outputs the correct function value, even when the malicious players treat. In Secure Multi-party Computation, we always assume that *semi-honest model* exists.

1. Support count among the common k-item sets privately using the homomorphic encryption scheme.

2. Using attribute-based encryption scheme, every party executes FP-tree construction and prepares for the global FP-tree construction.
3. Using the private matching scheme, every party merges the conditional FP-trees to get common frequent itemsets.
4. Secure global support count computation in the merged FP-trees.
5. Output the final result of association rules from the merged global FP-trees.

Initialization: A multiparty ABE system with homomorphic property is composed of K attribute authorities and one central authority. Each attribute authority is also assigned a value dk. The system uses the following algorithms: Setup : A randomized algorithm which must be run by some trusted party (e.g. central authority). Takes k as input the security parameter. Outputs a public key, secret key pair for each of the attribute authorities, and also outputs a system public key and master secret key which will be used by the central authority. (1)Attribute Key Generation : A randomized algorithm run by an attribute authority. Takes as input the authority's secret key, the authority's value d_k, a user's GID, and a set of attributes in the authority's domain A_C^k. (We will assume that the user's claim of these attributes has been verified before this algorithm is run). Output secret key for the user. (2) Central Key Generation : A randomized algorithm run by the central authority. Takes as input the master secret key and a user's GID and outputs secret key for the user. (3) Encryption : A randomized algorithm run by a sender. Takes as input a set of attributes for each authority, a message, and the system public key. Outputs the ciphertext. (4) Decryption : A deterministic algorithm run by a user. Takes as input a cipher- text, which was encrypted under attribute set AC and decryption keys for an attribute set A_u. Outputs a message m if $|A_C^k \cap A_u^k| > d_k$ for all authorities k.

3.3   Distributed Association Mining with FP-Tree

FP-growth is a divide-and-conquer methodology proposed by [8] which decomposes the association rules mining tasks into smaller ones. It only scans the database twice and does not generate candidate itemsets. The algorithm substantially reduces the search costs. At first, we let the parties build a global FP-tree together and then do the association rules mining on the global FP-tree. FP-growth, for mining the complete set of frequent patterns by pattern fragment growth. Efficiency of mining is achieved with three techniques: (1) a large database is compressed into a condensed, smaller data structure, FP-tree which avoids costly, repeated database scans, (2) our FP-tree-based mining adopts a pattern-fragment growth method to avoid the costly generation of a large number of candidate sets, and (3) a partitioning-based, divide-and-conquer method is used to decompose the mining task into a set of smaller tasks for mining confined patterns in conditional databases, which dramatically reduces the search space.

1. Since only the frequent items will play a role in the frequent-pattern mining, it is necessary to perform one scan of transaction database DB to identify the set of frequent items (with frequency count obtained as a by-product).

2. If the set of frequent items of each transaction can be stored in some compact structure, it may be possible to avoid repeatedly scanning the original transaction database.

3. If multiple transactions share a set of frequent items, it may be possible to merge the shared sets with the number of occurrences registered as count. It is easy to check whether two sets are identical if the frequent items in all of the transactions are listed according to a fixed order.

Given a transaction database DB and a minimum support threshold $MinSupp$, the problem of finding the complete set of frequent patterns is called the frequent-pattern mining problem. With the above observations, one may construct a frequent-pattern tree as follows. First, a scan of DB derives a list of frequent items, $\langle (f:4), (c:4), (a:3), (b:3), (m:3), (p:3) \rangle$ (the number after ":" indicates the support), in which items are ordered in frequency descending order.

Second, the root of a tree is created and labeled with "null". The FP-tree is constructed as follows by scanning the transaction database DB the second time.

1. The scan of the first transaction leads to the construction of the first branch of the tree: $\langle (f:1), (c:1), (a:1), (m:1), (p:1) \rangle$. Notice that the frequent items in the transaction are listed according to the order in the list of frequent items.

2. For the second transaction, since its (ordered) frequent item list $\langle f, c, a, b, m \rangle$ shares a common prefix $\langle f, c, a \rangle$ with the existing path $\langle f, c, a, m, p \rangle$, the count of each node along the prefix is incremented by 1, and one new node $(b:1)$ is created and linked as a child of $(a:2)$ and another new node $(m:1)$ is created and linked as the child of $(b:1)$.

3. For the third transaction, since its frequent item list $\langle f, b \rangle$ shares only the node $\langle f \rangle$ with the f-prefix subtree, f's s count is incremented by 1, and a new node $(b:1)$ is created and linked as a child of $(f:3)$.

4. The scan of the fourth transaction leads to the construction of the second branch of the tree, $\langle (c:1), (b:1), (p:1) \rangle$.

5. For the last transaction, since its frequent item list $\langle c, a, m, p \rangle$ is identical to the first one, the path is shared with the count of each node along the path incremented by 1.

A frequent-pattern tree (or FP-tree in short) is a tree structure defined below:

1. It consists of one root labeled as "null", a set of item-prefix sub-trees as the children of the root, and a frequent-item-header table.

2. Each node in the item-prefix sub-tree consists of three fields: item-name, count, and node-link, where item-name registers which item this node represents, count registers the number of transactions represented by the portion of the path reaching this node, and node-link links to the next node in the FP-tree carrying the same item-name, or null if there is none.

3. Each entry in the frequent-item-header table consists of two fields, (1) item-name and (2) head of node-link (a pointer pointing to the first node in the FP-tree carrying the item-name).

Based on this definition, we have the following FP-tree construction algorithm.

This property is directly from the FP-tree construction process, and it facilitates the access of all the frequent-pattern information related to a_i by traversing the FP-tree once following a_i's node-links. We can generate the conditional pattern-bases and the conditional FP-trees generated from the existing FP-tree. construction of a new FP-tree from a conditional pattern-base obtained during the mining of an FP-tree, the items in the frequent itemset should be ordered in the frequency descending order of node occurrence of each item instead of its support (which represents item occurrence). This is because each node in an FP-tree may represent many occurrences of an item but such a node represents a single unit (i.e., the itemset whose elements always occur together) in the construction of an item-associated FP-tree.

We can develop a distributed frequent-pattern mining algorithm with distributed FP-trees. When one party has received the tree string from another party, he generates new string by merging the received string and its own string.

4   The Details of Multi-party Mining Scheme

In our ABE scheme, we assume that the universe of attributes can be partitioned into K disjoint sets. Each will be monitored by a different authority. As mentioned above, we also have one trusted central authority who does not monitor any attributes.

4.1   Verifiable Secret Sharing

Secret-sharing schemes are used to divide a secret among a number of parties. The information given to a party is called the share (of the secret) for that party. It realizes some access structure that defines the sets of parties who should be able to reconstruct the secret by using their shares First, let's consider a very simplified scheme based on the Feldman Verifiable Secret Sharing scheme. Recall that, given d points $p(1), ..., p(d)$ on a $d - 1$ degree polynomial, we can use Lagrange interpolation to compute $p(i)$ for any i. However, given only $d - 1$ points, any other points are information theoretically hidden. According to the Lagrange formula, $p(i)$ can be computed as a linear combination of d known points. Let $\Delta_j(i)$ be the coefficient of $p(j)$ in the computation of $p(i)$. Then $p(i) = \sum_{j \in S} p(j) \Delta_j(i)$ where S is a set of any d known points and $\Delta_j(i) = \prod_{k \in S, j \neq k} (i - k)/(j - k)$. Note that any set of d random numbers defines a valid polynomial, and given these numbers we can find any other point on that polynomial.

4.2   Specifying Transaction's Attributes

If we take this approach, any user with any d attributes which are specified will be able to decrypt. But we want each encryptor to be able to give a specific subset of attributes such that at least d are necessary for decryption. In order to do this, we need an extra tool: bilinear maps, for bilinear map $e, g \in G_1$, and $a, b \in Zq$, $e(g^a, g^b) = e(g, g)^{ab}$. Now, suppose instead of giving each user $g^{p(i)}$ for each attribute i, we choose a random value t_i and give $g^{p(i)/t_i}$. If the user knew g^{t_i} for at least d of these attributes, he could compute $e(g, g)^{p(i)}$ for each i and then interpolate to find the secret $e(g, g)^{p(0)}$. Then if our encryption includes $e(g, g)^{p(0)}m$, the user would be able to find m. Thus, the encryptor can specify which attributes are relevant by providing g^{t_i} for each attribute i in the desired transaction set.

4.3   Multiple Encryptions

First, let's consider a very simplified scheme based on the Feldman Verifiable Secret Sharing scheme. Recall that, given d points $p(1), ..., p(d)$ on a $d - 1$ degree polynomial, we can use Lagrange interpolation to compute $p(i)$ for any i. However, given only $d - 1$ points, any other points are information theoretically hidden. According to the Lagrange formula, $p(i)$ can be computed as a linear combination of d known points. Let $\Delta_j(i)$ be the coefficient of $p(j)$ in the computation of $p(i)$. Then $p(i) = \sum_{j \in S} p(j) \Delta_j(i)$ where S is a set of any d known points and $\Delta_j(i) = \prod_{k \in S, j \neq k} (i - k)/(j - k)$. Note that any set of d random numbers defines a valid polynomial, and given these numbers we can find any other point on that polynomial. Thus our first attempt Multi-Authority Scheme is as follows:

Preparing for the Global FP-tree Construction

Init First fix $y_1...y_k$, $\{t_{k,i}\}_{i=1...n, k=1...K} \leftarrow Z_q$. Let $y_0 = \sum_{k=1}^{K} y_k$. **System Public Key** $Y_0 = e(g, g)_{y_0}$.

Attribute Authority k

Authority Secret Key The SW secret key: $y_k, t_{k,1}...t_{k,n}$.
Authority Public Key $T_{k,i}$ from the SW public key: $T_{k,1}...T_{k,n}$ where $T_{k,i} = g^{t_{k,i}}$.
Secret Key for User u from authority k Choose random $d - 1$ degree polynomial p with $p(0) = y_k$. Secret Key: $\left\{ D_{k,i} = g^{p(i)/t_{k,i}} \right\}_{i \in A_u}$.

Encryption for attribute set A_C

Choose random $s \leftarrow Z_q$.
Encryption: $E = Y_0^s m$, $\left\{ E_{k,i=T_{k,i}^s} \right\}_{i \in A_C^k, \forall k}$
Decryption: For each authority k, for d attributes $i \in A_C^k \cap A_u$, compute $e(E_{k,i}, D_{k,i}) = e(g, g)^{p(i)s}$. Interpolate to find $Y_k^s = e(g, g)^{p(0)s} = e(g, g)^{y_k^s}$. Combine these values to obtain $\prod_{k=1}^{K} Y_k^s = Y_0^s$. Then $m = E/Y_0^s$.

4.4   Private FP-Tree Matching

Here, we apply the secure matching protocol proposed by Freedman et al. [16] to merge the FP-tree between every two parties. We propose a framework whereby all parties participate to a secure aggregation mechanism without having access to the protected data. In order to ensure end to end confidentiality, the framework uses additive homomorphic encryption algorithms. All the count of the conditional FP-tree is merged in this step.

Private Merging Protocol

Input: Party A's input is a set $T_A = \{T_A^1, ..., T_A^k\}$, party B's input is a set $T_B = \{T_B^1, ..., T_B^l\}$. The elements in the input sets are taken from a domain of size N.

1. Party performs the following:
   (a) He chooses the secret-key parameters for a semantically-secure homomorphic encryption scheme, and publishes its public keys and parameters. The plaintexts are in a field that contains representations of the N elements of the input domain, but is exponentially larger.
   (b) She uses interpolation to compute the coefficients of the polynomial $P(y) = \sum_{i=0}^{k} \alpha_i T_B^i$ of degree k with roots $x_1, ..., x_k$.
   (c) She encrypts each of the $(k+1)$ coefficients by the semantically-secure homomorphic encryption scheme and sends to party B the resulting set of ciphertexts, $Enc(\alpha_0), ..., Enc(\alpha_k)$.
2. Party B performs the following for every $T_B^i \in T_B$:
   (a) He uses the homomorphic properties to evaluate the encrypted polynomial at T_B^i. That is, he computes $Enc(P(y)) = Enc(\sum_{i=0}^{k} \alpha_i T_B^i)$.
   (b) He chooses a random value r and computes $Enc(rP(y)+y)$. (One can also encrypt some additional payload data py by computing $Enc(rP(y)+ (T_B^i|p_B))$. Party obtains p_B iff T_B^i is in the intersection.) He randomly permutes this set of kS ciphertexts and sends the result back to the client
   .
3. Party A decrypts all l ciphertexts received. She locally outputs all values $x \in X$ for which there is a corresponding decrypted value .

Preventing Collusion. Note that we can easily extend this to prevent collusion: If we give all our users points from the same polynomial, any group with at least d transaction between them would be able to combine their keys to find p(0). However, if we instead give each user u a different polynomial p_u (but still with the same zero point $p_u(0) = p(0)$), then one user's points will give no information on the polynomial held by the other (as long as neither has more than d.1 points). To see this, note that, given any $d-1$ points on polynomial p_1 and any $d-1$ points on polynomial p_2, with the requirement that these polynomials must intersect at 0, it is still the case that any value for $y = p_1(0) = p_2(0)$ will define a valid pair of polynomials. Thus, y is information theoretically hidden.

Ideally, a public-key encryption scheme should be semantically secure against adaptive chosen-ciphertext attack. Informally, this means that an adversary can learn nothing about the plaintext corresponding to a given ciphertext c, even when the adversary is allowed to obtain the plaintext corresponding to ciphertexts of its choice. We henceforth denote this security notion as IND-CCA (indistinguishability against adaptive chosen-ciphertext attacks). that is to say that our scheme's security, which is under the semi-honest model, relies on the encryption's strength.

5   Conclusions

The main contribution of this paper is proposing a general framework for privacy preserving association rules mining. For that the randomization methodologies are not good enough to attain the high accuracy and protect clients' information from privacy breach and the malicious attack, we show that how association rules mining can be done in this framework and prove that is secure enough to keep the clients' privacy. We also show that our protocols works with less communication complexity and communication complexity compared to other related schemes.

In the future research, a common framework with more formal and reliable for privacy preservation will enable next generation data mining technology to make substantial advances in alleviating privacy concerns.

Acknowledgement

We would like to thank Dr. Bao Feng and Dr. Jianying Zhou from Cryptography & Security Department, Institute for Infocomm Research, Singapore and Dr. Guilin Wang from School of Computer Science, University of Birmingham, UK. We got some precious technical comments about private FP-tree merging from Dr. Bao and some editorial comments for Dr. Zhou and Dr. Wang.

References

1. Agrawal, R., Imielinski, T., Swami, A.N.: Mining association rules between sets of items in large databases. In: Proceedings of the ACM SIGMOD International Conference on Management of Data (1993)
2. Agrawal, R., Srikant, R.: Privacy-Preserving Data Mining. In: ACM SIGMOD Int'l Conf. on Management of Data, Dallas (May 2000)
3. Evfimievski, A., Srikant, R., Agrawal, R., Gehrke, J.: Privacy Preserving Mining of Association Rules. In: Proc. of 8th ACM SIGKDD Intl. Conf. on Knowledge Discovery and Data Mining (KDD) (2002)
4. Feldman, P.: A practical scheme for non-interactive verifiable secret sharing. In: Proc. of FOCS, pp. 427–437 (1987)

5. Fukazawa, T., Wang, J., Takata, T., Miyazak, M.: An Effective Distributed Privacy-Preserving Data Mining Algorithm. In: Fifth International Conference on Intelligent Data Engineering and Automated Learning, UK (2004)
6. Goldreich, O.: Foundations of Cryptography, vol. 2, ch.7. Cambridge Univ. Press, Cambridge (2004)
7. Goldreich, O., Micali, S., Wigderson, A.: How to play any mental game. In: Proceedings of the 19th annual ACM symposium on Theory of computing (1987)
8. Han, J., Pei, J., Yin, Y., Mao, R.: Mining Frequent Patterns without Candidate Generation: A Frequent-Pattern Tree Approach. Data Mining and Knowledge Discovery, 53–87 (2004)
9. Kantarcioglu, M., Clifton, C.: Privacy-Preserving Distributed Mining of association rules on horizontally partitioned data. In: Proceedings of the ACM SIGMOD Workshop on Research Issues on Data Mining and Knowledge Discovery (2002)
10. Lindell, Y., Pinkas, B.: Privacy preserving data mining. In: Bellare, M. (ed.) CRYPTO 2000. LNCS, vol. 1880, pp. 36–54. Springer, Heidelberg (2000)
11. Paillier, P.: Public-key cryptosystems based on composite degree residuosity classes. In: Stern, J. (ed.) EUROCRYPT 1999. LNCS, vol. 1592. Springer, Heidelberg (1999)
12. Shamir, A.: Identity-based cryptosystems and signature schemes. In: Blakely, G.R., Chaum, D. (eds.) CRYPTO 1984. LNCS, vol. 196, pp. 47–53. Springer, Heidelberg (1985)
13. Vaidya, J.S., Clifton, C.: Privacy Preserving Association Rule Mining in Vertically Partitioned Data. In: Proceedings of the Eighth ACM SIGKDD International Conference on Knowledge Discovery and Data Mining (2002)
14. Yao, A.C.: Protocols for Secure Computation. In: 23rd FOCS (1982)
15. Zhan, J.Z., Matwin, S., Chang, L.: Privacy-Preserving Collaborative Association Rule Mining. In: Procceding of DBSec 2005, pp. 153–165 (2005)
16. Freedman, M., Nissim, K., Pinkas, B.: Efficient Private Matching and Set Intersection. In: Cachin, C., Camenisch, J.L. (eds.) EUROCRYPT 2004. LNCS, vol. 3027, pp. 1–19. Springer, Heidelberg (2004)

Dichotomy Method toward
Interactive Testing-Based Fault Localization

Ji-Rong Sun[1], Zhi-Shu Li[1], and Jian-Cheng Ni[2]

[1] School of Computer Science, Sichuan University,
Chengdu, 610065, China
[2] School of Computer Science, Qufu Normal University,
Rizhao Shandong 276826,China
sunjirong@126.com, lzshu5@yahoo.com.cn, nijch@163.com

Abstract. A dichotomy method is presented to perform on test-based localization. First the test information itself is optimized from three aspects: searching scope localization using slice technique, redundant test case removal, and test suite reduction with nearest series. Secondly, the diagnosis matrix is set up according to the optimized test information and each code is prioritized accordingly. Thirdly, dichotomy method is iteratively applied to an interactive process for seeking the bug: the searching scope is cut in two by the checkpoint *cp*, which is of the highest priority; If *cp* is wrong, the bug is found; else we will ignore the codes before/after it according to the result of *cp*. Finally, we conduct three studies with Siemens suite of 132 program mutants. Our method scores 0.85 on average, which means we only need to check less than 15% of the program before finding out a bug.

Keywords: diagnosis matrix, dichotomy method, program slice, testing-based fault localization (TBFL), test suite optimization.

1 Introduction

To improve the quality of a program, we have to remove as many defects as possible in it without introducing new bugs at the same time. However, localizing a fault is a complex and time-consuming process. To reduce the cost on debugging, it is natural to locate a fault using information acquired from testing, which is referred as testing-based fault localization (TBFL). In practice, TBFL has become a research focus in recent years. The richer the information coming from testing, the more precise the diagnosis may be.

To reduce the human effort, many approaches have been proposed in recent years to automate fault localization based on the analysis of execution traces, such as ①Dicing[1],[2], ②TARTANTULA[3],[4], ③Interactive approach[5],[6], ④Nearest Neighbor Queries approach[7], ⑤SAFL[8],[9], ⑥Control-flow based Difference Metric approach [10], and ⑦Incremental approach[11] etc.

All approaches except ③ are automatic carried out to give a report of the most suspicious codes or the possibility of each code containing bug. While approach ③ is an interactive process, the information gathered from previous steps can be used to provide the ranking of suspicious statements for the current interaction step.

C. Tang et al. (Eds.): ADMA 2008, LNAI 5139, pp. 182–193, 2008.
© Springer-Verlag Berlin Heidelberg 2008

In approach ④ and ⑥, only one successful test case, most similar to the failed one, is selected out according to some metrics. Then the difference between these two execution traces will determine the report. In approach ① and ⑦, several successful traces will be picked up to prioritize the code. For each code, more times to appear in the successful slice, less impossible to contain any bug. In approach ②, ③ and⑤, an entire test suite is used to color the codes in the failed program, different color with different brightness stands for different possibility of containing bug.

Most of the TBFL tools have focused on how to compare the successful and failing execution traces. However, TBFL technique has an obvious shortcoming. Its effectiveness directly depends on the distribution of the test cases in the test suite. Thus how to maximize the utility of test information is above all the most important question in TBFL. Approaches ① to ④ will be compared with ours in this paper.

```
s1:  read(a,b,c);
s2:  class:=scalene;
s3:  if a=b or b=c
s4:            class:=isosceles;
s5:  if a=b and b=c
s6:            class:=equilateral;
s7:  if a*a=b*b+c*c
s8:       class:=right;
s9:  case class of
s10:    right:        area:=b*c/2;
s11:    equilateral: area:=a*2*sqrt(3)/4
s12:    otherwise:    s:=(a+b+c)/2;
s13:                  area:=sqrt(s*(s-a)(s-b)(s-c));
s14: write(class,area);
```

Fig. 1. Example program P

Table 1. Diagnosis matrix of program P

	t1 (2,2,2)	t2 (4,4,3)	t3 (5,4,3)	t4 (6,5,4)	t5 (3,3,3)	t6 (4,3,3)
s1	1	1	1	1	1	1
s2	1	1	1	1	1	1
s3	1	1	1	1	1	1
s4	1	1	0	0	1	1
s5	1	1	1	1	1	1
s6	1	0	0	0	1	0
s7	1	1	1	1	1	1
s8	0	0	1	0	0	0
s9	1	1	1	1	1	1
s10	0	0	1	0	0	0
s11	1	0	0	0	1	0
s12	0	1	0	1	0	1
s13	0	0	0	0	0	0
s14	1	1	1	1	1	1
S/F	1	1	1	1	0	1

2 Preliminary Work

Typically, the TBFL problem can be formalized as follows [5]:Given a program P under test, which is composed of a set of statements (denoted as $P=\{s_1,s_2,...,s_m\}$), and a test suite (denoted as $T=\{t_1,t_2,...,t_n\}$), the information acquired when running these test cases against P can be represented as a n*(m+1) Boolean execution matrix(called a **diagnosis matrix** in this paper), denoted as $E=(e_{ij})$ $(1\leq i\leq m+1,\ 1\leq j\leq n)$, where

$$e_{ij} = \begin{cases} 1 & statement\ s_i\ is\ executed\ by\ test\ t_j \quad (1\leq i\leq m) \\ 1 & test\ case\ t_j\ is\ successful \quad (i=m+1) \\ 0 & \end{cases} \qquad (1)$$

Thus, the TBFL problem can be viewed as the problem of calculating which statements are most suspicious based on the diagnosis matrix.

2.1 Sample Program

Let's have a sample program P in Fig. 1 and its diagnosis matrix in Table 1 to see how to use the test information; it will be further used to show how to prioritize the code and how to locate the bug in the following sections. Table 1 gives the test cases in T and its corresponding execution path. The program produces correct outputs on all test cases except t5, which is marked grey in Table 1. Because s11 uses the expression a*2 instead of a*a.

2.2 Using Slice to Cross Out Irrespective Statements

An execution slice with respect to a test case t is the set of code executed by t. If a statement is not executed under a test case, it cannot affect the program output for that test case. P's CFG is shown on the left in Fig. 2 and t5's execution slice is marked grey. Control didn't reach the statements 8,10,12,13 during the execution of t5, we can be sure that the error could not be brought by those statements.

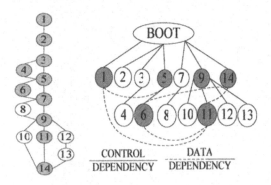

Fig. 2. Program P's DFD and CFG with respect to t5

A dynamic slice uses dynamic analysis to identify all and only the statements that contribute to the selected variables of interest on the particular anomalous execution trace. In this way, the dynamic slice technique prune away unrelated computation and the size of slice can be considerably reduced, thus allowing an easier location of the bugs [12]. P's CFG is shown on the right in Fig. 2 and t5's dynamic slice is marked grey, which can be obtained according to the dynamic control dependency and data dependency.Even statements 2,3,4,7 are executed but do not affect variable area. So the bug must exist in area's dynamic slice with respect to t5.

Let's use S_{wt} to stand for the slice of a particular failed test case wt, maybe execution or dynamic. We only need to focus on the statements in S_{wt}.

2.3 *Wrong* and *Right* Test Suite

Given such a failing run, fault localization often proceeds by comparing the failed run with successful run or runs. Because only one fault-revealing execution trace is considered in the manual fault localization process, then how to exploit multiple execution traces becomes the starting point of TBFL. Intuitively, the more test cases in test suite, the more accuracy of the TBFL report. But if several pieces of code in different places are executed by the same test cases (called indistinguishing statements), those codes will be given the same rank whatever approaches being taken. Experiments show more indistinguishing statements, less accurate diagnosis [8].

Let us use $Req(t,wt)$ to stand for the common statements both executed by the test case t and wt. Bigger $|Req(t,wt)|$ is, more codes in execution of t and wt are common, i.e, that means more "nearest" to wt [7].

$$Req(t,wt)=S_t \cap S_{wt} \tag{2}$$

We will create two subsets of T: *Right* and *Wrong*. All failed test cases are allocated to *Wrong*. Because all the failed test cases need fault localization, we only need to exclude the redundant successful test cases. Each successful test case will be allocated to *Right* according to the following rules:

1) If its execution is the same as anyone in *Wrong*, ignore it.
2) If several successful test cases' executions are the same, only one will be included in *Right* set. Thus test case t1, t6 will be ignored in diagnosis process.
3) At last the test cases in *Right* will be ordered according to the number of $|Req(t,wt)|$, the maximum is the first, the minimum is the last.

2.4 Test Suite Reduction Toward TBFL

An accurate bug diagnosis requires maximizing the information coming from testing process for a precise cross-checking and fault localization. However, experiments have shown that redundant test cases may bias the distribution of the test suite and harm TBFL [8]. We propose to use test suite reduction techniques to remove some harmful redundancy to boost TBFL.

Suppose we aim at finding one faulty statement each time. As described in previous section, we only need to check the code in S_{wt}. Given the initial diagnosis matrix E as input and the codes in S_{wt}, reduce the test suite T to T':

1) T'=Φ.
2) The test cases are allocated to *Right* or *Wrong* according to section 2.3.
3) Select the test case from *Right* in-sequence which means the nearest to *wt* into T' until all statements in S_{wt} are covered.
4) The test cases in *Wrong* must be existed in diagnosis process, so T'=T'+*Wrong*.

3 Diagnosis Matrix Optimization

Since some irrespective statements have been ruled out by slice technique and some harmful redundant test cases are got rid off from T, we need to build up a new diagnosis matrix E' aiding to rank the statements in S_{wt} toward TBFL. The test cases in T' and the statements in S_{wt} will only be evolved in E'.

For example, if we take up the dynamic slice technique with t5, then we can obtain a new optimized diagnosis matrix as shown in the left of Table 2.

Table 2. Optimized diagnosis matrix E' and Priority(s_i) of S_{t5}

	optimized diagnosis matrix E'				%S	%F	Priority(si)
	t2 (4,4,3)	t3 (5,4,3)	t4 (6,5,4)	t5 (3,3,3)			
s1	1	1	1	1	100%	100%	0.5
s5	1	1	1	1	100%	100%	0.5
s6	0	0	0	1	0	100%	1
s9	1	1	1	1	100%	100%	0.5
s11	0	0	0	1	0	100%	1
s14	1	1	1	1	100%	100%	0.5
S/F	1	1	1	0			

4 Dichotomy Method in TBFL

Experimental results show that even the automatic TBFL report is efficient, the developer needs to examine up to 20% of the total statements for less than 60% of faults and examine more statements for other faults [3],[7],[10]. Therefore, current TBFL approaches still can hardly serve as an effective substitute of manual fault localization. We focus on how to combine the merit of manual fault localization and TBFL. To achieve this, we proposed a **Dichotomy Method** in TBFL.

4.1 Code Prioritization

Let's use N_f to be the number of failed test cases and $N_f(s)$ to be the number of test cases in N_f which execute the statement s. We use *%Failed(s)* to stand for the ratio of failed test cases that execute s, which means the error possibility of s.

$$\% \, Failed(s) = \frac{N_f(s)}{N_f} \times 100\% \tag{3}$$

Similarly, let's use N_s, $N_s(s)$, $\%Successful(s)$ to be the number of successful test cases, the number of test cases in N_s which execute the statement s and the ratio of successful test cases that execute s.

$$\% \, Successful \; (s) = \frac{N_s(s)}{N_s} \times 100\% \tag{4}$$

Let's use $Priority(s)$ stand for the possibility of statement s containing a bug. It can be obtained by combining the equation (3) and (4) as follows:

$$Priority(s \,) = \frac{\% \, Failed(s)}{\% \, Failed(s) \; + \% \; Successful \; (s)} \tag{5}$$

Diagnosis matrix E may be the initial one or the optimized one. If E is an optimized one, only the statements in S_{wt} are to be ranked with a priority. $\%Successful \; (s)$, $\%Failed(s)$ and $Priority(s)$ of each code in S_{t5} are listed in the right of Table 2.

4.2 Dichotomizing Search Method in TBFL

Any TBFL tool described above ranks the statement directly without optimizing the testing information and will be ceased to turn in a report with a list of code's priority. Then the code will be checked one by one from the highest priority to the least. While our TBFL tool is a semi-automatic, each time which statement is to be checked depends on the checking result last time. The architecture of our dichotomizing search method toward TBFL is illustrated in Fig. 3.

The whole process can be elaborated as follows:

① Acquiring diagnosis matrix: Given the traces and results of each test case obtained from testing process as input, it will output the diagnosis matrix E.

② Acquiring slice of wt: We can preliminary conclude that the bug exists in S_{wt}. Suppose we aim at one default at a time. If use execution slice technique, no other resource needed and the trace of wt is S_{wt}; If use dynamic slice, the dynamic slice S_{wt} will be acquired with the help of slicing tools.

③ Acquiring $Right$ and $Wrong$: Allocating each test case in the initial test suite T to $Right$ and $Wrong$ individually according to the rules elaborated in section 2.3.

④ Test suite reduction: We use the greedy algorithm to select out nearest test cases from T to T' as described in section 2.4.

⑤ Acquiring optimized diagnosis matrix: After some redundant information cross out from testing process, a new diagnosis matrix is required to rank the code in S_{wt}.

⑥ Prioritizing code: Given an initial or optimized diagnosis matrix E as input, each code in E will be evaluated with a priority according to section 4.1. Then a report will be turned in with the ranked code list. We let a=0, b=|E|. The index a, b are used to present the searching range. The bug must exist in the statements between a and b.

⑦ Setting the checkpoint cp: Looking up the report, find a statement with maximum $Priority(cp)$ from a to b and make it a checkpoint cp. We use **pred(cp)** and *succ(cp)* to stand for the variables before and after *cp* separately. We are sure that *cp* is the most possible of containing fault. The variables accessed by the checkpoint *cp* are examined carefully. If there are several statements ranked with the same highest priority, then we pick the last one as checkpoint. Because we think the code in the earlier has been checked more times, it is less to be faulty. Variable *k* is used to count the iteration times, which means how many statements have been examined before the bug found. In table 2, s6 and s14 are ranked the same, so s14 is first set as *cp*. And it is faulty, the algorithm terminates.

⑧Dichotomizing the searching range: The different conditions are to be analyzed: **1)**If these values are already incorrect before executing *cp*, i.e. *pred(cp)* is error, we can assume that there should be a faulty statement before *cp*. Thus the codes after *cp* are innocent to the bug, b=*cp*-1; **2)** If both *pred(cp)* and *succ(cp)* are correct, we would assume that no faulty statement has been executed yet, a=*cp*+1. **3)** If *pred(cp)* is correct and *succ(cp)* is incorrect, we may determine that the statement *cp* is a faulty one, thus the algorithm terminates and the bug is found. Otherwise go to ⑦ for next iteration.

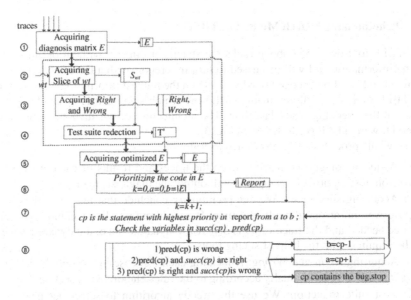

Fig. 3. Architecture of dichotomy method in TBFL

From the beginning, we have supposed to find out one bug a time. We can use the *dichotomy method* to gradually narrow down the searching range. Steps ② to ④ are marked within dashed rectangle in Fig.3. Those steps aim to maximize the utility of testing information and to give an accurate report. Steps ⑥ to ⑧ are used to dichotomize the searching range. Using the statement with highest rank (i.e. *cp*) to split the suspect range in two, we look into the variables accessed by *cp* to see whether abnormal occurs. Thus the next binary search range is determined.

5 Experiment

To investigate the effectiveness of our *dichotomy method* in finding out the faulty statements, we have designed a number of studies together with Approach ① to ④. Among them, ①, ②and ④ are automatic and end with a report of ranking list, while ③and ours are semi-automatic to continue with the report for further localization. To investigate the effectiveness of our technique and guide our future work, we considered three questions: (1)How many checkpoints have been set before finding out the faulty code with different slice technique? (2)Does diagnosis matrix optimization really work? How does the quality of test suite itself influence the effect of TBFL tool? (3)Does our method really overwhelm others in quality?

5.1 Programs Under Test

The target programs used in our experiment are the Siemens programs, which were first collected and used by Hutchins et al. [13] and were also used in [5],[7],[10].

The Siemens programs consist of 132 versions of seven programs in C with injected faults, as shown in Table 3. The last four columns show LOC (lines of code), the number of test cases in T and failed test cases in *Wrong*, the number of faulty versions, respectively. Each faulty version has exactly one injected fault. Some of the faults are code omissions; some are stricter or looser conditions in the statements; some focus on the type faults of variables, and so on. For each program, its initial test suite T is first created by the black-box test suite and then more test cases are manually added in to ensure that each executable statement, edge, and definition-use pair in the is covered by at least 30 different test cases. In our experiment, we use the initial test suite T of each Siemens programs to execute all faulty versions. For each faulty version, record the corresponding execution matrix E.

Table 3. Relative data of the experimental program

Program	Descption	LOC	ITI	IWrongI	NoV
Replace	Pattern replacement	516	5,542	3–309	32
Printtokens	Lexical analyzer	402	4,130	6–186	7
Printtokens2	Lexical analyzer	483	4,115	33–518	20
Schedule1	Priority scheduler	299	2,650	7–293	9
Schedule2	Priority scheduler	297	2,710	2–65	10
Tot_info	Information measure	346	1,052	3–251	23
Tcas	Altitude separation4	138	1,608	1–131	41

5.2 Evaluation Framework

Because the faulty statement is injected manually, we can know where it is before hand. Thus from the report, we can directly know how many codes will be examined or how many checkpoints will be set before the bug has been found.

To evaluate the performance of these different TBFL tools, we need a quantitative measure of a fault localizer's report quality. Formally, given a report of a mutant, that is, a list of program features the localizer indicates as possible locations of the bug, we want to compute and assign a score to it. We adapt the evaluation technique that was originally proposed by Renieris and Reiss [7] and later adopted in [5], [10]. For each fault, this measure defines a score that indicates how much portion of code does not need to be examined for finding its location. For example, for a faulty program consisting of 100 statements, if we need to examine 5 statements before we find the faulty one, the score is 0.95.

We use *Score(wt)* to stand for the effectiveness of a method with respect to *wt* when checking the bug in a given version. Using all mutants of a program, the average diagnosis accuracy is computed, it estimates the quality of the diagnosis method. Thus the score of a method for *P* is the average of scores of all versions, which can be calculated by equation (6).

$$Score(P) = \frac{\sum Score(wt)}{\mid NoV \mid} \tag{6}$$

5.3   Study 1: Execution Slice vs. Dynamic Slice

We conduct the experiment in this study with the initial test suite, aiming at comparing the effectiveness of slice technique in finding the bug.

First Steps ②,③,④,⑤ are ignored, we only use *dichotomy method* to seek the bug in the whole program from initial diagnosis matrix. The score's distribution of the report is listed in Table 4 column Program(T). And then step ② is added, execution slice and dynamic slice are applied on *wt* individually and the codes in S_{wt} only need be examined for each version. The results are shown in last two columns of Table 4.

Table 4 compares the distribution of scores with non-slice, execution slice and dynamic slice over the percentage of total versions. We found that slice technique really does work in comparing with non-slice and dynamic slice technique do performs better than execution one. When examining less than 20% statements of the program, only 62.12% fault can be found with non-slice technique, while 77.27% faults with execution slice, and 84.09% with dynamic slice.

For a given failed test case *wt* in relation to one version, there maybe more than one failed test case at the same time. The codes in *P* but out of S_{wt} can also be executed by other failed test cases, thus can be ranked with a higher priority, which may mislead the diagnosis when the searching range is not limited to S_{wt}. So first to local the searching range in S_{wt} is very essential.

Table 4. Versions(%) of average Score distribution

Score	Program(T)	Execution(T)	Dynamic (T)
0-0.1	3.03	2.27	2.27
0.1-0.2	9.09	1.52	1.52
0.2-0.3	1.52	0.00	0.00
0.3-0.4	1.52	0.00	0.00
0.4-0.5	0.76	0.00	0.00
0.5-0.6	4.55	0.76	0.76
0.6-0.7	6.06	5.30	3.79
0.7-0.8	11.36	12.88	7.58
0.8-0.9	19.70	25.00	28.79
0.9-1.0	42.42	52.27	55.30

5.4 Study 2: T vs. T'

The second set of studies evaluates the effectiveness of diagnosis optimization. From steps ③ to ⑤, we have tried to get rid of the harmful information and furthest utilize the information from testing process. In this study, we try to estimate how those steps contribute to the scores of our *dichotomy method*. Based on study 1, steps ③ to ⑤ are added in to acquire T' of each version. When optimizing the diagnosis matrix in step ⑤, we adopt the execution and dynamic slice separately.

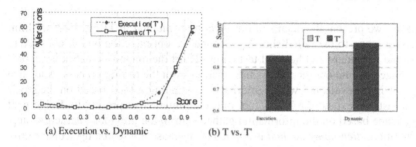

(a) Execution vs. Dynamic   (b) T vs. T'

Fig. 4. Effectiveness of test suite reduction in dichotomy method

Thus the score of each version can be calculated with optimized E' and its distribution is shown in Fig. 4(a), where execution and dynamic slice technique is in comparison. With either slice technique, more than 50% bugs can be found in less than 10% of the program and more than 80% bugs can be found in less than 20% of the program.

Combine with the result in study 1, the scores of *dichotomy method* regarding T and T' can be acquired respectively, which are illustrated in Fig.4(b). The test suite optimization really works, which promote about 4% diagnosis accuracy.

5.5 Study 3: Dichotomy Method vs. Other TBFL Tool

The third set of studies compares the accuracy of our method with other methods. As acquiring dynamic slice needs more resources and the execution trace has already

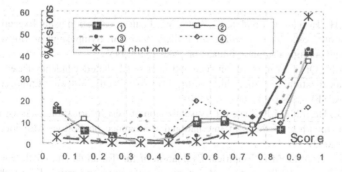

Fig. 5. Effectiveness of different TBFL tool

existed and also be used in other TBFL tools, to be fair, we will take the execution slice of *wt* for contrast.

The scores of Approach ① to ④ can be obtained from reference [5],[7],[10]. Then the effectiveness of these 5 TBFL tools is illustrated in Fig. 5. The score of our method outperforms the others at least by 30%.

We have also found that there exist some bugs which would be located nearly whole program having been examined, whatever approach adopted.

6   Conclusion and Future Work

In this paper, we present the details of our *dichotomy method* in TBFL. First we limit the searching scope to the failed slice S_{wt}. Second we optimize the initial test suite to exclude some redundant and harmful test cases. Third the diagnosis matrix is accordingly optimized to rule out the useless information from the testing process. And each code in S_{wt} will be evaluated with a priority of containing a fault based on diagnosis matrix. At last, we extend the TBFL tool to use an interactive process to decide next searching scope based on the information gathered from the previous interaction step. In each iteration, *dichotomy method* is applied to decrease the searching scope: Looking into the diagnosis matrix, select out a statement with highest priority as checkpoint *cp* within the searching scope, and inspect the variables before and after *cp* carefully. If the variables before *cp* is right and after *cp* is wrong, then *cp* is the faulty code, algorithm terminates; If the variables before *cp* is wrong, then checking scope will be set before *cp*; If the variables before and after *cp* both are right, then checking scope will be set after *cp*.

Based on the results of three studies that evaluate the effectiveness of dichotomy method, we find that each step in our technique does contribute to helping locate suspicious statements and our technique does outperform the others at least by 30% in score.

The studies also suggest some directions for our future work: (1) what kind of fault is always with a low score nearly to 0? (2) When several faults are injected to a version at the same time, could our method preserve to be superior to others?

References

1. Agrawal, H., Horgan, J., London, S., Wong, W.: Fault Localization using Execution Slices and Dataflow Tests. In: Proceedings of ISSRE 1995 (Int. Symposium on Software Reliability Engineering), Toulouse, France, pp. 143–151 (1995)
2. Wong, W.E., Qi, Y.: An execution slice and inter-block data dependency-based approach for fault localization. In: Proceedings of the 11th Asia-Pacific Software Engineering Conference (APSEC 2004), pp. 366–373 (2004)
3. Jones, J.A., Harrold, M.J., Stasko, J.: Visualization of Test Information to Assist Fault Localization. In: Proc. of the 24th International Conference on Software Engineering, pp. 467–477 (2002)
4. Jones, J.A., Harrold, M.J.: Empirical Evaluation of the Tarantula Automatic Fault Localization Technique. In: Proceedings of Automated Software Engineering, USA (2005)

5. Hao, D., Zhang, L., Zhong, H., Mei, H., Sun, J.: Towards Interactive Fault Localization Using Test Information. In: Proc. of the 13th Asia Pacific Software Engineering Conference (APSEC 2006), pp. 277–284 (2006)
6. Hao, D.: Testing-Based Interactive Fault Localization. In: Proc. of the 28th international conference on Software engineering 2006, pp. 957–960 (2006)
7. Renieris, M., Reiss, S.P.: Fault Localization with Nearest Neighbor Queries. In: Proc. of International Conference on Automated Software Engineering, pp. 30–39 (2003)
8. Hao, D., Zhang, L., Zhong, H., Mei, H., Sun, J.: Eliminating Harmful Redundancy for Test-Based Fault Localization using Test Suite Reduction: An Experimental Study. In: Proc. of the 21th International Conference on Software Maintenance, pp. 683–686 (2005)
9. Hao, D., Pan, Y., Zhang, L., Zhao, W., Mei, H., Sun, J.: A Similarity-Aware Approach to Testing Based Fault Localization. In: Proc. of the 20th IEEE International Conference on Automated Software Engineering, November, pp. 291–294 (2005)
10. Guo, L., Roychoudhury, A., Wang, T.: Accurately choosing execution runs for software fault localization. In: International Conference on Compiler Construction, pp. 80–95 (2006)
11. Jirong, S., Zhishu, L., Jiancheng, N., Feng, Y.: Priority Strategy of Software Fault Localization. In: Proc. of the 6th WSEAS International Conference on Applied Computer Science (ACOS 2007), pp. 500–506 (2007)
12. Agrawal, H., DeMillo, R.A., Spafford, E.H.: Debugging with Dynamic Slicing and Backtracking. Software-Practice & Experience 23(6), 589–616 (1996)
13. Hutchins, M., Foster, H., Goradia, T., Ostrand, T.: Experiments on the effectiveness of dataflow and control flow-based test adequacy criterions. In: Proc. of the 16th International Conf. on software. Eng., pp. 191–200 (1994)

Maintaining the Maximum Normalized Mean and Applications in Data Stream Mining

Jan Peter Patist

Artificial Intelligence,
Vrije universiteit Amsterdam, De Boelelaan 1081a,
1081 HV Amsterdam,
The Netherlands
jpp@few.vu.nl

Abstract. In data stream mining many algorithms are based on fixed size sliding windows to cope with the aging of data. This despite of some flaws of fixed size windows. Namely, it is difficult to set the size of the window and there does not exist an optimal window size due to different types of changes in the underlying distribution of the data stream. Because of these reasons the algorithm performance degrades. We propose some initial steps toward efficiently equipping sliding window algorithms with flexible windowing. This is done by the efficient maintenance of a statistic called, the maximum normalized mean. This statistic is maximized over all time windows and thus uses flexible windowing. We show that several algorithms can be restated such that it uses the maximum normalized mean as a building block. The usefulness of the normalized mean in the context of these algorithms is shown by means of experiments.

1 Introduction

In the last decade there has been a large increase of data, of which examples are internet/intranet data, network traffic, etc.. This large increase in the amount of data resulted in the understanding of the need for and consequently the development of new algorithms, frameworks and methodologies to cope with new problems arising due to the high speed and volume of the data. With the increase of the importance of data streams and consequently the analysis of streams a new sub domain in data mining, called data stream mining was born.

Analysis of streams is different from the analysis of static data sets. First of all, the computational and space requirements are more demanding due to the continuous flow of data. Secondly, the relevance of the data is variable over time caused by changes in the underlying data generating process.

An overview of the research performed on the data streams can be found in [1] [2]. Examples of developed algorithms are: approximate calculation of statistics, sampling, model updating in the context concept drift, data stream querying, etc..

In data stream mining many algorithms are based on fixed size sliding windows to cope with the aging of data. A sliding window is a buffer of a fixed capacity.

C. Tang et al. (Eds.): ADMA 2008, LNAI 5139, pp. 194–206, 2008.

Incoming data points are added to the buffer for which the oldest data points are removed. A clear flaw is that no any-time optimal window exists due to different types of changes in the data, and consequently the system performance is sub-optimal.

In this paper we propose an algorithm for the maintenance of a statistic, which we call the maximum normalized mean. This statistic is the mean, normalized by the number points used in its estimation, maximized over the n most recent data points in the stream. The flexible windowing is due to the maximization over all time windows reaching the most recent data point x_c.

To incorporate information about the uncertainty in the estimation of the mean, the mean is multiplied by a normalization function, which is only dependent on the number of data points in the window.

In classical hypothesis testing, statistics are often rescaled by the number of data points used in the estimation of the statistic. For example the Kolmogorov statistic D, in the two sample context, is rescaled by $\sqrt{\frac{na}{n+a}}$, where n is the length of the window and a is a constant. Note that the maximum normalized mean can also be maintained over a transformed stream $g(x_n), \ldots, g(x_c)$ by function g. Consequently the maintenance of the maximum normalized mean can be used as a building block by different data stream algorithms.

Applications appearing in the literature using instantiations of the maximum normalized mean are [3][4]. In [4] an algorithm is proposed to find frequent item sets over a data stream. The authors advocate that the maximum mean is a better translation of the term frequent than frequency estimates based on a sliding window or an exponentially weighting scheme. In the paper [3] the maximum normalized mean is used in a change detection algorithm. The maximum normalized mean is used to approximate the Kolmogorov-Smirnov (KS) two sample test, which is maximized over the time. To obtain the z-value the KS statistic is normalized by $\sqrt{\frac{na}{n+a}}$. In the standard application of the KS test the constants n and a refer to sample sizes.

Our contribution is that we show that the maximum normalized mean, for a general normalization function, can be maintained efficiently with respect to time and space. Furthermore we show that the already mentioned applications can be embedded within this framework. As a consequence, the result in the paper [3] is improved. Namely in the paper it is assumed that $a >> n$, a constraint on the sizes of the samples, which can be an unreasonable assumption.

Essentially the maintenance algorithm is the same as in [3], however it is proved for a more general normalization function, which makes the assumption, $a >> n$, unnecessary. Furthermore we give another example of the embedding of a two sample test in our framework. This two sample test is the Mann-Whitney two sample test. The validity of our approach is proved theoretically. Whereas the efficiency of the method is shown empirically.

In the following section we discuss first the related work, then we address the algorithm to maintain the maximum normalized mean. Hereafter we give a theoretical proof of the correctness of the algorithm. Then we demonstrate the embedding of the two change detection algorithms and the frequent item set algorithm. The usefulness of the change detection algorithms is shown by means of experiments.

2   Related Work

Maintenance of statistics. In this section we summarize important work in the area of change detection and the maintenance of statistics. The importance of these two topics with respect to this paper is evident. Namely, change detection is one of the applications which can benefit from the use of the maximum normalized mean. Work on the maintenance of the statistics is important because perhaps it offers possibilities to further improve upon the efficiency of our maintenance method.

There is a lot of research performed on the maintenance of statistics over data streams. The research covers mainly general efficient approximate maintenance methods, efficient maintenance of particular statistics and maintenance methods of statistics in the context of decreasing data relevance over time.

Examples of efficient general approximate maintenance methods are sampling [5], smart data structures [6] and random sketches [7]. Work on the efficient maintenance of particular statistics are on the variance, norms, entropy, k-means clusters, etc.. Furthermore, methods differ in calculations over the whole stream or over a sliding window [6]. All methods are approximate methods with probabilistic guarantees on the accuracy of the estimation. See for an overview of these methods [2] and [8].

Change detection. Early work in the domain of statistics is the work [9] and [10] on the CUSUM algorithm and the sequential probability ratio test. Both methods are statistical in nature using probability distributions to detect changes. A possible disadvantage of these methods could be the difficulty of finding the appropriate family of distribution as well estimating accurately the parameters of this distribution. For an instructive overview on statistical change detection of abrupt changes, see [11].

In [12] the author proposes a change detection framework based on the martingale framework. Their approach is claimed to be an efficient one-pass incremental algorithm, like most data stream algorithms. The algorithm does not require a sliding window on the data stream, and works also for high dimensional and multi-class data streams. In the paper, martingales are used to test exchangeability. Exchangeability means that the data is invariant under permutations. Whenever the exchangeability property is violated it likely that a change has occurred. In practice the framework can be used after transforming the data stream to a stream, where the independence assumption holds.

A sketch based detection algorithm is proposed in [13], for the purpose of the detection of attacks and failures in network traffic. Sketches are data structures for efficiently compressing the data. Change is detected by monitoring the errors of forecast models build upon these sketches.

The sequential hypothesis testing method [10] is adopted in [14] for the problem of change detection in which the independence assumption is violated. This results in time and space efficient algorithms. The method is not dependent on window assumptions and has shorter delays than window-based solutions.

In [4] an algorithm is proposed for the estimation of frequent item sets. One of the key points of the paper is the translation of what is 'frequent'. The authors are of the opinion the mean frequency maximized over the most recent points is a better translation of 'frequent' than the frequency estimate over a sliding window or based upon an exponential weighting scheme. This paper is relevant to this paper because it can be formulated such that the frequency estimation is equal to the maintenance of the maximum normalized mean, for which the normalization function is a constant function.

In [15] a change detection framework is proposed, for the environment of data streams, based upon non-parametric two sample tests. A fixed reference sample is successively compared with the last 'received' n data points, also called a sliding window of size n. When a new data point 'flows' in it is added to the window for which the oldest data point is removed.

Non-parametric two sample tests are used two detect significant deviation in the stream. Several statistical tests are proposed and compared, based upon Kolmogorov-Smirnov, Relativized Discrepancy and the Mann-Whitney two sample test. I should be noted that in the paper the authors also show that KS-statistic can be maintained efficiently using balanced trees with a time complexity per data point of $\log(a + n)$. The constants a and n are the sizes of the reference fixed sample and the sliding window. In the context of this paper this is important work, because essentially this framework is the basis of one of the applications of the maintenance of the maximum normalized mean.

The above described framework is extended in [3], by two sample testing in a data stream environment using a variable window instead of a fixed sliding window. In the paper this is done for the case of the Kolmogorov-Smirnov two sample test, in which the KS statistic is approximated. Empirically is shown that this can be done efficiently in space and time. This paper is important to the current paper because of two reasons. Firstly, like in [3] it is an application of the maintenance of the maximum normalized mean. Secondly, essentially the algorithm for maintenance of the maximum normalized mean is equivalent to the algorithm described in [3]. As a consequence the results on the time and space efficiency of the maintenance of the maximum normalized mean are already investigated in [3].

3   Problem Formulation

Let us define a data stream s as a possibly infinite sequence $(x_0^d, \ldots, x_i^d, \ldots)$ of data points x_i's from some domain D^d. In this paper, when we refer to the data stream, it is 1-dimensional and from the real domain. the data 'flows' in, at different rate and possibly indefinitely. We refer to x_0 and x_c as the starting point the last data point 'received'.

One of the objectives of this paper is to propose an efficient algorithm for the maintenance of the maximum normalized mean. The maximum normalized mean is the mean which is normalized, only dependent on the number of data points, and maximized over all time windows.

The maximum normalized mean, at time c, is defined by:

$$MNM = \max_n f(n) \cdot \mu_n, \quad \mu_n = \frac{1}{c-n} \sum_{i=(c-n)}^{c} x_i,$$

where $f(n)$ is a normalization function independent of data, only dependent on the number of data points used in estimating the mean μ_n. The indices n,c are time indices of which c is the last 'received' data point.

Data streams are often associated with high data rates. At rates such that storage is impossible and efficient time and space algorithms have to be developed. Consequently, our second objective is to show that the proposed method is time and space efficient.

The motivation of the multiplication of the mean with a normalization function is to express uncertainty. this is evidently important in comparing statistics estimated on different sized windows. An example of the use of the normalization function are weighting functions in distance functions and statistics used in hypothesis testing.

An important reason of the usefulness of the statistic is the re-usability of the maintenance algorithm in different data stream mining algorithms. For example [4], in which the statistic is used in the maintenance of frequent items and sets. The authors advocate that the maximum mean statistic is a better translation of what is 'frequent'.

In the paper an item I is frequent when

$$\max_n \hat{f}_I(x_{(c-n),\dots,x_c}),$$

where $\hat{f}$ is the observed relative frequency of item I over the last n points, and s an user defined support threshold. Clearly the function $\hat{f}_I$ is equivalent to $f \cdot \mu$, where f is a constant function and μ the relative frequency of item I.

Another example application is change detection [3]. The paper extends the framework in which change is detected using two buffers, called reference buffer, and a sliding window buffer of the n most recent points. The reference buffer is filled with data and remains fixed until change is detected. After the detection of change the procedure is restarted. A 'distance' function is used to express the 'distance' between the buffers. Whenever the 'distance' is larger than a user defined threshold an alarm is signaled. In the paper [15] the 'distance' function is a two sample test. Using a fixed window size algorithm is not optimal. A fixed window leads to either detection delay or loss of detection power compared to the optimal window size. The optimal window is approximated by maximizing the 'distance' over the time window.

The formulation of change detection can be restated as:

$$S = \max_n d(R_{ref}, W_{c-n}^c),$$

An alarm is signaled when $S > t$, where t is an user defined threshold, R is the reference set, d a 'distance' function, and window W equals $\cup_{i=(c-n)}^{c} x_i$. Clearly, the formulation of change detection can be restated as the maintenance of the maximum normalized mean, when the distance function can be decomposed into a product of a normalization function and the mean over the time window. Furthermore the normalization function is constraint to the class of continuous monotonically increasing concave functions. An example of a normalization function is $f(n) = \sqrt{n}$.

4   Maintenance Algorithm

As mentioned earlier the maintenance algorithm of our statistic is equivalent to the algorithm described in [3]. the only difference is that in this paper it is proved that the maintenance algorithm can be used in case of a more general normalization function, instead of $f(n) = \sqrt{n}$. A consequence of using the same maintenance algorithm is that the efficiency results, obtained in [3], holds also for our case.

For a better understanding we summarize the results of the paper. The maintenance algorithm works as follows: statistics are stored for every incoming point in a buffer B. These statistics are the cumulative sum $\sum_{i=0}^{n} x_i$ over the data points seen so far and the time index n. From these statistics, for every point in B we can calculate μ_m and f_n and thus MNM. We obtain the maximum by calculating MNM for every point in B and selecting the maximum.

For a certain point p_m in B under certain conditions it holds that MNM_p is always smaller than MNM_i for another point i in B, independent of the further development of the stream. Consequently it is not necessary to maintain point p in the buffer. These conditions are: $\mu_{nm} < 0$ and $\mu_{nm} > \mu_m k$ for which $n > m > k$. In both cases we can remove point p_m. These conditions are used to formulate pruning rules and validity is proved in the following section.

By the possibility of keeping the buffer small we obtain an efficient algorithm. It is empirically shown [3] that the pruning rules can be efficiently applied ($c <<$ $|B|$) on a buffer with a 'maximum' observed size of ≈ 20. This result is also observed in [4]. In the paper [4] a worst space scenario is given by means of sorted Farey sequences. However in practice this is never observed.

4.1   Proof

Before we enter technicalities we fix the notation. The statistic $d_n = f(n)\frac{1}{n}\sum_{i}^{c} x_i$, is the normalized mean at the n-th point back in time. In the following section we assume $n > m > k$, thus x_n is a point in time earlier received than x_k. The data point x_c is the last received data point. The value f_n is the normalization function applied to n, thus $f(n)$. The mean μ_{nm} is equal to $\frac{1}{n-m}\sum_{n+1}^{m} x_i$.

In this section we proof the following two statements:

1. $(\mu_{nm} < 0) \wedge (n > m) \rightarrow (d_n > d_m)$
2. $(\mu_{nm} > \mu_{mk}) \wedge (n > m > k) \rightarrow (d_n > d_m) \vee (d_k > d_m)$

Proof of 1. Let us assume $\mu_{nm} < 0$ and $n > m$. Note that $d_{nf} = \sigma_n \sum_n^f x_i$ and $d_{mf} = \sigma_m \sum_m^f x_i$, where $\sigma_i = \frac{f(i)}{i}$ for a arbitrary data point f, $f < m < n$. By the definition of μ_{nm} and the fact that $\mu_{nm} < 0$ we obtain $\sum_n^f x_i < \sum_m^f x_i$. From the concavity of f it holds that $\sigma_n < \sigma_m$. We conclude $(\mu_{nm} < 0) \wedge (n > m) \rightarrow (d_n < d_m)$, because $(d_n < d_m) \equiv \sigma_n \sum_n^f x_i < \sigma_m \sum_m^f x_i$ where $\sigma_n < \sigma_m$ and $\sum_n^f x_i < \sum_m^f x_i$.

Proof of 2. Statement 2 is proved by deriving contradiction from the negation of statement 2. By negating statement 2, we obtain $\mu_{nm} > \mu_{mk} \wedge d_m > d_n \wedge d_m > d_k \wedge n > m > k$. From $d_m > d_n$ and $d_m > d_k$ we derive constraints on μ_{mf} for an arbitrary point f, for which $f < k < m < n$. By combining the constraints, $\mu_{nm} > \mu_{mk}$ and the concavity and monotonicity of f we derive a contradiction.

Consequences of $d_m > d_n$. By definition, $d_n < d_m \equiv f_n \mu_{nf} < f_m \mu_{mf}$, where $\mu_{nf} = \alpha \mu_{nm} + (1-\alpha)\mu_{mf}$ and $(1-\alpha) = \frac{m}{n}$. From this we obtain: $(d_m > d_n) \equiv f_n(\alpha\mu_{nm} + (1-\alpha)\mu_{mf}) < f_m \mu_{mf}$. After some simple rewriting and substitution of α by $\frac{m}{n}$ we obtain conditions on μ_{mf} : $(d_m > d_n) \equiv \mu_{nm} \frac{\frac{n}{m}-1}{\frac{f_m}{f_n}\frac{n}{m}-1} < \mu_{mf}$.

Consequences of $d_m > d_k$. By similar reasoning we can derive conditions on μ_{mf} from $(d_m > d_k)$. We obtain $(d_m > d_k) \equiv \mu_{mk} \frac{1-\frac{k}{m}}{1-\frac{f_m}{f_k}\frac{k}{m}} > \mu_{mf}$.

Combining results. From the consequences we obtained: $(d_m > d_n) \equiv \mu_{nm} \frac{\frac{n}{m}-1}{\frac{f_m}{f_n}\frac{n}{m}-1} < \mu_{mf}$ and $(d_m > d_k) \equiv \mu_{mk} \frac{1-\frac{k}{m}}{1-\frac{f_m}{f_k}\frac{k}{m}} > \mu_{mf}$. From the conditions on μ_{mf} and $d_m > d_n \wedge d_m > d_k$ it follows that $\mu_{nm} \frac{\frac{n}{m}-1}{\frac{f_m}{f_n}\frac{n}{m}-1} < \mu_{mk} \frac{1-\frac{k}{m}}{1-\frac{f_m}{f_k}\frac{k}{m}}$. Now we derive contradiction using $\mu_{nm} > \mu_{mk}$ and show that $\frac{\frac{n}{m}-1}{\frac{f_m}{f_n}\frac{n}{m}-1} > \frac{1-\frac{k}{m}}{1-\frac{f_m}{f_k}\frac{k}{m}}$. By some simple rewriting:

$$\frac{\frac{n}{m}-1}{\frac{f_m}{f_n}\frac{n}{m}-1} > \frac{1-\frac{m}{k}}{1-\frac{f_m}{f_k}\frac{k}{m}} = \frac{n-m}{\frac{n}{f_n}-\frac{m}{f_m}} > \frac{m-k}{\frac{m}{f_m}-\frac{k}{f_k}} = \frac{\frac{1}{\sigma_m}-\frac{1}{\sigma_k}}{m-k} > \frac{\frac{1}{\sigma_n}-\frac{1}{\sigma_m}}{n-m}$$

Because f is a monotonically increasing and concave function we have $f_n > f_m > f_k$ and $\sigma_n < \sigma_m < \sigma_k$ and $\frac{1}{\sigma_n} > \frac{1}{\sigma_m} > \frac{1}{\sigma_k}$.
By this,

$$\frac{n-m}{\frac{n}{f_n}-\frac{m}{f_m}} > \frac{m-k}{\frac{m}{f_m}-\frac{k}{f_k}} = \frac{\frac{1}{\sigma_m}-\frac{1}{\sigma_k}}{m-k} > \frac{\frac{1}{\sigma_n}-\frac{1}{\sigma_m}}{n-m} = \frac{g_m-g_k}{m-k} < \frac{g_n-g_m}{n-m},$$

where $g_i = \frac{1}{\sigma_i}$ and g is a monotonically increasing concave function. The fractions $\frac{g_m-g_k}{m-k}$ and $\frac{g_n-g_m}{n-m}$ are gradients Δ_{mk}, Δ_{nm} over intervals n, m and m, k. We obtain:

$$\frac{g_m-g_k}{m-k} < \frac{g_n-g_m}{n-m} = \Delta_{mk} > \Delta_{nm} = f'_{mk} > f'_{nm}$$

By the continuity of g and the application of the mean value theorem there exist points i, j for which $n < i < m$ and $m < j < k$ such that $f'(i) = \Delta_{nm}$

and $g'(j) = \Delta_{mk}$. Then by the concavity and monotonicity: $f'_{mk} > f'_{nm}$. From this it follows that $\frac{1-\frac{m}{n}}{\frac{I_m}{f_n}\frac{n}{m}-1} > \frac{1-\frac{k}{m}}{1-\frac{I_m}{f_k}\frac{k}{m}}$. Concluding, we showed that $\frac{1-\frac{m}{n}}{\frac{I_m}{f_n}\frac{n}{m}-1} >$ $\frac{1-\frac{k}{m}}{1-\frac{I_m}{f_k}\frac{k}{m}}$ and $\mu_{nm} > \mu_{mk}$ follows from negating statement 2. From this follows:

$F : \mu_{nm}\frac{1-\frac{m}{n}}{\frac{I_m}{f_n}\frac{n}{m}-1} > \mu_{mk}\frac{1-\frac{k}{m}}{1-\frac{I_m}{f_k}\frac{k}{m}}$. A consequence of $d_m > d_k$ and $d_m > d_n$ is

$\mu_{nm}\frac{1-\frac{m}{n}}{\frac{I_m}{f_n}\frac{n}{m}-1} < \mu_{mk}\frac{1-\frac{k}{m}}{1-\frac{I_m}{f_k}\frac{k}{m}}$ which contradicts F and proofs statement 2.

5   Example Applications of the MNM Statistic

In this section we show how two change detection algorithms and an algorithm for the maintenance of frequent item sets can be transformed into the maintenance of the MNM statistic. Furthermore effectiveness is investigated.

5.1   Example 1: Kolmogorov-Smirnov Two Sample Test

The Kolmogorov-Smirnov (KS) two sample non-parametric test, tests whether two samples are drawn from the same continuous distribution, and is independent of distribution. The KS-statistic is a function of the cumulative distribution of two samples. The maximum distance between the cumulative distribution functions of these two samples defines the KS D statistic.

The D statistic is normalized by the sizes of the two samples and transformed into a p-value using an asymptotic distribution. The test determines whether we can reject the hypothesis that the two samples are from the same distribution by comparison of the p-value with a user defined critical value.

In the context of data streams the test is used to compare two samples, namely a reference set, ref, and a sliding window, w. Every time a data point flows in, the sliding window is changed and the test is performed on the two samples to detect possible change in the underlying data distribution. When change is detected the reference set is refilled and the process is repeated.

The Kolmogorov statistic D is defined by:

$$D = \max_x | ecdf_{ref}(x) - ecdf_n(x) |, x \in (S_{ref} \bigcup S_w),$$

where x is element of the union of the reference set and the sliding window w. The empirical cumulative distribution function of a sample s is defined by: $ecdf(x) = \frac{1}{|s|}\sum_{i=1}^{|s|} \delta(x_i \leq x)$, where δ is the indicator function. The KS-statistic is normalized by a factor dependent on sizes $|ref|$ and $|w|$. In the case of a fixed window this factor is a constant and does not change the point of the maximum. However in the context of our flexible windowing, we want to maximize the normalized KS-statistic over all time windows and this complicates matters.

$$D_{norm} = \sqrt{\frac{|ref||w|}{(|ref| + |w|)}}D,$$

Note that in this context $|ref|$ is a constant and w variable.

We are interested in the $n - th$ most recent point that maximizes the normalized KS. The maximum is called F.

$$F = \max_w KS_{norm} \tag{1}$$

$$\approx \max_q \max_w \sqrt{\tfrac{|ref||w|}{(|ref|+|w|)}} \mid ecdf_{ref}(q) - ecdf_w(q) \mid, q \in Q \tag{2}$$

We approximate the KS statistic by restricting the maximization of D over a subset Q. When Q equals $(ref \cup w)$ the $\max_q \mid ecdf_{ref}(q) - ecdf_w(q) \mid$ equals the original D-statistic. Of course the larger Q the better the approximation. By fixing the set Q the functions $ecdf_{ref}$ and $ecdf_w$ are fixed. To maintain the F statistic we maintain two buffers for every $q \in Q$. One buffer for the maximization of a positive and one for a negative deviation. To calculated F we maximize for every q, the term 2 and maximize over all these maxima. Note that for the maximization of term 2 the term $c := ecdf_{ref}(q)$ is a constant, α_q. Furthermore the $ecdf_w$ at point q equals $\frac{1}{|w|} \sum_{i=1}^{|w|} \delta(x_i \le q)$. Then F can be reduced to:

$$F \approx \max_q \max_w f_w \mu_w,$$

where

$$f_w = \sqrt{\frac{|ref||w|}{(|ref| + |w|)}}, \mu_w = \frac{1}{|w|} \sum_{i=1}^{|w|} |\alpha_q - \delta(x_i \le q)|$$

As can be seen the F statistic uses the maximum normalized mean as a building block. To maintain F we maintain buffers for every q two buffer. Two buffers are used for every q to eliminate the abs function in $|\alpha_q - \delta(x_i \le q)|$.

Power Investigation 1. In this section we investigate the power of the approximation of the KS-statistic, by fixing the subset Q. The power of approximation is investigated by simulation of synthetic data and compared to the original KS-test, under different magnitude jumps in the mean and variation, the resolution of the approximation, thus the size of Q, and the size of the reference set.

Certainly, there are distributions constituting for the alternative hypothesis, for which the KS-test approaches 100% detections and the approximate KS-test 0%. This alternative distribution is created by a local deviation in density between two q-values. However this is no problem because of two reasons. Firstly, with a sufficient number of q-values the probability that the local deviation is exactly between two q-values goes to zero. Secondly, we are maybe not interested in very small local deviations.

The objective of the experiments is to give insight into the loss caused by the approximation. We experimented with jumps in the mean and variance of a normal distribution. Furthermore we investigated the power as a function of the resolution of the approximation and the size of the reference set. The q-values are selected using the equal probability principle based on the empirical distribution of the reference set. The false positive rate is set to 0.01.

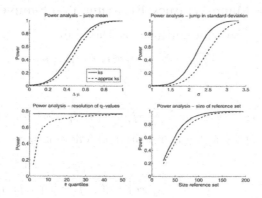

Fig. 1. Power analysis of the standard two sample KS-test and the approximate KS-test. In the top left corner the detection power is measured as a function of the magnitude of a jump in the mean of the standard normal distribution, $H_0 = N(0,1)$, $H_1 = N(0 + \Delta\mu, 1)$. In the top right figure is shown the power as a function of a jump in the variance of the standard normal distribution, $H_0 = N(0,1)$, $H_1 = N(0, 1 + \Delta\sigma)$. In the left bottom corner the power is shown as a function of the resolution of the q-values, $H_0 = N(0,1)$, $H_1 = N(0.5, 3)$. In the right bottom figure is shown the power as a function of the size of the reference window, $H_0 = N(0,1)$, $H_1 = N(.5, 2)$.

The results of the experiments are shown in figure 1. The approximation in top figures are based on 10 q-values. The left upper figure shows the power as a function of a jump in the mean. Clearly for a approximation of 10 q-values the power of the approximate KS-test and the standard KS-test is minimal. The bottom figures show in a increase in the power as a function of the number of q-values and the size of the reference set.

Power Investigation 2. In this section we give an example of the improvement obtained by maximizing the normalized KS statistic instead of using a fixed size sliding window. We compare the performance of the maximum normalized KS to sliding windows of fixed size. The number of q-values was 10, selected using equal frequency principle on the reference set of 100.

A data stream of size 200 is generated from of which the first half is generated from a standard normal distribution $N(0,1)$ and the second half by an alternate normal distribution $N(0.25, 1)$. The performance is measured by means of the false alarm rate, detection rate and the mean detection delay. In Table 1 is shown the false alarm rate per 100 data points as a function of the detection rate and the delay as a function of the false alarm rate for different change detection algorithms.

On the left top figure the detection power is approximately equal for all methods for all false alarm rates. On the right top figure we observe a shorter mean delay for the maximum normalized KS-test. The maximum normalized KS results in the lowest delay for all false alarm rates.

5.2 Example 2: Mann-Whitney Ranksum Two Sample Test

The Mann-Whitney ranksum statistic U is defined by,

$$U = \frac{\sum_{x_j \in w} \sum_{x_i \in ref} \delta(x_i < x_j) - \mu}{\sigma},$$

where

$$\mu = |ref||w|/2, \quad \sigma = \sqrt{|ref||w| \cdot (|ref| + |w| + 1)/12}$$

The normalized U statistic can be rewritten in following way:

$$U = \frac{\sum_{x \in w} \sum_{y \in ref} \delta(y < x) - \frac{|ref| \cdot |w|}{2}}{\sqrt{|ref||w|(|ref| + |w| + 1)/12}} =$$

$$= f_w \cdot \mu, f = \sqrt{\frac{|ref||w|}{(|ref| + |w| + 1)/12}}, \mu = \frac{1}{|w|} \sum_{|x \in w|} \{\alpha_x - 0.5\}$$

We have rewritten the U statistic as the normalized mean. Maximization of the U statistic over the time window is performed by maximization over the normalized mean, what our framework supports. We maintain two buffers for positive and negative deviation and maximize over the maximum 'distance' calculated over these buffers.

Power Investigation. The improvement of using the normalized Mann-Whitney statistic is shown in a same way as for the approximate KS-test. The maximized normalized Mann-Whitney is compared to sliding window algorithms. A data stream of size 200 is generated from of which the first half is generated from a standard normal distribution $N(0, 1)$ and the second half by an alternate normal distribution $N(0.25, 1)$. The performance is measured by means of the false alarm rate, detection rate and the mean detection delay. In Table 1 is shown the false alarm rate per 100 data points as a function of the detection rate and the delay as a function of the false alarm rate for different change detection algorithms.

On the left bottom figure the detection power is largest for the maximum normalized Mann-Whitney for all false alarm rates. The magnitude of the improvement is dependent on the choice of the expected false alarm and detection rate. A false alarm rate of 0.2 means a probability of 0.2 of observing a false alarm within 100 data points. On the right bottom figure we observe a shorter mean delay for the maximum normalized Mann-Whitney. The maximum normalized Mann-Whitney results in the lowest delay for all false alarm rates. This, despite of the increase of power. Usually, when detecting smaller deviations, which other methods miss, lowers the mean delay.

5.3 Example 3: Maximum Frequency

As mentioned earlier the translation of what is frequent in [4] is $\max_w f \mu_w$, where f is constant function. This interpretation can be embedded in the framework of the maximum normalized mean by setting f to for example $c + \sqrt{|w|}$,

Table 1. Left: the false alarm rate as a function of the detection rate. Right: the mean delay as a function of the false alarm rate for different change detection algorithms. The methods $w = 20$, $w = 30$, $w = 40$, $w = 50$ correspond to sliding window algorithms of size w. In the top figures max_d equals the maximum normalized approximate KS algorithm and the bottom the maximum normalized MW test.

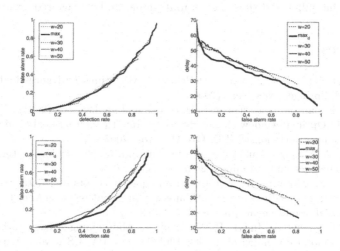

where constant $c \to \infty$. For further implementation of the use of the maximum frequency in the maintenance of frequent item sets we refer to [4].

5.4   Kolmogorov-Smirnov and Mann-Whitney

A constraint on the possibility of the maintenance of the maximum normalized mean is that the normalization function must be a positive monotonically increasing concave function for the positive real domain. In case of the Kolmogorov-Smirnov statistic the normalization function equals $\sqrt{\frac{|ref||w|}{|ref|+|w|}}$ and for Mann-Whitney it is equal to $\sqrt{\frac{|ref||w|}{(|ref|+|w|+1)/12)}}$. Both functions have negative second derivative functions and are monotonically increasing functions.

6   Conclusion and Future Work

We can conclude that the maximum normalized mean is an important statistic in certain data stream applications, where recognized applications are frequency estimation and change detection. It is shown that the maximum normalized mean can be efficiently maintained over data streams for a broad family of normalization functions. We further gave examples of using the maximum mean statistic in approximating the Kolmogorov-Smirnoff 'distance' as well the ranksum test and examples of improvements over sliding windows. Furthermore, in the case of the approximate KS-test, the balance is shown between the resolution which determines the approximation and the detection power gained by the optimal window size.

Future research will incorporate the search for more applications which can be translated in a similar way as the problems of the two-sample tests and frequent item sets. Furthermore is would be nice to have the theoretical guarantees on the size of the buffer and thus the computational and storage requirements.

References

1. Aggarwal, C.C.: Data Streams: Models and Algorithms (Advances in Database Systems). Springer, New York (2006)
2. Muthukrishnan, S.: Data streams: algorithms and applications (2003)
3. Patist, J.: Optimal window change detection. In: 7th International Conference on Data Mining - workshops. IEEE, Los Alamitos (2007)
4. Calders, T.: Mining frequent itemsets in a stream. In: Proceedings of the international conference on data mining 2007, pp. 83–92 (2007)
5. Manku, G.S., Motwani, R.: Approximate frequency counts over data streams. In: VLDB 2002: Proceedings of the 28th international conference on Very Large Data Bases, VLDB Endowment, pp. 346–357 (2002)
6. Datar, M., Gionis, A., Indyk, P., Motwani, R.: Maintaining stream statistics over sliding windows (extended abstract), Philadelphia, PA, USA, vol. 31, pp. 1794–1813. Society for Industrial and Applied Mathematics (2002)
7. Indyk, P.: Stable distributions, pseudorandom generators, embeddings, and data stream computation. J. ACM 53, 307–323 (2006)
8. Aggarwal, C.: A framework for diagnosing changes in evolving data streams. In: Sigkdd Explorations, vol. 3 (2003)
9. Page, E.: Continuous inspection schemes. In: Biometrika, vol. 41, pp. 100–115
10. Wald: Sequential analysis. John Wiley and Sons, New York (1947)
11. Basseville, M., Nikiforov, I.V.: Detection of Abrupt Changes: Theory and Application: Theory and application. Prentice Hall, Englewood Cliffs (1993)
12. Ho, S.S.: A martingale framework for concept change detection in time-varying data streams. In: Proc. 22nd International Conference on Machine Learning, pp. 321–327 (2005)
13. Krishnamurthy, B., Chen, Y.: Sketch-based change detection: Methods, evaluation, and applications. In: IMC 2003 (2003)
14. Muthukrishnan, S., Berg, E., Wu, Y.: Sequential change detection on data streams. In: 7th International Conference on Data Mining - workshops. IEEE, Los Alamitos (2007)
15. Ben-David, S., Gehrke, J., Kifer, D.: Detecting change in data streams. In: International Conference on Very Large Databases 2004, vol. 30, pp. 180–191 (2004)

Identification of Interface Residues Involved in Protein-Protein Interactions Using Naïve Bayes Classifier

Chishe Wang[1,2], Jiaxing Cheng[1], Shoubao Su[1], and Dongzhe Xu[3]

[1] Key Laboratory of Intelligent Computing & Signal Processing, Ministry of Education,
Anhui University, Hefei 230039, China
[2] Department of Computer Science and Technology, Chaohu College, Chaohu 238000, China
[3] Department of Mordern Mechanics,University of Science and Technology of China,
Hefei 230026, China
wyxcs@163.com

Abstract. The identification of interface residues involved in protein-protein interactions(PPIs) has broad application in rational drug design and metabolic etc. Here a Naïve Bayes classifier for PPIs prediction with features including protein sequence profile and residue accessible surface area was proposed. This method adequately used the character of Naïve Bayes classifier which assumed independence of the attributes given the class. Our test results on a diversity dataset made up of only hetero-complex proteins achieved 68.1% overall accuracy with a correlation coefficient of 0.201, 40.2% specificity and 49.9% sensitivity in identify interface residues as estimated by leave-one-out cross-validation. This result indicated that the method performed substantially better than chance (zero correlation). Examination of the predictions in the context of 3-dimensional structures of proteins demonstrated the effectiveness of this method in identifying protein-protein sites.

Keywords: Naïve Bayes classifier, Protein-protein interactions, Sequence profile, Residue accessible surface area.

1 Introduction

Protein-protein interactions play a pivotal role in biological systems such as disease-causing mutations often occur in protein interfaces. Interface prediction can thus directly contribute to the understanding of disease mechanisms and help the design of therapeutic agents. Interface site predict also has applications in DNA-binding sites, functional sites and protein docking [1]. Identification of protein-protein interaction sites and detection of specific amino acid residues that contribute to the specificity and strength of protein interactions have become a critical challenge in functional genomics.

Various experimental methods have been used to identify interface residues involved in protein-protein interactions [2,3,4]. But all of these experimental methods have a common disadvantage: laborious and time-consuming. Based on this reason, more and more computational methods are provided. These are main include two kinds of methods. At the level of individual residues, Asako Koike and Toshihisa Takagi [5], Jo-Lan Chung et al. [6] use SVM method, Changhui Yan et al. use a

C. Tang et al. (Eds.): ADMA 2008, LNAI 5139, pp. 207–216, 2008.
© Springer-Verlag Berlin Heidelberg 2008

two-stage classifier [7], Yanay Ofran and Burkhard Rost, Huiling Chen and Huan-Xiang Zhou use neural network method [8,9], Ming-Hui Li et al. use conditional random fields method [10] to predict interact residue. At the level of surface patches, James R. Bradford et al. use Bayesian network and SVM method to predict interact sites[11,12].

Among these methods, some use structure and sequence information of proteins and another only use sequence information. By now (January 10, 2008), it has 48,395 structures in Protein Data Bank(PDB) [13] while it only has 19585 protein-protein interact information in DIP database [14]. Base on this reason, computational methods that can identify interface residues are urgently needed and can be used to guide biologists to make specific experiments on proteins.

The Bayesian network method has been shown to be quite successful in bioinformatics [1]. The advantage of Bayesian network method is that it can process uncertain data efficiently. Especially, the naïve bayes classifier has high efficient in processing data which has independence each other. In this article, we put forward a naïve bayes classifier that identifies interface residues primarily on the basis of sequence profile and residue accessible surface area(ASA) at the level of individual residues. Each surface residue needs to be labeled as an interface residue or non-interface residue. The input to the naïve bayes classifier is ASA and profile which consists of 21 values. Each value of profile expresses a kind of residue's conservation frequency and ASA expresses the structure-derived information. Obviously, these 21 values have high independence each other. According this agreement between Naïve bayes classifier and these 21 values, we choose naïve bayes classifier to predict the protein-protein interact sites. Our test result denotes our method is an efficient method in this aspect.

2 Materials and Methods

2.1 Generation of the Data Set

Till now, no standard dataset can be chosen as standard dataset to predict protein-protein interface sites. Different methods have different dataset. Here we choose our training dataset from the set of 70 protein hetero-complexes used in the work of Chakabarti and Janin [15]. This dataset has eight kinds of proteins and also used by I. Res et al. [7,16].

Based on this dataset, we get our own dataset using a number of stringent filtering steps in order to make our dataset has more challenge. We remove the proteins whose resolution was >3.0Å and eliminated protein with fewer than 20 residues. Low sequence identity makes it more challenging than the sets which have high sequence according to article [16]. Two chains were considered to have high homology [6,17] if (1) over 90% of their sequence were matched and (2) the sequence identity over the matched region was greater than 25%. According to this criterion, we get our own dataset. This dataset include 90 protein chains in 57 protein complexes. All of this protein chains are list in the Table 1:

Table 1. Dataset of protein-protein hetero-complex

A. proteaseinhibitor complexes (19)				1BRS_A	1BRS_D	1DFJ_E	1DFJ_J
1AVW_E	1CHC_F	1CHC_G	1CSE_E	1DHK_A	1DHK_B	1FSS_A	1FSS_B
1CSE_I	1FLE_I	1HIA_A	1HIA_I	1GLA_F	1GLA_G	1UDI_E	1UDI_I
1MCT_I	1PPF_I	1STF_E	1STF_I	1YDR_E	2PCC_A	2PCC_B	
1TGS_I	2PTC_I	2SIC_I	2SNI_I	E . G- protein, cell cycle signal transduction complexes (18)			
3SGB_E	4CPA_A	4CPA_I		1ACO_A	1ACO_B	1A2K_A	1A2K_C
B . Large protease complexes (5)				1AGR_A	1AGR_E	1AIF_C	1EFU_A
1BTH_L	1DAN_L	1DAN_T	1DAN_U	1EFU_B	1FIN_A	1FIN_B	1GG2_B
4HTC_I				1GG2_G	1GOT_G	1GUA_A	1GUA_B
C. Antibodyantigen complexes (16)				1TX4_A	2TRC_P		
1AC7_A	1AC7_B	1AC7_D	1JHL_A	F .Miscellaneous complexes (17)			
1JHL_L	1KB5_B	1MEL_A	1NCA_N	1AK4_A	1AK4_C	1ATN_A	1ATN_D
1NFD_E	1NSN_L	1NSN_S	1OSP_O	1DKG_A	1DKG_D	1EFN_A	1EFN_B
1QFU_A	1QFU_B	1VFB_B	2JEL_P	1FC2_C	1FC2_D	1HWG_A	1HWG_B
D. Enzyme complexes (15)				1IGC_A	1SEB_D	1YCS_A	1YCS_B / 2BTF_P

2.2 Surface and Interface Residues Definitions

Interfaces are formed mostly by residues that are exposed to the solvent. Therefore, we focused on those residues with accessible surface areas above certain thresholds. Solvent exposure is separately computed for each chain, using the DSSP program [18]. Each complex is split in different files containing only the coordinates of a single chain.

If the ratio of the surface area of each residue to the nominal maximum area [19] exceeded a threshold, it was defined as a surface residue. This threshold is different in different article. We adopt 25% as our threshold according to Changhui Yan et al [7,17,20, 21].

According to the aforementioned criterion, we have 8266 surface residues from 90 proteins. Its percentage of the total 16325 residues is 50.63%. During these surface residues, I get 2476 interface residues, its percentage of the surface residues is 29.95%.

2.3 Character Vector

Interface prediction relies on characteristics of residues found in interfaces of protein complexes. The characteristics of interface residues are different. The most prominent involve: sequence conservation; proportions of the 20 types of amino acids; secondary structure; solvent accessibility; side-chain conformational entropy etc. Most of these characters are structure information. In this article, we choose sequence profile and residue accessible surface area as our test character. Profile is sequence information which denotes its potential structural homolog. Each residue is coded as a vector of 20 elements, whose values are taken from the corresponding frequencies in the multiple sequence alignment of the protein as extracted from the HSSP file [22]. Accessible surface area(ASA) feature represents the relative accessible surface area. ASA of each residue is calculated using DSSP program [18].

2.4 Naïve Bayes Classifier

We used the naïve Bayes classifier to address a binary classification problem: residues have to be classified as interacting ('positive' examples) or non-interacting('negative' examples). Each instance(residue) is described by an input vector of attributes.

Naïve bayes classifiers use a probabilistic approach to classify data: they try to compute conditional class probabilities and then predict the most probable class. Let C denote a class attribute with a finite domain of m class, let $A_1,..., A_n$ be a set of other attributes used to describe a case of an object of the universe of discourse, and let $a_{i_j}^{(j)}$ for a value of an attribute A_j. The Naïve Bayes classifier assumes independence of the attributes given the class. For a given instantiation ω, a naïve bayes classifier tries to compute the conditional probability

$$P(C = c_i \mid \omega) = P(C = c_i \mid A_1 = a_{i_1}^{(1)},..., A_n = a_{i_n}^{(n)})$$

For all c_i and then predicts the class for which this probability is highest. The implementation of the BN algorithm used here is the Christian Borgelt's package [23].

2.5 Performance Measures

The results reported in this work concern the evaluation of residue classification based on the following quantities: let TP is the number of true positives (residues predicted to be interface residues that actually are interface residues); FP the number of false positives (residues predicted to be interface residues that are in fact not interface residues); TN the number of true negatives; FN the number of false negatives; N=TP+TN+FP+FN(the total number of examples). Then we have:

$$Sensitivity^+ = \frac{TP}{TP + FN}, \text{ also called Recall}$$

$$Specificity^+ = \frac{TP}{TP + FP}, \text{ also called Precision}$$

$$Accuracy = \frac{TP + TN}{N},$$

$$CC = \frac{TP \times TN - FP \times FN}{\sqrt{(TP + FN)(TP + FP)(TN + FP)(TN + FN)}}$$

In brief, sensitivity is equal to the fraction of interface residues found, specificity equals the fraction of determined non-interface residues, accuracy is to measure the performance for labeling or classifying the whole test data set. Correlation coefficient(CC) is to measure the correlation between predictions and actual test data, which ranges from -1(perfect anti-correlation) to 1 (perfect correlation).

3 Experiments and Results

3.1 Cross-Validation

The naïve bayes classifier was trained to predict whether or not a surface residue is located in the interface based on the identity of the target residue and its sequence neighbors.

The effectiveness of the approach was evaluated using 90 leave-one-out cross validation (jack-knife) experiments. The fact that there are more non-interface residues than interface residues in the training set leads to higher precision and lower recall for many classifiers. To obtain a balanced training set from each chain that is to be used for training we extracted interacting residues and an equal number of randomly sampled non-interacting residues. We trained our classifier on profile and ASA feature of protein. In six kinds of protein hetero-complexes, we get test result listed in table 2.

Table 2. Test result in six kinds of protein hetero-complexes

Complexes type	Accuracy %	Sensitivity %	Specifity %	CC
Protease-inhibitor complexes	68.8	62.1	39.0	0.263
Large protease complexes	56.4	79.8	45.3	0.217
Antibody-antigen complexes	64.6	45.3	35.7	0.131
Enzyme complexes	73.0	41.0	37.4	0.192
G-protein,cell cycle,signal transduction complexes	69.1	52.3	42.1	0.221
Miscellaneous complexes	68.5	37.1	45.0	0.178

From this result, we find our classifier has good performance in diversity dataset. In 42% of the proteins, the classifier recognized the interaction surface by identifying at least half of the interface residues, and in 87% of the proteins, at least 20% of the interface residues were correctly identified.

According to the article, close neighbors of an interface reside have a high likelihood of being interface residues. The closer a sequence neighbor is to an interface residue, the greater is its likelihood of being an interface residue. When the distance increases to 16 residues, the likelihood drops to 0. The observation that the interface residues tend to form clusters on the primary sequence suggests the possibility of detecting protein-protein interface residues from local sequence information. So we test our dataset on different window. Sizes between 3 and 9 were tested and all of these test results are listed in Table 3.

Table 3. Test result on different window size

	Accuracy %	Sensitivity %	Specifity %	CC
Profile*	68.1	49.9	40.2	0.201
Profile(3)	64.6	44.0	35.4	0.131
Profile(5)	62.9	42.5	39.1	0.116
Profile(7)	61.7	41.7	41.2	0.105
Profile(9)	61.3	41.6	42.7	0.104

From this result, we can see when we use different window sizes the result change a little. This performance also denotes our classifier is superior in independence character but turn bad when this independence is changed.

3.2 Comparison with Other Studies

Comparison with other methods is difficult because of the variety of data sets used and the difference in definitions of interface and surface residues.

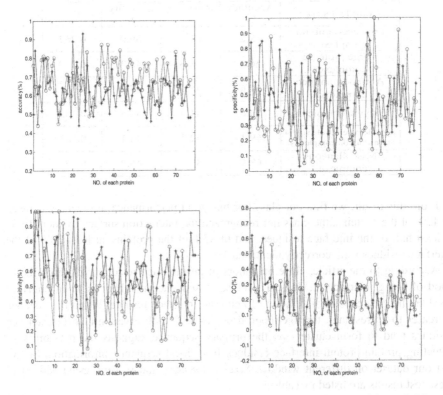

Fig. 1. Compare with Changhui Yan's result in accuracy, specificity,sensitivity and CC

Changhui Yan's research [24] also use the dataset which was chosen from the set of 70 protein hetero-complexes used in the work of Chakabarti and Janin. It has 115 proteins and we have 90 proteins. They use SVM method to predict the interact sites and use the resemble method to define the character of proteins. In order to compare, we choose the same 77 proteins from this two dataset. It has average 68% accuracy in our dataset and 62% accuracy in Changhui Yan's dataset with 46.7 to 40.2 in specificity, 58.9 to 49.9 in sensitivity, 0.215 to 0.201 in CC. All of these 77 proteins are listed in Figure 1.

In these four figs, red denotes our test result while blue denotes Changhui Yan's research. Obviously these two method have resemble result in 77 proteins. Especifially in accuracy our result 6% higher than SVM method in average and 53 proteins(69% in all) are higher than SVM method. This also proved our method's validity.

3.3 Some Predicted Examples

Here we give some examples that are predicted by naive bayes classifier trained on trimed dataset. The first example is the refined 2.4 angstroms x-ray crystal structure of recombinant human stefin b in complex with the cysteine proteinase papain [25]. We use our classifier predict 9 residues to be interface with 75% sensitivity and 53% specificity(Fig. 2b) while the actual interface residues is 17(Fig. 2a).

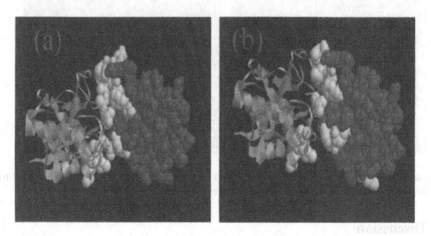

Fig. 2. Predicted interface residue (yellow color) on protein(PDB code 1STF_I) identified by (a) the actual interface residues (b) the naive bayes classifier

The second example is refined crystal structure of the potato inhibitor complex [26]. We use our classifier predict 14 residues to be interface with 82% sensitivity and 88% specificity(Fig. 3b) while the actual interface residues is 16(Fig. 3a).

The last example given by us is crystallographic refinement and atomic models of a human fc fragment and its complex [27]. We use our classifier predict 7 residues to be interface with 50% sensitivity and 58% specificity(Fig.4a) while the actual interface residues in 12(Fig. 4b).

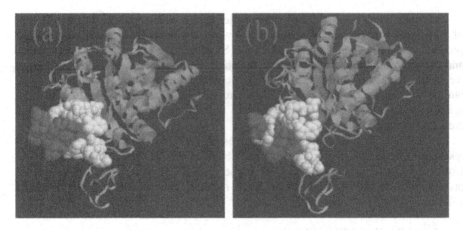

Fig. 3. Predicted interface residue (yellow color) on protein(PDB code 4CPA_I) identified by (a) the actual interface residues (b) the naive bayes classifier

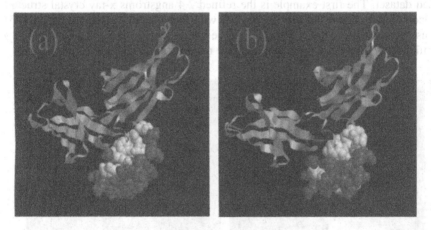

Fig. 4. Predicted interface residue(yellow color) on protein(PDB code 1FC2_C) identified by (a) the actual interface residues (b) the naïve bayes classifier

4   Discussion

Interface prediction has become more and more successful. The predicted interface residues can be directly used to guide experimental studies. For example, they may direct experimental efforts toward a particular region on a protein surface in studying its interactions with another protein. They may also be used to help solve the docking problem by vastly reducing the amount of configurational space needed to be searched to build a stuctural model for the protein complex.

In this study, we select naive bayes classifier as our predictor to predict protein-protein interact sites. This method use profile of protein and ASA as input vector. Because each value of profile denote a kind of residue's conservation, it has high independence each other. The ASA of each residue is structure character of protein while profile is squence character of protein. Obviously, these two character has high independence too. It is agree with the naive bayes's independence of the attributes. Our test result validates this feature. But we also know not only the target residue has influnce the result alone, the neighbour residues of each target residue also have important influnce in the result. Our test result proved the naive bayes can not solve this problem efficiently. The TAN(Tree Augmented Naive Bayes Classifier) maybe solve this problem efficiently. Of course, choose diffient characters of each protein also have influnce in the predicted result. Moreover, analysis of the binding site "rules" generated by classifiers may provide valuable insight into the protein-protein interact sites recognition.

Acknowledgments

This work was supported partially by the Projects of Provincial Natural Scientific Fund from the Bureau of Education of AnHui Province(Nos. KJ2007B066, KJ2007A087, KJ2008B38ZC) and the Science and Research Fund from the Bureau of Anhui Province for young teachers(No. 2007jql140).

References

1. Zhou, H.-X., Qin, S.: Interaction-site prediction for protein complexes: a critical assessment. Bioinformatics 23(17), 2203–2209 (2007)
2. Ben-Shem, A., Frolow, F., Nelson, N.: Crystal structure of plant photosystem I. Nature 426, 630–635 (2003)
3. Lanman, J., Lam, T.T., Bames, S., Sakalian, M., Emmett, M.R., Marshall, A.G., Prevelige, J., Peter, E.: Identification of novel interactions in HIV-1 capsid protein assembly by high-resolution mass Spectrometry. J. Mol. Biol. 325, 759–772 (2003)
4. Trester-Zedlitz, M., Kamada, K., Burley, S.K., Fenyo, D., Chait, B.T., Muir, T.W.: A modular cross-linking approach for exploring protein interactions. J. Am. Chem. Soc. 125, 2416–2425 (2003)
5. Koike, A., Takagi, T.: Prediction of protein-protein interaction sites using support vector machines. Protein Engineering, Design & Selection 17(2), 165–173 (2004)
6. Chung, J.-L., Wang, W., Bourne, P.E.: Exploiting sequence and structure homologs to identify protein-protein binding sites. PROTEINS:Structure, Function, and Bioinformatics 62, 630–640 (2006)
7. Yan, C., Dobbs, D., Honavar, V.: A two-stage classifier for identification of protein-protein interface residues. Bioinformatics 20 (suppl. 1), i371-i378 (2004)
8. Ofran, Y., Rost, B.: Predicted protein-protein interaction sites from local sequence information. FEBS Letters 544, 236–239 (2003)
9. Chen, H., Zhou, H.-X.: Prediction of Interface residues in protein-protein complexes by a consensus neural network method: test against NMR data. PROTEINS: Structure, Function, and Bioinformatics 61, 21–35 (2005)
10. LI, M.-H., Lin, L., Wang, X.-L., Liu, T.: Protein-protein interaction site prediction based on conditional random fields. Bioinformatics 23(5), 597–604 (2007)
11. James, R., Bradford, C.J., Needham, A.J., Bulpitt, D.R.: Westhead: Insights into protein-protein interfaces using a Bayesian network prediction method. J. Mol. Biol. 362, 365–386 (2006)

12. Bradford, J.R., Westhead, D.R.: Improved prediction of protein-protein binding sites using a support vector machines approach. Bioinformatics 21(8), 1487–1494 (2005)
13. Berman, H.M., Westbrook, J., Feng, Z., Gilliland, G., Bhat, T.N., Weissig, H., Shindyalov, I.N., Bourne, P.E.: The Protein Data Bank. Nucleic Acids Res. 28, 235–242 (2000)
14. Xennarios, I., Salwinski, L., Duan, X.J., Higney, P., Kim, S., Eisenberg, D.: DIP: The Database of Interacting Proteins. A research tool for studying cellular networks of protein interactions. Nucleic Acids Res. 30, 303–305 (2002)
15. Chakrabarti, P., Janin, J.: Dissecting protein-protein recognition sites. PROTEINS: Structure, Function, and Genetics 47, 334–343 (2002)
16. Res, I., Mihalek, I., Lichtarge, O.: An evolution based classifier for prediction of protein interfaces without using protein structures. Bioinformatics 21(10), 2496–2501 (2005)
17. Dong, Q., Wang, X., Lin, L., Guan, Y.: Exploiting residue-level and profile-level interface propensities for usage in binding sites prediction of proteins. BMC Bioinformatics 8(147), 1–13 (2007)
18. Kabsch, W., Sander, C.: Dictionary of protein secondary structure: pattern of hydrogen-bonded and geometrical features. Biopolymers 22, 2577–2637 (1983)
19. Rost, B., Sander, C.: Conservation and prediction of solvent accessibility in protein families. PROTEINS: Structure, Function, and Genetics 20, 216–226 (1994)
20. Jones, S., Thornton, J.M.: Principles of protein-protein interactions. Proc. Natl. Acad. Sci. USA 93, 13–20 (1996)
21. Yan, C., Honavar, V., Dobbs, D.: Identification of interface residues in protease-inhibitor and antigen-antibody complexes: a support vector machine approach. Neural Comput. & Applic. 13, 123–129 (2004)
22. Dodge, C., Schneider, R., Sander, C.: The HSSP database of protein structure-sequence alignments and family profiles. Nucleic Acids Res. 26, 313–315 (1998)
23. Christian Borgelt's Webpages, http://www.borgelt.net//bayes.html
24. Honavar, V., Yan, C., Dobbs, D.: Predicting protein-protein interaction sites from amino acid sequence. Technical report ISU-CS-TR 02-11, Department of Computer Science, Iowa State University, pp. 2–11 (2002), http://archives.cs.iastate.edu/documents/disk0/00/00/02/88/index.html
25. Stubbs, M.T., Laber, B., Bode, W., Huber, R., Jerala, R., Lenarcic, B., Turk, V.: The refined 2.4 A X-ray crystal structure of recombinant human stefin B in complex with the cysteine proteinase papain: a novel type of proteinase inhibitor interaction. EMBO J. 9, 1939–1947 (1990)
26. Rees, D.C., Lipscomb, W.N.: Refined crystal structure of the potato inhibitor complex of carboxypeptidase A at 2.5 A resolution. J. Mol. Biol. 160, 475–498 (1982)
27. Deisenhofer, J.: Crystallographic refinement and atomic models of a human Fc fragment and its complex with fragment B of protein A from Staphylococcus aureus at 2.9- and 2.8-A resolution. Biochemistry 20, 2361–2370 (1981)

Negative Generator Border for Effective Pattern Maintenance

Mengling Feng,[1] Jinyan Li,[1] Limsoon Wong[2], and Yap-Peng Tan[1]

[1] Nanyang Technological University
[2] National University of Singapore
{feng0010,jyli,eyptan}@ntu.edu.sg, wongls@comp.nus.edu.sg

Abstract. In this paper, we study the maintenance of frequent patterns in the context of the generator representation. The generator representation is a concise and lossless representation of frequent patterns. We effectively maintain the generator representation by systematically expanding its *Negative Generator Border*. In the literature, very few work has addressed the maintenance of the generator representation. To illustrate the proposed maintenance idea, a new algorithm is developed to maintain the generator representation for support threshold adjustment. Our experimental results show that the proposed algorithm is significantly faster than other state-of-the-art algorithms. This proposed maintenance idea can also be extended to other representations of frequent patterns as demonstrated in this paper [1].

1 Introduction

Frequent patterns, also called frequent itemsets, refer to patterns that appear frequently in a particular dataset [1]. The discovery of frequent patterns can be formally defined as follows. Let $\mathcal{I} = \{i_1, i_2, ..., i_m\}$ be a set of distinct literals called "items", and also let $\mathcal{D} = \{t_1, t_2, ..., t_n\}$ be a transactional "dataset", where t_i ($i \in [1, n]$) is a "transaction" that contains a non-empty set of items. Each subset of $\mathcal{I}$ is called a "pattern" or an "itemset". The "support" of a pattern P in a dataset $\mathcal{D}$ is defined as $sup(P, \mathcal{D}) = |\{t | t \in \mathcal{D} \wedge P \subseteq t\}|$. A pattern P is said to be *frequent* in a dataset $\mathcal{D}$ if $sup(P, \mathcal{D})$ is greater than or equal to a pre-specified support threshold ms. The support threshold, ms, can also be defined in terms of percentage, in which a pattern P is said to be *frequent* in a dataset $\mathcal{D}$ if $sup(P, \mathcal{D}) \geq ms \times |\mathcal{D}|$. The collection of all frequent patterns in $\mathcal{D}$ is called the "space of frequent patterns" and is denoted as $\mathcal{F}(\mathcal{D}, ms)$. The task of frequent pattern discovery is to find all the patterns in $\mathcal{F}(\mathcal{D}, ms)$. Figure 1 shows an example of transactional dataset and the corresponding frequent pattern space when $ms = 1$.

Datasets are dynamic in nature. From time to time, new transactions/items may be inserted; old and invalid transactions/items may be removed; and the

---

[1] This work is partially supported by an A*STAR SERC PSF grant, a MOE AcRF Tier 1 grant, and an A*STAR AGS scholarship.

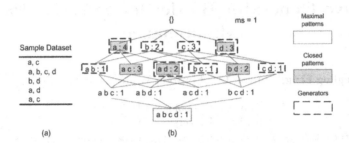

Fig. 1. (a) An example of transactional dataset. (b) The pattern space of the sample dataset in (a), and the concise representations of the pattern space.

support threshold may be adjusted to obtain the desirable sets of frequent patterns. Repeating the discovery process every time the dataset is updated is a naive and definitely inefficient solution. Thus, there is a strong demand for effective algorithms to maintain frequent patterns for data updates and support threshold adjustment.

Most of the current maintenance algorithms can be grouped into two major categories: *Apriori*-based and sliding window filtering *(SWF)*. Both the *Apriori*-based and *SWF* approaches are developed based on the candidate-enumeration-and-elimination framework. *Apriori*-based algorithms [2, 6] enumerate new candidates iteratively based on the *a priori* property. *SWF* algorithms [5, 11] slice a dataset into several partitions and then employ a filtering threshold in each partition to generate candidate patterns. The *Apriori*-based algorithms and *SWF* algorithms aim to update and maintain the entire frequent pattern space. However, the undesirable large number of frequent patterns greatly limits their performance. To break the bottleneck, concise representations of frequent patterns, more importantly, efficient maintenance of the concise representations are highly desired. In this paper, we focus our investigation on the maintenance of the generator representation [14] — a concise and lossless [2] representation of frequent patterns.

In the literature, algorithms have been proposed to maintain two types of concise representations under some unfavorable restrictions. Moment [7] is one example. Moment dynamically maintains the frequent closed patterns [14]. However, Moment is proposed on the hypothesis that there are only *small changes* to the frequent closed patterns given a small amount of updates. Due to this strict constraint, the performance of Moment degrades dramatically when the amount of updates gets large. ZIGZAG [16] is another example, which effectively maintains the maximal patterns [3]. ZIGZAG updates the maximal patterns by a backtracking search, which is guided by the outcomes of the previous maintenance iteration. Although the maximal patterns can concisely represent frequent patterns, they do not provide support information for other frequent patterns.

---

[2] We say a representation is lossless if it is sufficient to derive and determine the support of all frequent patterns without accessing the datasets.

That is, the maximal pattern is a lossy representation. In this work, unlike ZIGZAG for the maximal patterns, our maintenance algorithm is for a lossless representation; unlike Moment which bears some unfavorable assumptions, our maintenance algorithm aims to handle wide range of changes efficiently.

We propose to maintain the generator representation by expanding the *Negative Generator Border*. The expansion of the negative generator border is guided by a systematic technique, which ensures the expansion is complete and yet involves no redundancy. To better illustrate the idea, we focus on the update scenario where the support threshold is adjusted. A novel algorithm — Support Threshold Update Maintainer (STUM) — is proposed. Although support thresholds can be defined in terms of either counts or percentages, (STUM) applies to both definitions. We further show that the proposed maintenance idea can be extended to other concise representations that share common characteristics with the generator representation.

2 Generators and Negative Generator Border: A Concise Representation

The concept of **generator**, also known as the **key pattern**, is first introduced in [14]. The generators, together with the close patterns and maximal patterns, are commonly used concise representations of the frequent pattern space. Figure 1 (b) demonstrates how these representations are applied to the frequent pattern space of the sample dataset in Figure 1 (a). Other types of frequent pattern representations are also available such as the free-sets [4] and the disjunctive-free sets [10]. But the support inference by these representations is very complicated. Details of these representations can be found in the Appendix (http://www.ntu.edu.sg/home5/feng0010/appendix.pdf).

To effectively maintain the frequent patterns, we propose to represent the space of frequent patterns with both the frequent generators and the negative generator border. For ease of discussion, this representation is referred as *the generator representation* for the rest of the paper.

Definition 1 (Generator). *Given a dataset $\mathcal{D}$ and support threshold ms, a pattern P is a "generator" iff for every $P' \subset P$, it is the case that $sup(P', \mathcal{D}) > sup(P, \mathcal{D})$; and a pattern P is a frequent "generator" iff P is a "generator" and $sup(P, \mathcal{D}) \geq ms$.*

For a dataset $\mathcal{D}$ and support threshold ms, the set of frequent generators, $\mathcal{FG}(\mathcal{D}, ms)$, includes all generators that are frequent. On the other hand, the **negative generator border**, $NBd(\mathcal{FG}(\mathcal{D}, ms))$, refers to the set of the minimal infrequent generators, and it is formally defined as:

Definition 2 (Negative Generator Border). *Given a dataset $\mathcal{D}$ and support threshold ms, $NBd(\mathcal{FG}(\mathcal{D}, ms)) = \{G | G \notin \mathcal{FG}(\mathcal{D}, ms) \wedge (\forall G' \subset G, G' \in \mathcal{FG}(\mathcal{D}, ms))\}$.*

Generators in the negative generator border are named **negative border generators**. For a dataset $\mathcal{D}$ and support threshold ms, the generator representation includes: the set of frequent generators, $\mathcal{FG}(\mathcal{D}, ms)$, the negative generator border, $NBd(\mathcal{FG}(\mathcal{D}, ms))$, and their corresponding support values. Following Definition 1,2 and the *a priori* property of frequent patterns, we have the following corollary.

Corollary 1. *Given a dataset $\mathcal{D}$ and support threshold ms, (1) a pattern P is infrequent iff $\exists G | P \supseteq G \wedge G \in NBd(\mathcal{FG}(\mathcal{D}, ms))$; (2) a pattern P is frequent iff $\nexists G | P \supseteq G \wedge G \in NBd(\mathcal{FG}(\mathcal{D}, ms))$; and (3) for any frequent pattern P, $sup(P, \mathcal{D}) = min\{sup(G, \mathcal{D}) | G \subseteq P, G \in \mathcal{FG}(\mathcal{D}, ms)\}$.*

Corollary 1 implies that the generator representation is sufficient to determine all frequent patterns and their support values. Therefore, the generator representation is a lossless concise representation. We also observe that generators follow the *a priori* property as stated in FACT 3. When datasets are updated, the *a priori* characteristic of generators allows us to effectively enumerate newly emerged generators from the negative generator border. The negative generator border acts conveniently as a start point for us to resume the pattern enumerations.

Fact 3 (Cf. [12]). *Let P be a pattern in $\mathcal{D}$. If P is a generator, then every subset of P is also a generator in $\mathcal{D}$. Furthermore, if P is a frequent generator, then every subset of P is also a frequent generator in $\mathcal{D}$.*

Another advantage of the generator representation is that it can derive maximal patterns and closed patterns easily. One can derive frequent closed patterns from the frequent generators with the "closure" operation [14]. For a particular generator G, the "closure" operation is to find the maximal pattern C such that C and G always appear together in the dataset. Li. et al [12] have proposed some efficient techniques to conduct the "closure" operation. For frequent maximal patterns, they are basically the longest frequent closed patterns. Therefore, following the similar procedure as the derivation of closed patterns, one can also derive frequent maximal patterns easily from the frequent generators.

By concisely representing the frequent patterns using the generator representation, we greatly reduce the number of involved patterns and thus the complexity of the frequent pattern maintenance problem. Instead of maintaining the large number of frequent patterns, we only need to maintain the generators and the negative generator border. Moreover, the *a priori* characteristic of generators allows us to generate new generators and update the negative generator border effectively by expanding the exiting border.

3   Negative Generator Border in Pattern Maintenance

We investigate in this section how the concept of negative generator border can be employed to facilitate the maintenance of the generator representation. We focus on the update scenario where the support threshold is adjusted. We also introduce systematic enumeration data structure and techniques to ensure the maintenance process with the negative generator border is complete and efficient. It is also discovered that the proposed maintenance idea can be generalized to other more complicated representations of frequent patterns, e.q. the free-sets [4] and the disjunctive-free sets [10].

3.1 Support Threshold Adjustment Maintenance

Setting the right support threshold is crucial in frequent pattern mining. Inadequate support threshold may produce too few patterns to be meaningful or too many to be processed. It is unlikely to set the appropriate threshold at the first time. Thus the support threshold is often adjusted to obtain desirable knowledge. Moreover, in the case where the support threshold ms is defined in terms of percentage, data updates, such as transaction insertion and deletion, also induce changes in the absolute support threshold. Transaction insertions cause increases in the data size $|\mathcal{D}|$ and thus increases in the absolute support threshold, which is calculated as $ms \times |\mathcal{D}|$. Likewise, transaction deletions lead to decreases in the absolute support threshold.

When the support threshold increases, some existing frequent generators become infrequent, and the frequent pattern space shrinks. The generator representation of frequent patterns can be maintained by removing the existing generators that are no longer frequent and reconstructing the negative generator border with the minimal patterns among the newly infrequent generators and the original negative border generators. The maintenance process is quite straightforward, and thus it is not the focus of this paper and will be omitted for the subsequent discussion.

When the threshold decreases, new frequent generators may emerge, and the frequent pattern space expands. In this case, the maintenance problem becomes more challenging, as little is known about the newly emerged generators. We resolve this challenge efficiently based on the concept of negative generator border.

Negative Generator Border. is defined based on the the idea of *negative border*. The notion of negative border is first introduced in [13]. The negative border of frequent patterns refers to the set of minimal infrequent patterns. Maintenance algorithm **Border** [2] is proposed based on the idea of negative border. In **Border**, newly emerged frequent patterns are enumerated level-by-level from the negative border. However, **Border** aims to maintain the whole set of frequent patterns and thus suffers from the tremendous size of frequent patterns.

On the other hand, the negative generator border, as formally defined in Definition 2, refers to the set of minimal infrequent generators. The negative generator border records the nodes, where the previous enumeration of generator stops, as shown in Figure 2 (b). It thus serves as a convenient starting point for further enumeration of newly emerged generators when the support threshold decreases.

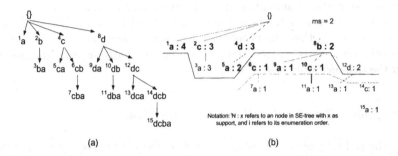

(a)   (b)

Fig. 2. (a)A set-enumeration tree of items $\{a, b, c, d\}$ with ordering $d <_0 c <_0 b <_0 a$. (b)The set-enumeration tree for the sample dataset with suppose threshold $ms = 2$; the solid line separates the frequent patterns from the infrequent ones; the patterns in bold form the generator representation; and the generators between the solid and the dotted lines form the negative generator border

This allows us to utilize previously obtained information to avoid redundant generation of existing generator and enumeration of unnecessary candidates.

Proposition 1. *Given a dataset $\mathcal{D}$ and a support threshold ms, let $\mathcal{FG}(\mathcal{D}, ms)$ denote the set of frequent generators and $NBd(\mathcal{FG}(\mathcal{D}, ms))$ be the corresponding negative generator border. Suppose the support threshold is adjusted to ms_{upd}, where $ms_{upd} < ms$. For every newly emerged generator G ($G \notin \mathcal{FG}(\mathcal{D}, ms) \wedge G \in \mathcal{FG}(\mathcal{D}, ms_{upd})$), there exists $G' \in NBd(\mathcal{FG}(\mathcal{D}, ms))$ and $G'' \in NBd(\mathcal{FG}(\mathcal{D}, ms_{upd}))$ such that $G' \subseteq G \subseteq G''$.*

Proof. The proposition can be proven easily based on the a priori *property of generators, and thus it is not included here.*

Proposition 1 shows that, when the support threshold decreases, every newly emerged generator falls in between the original and the updated negative generator border. This implies that all newly emerged generators can be generated without extra overhead, as we enumerate the updated negative generator border from the original border. This further simplifies the maintenance task to the update of the negative generator border.

We update the negative generator border based on the candidate-enumeration-elimination framework. Candidates of new frequent generators and border generators are enumerated iteratively based on the a priori characteristic of generators. Thus the next question is: how we can efficiently enumerate candidates?

Systematic Pattern Enumeration. method is the answer to this question. In this paper, we employ the "Set-enumeration Tree" [15], a conceptual data structure, to facilitate the candidate enumeration for the update of the negative generator border.

Let the set $I = \{i_1, ..., i_m\}$ of items be ordered according to an arbitrary ordering $<_0$ so that $i_1 <_0 i_2 <_0 \cdots <_0 i_m$. For itemsets $X, Y \subseteq I$, we write

$X <_0 Y$ iff X is lexicographically "before" Y according to the order $<_0$. We say an itemset X is a "prefix" of an itemset Y iff $X \subseteq Y$ and $X <_0 Y$. We write $last(X)$ for the item $\alpha \in X$, if the items in X are $\alpha_1 <_0 \alpha_2 <_0 \cdots <_0 \alpha$. We say an itemset X is the "precedent" of an itemset Y iff $X = Y - last(Y)$.

A set-enumeration tree (SE-$Tree$) is a conceptual organization on the subsets of I so that $\{\}$ is its root node; for each node X such that $Y_1, ..., Y_k$ are all its children from right to left, then $Y_1 <_0 \cdots <_0 Y_k$; for each node X in the set-enumeration tree such that $X_1, ..., X_k$ are siblings to its left, we make $X \cup X_1, ..., X \cup X_k$ the children of X; $|X \cup X_i| = |X| + 1 = |X_i| + 1$; and $|X| = |X_i| = |X \cap X_i| + 1$.

We also induce an enumeration ordering on the nodes of this SE-$Tree$ so that given two nodes X and Y, we say $X <_1 Y$ iff X would be visited before Y when we visit the set-enumeration tree in a left-to-right top-down manner. Since this visit order is a bit unusual, we illustrate it in Figure 2 (a). Here, the number besides the node indicates the time at which the node is visited. Note that; although SE-$tree$ is defined with an arbitrary item order $<_0$, to reduce the number of nodes to be generated and visited in the SE-$tree$ and thus the time complexity of the enumeration, we, as shown in Figure2 (b), organize items in ascending frequency order.

As shown in Figure 2, the SE-$tree$ not only effectively ensures that the enumeration of the new frequent generators and the negative border generators is complete. The SE-$tree$ also provides an efficient way to enumerate patterns, in which no repeated enumerations and thus redundancy are involved. Take the node "^6c" in Figure 2 (b) as an example. Suppose the corresponding negative border generator of node "^6c" — $\{c, d\}$ — becomes frequent after the support threshold adjustment. Node "^6c" now acts as a starting point for further enumeration of the newly emerged frequent generators. From Figure 2 (b), it can been seen that node "^6c" has only one sibling node on its left — node "^5a". Therefore, according to the SE-$tree$ enumeration order, we conveniently know that only one candidate pattern $\{a, c, d\}$ are required to be enumerated from node "^6c". Furthermore, we are also sure that the pattern $\{a, c, d\}$ will not be enumerated again from any other nodes.

Another advantage of SE-$tree$ is that: for every pattern P, all its subsets are enumerated before it. Together with FACT 3, this allows us to judge whether any pattern P is a generator as P is enumerated. Take pattern $\{a, c, d\}$ in Figure 2 (b) as an example. As shown, all subsets of $\{a, c, d\}$, including $\{a\}$, $\{c\}$, $\{d\}$, $\{a, c\}$, $\{a, d\}$ and $\{c, d\}$, are enumerated before $\{a, c, d\}$. When $\{a, c, d\}$ is enumerated, we can decide immediately that it is not a generator, since one of its subset, $\{a, c\}$, is not a generator. In addition, the SE-$tree$ can also serve as an efficient storage structure for the generator representation, as shown in Figure 2 (b).

Combining the above findings, a novel algorithm is proposed to maintain the generator representation of frequent patterns for support threshold adjustment. The proposed algorithm is named as the "Support Threshold Update Maintainer" (STUM), and it is discussed in Section 4.

Algorithm 1. Proposed algorithm STUM

Input: $\mathcal{N} = \{G_1, G_2, ..., G_m\}$, the negative generator border, where $G_1 >_0 G_2 >_0 ... >_0 G_m$; $\mathcal{FG}$, the existing frequent generators; and ms', the new support threshold.
Output: $\mathcal{FG}'$ the updated frequent generators; and $\mathcal{N}'$ the updated negative generator border.
Method:
1: $\mathcal{FG}' := \mathcal{FG}$; {Initialization.}
2: **for all** $G_i \in \mathcal{N}$ **do**
3:　　ExpandNBGenerator(G_i, ms');
　　　{Expand from the negative border generators.}
4: **end for**
5: **return** $\mathcal{FG}'$ and $\mathcal{N}'$;

3.2 Generalization and Extension

It is discovered that the proposed maintenance method can be generalized to other types of frequent pattern representations. This holds true as far as the representation follows the following characteristics:

- the representation is composed with both the frequent representation patterns (e.q. frequent generators) and its corresponding negative border (e.q. negative generator border), and
- the representation pattern follows the *a priori* property.

Among previously proposed frequent pattern representations, the free-sets [4] and the disjunctive-free sets [10] are two examples that follow the above characteristics. The detailed definitions of these two representations are included in the Appendix (http://www.ntu.edu.sg/home5/feng0010/appendix.pdf).

4 Support Threshold Update Maintainer (STUM)

The proposed maintenance algorithm, STUM, is presented in Algorithm 1 and Procedure 2. When the support threshold decreases, some negative border generators emerge to be frequent. We treat these border generators as starting points. The basic idea of STUM is to expand the frequent pattern space from these starting points. For a particular negative border generator G, the expand process is to enumerate new frequent generators from G. The enumeration follows the enumeration order of *SE-tree*, which ensures to be complete and efficient.

4.1 Complexity Analysis

According to Algorithm 1 and Procedure 2, the time complexity of STUM is proportional to the number of candidates enumerated during the generation of newly emerged frequent generators. Thus the complexity of the proposed algorithm can be modelled as $O(N_{GenCan})$, where N_{GenCan} refers to the number of enumerated generator candidates. According to the complexity study, we foresee that STUM is more efficient than some of the previous algorithms, such as Border [2]. The computational complexity of Border is $O(N_{FreqCan})$, where $N_{FreqCan}$ refers to the number of candidates enumerated during the generation of newly emerged frequent patterns. In general, $N_{GenCan} \ll N_{FreqCan}$, as shown in Table 1.

Procedure 2. ExpandNBGenerator

Input: G, a negative border generator or a newly emerged frequent generator; ms', the new support threshold.
Output: $\mathcal{FG}'$ the updated frequent generators; and $\mathcal{N}'$ the updated negative generator border.
Method:
1: **if** $sup(G) >= ms'$ **then**
2:     $G \rightarrow \mathcal{FG}'$ {Newly emerged generator}
       {Enumerate new generators from G}
3:     **for all** $i >_0 last(G)$ **do**
4:       $G' := G \cup i$;
5:       **if** G' is a generator **then**
6:          ExpandNBGenerator(G', ms')
7:       **end if**
8:     **end for**
9: **else**
10:     $G \rightarrow \mathcal{N}'$ {Update negative generator border.}
11: **end if**
12: **return** $\mathcal{FG}'$ and $\mathcal{N}'$;

Table 1. Approximate number of enumerated candidates by STUM and Border when the support threshold is adjusted to half of the original one. Here ms denotes the original support threshold.

	accidents $ms = 50\%$	gazelle $ms = 0.5\%$	mushroom $ms = 0.5\%$	T10I4D100K $ms = 1\%$	BMS-POS $ms = 0.5\%$	pumsb_star $ms = 20\%$
STUM	5K	58	27K	173	8K	100K
Border	36K	3K	533K	16K	30K	122K

4.2 Implementation

As shown in Procedure 2, for every enumerated generator candidates, we need to retrieve its support value. To avoid multiple scans of datasets, we employ a prefix-tree and a header table to summarize the dataset. Figure 3 (a) demonstrates how the sample dataset is compressed and stored in a prefix tree. (Details on the construction of prefix tree can be found in [9].) With the prefix tree and the header table, support values of patterns can be retrieved without data scanning. Let us take the sample dataset in Figure 3 as an example. Suppose we need to obtain the support of pattern $\{a, b\}$. We first need to look for all the paths that contain item b based on the linked list pointers in the header table. Then, for each path that contains b, we travel up and search for item a. In this case, only one path contains both items b and a, and the support of the path is 1. Therefore, we have $sup(\{a, b\}, \mathcal{D}) = 1$.

The prefix tree structure also facilitates effective candidate pruning. According to Procedure 2, the generator candidates are produced based on the enumeration order of *SE-tree*. Given a generator G, only items $i >_0 last(G)$ are enumerated. This greatly reduces the number of unnecessary enumerations. On top of that, with the concept of local prefix tree, we can completely avoid generating unnecessary candidates. For example, Figure 3 (b) shows the local prefix tree for generator $\{d\}$. Suppose $ms = 2$. Based on the local prefix tree, we know immediately that the enumeration of candidate $\{c, d\}$ is not necessary, for its support is below ms.

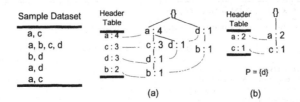

Fig. 3. (a) Global prefix tree and header table for the sample dataset with ordering $b <_0 d <_0 c <_0 a$; and (b) local prefix tree and header table for pattern $\{d\}$

5   Experimental Evaluation

The computational effectiveness of the proposed algorithm, STUM, is tested on several benchmark datasets from the *FIMI* Repository [8]. STUM is evaluated with various degrees of support threshold adjustment.

STUM is compared with some state-of-the-art frequent pattern discovery and maintenance methods, including GC-growth [12], ZIGZAG [16] and Border [2]. GC-growth is an effective algorithm that generates frequent generators. ZIGZAG is one of the recently proposed frequent maximal pattern maintenance algorithm. Border is a frequent pattern maintenance algorithm proposed based on the concept of negative border. The original implementation of Border requires multiple data scans. This induces heavy I/O overhead. To have a better comparison with the proposed method, we improved the implementation of Border. We employ a prefix-tree structure in Border to summarize the dataset and thus to avoid multiple data scans. We name the improved implementation of Border as Border(prefixTree). All the experiments are run on a PC with 2.8 GHz processor and 2 GB RAM.

Figure 4 compares the computational time of STUM against the one of other methods. We observe that, in general, STUM outperforms the rest considerably. However, it is also observed that, compared to the frequent generator discovery algorithm GC-growth, the advantage of STUM drops as the change of support threshold gets larger. This is because large variation in support threshold logically leads to dramatic changes in the frequent pattern space. Thus it is more expensive to update. Therefore, the advantage of STUM is found to diminish when the change of support threshold gets larger. It is inevitable that when the support threshold is adjusted to a certain extent, the change induced to the pattern space becomes so significant that it becomes more efficient to re-discover the patterns than to maintain and update them.

We also measure the "speed-up" achieved by STUM against other methods. The speed-up is calculated as the ratio between the computational time of the comparing method and that of the proposed method. Table 2 summarizes the average speed-up we have achieved on various datasets. Since Border suffers from heavy I/O overhead, STUM outperforms Border significantly. It can also been seen that, by employing the prefix-tree structure, the improved implementation of Border is much faster than the original implementation. STUM performs the best on dataset $T10I4D100K$. It is faster than the other methods by at least an order of magnitude.

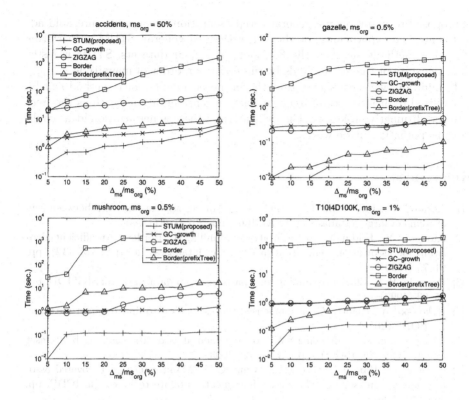

Fig. 4. Comparison of computation time of the proposed algorithm — STUM, GC-growth, ZIGZAG, Border and Border(prefixTree)

Table 2. Average speed-up achieved by STUM. T_{comp} denotes the computational time of the comparing algorithms, and T_{STUM} is that of the proposed algorithm

T_{comp}/T_{STUM}	accidents $ms_\% = 50\%$	gazelle $ms_\% = 0.5\%$	mushroom $ms_\% = 0.5\%$	T10I4D100K $ms_\% = 1\%$
ZIGZAG	2.8	19.4	10.8	19.5
GC-growth	31	17.2	11.6	31.5
Border	230	828	1334	927
Border(prefixTree)	3.7	2.5	4.4	87.8

6 Closing Remarks

In this paper, we compressed the frequent pattern space with the generator representation, which includes the set of frequent generators, the negative generator border and their support values. We observed that generators follow the *a priori* property. Based on this property, we proposed to maintain the generator representation by expanding the negative generator border. Systematic enumeration methods are developed to ensure the expansion of the negative border is complete and non-redundant. Based on the above findings, a new algorithm, STUM, is proposed to maintain the generator representation for support threshold adjustment. The experimental studies show that, in general, STUM outperforms the other methods significantly. For some particular datasets, STUM is faster than the state-of-the-art methods by more than an order of magnitude.

In addition, we have shown that the proposed maintenance method can be generalized to other types of frequent pattern representations, such as the freesets and disjunctive-free sets. The realization of these generalization ideas could serve as potential future works.

References

[1] Agrawal, R., Imielinski, T., Swami, A.N.: Mining association rules between sets of items in large databases. In: SIGMOD, pp. 207–216 (1993)

[2] Aumann, Y., Feldman, R., Lipshtat, O., Manilla, H.: Borders: An efficient algorithm for association generation in dynamic databases. In: JIIS, vol. (12), pp. 61–73 (1999)

[3] Bayardo, R.J.: Efficiently mining long patterns from databases. In: SIGMOD, pp. 85–93 (1998)

[4] Bykowski, A., Rigotti, C.: A condensed representation to find frequent patterns. In: PODS (2001)

[5] Chang, C., et al.: Enhancing SWF for incremental association mining by itemset maintenance. In: PAKDD, pp. 301–312 (2003)

[6] Cheung, D., Han, J., Ng, V.T.Y., Wong, C.Y.: Maintenance of discovered association rules in large databases: an incremental update technieq. In: ICDE, pp. 106–114 (1996)

[7] Chi, Y., Wang, H., Yu, P.S., Muntz, R.R.: Moment: Maintaining closed frequent itemsets over a stream sliding window. In: Perner, P. (ed.) ICDM 2004. LNCS (LNAI), vol. 3275, pp. 59–66. Springer, Heidelberg (2004)

[8] Frequent Itemset Mining Dataset Repository, http://fimi.cs.helsinki.fi

[9] Han, J., Pei, J., Yin, Y.: Mining frequent patterns without candidates generation. In: SIGMOD, pp. 1–12 (2000)

[10] Kryszkiewicz, M.: Concise representation of frequent patterns based on disjunction-free generators. In: ICDM, pp. 305–312 (2001)

[11] Lee, C.-H., Lin, C.-R., Chen, M.-S.: Sliding window filtering: An efficient method for incremental mining on a time-variant database. Information Systems 30(3), 227–244 (2005)

[12] Li, H., Li, J., Wong, L., Feng, M., Tan, Y.-P.: Relative risk and odds ratio: A data mining perspective. In: PODS, pp. 368–377 (2005)

[13] Mannila, H., Toivonen, H.: Levelwise search and borders of theories in knowledge discovery. Data Mining and Knowledge Discovery 1(2), 241–258 (1997)

[14] Pasquier, N., Bastide, Y., Taouil, R., Lakhal, L.: Discovering frequent closed itemsets for association rules. In: Beeri, C., Bruneman, P. (eds.) ICDT 1999. LNCS, vol. 1540, pp. 398–416. Springer, Heidelberg (1998)

[15] Rymon, R.: Search through systemactic set enumeration. In: KR 1992, pp. 539–550 (1992)

[16] Veloso, A.A., Meira Jr., W., de Carvalho, M.B., Possas, B., Parthasarathy, S., Zaki, M.J.: Mining frequent itemsets in evolving databases. SIAM, Philadelphia (2002)

CommTracker: A Core-Based Algorithm of Tracking Community Evolution*

Yi Wang, Bin Wu, and Xin Pei

Beijing Key Laboratory of Intelligent Telecommunications Software and Multimedia,
Beijing University of Posts and Telecommunications, Beijing
{wangyi.tseg,peixin11}@gmail.com
wubin@bupt.edu.cn

Abstract. Social network analysis has been a hot topic in the field of graph mining. After people have achieved the goal of detecting communities from various networks, now they are interested in how these explored communities change as time passes by. In other words, people focus on the problem of community evolution and further discover those dynamic characteristics of kinds of networks. Here, we propose Comm-Tracker, a novel and parameter-free algorithm of tracking community evolution, which utilizes the representative quality of core nodes in a community to establish the evolving relationship between two communities in consecutive time snapshots. With such a distinct strategy, it is suitable for analyzing large scale datasets. Depending on relationships established from CommTracker, it is feasible to identify *community split* and *mergence*. In addition, one relationship amongst evolution traces, *evolution traces intersection*, is also studied. At last, we demonstrate the correctness and effectiveness of our algorithm on 4 real datasets.

1   Introduction

In the field of graph mining, more and more researchers are attracted by social network analysis where persons are abstracted to nodes and their associations to edges. They devote themselves to mining valuable information from those special networks, especially detecting community structures. The vertices within communities have higher density of edges while vertices between communities have lower density of edges. After community structures have been discovered by many algorithms, people are interested in not only a community in a single snapshot but also its associated developing trend in several successive ones. For example, there exists a community in snapshot t, and what about its state in the next snapshot $t+1$? Does it split into smaller ones or merge into a larger one with another community? Moreover, during community evolution, some members will join or leave a community.

---

* This work is supported by the National Natural Science Foundation of China under Grant 60402011 and National Eleven Five-Year Scientific and Technical Support Plans under Grant 2006BAH03B05.

C. Tang et al. (Eds.): ADMA 2008, LNAI 5139, pp. 229–240, 2008.

In order to observe how a group of persons evolves, we propose a novel algorithm, which takes advantage of core nodes and it is quite different from many existing ones. As uncovered in [1], real networks follow a power-law distribution, indicating that some nodes act as central ones, and others ordinary ones. Shaojie Qiao and Qihong Liu concentrate on mining core members of a crime community [2][3]. Nan Du successfully rests on attributes of core nodes to represent those of a whole community [4]. We notice the capability of core nodes and therefore make them play a key role in our algorithm to find out successors or predecessors of a community as well as related change points. Additionally, the algorithm requires no user-defined parameters, and operates automatically without prejudices or presumptions.

Now how to effectively detect core nodes in a community is a problem to be addressed. In the paper, a parameter-free method has also been developed, adaptive to different community structures.

Contributions. Our core-based algorithm of tracking community evolution has the following key properties:

- *Parameter − free*: Our algorithm requires no parameters from users, nor a threshold to confirm the evolving relationship between two communities.
- *Large − scale accommodative*: Getting rid of node/edge matching reduces calculation and therefore it is a good candidate for tracking large-scale community evolution.
- *Straightforward*: Depending on the algorithm, it offers a straightforward way to identify *community split* and *mergence*. To the best of our knowledge, few algorithms have such a capability.

The rest of the paper is organized as follows: Section 2 reviews the related work. Section 3 introduces some necessary definitions. Section 4 presents the parameter-free core detection algorithm and Section 5 presents our core-based algorithm of tracking community evolution. Section 6 introduces evolution trace intersection. Section 7 shows the experimental evaluations and Section 8 concludes.

2   Related Work

Graph mining has been a very active area in the data mining field, not only limited to static graph mining but also expanding gradually into the realm of dynamic graph.

Within static graph mining, community detection has been paid much attention. Various methods have been utilized to detect these structures. Among them, there are Newman's betweenness algorithm [5], Nan Du's clique-based algorithm[4] and CPM[6] that focuses on finding overlapping communities. Clustering is another technique to group similar nodes into large communities, including L. Donetti and M. Munoz's method[7] which exploits spectral properties of the graph as well as J. Hopcroft's "natural community" approach[8].

With respect to core node detection, R. Guimera and L.A.N. Amaral propose a methodology that classifies nodes into universal roles according to their pattern of intra- and inter-module connections [9]. B. Wu offers a method to detect core nodes with a threshold [10]. S. Qiao and Q. Liu dedicate themselves to mining core members of a crime community [2][3].

As to dynamic graph mining, T.Y. Berger-Wolf and J. Saia study community evolution based on node overlapping [11]; J. Hopcroft and O. Khan propose a method which utilizes "nature community" to track evolution[12]. However, both methods have to set some parameters, which is too difficult to be adaptive to various situations. In contrast, E. Keogh suggests the notion of parameter free data mining[13]. Both our methods in the paper share the same spirit.

Moreover, G. Palla and A.L. Barabási provide a method which effectively utilizes edge overlapping to build evolving relationship[14]. J. Sun's GraphScope is a parameter-free mining method of large time-evolving graphs[15], using information theoretic principles. Many other methods have been accomplished to concentrate on community change[16][17][18].

3   Problem Definition

The table below lists almost all the symbols used in the paper.

Sym.	Definition
$C_i^{(t)}$	Community of index i in snapshot t
$N_i^{(t)}$	Node of index i in snapshot t
$W(N_i^{(t)})$	Weight of a node of index i in snapshot t
$Cen(N_i^{(t)})$	Central degree of node $N_i^{(t)}$
$Core(C_i^{(t)})$	Core node set of $C_i^{(t)}$
$Node(C_i^{(t)})$	Node set of $C_i^{(t)}$
$Edge(C_i^{(t)})$	Edge set of $C_i^{(t)}$
$|Node(C)|$	community C size
$C_i^{(t)} \to C_j^{(t+1)}$	$C_i^{(t)}$ is a predecessor of $C_j^{(t+1)}$ or $C_j^{(t+1)}$ is a successor of $C_i^{(t)}$
$C_i^{(t-k)} \Rightarrow C_j^{(t)}$	$C_i^{(t-k)}$ is an ancestor of $C_j^{(t)}$
$Evol(C_i^{(t)})$	Evolution trace of $C_i^{(t)}$
$|Evol(C_i^{(t)})|$	Span of evolution trace of $C_i^{(t)}$

Definition 1. *(COMMUNITY EVOLUTION TRACE). An evolution trace $Evol(C_x^{(t)})$ is a time-series of $C^{(t+n)}$ as follows:*

$$Evol(C_x^{(t)}) := \{C_x^{(t)}, C_x^{(t+1)}, C_y^{(t+1)}, C_x^{(t+2)} \ldots, C_x^{(t+n)}\}(n \geq 0)$$

where each community $C_x^{(t+i)}, i \in [1, n]$ satisfies the condition that there exists at least one community $C_x^{(t+i-1)}$, and then $C_x^{(t+i-1)} \to C_x^{(t+i)}$. Note that more than one community is allowed to appear in the same snapshot $t+i$, like $C_x^{(t+1)}, C_y^{(t+1)}$ both locating in the snapshot $t + 1$. $|Evol(C_x^{(t)})|$ is $n + 1$

Definition 2. *(ANCESTOR OF A COMMUNITY). The definition of a community's ancestor is as follows:* $C_i^{(t-k)} \Rightarrow C_j^{(t)}$ *if there is an evolving chain* $C_i^{(t-k)} \rightarrow C_x^{(t-k+1)}, \ldots, \rightarrow C_j^{(t)} (k \geq 1)$

4 Core Node Detection Algorithm

As discussed above, core nodes are of greatest importance in our evolution algorithm, so its preparation work, selecting core nodes from a community, is a key step. The structure of a community is too dynamic and unpredictable to set an empirical threshold to distinguish core nodes from ordinary ones. Unlike [10], the following method concentrates on not only effectiveness but also parameter free.

A node can be weighed in terms of many aspects, such as degree, betweenness, Page Rank and so on. Generally, the higher a node's weight is, the more important it is in a community. One of these methods can be chosen to give a node N_i a weight value $W(N_i)$ according to practical requirements.

In our algorithm, both the community topology and the node weight are considered as critical factors to distinguish core nodes from ordinary ones. In Algorithm 1, we present the whole algorithm.

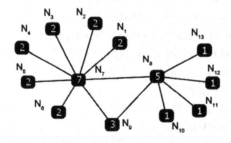

Fig. 1. Core detection illustration. Note that a node weight is not equal to its degree.

The basic idea behind the algorithm is similar to a vote strategy. For each node N_i, its centrality is evaluated by those nodes linked with it. Assuming that $W(N_i)$ is higher than the weight of a linked node, $W(N_j)$, then N_i is considered as a more important node than N_j, so N_i's centrality value should be incremented by a specified value while N_j's value is reduced by a specified value. Here, $|W(N_i) - W(N_j)|$ is employed to represent the centrality difference between two nodes. Through the "vote" of all round nodes, if N_i's centrality is nonnegative, it is regarded as a core node. Otherwise, it is just an ordinary node.

As Fig. 1 shows, the number in a node indicates the node weight, eg. $W(N_8) = 5$. The running result is that $Cen(N_7) = 36, Cen(N_8) = 16$ whereas $Cen(N_9) = -6, Cen(N_i) = -5, i \in [1,6], Cen(N_j) = -4, j \in [10,13]$. Therefore, the core set are $\{N_7, N_8\}$.

Algorithm 1. Core Detection Algorithm

Require: a community C with n nodes
Ensure: $Core(C)$
1: **procedure** CoreDetection
2:     **if** $W(N_1) = W(N_2) = \ldots = W(N_n)$ **then**
3:         return C
4:     **end if**
5:     $Cen(N_i) = 0, i \in [1, n]$
6:     **for** every edge $e \in Edge(C)$ **do**
7:         N_i, N_j are nodes connected with e
8:         **if** $W(N_i) < W(N_j)$ **then**
9:             $Cen(N_i) = Cen(N_i) - |W(N_i) - W(N_j)|$
10:            $Cen(N_j) = Cen(N_j) + |W(N_i) - W(N_j)|$
11:        **end if**
12:        **if** $W(N_i) \geq W(N_j)$ **then**
13:            $Cen(N_i) = Cen(N_i) + |W(N_i) - W(N_j)|$
14:            $Cen(N_j) = Cen(N_j) - |W(N_i) - W(N_j)|$
15:        **end if**
16:    **end for**
17:    coreset $= \{\}$
18:    **for** every node $N_i \in Node(C)$ **do**
19:        **if** $Cen(N_i) \geq 0$ **then**
20:            input N_i into coreset;
21:        **end if**
22:    **end for**
23:    return coreset
24: **end procedure**

In general, Algorithm 1 is effective to detect core nodes in a small network scope, like community, where node distances are no more than 3 hops and each node has large probability to connect to all other ones. The core detection algorithm requires $O(Edge(C))$ for each community.

5   Core-Based Algorithm of Tracking Community Evolution

Our algorithm to be introduced heavily relies on core nodes instead of the overlapping level of nodes or edges between two communities. A good example is the co-authorship community where core nodes represent famous professors and ordinary ones are other students. The research interest of professors is usually that of a whole community. Moreover, it is harder for professors to change their research interest than for those ordinary students. Thus, taking advantage of not all nodes that include those high fluctuating ones but these representative and reliable core nodes, will be more accurate and effective to track community evolution.

T. Y. Berger-Wolf and J. Saia propose a method based on the overlapping level of nodes that $C^{(t+1)}$ is a successor of $C^{(t)}$ if $nodeoverlap(C^{(t)}, C^{(t+1)}) \geq s$ [11]. However, to set a proper s is challenging for users. When members of a community change dramatically and s is given a higher value, $C^{(t+1)}$ will be considered to disappear because of too low overlapping level between them, but in fact $C^{(t+1)}$ still exists. Otherwise, if s is set a bit low, doing so will give irrelevant communities more opportunities to become the successors of $C^{(t)}$, leading to "successors explosion" and masking those real successors.

G. Palla and A. L. Barabási provide an approach utilizing the overlapping of edge between two communities[14], but it fails to deal with split and mergence amongst communities. As there are one $C^{(t)}$ and two $C_i^{(t+1)}$, $C_j^{(t+1)}$, in snapshot t and $t + 1$ respectively, if the edge overlapping level between $C^{(t)}$ and $C_i^{(t+1)}$ is higher than that between $C^{(t)}$ and $C_j^{(t+1)}$, $C_i^{(t+1)}$ becomes the successor of $C^{(t)}$ while $C_j^{(t+1)}$ is considered as a new born community. Actually, $C^{(t)}$ may split into two parts. The similar problem also exists in the process of community mergence.

The disadvantage of both methods discussed above is to treat all nodes or edges in an unprejudiced way and it is not accorded with the reality where different nodes or edges have different influences. Our method has deeply paid attention to such a difference so that it puts emphasis on core nodes.

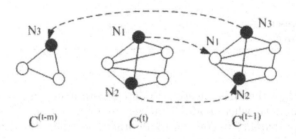

Fig. 2. Community Evolution illustration: core nodes are dark and ordinary ones light. As we seen, (1) in snapshot $t + 1$, $C^{(t+1)}$ contains two core node N_1, N_2 of $C^{(t)}$. (2) Node N_3 has also been in $C^{(t-m)}$, an ancestor of $C^{(t)}$. Therefore, $C^{(t+1)}$ becomes the succeeding community of $C^{(t)}$. In practice, if $C^{(t)}$ has no ancestor, then communities satisfying the first condition will become $C^{(t)}$'s successors automatically.

The basic thought of our algorithm can be described as:

$C_i^{(t)} \rightarrow C_j^{(t+1)}$ if and only if (1) at least one core node of $C_i^{(t)}$ appears in $C_j^{(t+1)}$, that is, $Core(C_i^{(t)}) \cap Node(C_j^{(t+1)}) \neq \emptyset$ (2) at least one core node of $C_j^{(t+1)}$ must appear in some ancestor community of $C_i^{(t)}$, that is, there exists one $C_k^{(t-m)}$, $C_k^{(t-m)} \Rightarrow C_i^{(t)}$, $Node(C_k^{(t-m)}) \cap Core(C_j^{(t+1)}) \neq \emptyset$. (see Fig. 2)

For the first condition, it is reasonable to consider $C_i^{(t)}$'s core nodes appear in some succeeding community $C_j^{(t+1)}$, due to the representative quality of core

---

Algorithm 2. Community Evolution Algorithm

Require: a specified community $C_i^{(t)}$ and all the communities in the snapshot $t+1$
Ensure: $Evol(C_i^{(t)})$
 1: **procedure** COMMUNITY EVOLUTION
 2:     $Evol(C_i^{(t)}) = \{C_i^{(t)}\}$
 3:     $Core(C_i^{(t)}) = \text{CoreDetection}(C_i^{(t)})$
 4:     **for** every community $C_j^{(t+1)}$ in snapshot $t+1$ **do**
 5:         $Core(C_j^{(t+1)}) = \text{CoreDetection}(C_j^{(t+1)})$
 6:         **if** $Core(C_i^{(t)}) \cap Node(C_j^{(t+1)}) \neq \emptyset$ and $Node(C_k^{(t-m)}) \cap Core(C_j^{(t+1)}) \neq \emptyset$
    and $C_k^{(t-m)} \Rightarrow C_i^{(t)}$ **then**
 7:             establish the relationship $C_i^{(t)} \rightarrow C_j^{(t+1)}$
 8:             $Evol(C_j^{(t+1)}) = \text{Community Evolution}(C_j^{(t+1)})$
 9:             $Evol(C_i^{(t)}) = Evol(C_i^{(t)}) \cup Evol(C_j^{(t+1)})$
10:         **end if**
11:     **end for**
12:     **return** $Evol(C_i^{(t)})$
13: **end procedure**

---

nodes. As to the second condition, if some community $C_j^{(t+1)}$ wants to become the succeeding one of a specified community $C_i^{(t)}$, it must suffice that its core nodes appear in some ancestor of $C_i^{(t)}$, because of the stable quality of core nodes, that is , core nodes do not appear suddenly without any evidence in the past snapshots.

We describe the whole algorithm in Algorithm 2.

From the aspect of successors and predecessors, we provide a very straight-forward way to identify *community split, community mergence, community birth* and *community death*. Note that they are four phenomena that occurs in a single evolution trace.

- Community Split: a community has more than one successor.
- Community Mergence: a community owns more than one predecessor.
- Community Birth: a community has no predecessor.
- Community Death: a community has no successor.

Under the precondition that there is an index table which maps a node to those communities containing it, the running time of CommTracker requires about $O(Q_{com} \cdot R_{max} + Q_{com} \cdot R_{max} \cdot S) = O(Q_{com} \cdot R_{max} \cdot S)$, where Q_{com} is the quantity of all communities, R_{max} means the maximum quantity of core nodes in a community and S is snapshot quantity.

6   Evolution Traces Intersection

It is rare that a community evolves alone, without any intersection with other communities. In general, one research community will frequently communicate with others of a similar domain to obtain relevant information. From the aspect of evolution traces, if a community $C_i^{(t)}$ appears in two or more evolution traces, such a community is regarded as a shared community. Performing the statistics of the quantity of shared community accurately is helpful for us to make knowledge of events happened among community evolutions. In the co-authorship network, shared communities are reflected as the collaboration events of research groups in a specified time. As Fig. 3 shows, we discover two evolution traces, $Evol(C_1^{(t+1)}) = \{C_1^{(t+1)}, C_2^{(t+2)}, C_3^{(t+3)}, C_1^{(t+4)}, C_2^{(t+5)}\}$ and $Evol(C_1^{(t+2)}) = \{C_1^{(t+2)}, C_1^{(t+3)}, C_2^{(t+3)}, C_1^{(t+4)}, C_1^{(t+5)}\}$. Obviously, $C_1^{(t+4)}$ is a shared community locating in both $Evol(C_1^{(t+1)})$ and $Evol(C_1^{(t+2)})$ but $C_1^{(t+4)}$ can not be considered as a mergence community because it lies in two different traces.

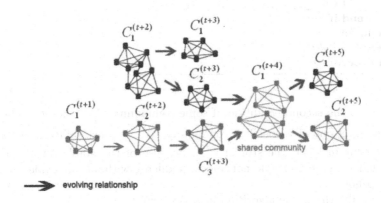

Fig. 3. Evolution traces intersection

Here, we give the definition of community age as follows:

Definition 3. *(COMMUNITY AGE). For a community lying in a single evolution trace, its age is time span between the birth snapshot and the current snapshot. But for a community locating in two or more traces, that is, a shared community, the longest value of its time spans is set as its age.*

For example, in Fig. 3, $C_3^{(t+3)}$'s age is 3. $C_1^{(t+4)}$ is a shared community, whose ages are 4 and 3 in $Evol(C_1^{(t+1)})$ and $Evol(C_1^{(t+2)})$ respectively. Thus, we set 4 as $C_1^{(t+4)}$'s age.

7   Experimental Evaluation

The datasets we consider are (1) the half year list of articles in Cornell University Library e-print condensed matter (cond-mat) archive spanning 14 years, over 30,000 communities (http://cn.arxiv.org); (2) the controlled terms related to computer in EI village from 1993 to 2006 (http://www.engineeringvillage2.org.cn);

(3) ENRON email dataset over 3 years (http://www.cs.cmu.edu/enron/); (4) the records of phone calls between customers of a mobile phone company spanning 20 weeks in one province. Nan Du's *ComTector* is employed to detect communities [4]. (The detailed information is seen in Table 1)

Table 1. Dataset summary

dataset	cond-mat	EI terms	Enron	mobile phone
time span	14 years	14 years	144 weeks	20 weeks
snapshot	0.5 year	1 year	1 week	2 weeks
average community number per snapshot	1164	133	60	5794
evolution trace number	20101	979	5023	14177
average community size	5	13	11	100
core number per community	2	4	2	6
running time	8s	2s	23s	1551s
node construction	authors	controlled terms	persons	persons
edge construction	collaboration events	appearances in the same article	email events	call events

7.1   The Cond-Mat Dataset

The weight of each node is calculated in a rational way that if one paper has n authors, then each of them will get the weight of $1/n$.

To make knowledge of community member stability, we use a function MS, similarly defined in [14], to quantify the relative member stability rate between two success communities:

$$MS(C^{(t)}) = \frac{C^{(t)} \cap (C_1^{(t+1)} \cup C_2^{(t+1)} \ldots \cup C_n^{(t+1)})}{C^{(t)} \cup (C_1^{(t+1)} \cup C_2^{(t+1)} \ldots \cup C_n^{(t+1)})} \qquad (1)$$

where $C^{(t)} \rightarrow C_i^{(t+1)}$ ($i \in [1, n]$) and $C^{(t)}$ represents $Node(C^{(t)})$ in brief. The member stability of an evolution trace is the average value of all contained communities' MS, except those without successors.

Fig. 4 a(1) indicates that longer life evolution traces change at a higher rate while those with shorter life span alter at a lower rate. The result above suggests that if a community is too stable to absorb new members, it will die very quickly, while a community persists for a longer duration if it is capable of dynamically altering their memberships. From Fig. 4 a(2), it is obvious that larger communities trend to live a longer lives. Two conclusions above are consistent with those revealed in [14] under the same dataset.

Fig. 4 a(3) and (4) uncover what communities are likely to split or merge. Here, we first define a criterion called "core united coefficient"(CUC) to measure the cluster degree amongst core nodes. Its definition is as follows:

$$CUC = \frac{2 \times |\{e|e \text{ is a edge and both its nodes are core}\}|}{|Core(C)| \times (|Core(C)| - 1)} \qquad (2)$$

A low CUC somewhat suggests that leaders in the community actually work in a mutual independent way, leading to some sub-communities within it while a high CUC indicates leaders collaborate with each other. As Fig. 4 a(3) shows, a community whose CUC is high has a low probability to split or merge while a community with a lower CUC has a higher likelihood of split and mergence in the next snapshot. In Fig. 4 a(4), the larger size a community has, the higher probability it will split or merge with. Two phenomena are in accordance with people 's predictions. Assuming a large community contains small sub-communities, its structure is so instable as to disintegrate into independent ones in the next snapshot whereas it is not likely for a small cohesive community to change its state.

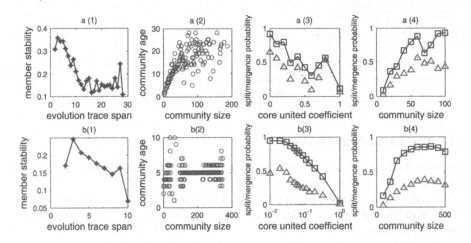

Fig. 4. Cond-mat dataset and mobile phone dataset. Here, in a(3),a(4),b(3),b(4), the rectangle line represents split condition and the triangle line represents mergence condition.

7.2   Mobile Phone Dataset

The enormous dataset contains more than 500 million calling records, from which we can discover more than 5000 communities in the snapshot of every two week. The weight of a node is equal to its degree in this case. Four same experiments of cond-mat dataset are performed and we obtain similar results (See Fig. 4 from b(1) to b(4)). Again, the first two experiment results coincide with those from [14] and the correctness of our algorithm is further validated.

7.3   The EI Controlled Term Dataset of Computer

The weight of a controlled term increases by 1 if it appears in one article. A community of controlled terms largely represents a research domain, so some community evolution partly reflects the development situation of a corresponding domain. Fig. 5 (a) lists some computer research domains and their research durations.

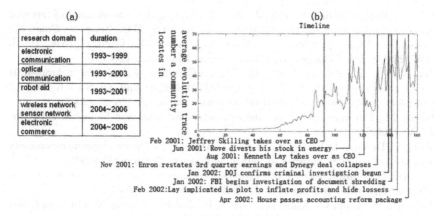

Fig. 5. Research domains with their durations and Enron key events

7.4   Enron Dataset

In this case, the weight of a node is equal to its degree. As we discuss above, the emergence of a community shared by several evolution traces partially reflects those traces' activeness. In a snapshot, the more shared communities appear, the more highly active evolution traces will be. Here, we use average evolution trace number a community locates in to estimate the activeness of a whole network in some snapshot. For instance, in Fig. 3, values are 1,2 in the snapshot $t+3$ and $t+4$ respectively. Such a measure helps us to discover those key events of Enron (See Fig. 5 (b)).

8   Conclusions

We propose a core-based evolution tracking algorithm, which has all of the following properties: (1) it is parameter free; (2) It effectively tracks evolution traces and further discovers split/mergence points. (3) It is efficient and correct. We also perform experiments on four real networks (co-authorship network, vocabulary network, email network and mobile call network), by the validation of which, our algorithm reveals diverse dynamic characteristics of different domains and discovers key events and research domains.

References

1. Barabási, A.L., Albert, R.: Emergence of scaling in random networks. Science 286, 509 (1999)
2. Qiao, S., Tang, C., Peng, J., Fan, H., Xiang, Y.: Vccm mining: Mining virtual community core members based on gene expression programming. In: Chen, H., Wang, F.-Y., Yang, C.C., Zeng, D., Chau, M., Chang, K. (eds.) WISI 2006. LNCS, vol. 3917, pp. 133–138. Springer, Heidelberg (2006)

3. Liu, Q., Tang, C., Qiao, S., Liu, Q., Wen, F.: Mining the core member of terrorist crime group based on social network analysis. In: Yang, C.C., Zeng, D., Chau, M., Chang, K., Yang, Q., Cheng, X., Wang, J., Wang, F.-Y., Chen, H. (eds.) PAISI 2007. LNCS, vol. 4430, pp. 311–313. Springer, Heidelberg (2007)

4. Du, N., Wu, B., Pei, X., Wang, B., Xu, L.: Community detection in large-scale social networks. In: Proceedings of the 9th WebKDD and 1st SNA-KDD 2007 workshop on Web mining and social network analysis, pp. 16–25 (2007)

5. Givan, M., Newman, M.: Community structure in social and biological networks. PNAS (2002)

6. Palla, J., Derényi, I., Farkas, I., Vicsek, T.: Uncovering the overlapping community structure of complex network in nature and society. Nature 435 (2005)

7. Donetti, L., Munoz, M.: Detecting network communities: a new systematic and efficient algorithm. Journal of Statistical Mechanics 443 (2004)

8. Hopcroft, J., Khan, O., Kulis, B., Selman, B.: Natural communities in large linked networks. In: Proceedings of ACM SIGKDD, pp. 541–546 (2003)

9. Guimera, R., Amaral, L.A.N.: Functional cartography of complex metabolic networks. Functional cartography of complex metabolic networks 443 (2005)

10. Wu, B., Pei, X., Tan, J., Wang, Y.: Resume mining of communities in social network. In: ICDM workshop, pp. 435–440 (2007)

11. Berger-Wolf, T.Y., Saia, J.: A framework for analysis of dynamic social networks. In: Proceedings of ACM SIGKDD, pp. 523–528 (2006)

12. Hopcroft, J., Khan, O., Kulis, B., Selman, B.: Tracking evolving communities in large linked networks. PNAS (2004)

13. Keogh, E., Lonardi, S., Ratanamahatana, C.A.: Towards parameter-free data mining. In: Proceedings of ACM SIGKDD, pp. 206–215 (2004)

14. Palla, G., Barabási, A., Vicsec, T.: Quantifying social group evolution. Nature 446 (2007)

15. Sun, J., Faloutsos, C., Papadimitriou, S., Yu, P.S.: Graphscope: parameter-free mining of large time-evolving graphs. In: Proceedings of ACM SIGKDD, pp. 687–696 (2007)

16. Backstrom, L., Huttenlocher, D., Kleinberg, J., Lan, X.: Group formation in large social networks: membership, growth, and evolution. In: Proceedings of ACM SIGKDD, pp. 44–54 (2006)

17. Leskovec, J., Kleinberg, J., Faloutsos, C.: Graphs over time:densification laws, shrinking diameters and possible explanations. In: Proceedings of ACM SIGKDD (2005)

18. Zhou, D., Councill, I.G., Zha, H., Giles, C.L.: Discovering temporal communities from social network documents. In: Perner, P. (ed.) ICDM 2007. LNCS (LNAI), vol. 4597, pp. 745–750. Springer, Heidelberg (2007)

Face Recognition Using Clustering Based Optimal Linear Discriminant Analysis

Wenxin Yang[1], Shuqin Rao[1], Jina Wang[1], Jian Yin[1], and Jian Chen[2]

[1] Department of Computer Science,
Sun Yat-Sen University, Guangzhou, 510275, China
soloistyang@gmail.com
[2] School of Software,
South China University of Technology,
Guangzhou, 510006, China

Abstract. Recently, A. M. Martinez indicated that, the angle between the eigenvector corresponding to the largest eigenvalue of the inter-class covariance and the eigenvector corresponding to the largest eigenvalue of the intra-class covariance is more crucial to the performance of traditional linear discriminant methods, furthermore, if the two eigenvectors are parallel, the final results may be disputable. However, upon careful scrutiny on his assertion, we concluded that the angle between the two eigenvectors is less decisive to the performance, moreover, the main drawback of traditional linear methods is the inter-class covariance cannot precisely reflect the discriminant information. Simply maximizing the inter-class covariance in the principle component space may induce the losing of adjacent class-pair's contribution. Therefore,we propose the **Optimal Linear Discriminant Analysis**(henceforth OLDA)method, which distributes equivalent authority for each class-pair by employing "discriminative power". Besides, we employ the gradient scheme to derive the feature vectors. Thirdly, to address the multimodal problem, the pre-clustering mechanism is adopted to ameliorate the nonlinear structure. We apply our method on a practical face database and a virtual database, the experimental results show the promise of our method.

1 Introduction

Fast and simple to implement, linear dimension reduction methods have been widely accepted in the fields of pattern recognition and machine learning for decades. For example, Principal Component Analysis(henceforth PCA) [1] is to find the optimal projection directions in the sample space that will maximize the total scatter across all data points, and Linear Discriminant Analysis(LDA) [2] tries to maximize S_B, the inter-class covariance scatter matrix, and minimize S_W, the intra-class covariance simultaneously. So the data from different classes are as well separated as possible in a low dimensional space. However, the LDA method always suffers from the small sample size problem, then the PCA process is introduced primarily for pre dimension reduction. The null space based linear discriminant analysis [3]tries to diminish the scatter within all samples, which can also approach the small sample size problem and get higher performance, but the huge computational complexity is really insufferable.

C. Tang et al. (Eds.): ADMA 2008, LNAI 5139, pp. 241–249, 2008.
© Springer-Verlag Berlin Heidelberg 2008

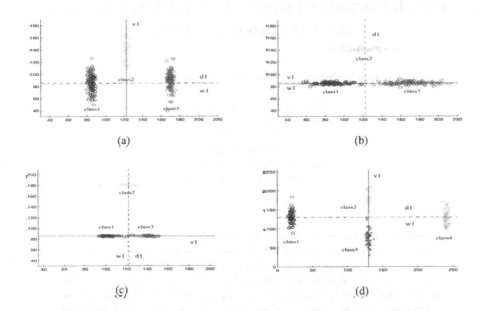

Fig. 1. In all the figures, the blue solid line represents the first eigenvector of the intra-class covariance, labeled as v1, while the blue dash line denotes the first eigenvector of the inter-class covariance, labeled as w1. The final discriminant direction is shown as the red dashdot line, labeled as d1.

Unfortunately, in spite of being accepted for decades, those linear methods are incompetent in perfectly approaching even linear problems. A. M. Martinez proposed that, when the eigenvector corresponding to the largest eigenvalue of the inter-class covariance and the eigenvector corresponding to the largest eigenvalue of the intra-class covariance are parallel, the linear methods may become invalidate [4]. Fig.1 illustrates their conception, In Fig.1(a), the angle between $v1$ and $w1$ is orthonormal, the classification result $d1$ is correct, however, in Fig.1(b), the angle between $v1$ and $w1$ is nearly zero, $d1$ is no longer competent for classification. They also employ this conclusion to data clustering analysis [5] and principle components selection scheme [6].

However, after a careful scrutiny on Martinez's conclusion, there are still some problems. Firstly, their conclusion neglects the significant function of the eigenvalues, which signify the extent corresponding to class scatter, and play more important roles than the angle relationship of eigenvectors. Secondly, even if their contention is true, whether the angle is orthonormal is definitely not a feasible quantitative rule to be embedded in relative discriminant algorithms. Return to Fig.1, a three classes problem in Fig.1(c) and a four classes problem in Fig.1(d) are counterexamples to Martinez's viewpoint. In both figures, $v1$ and $w1$ are orthonormal, meeting their condition, however, the final discriminant direction $d1$ is also incorrect. From Fig.1, we can assert that the angle between the eigenvectors of the intra-class covariance and the eigenvectors of the inter-class covariance makes little impact to the robustness of the traditional linear methods.

Why does LDA invalidate? On intuitional analysis of Fig.1, in kind of similarity, the final discriminant direction both can't classify the two mean value adjacent classes. Upon this perception, simply summing up each inter-class covariance as LDA does can't reflect the optimal discriminant information, linear summation of these covariances may induce unjustness of each adjacent class-pair's contribution. In this paper, we propose the Optimal Linear Discriminant Analysis method, which employs the **discriminative power**(defined in Sec.2) to illustrate the discriminant information, it expresses more precisely on class distinction, and moreover, an upper limit can balance each class-pair's contribution to the final discriminant direction. Successively, a gradient based iterative scheme is introduced to get the optimal transformation vector.

The following part of this paper is organized as below: Section 2 redefines the cost function by introducing the discriminative power. In Section 3, we employ an iterative scheme to derive the feature vectors. To address the multimodal problems, we combine the clustering method in Section 4. Section 5 gives the experimental results on a practical database and a virtual one.

2   The Optimal Discriminant Direction

Simply maximize the inter-class covariance in the principal component space, as LDA does, can't derive the optimal classification. Therefore, it is necessary to employ another expression to reveal the relationship between the optimal discriminant direction and each class-pair's contribution. In this paper, we introduce "discriminative power", which is defined as:

Definition. *The class-pair's inter-class covariance, after eliminating each intra-class covariance's influence, versus its original scatter power in the projection space, can precisely measure each class-pair's contribution to the final discriminant direction, and it is defined as "discriminative power".*

Upon the definition above, we propose the mathematical expression of the item "discriminative power" D_{ij} of class i and class j as below:

$$
\begin{aligned}
D_{ij} &= \frac{V^T((\mu_i - \mu_j)(\mu_i - \mu_j)^T - \Sigma_i - \Sigma_j)V}{(\mu_i - \mu_j)^T V V^T (\mu_i - \mu_j)} \\
&= \frac{V^T((\mu_i - \mu_j)(\mu_i - \mu_j)^T)V}{(\mu_i - \mu_j)^T V V^T (\mu_i - \mu_j)} - \frac{\Sigma_i}{(\mu_i - \mu_j)^T V V^T (\mu_i - \mu_j)} \\
&\quad - \frac{\Sigma_j}{(\mu_i - \mu_j)^T V V^T (\mu_i - \mu_j)} \\
&= D_s - D_f - D_g
\end{aligned}
\tag{1}
$$

where Σ_i and Σ_j denote the intra-class covariance of class i and j, μ is the mean vector, V denotes the feature vectors.

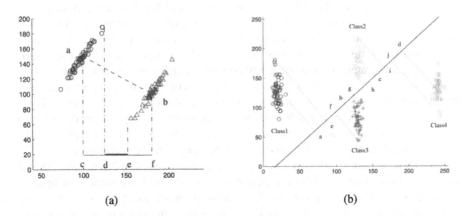

(a)   (b)

Fig. 2. Fig.2(a) shows two classes, a and b are the central points of each class, cf is the momentary classification direction during the searching process, cf is the class-pair's scatter in the projected low-dimensional space, cd and ef indicate each class's scatter in the reconstructed space. In Fig.2, the black solid line denotes the optimal discriminant direction, a, b, c, d are the central points of each class in the low-dimensional space, individually, moreover, e, f, g, h, i, j are the corresponding class margin's mapping on the discriminant direction.

For further understanding of our intention, return to Fig.2(a). LDA utilizes the mean distance ab in the principle component space to express the discriminant information, however, this makes the adjacent class-pair unsensible to the direction selecting. While, the discriminative power tries to select the unoverlapped area de from the total extension cf of each class-pair. For linear separable data, despite of the class distribution and lying direction, the length of de is always less than cf, which ensures the upper limit of class-pair's discriminative power is no more than 1. Therefore, no matter distant or adjacent class-pair, their contributions are equivalent to the final discriminant direction.

In LDA, the inter-class covariance can partly reflect the discriminative power, but not precisely, the simply linear summation may induce the ineffectiveness of the adjacent class-pair. Furthermore, although LDA process tries to avoid the intra-class covariance's disturbance by projecting each point to the principle component space, some unusual intra-class can't be minimized by the holistic PCA preprocess, it will affect the performance more or less. According to Theorem.2, the discriminative power can indeed eliminate the influence of each intra-class covariance, and moreover, makes each class-pair contribute equivalently. According to the discussion above, we propose the prerequisite for deriving the optimal discriminant direction:

Remark. *The discriminative power can reflect the discriminant information more precisely, therefore, the optimal discriminant direction can be derived by maximizing each class-pair's discriminative power.*

Upon the discussion above, we propose our definition of the objective function, the optimal discriminant vector V can be derived from the equation below:

$$V = \arg\max_V \| \sum_{i=1}^{C-1} \sum_{j=i+1}^{C} \frac{V^T((\mu_i - \mu_j)(\mu_i - \mu_j)^T - \Sigma_i - \Sigma_j)V}{(\mu_i - \mu_j)^T VV^T(\mu_i - \mu_j)} \|$$

$$= \arg\max_V \| \sum_{i=1}^{C-1} \sum_{j=i+1}^{C} D_{ij} \| \tag{2}$$

After improving the cost function, avoid being sensible to the distant class-pair's distribution, the final discriminant direction is always decided by the data's integral distribution. Fig.2 illustrates the synergetic effect of each class-pair's discriminative power. Where $\frac{gh}{bc}$ denotes the discriminative power of class2 and class3, similarly, $\frac{cj}{ad}$ for class1 and class4. In spite of huge disparity in mean distance, the contributions of this two class-pairs' are confined by a consistent upper bound 1. Moreover, if the iterative process is prone to diminish the ratio $\frac{gh}{bc}$ for maximizing $\frac{cj}{ad}$, the numerator part of D_{ij} will be negative in certain condition, and the denominator part of D_{ij} is nearly zero simultaneously, the co-effect may result D_{ij} in a considerable negative value, hence the relative direction is hardly be selected. Therefore, maximizing the summation of all those class-pairs' discriminative power pays nearly equivalent attention to each one, instead of mainly the distant ones.

3 Our Solution

Our OLDA method can address the drawbacks of the traditional methods and find the optimal objective space for linear separable data. However, due to the influence of the vector V in the denominator part, we can't introduce the eigen solution method as before. Therefore, the gradient descent algorithm has been employed for feature extraction, this method has been accepted in many fields of both practical and mathematical optimization processes.

First, for simplification, let $A_{ij} = d_{ij}d_{ij}^T - \Sigma_i - \Sigma_j$, and $d_{ij} = \mu_i - \mu_j$, then we have

$$D_{ij} = \frac{V^T A_{ij} V}{d_{ij}^T VV^T d_{ij}}$$

The iterative algorithm are listed as:

---

1. Randomly initialize V^0.
2. Calculate each discriminative power's derivative towards vector V.
   $$\frac{\partial D_{ij}}{\partial V} = \left(\frac{2A_{ij}}{(d_{ij})^T VV^T d_{ij}} - \frac{2V^T A_{ij} V d_{ij}(d_{ij})^T}{((d_{ij})^T VV^T(d_{ij}))^2} \right) V$$
3. Accumulate the derivatives of each class-pair.
   $$\nabla = \sum_{i=1}^{C-1} \sum_{j=i+1}^{C} \frac{\partial D_{ij}}{\partial V}$$
4. Select the proper step value η to adjust the vector V.
   $$V^{n+1} = V^n + \eta \nabla$$
5. Normalize the vector V^{n+1} by
   $$V^{n+1} = \frac{V^{n+1}}{\|V^{n+1}\|}$$
6. Update D^n to D^{n+1} with V^{n+1}, if D is convergence, $V_{opt} = V^{n+1}$, else go to step 2.

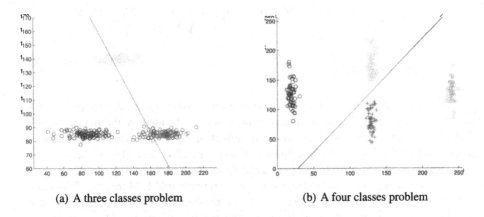

(a) A three classes problem   (b) A four classes problem

Fig. 3. The OLDA method is employed for solving the problems in Fig.1

It should be pointed out that, the restriction we introduced for accelerating the iterative process can also help us avoid the local minimum problem. Different from the step value fixed strategy, the self-adaptive step is generated upon the global gradient, which can find the fastest descending direction in each current position. Furthermore, the restriction tries to select the step value by the global gradient, which avoids local minimum problem. Fig.3 illustrates the experimental results on the three class problem and the four classes problem which LDA is incapable to solve.

4   Solving the Nonlinear Problems

Unfortunately, due to the complexity and diversity, our OLDA method is not suitable for all nonlinear problems. However, with the perfect solution of the linear separable data, we can firstly apply the traditional clustering approach to divide each nonlinear class into several single Gaussian distributions, and then perform our OLDA method for solving linear problems.

Generally speaking, an underlying distribution of data can be properly approximated by a mixture of Gaussian models with cluster analysis. To divide each class into several single Gaussian subclasses, a new spectral clustering method proposed by Lihi Z.M. & Pietro P. [7] is introduced. Assuming that the eigenvector $X \in \Re^{n \times C}$ in an ideal case is polluted by a linear transformation $R \in \Re^{C \times C}$, the method can recover the rotation R through a gradient descent scheme, the corresponding cost function J to be minimized is defined as:

$$J = \sum_{i=1}^{n} \sum_{j=1}^{C} \frac{Z_{ij}^2}{M_i^2} \tag{3}$$

Where Z is the rotated eigenvector, n is the number of points, C means the possible group number, $M_i = \max_j Z_{ij}$, i and j denote the row and the column of matrix Z, respectively. As a result, the number of clusters in each class could be automatically estimated without local minimum. It is noticeable that the spectral clustering method can perform quite well even for small sample sizes. The details about the method can be seen in [7].

5 Experiments and Results

In this section, the FERET face database and a simulated database are used for evaluating the performance of the proposed algorithm.

5.1 Performance on FERET Database

The FERET database is constituted by 40 different persons, each of them with 10 images of the face. The FERET database is mainly composed of frontal images, and in this experiment, all the images are cropped to 30×30 pixels for removing the influences of background and hairstyle. Meanwhile, all the face images are roughly and manually aligned. For all the experiments, each database is randomly divided into a training set and a test set without overlapping. The 1-NN (nearest neighbor) classifier will be employed for classification as soon as the data is reduced to the discriminant subspace. All the reported results are the average of 100 repetitions under the mentioned procedure. The experimental results are shown in Fig.4.

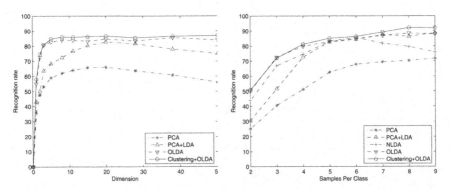

(a) Performance On Different Dimensions (b) Performance On Different Training Samples

Fig. 4. Experiments on FERET database

In Fig.4(a), we try to evaluate the OLDA method's competence in dimension reduction, we give a comparison of each discriminant algorithm, such as PCA, LDA, with the proposed OLDA and clustering based OLDA method. The number of training samples per class is manually set as 5, the others are for testing. In our experiment, the dimension in reconstructed space is designated from 1 to 50, nonlinearly. It is not difficult to see that the accuracy based on the proposed OLDA algorithm always outperforms the other two algorithms, especially when projected to the low dimensional space. Fig.4(b) evaluates the influence of variable training samples. In this experiment, the training samples per class is manually set from 2 to 9 gradually, for recognition. Totally, the OLDA algorithm obtains a considerable improvement compared to other linear algorithms. However, with the increasing of training samples, the superiority of OLDA fades a little, that is mainly because of the single Gaussian assumption of OLDA method. To conquer the disadvantage of the OLDA method, we can introduce the cluster analysis scheme like Clustering based OLDA method does, whose self tuning clustering scheme can precisely divided each class into single Gaussian clusters.

5.2 Performance on Synthetic Database

For further evaluation on the discriminant ability of the proposed OLDA algorithm under the non-single Gaussian situation, a simulated database is introduced for test. Here 200 samples from five different 40-dimensional ($d = 40$) Gaussian classes were generated. The i-th sample of the c-th class is generated as $x_i = B_c c + \mu_c + n$, where $x_i \in \Re^{40}$. And each element of random matrix $B_c \in \Re^{40 \times 30}$ is generated from $\mathcal{N}(0, I)$, $c \in \mathcal{N}_{30}(0, I)$, $n \in \mathcal{N}_{40}(0, I)$. The mean of five classes are $\mu_1 \in 4[\overrightarrow{1}_{40}]^T$, $\mu_2 \in 4[\overrightarrow{0}_{40}]^T$, $\mu_3 \in -4[\overrightarrow{0}_{20} \overrightarrow{1}_{20}]^T$, $\mu_4 \in 4[\overrightarrow{1}_{20} \overrightarrow{0}_{20}]^T$, $\mu_5 \in -4[\overrightarrow{1}_{10} \overrightarrow{0}_{10} \overrightarrow{1}_{10} \overrightarrow{0}_{10}]^T$ respectively. To delicate the performance on no-Gaussian covariance, we give a contrast of the classical LDA algorithm and the OLDA algorithm. The experimental results are shown in Fig.5.

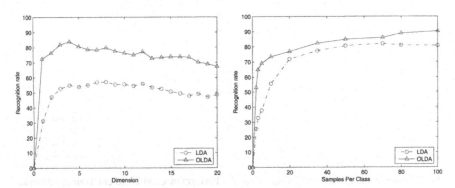

(a) Performance On Different Dimensions   (b) Performance On Different Training Samples

Fig. 5. Experiments on virtual database

In Fig.5(a), both the performance of LDA and OLDA algorithm doesn't fluctuate much with the change of dimension, and, they all reach stable performance when the reconstructed dimension is about 4. But, in general, our OLDA method can get a 20% higher recognition rate compared with LDA . Fig.5(b) gives a intuitional expression of the two algorithm's performance with the increasing of training samples per class. In most of the conditions, our OLDA method can outperform LDA in about 15% , especially when the number of training samples per class is less than 10, the OLDA can get a higher classification rate at nearly 70%, while, LDA only gives about 35%. Therefore, even when dealing with non-Gaussian covariance problems, our OLDA method can also outperform LDA in most situations.

6 Conclusion

In this paper, we elaborate why LDA invalidates in some particular situations, the main reason is that it overly emphasizes on the distant class-pair's contribution to the final discriminant direction. According to the analysis, we redefine the criterion for classification, each class-pair's weight is equally concerned by employing the discriminative power. Furthermore, a gradient based scheme is introduced for iterative solution. Upon experiments on both virtual and face database, we can conclude that, our OLDA method can outperform the other linear methods, especially when the training samples are not sufficient.

Acknowledgment

This work is supported by the National Natural Science Foundation of China (60573097, 60773198, 60703111), Natural Science Foundation of Guangdong Province (05200302, 06104916), Specialized Research Fund for the Doctoral Program of Higher Education(20050558017), Program for New Century Excellent Talents in University of China(NCET-06-0727)

References

1. Turk, M., Pentland, A.P.: Eigenfaces for Recognition. J. Cognitive Neuroscience 3(1), 71–86 (1991)
2. Belhumeur, P.N., Hespanha, J.P., Kriegman, D.J.: Eigenfaces vs. Fisherfaces: Recognition Using Class Specific Linear Projection. IEEE Trans. Pattern Analysis and Machine Intelligence 19(7), 711–720 (1997)
3. Chen, L.F., Liao, H.Y., Ko, M.T., Lin, J.C., Yu, G.J.: A New LDA-Based Face Recognition System Which Can Solve the Small Sample Size Problem. Pattern Recognition 33, 1713–1726 (2000)
4. Martinez, A.M., Zhu, M.L.: Where are linear feature extraction methods applicable? IEEE Transactions on Pattern Analysis and Machine Intelligence 27(12), 1934–1944 (2005)
5. Zhu, M.L., Martinez, A.M.: Subclass discriminant analysis. IEEE Transactions on Pattern Analysis and Machine Intelligence 28, 1274–1286 (2006)
6. Zhu, M.L., Martinez, A.M.: Selecting Principal Components in a Two-Stage LDA Algorithm. In: IEEE Computer Society Conference on Computer Vision and Pattern Recognition 2006, June 17-22, 2006, vol. 1, pp. 132–137 (2006)
7. Zelnik-Manor, L., Perona, P.: Self-tuning spectral clustering. In: Saul, L.K., Weiss, Y., Bottou, L. (eds.) Advances in Neural Information Processing Systems, vol. 17, pp. 1601–1608. MIT Press, Cambridge (2005)

A Novel Immune Based Approach for Detection of Windows PE Virus

Yu Zhang[1], Tao Li[1], Jia Sun[2], and Renchao Qin[1]

[1] School of Computer Science, Sichuan University, Chengdu 610065, China
bullzhangyu@yahoo.com.cn
[2] Department of humanism education, Huaihua University, Huaihua 418000, China
tomsunjia@yahoo.com.cn

Abstract. Generic computer virus detection is the absolute need of the hour as most commercial antivirus products fail to detect unknown and new Windows PE viruses. Motivated by the success of immune-based techniques in intrusion detection systems, recent research in detecting computer viruses is directed towards devising efficient non-signature-based techniques. We observe that each Windows PE virus whether or not it is encrypted must have a relocation module to relocate its variables or constants in the infected programs. Due to its unique characteristic, the virus relocation module can be extracted as an antibody in the immune systems to detect the specific antigens. In this paper, we presented a novel Windows PE virus detection approach that draws inspiration from artificial immune system and the structure of the relocation module of the virus. The structure of Windows PE virus is sufficiently analyzed. The dynamic evolution of self and nonself, the presentation of the antigen, and the generation of the antibody are proposed. The experiment is conducted and its results indicate that this approach not only has relatively higher detection rate of unknown Windows PE virus than the earlier known methods, but also has better capability of self-adaptive and self-learning.

Keywords: computer immune system, PE virus detection, relocation module, virus gene pool.

1 Introduction

The ever-increasing computer viruses have caused huge economic losses since the advent of computer viruses [1] [2]. Most signature-based antivirus products are effective to detect known viruses but not unknown viruses or viruses' variants, which makes them often lag behind viruses. In other words, antivirus often takes remedial measures to recuperate damage caused by viruses, not preventive measures to control viruses before they occur, and not strictly effective measures to block viruses' propagation during their epidemic.

Since most computer viruses are platform-dependent, they can operate only on a single operating system. With the operating system transforming from DOS to Windows, most previously DOS computer viruses cannot work in the new environment and Windows viruses including Windows macro virus, Windows script virus, and Windows PE virus are becoming more and more popular. However, Windows macro

C. Tang et al. (Eds.): ADMA 2008, LNAI 5139, pp. 250–259, 2008.
© Springer-Verlag Berlin Heidelberg 2008

viruses gradually decrease with the security enhancements of Microsoft's Office suite, and so do Windows script viruses because of the security enhancements of IE browser. Unlike them, the ever-growing PE (Portable Executable) viruses are easy to propagate between different platforms and are difficult to detect by antivirus because of their portable file format. In addition, PE viruses have become the favorite target of most virus writers who exhibit their techniques in the virus community. All these actions led to the development and upgrade of PE viruses, which makes the antivirus more and more difficult to detect them, let alone to remove them.

As for Windows PE virus detection, antivirus researchers put forth different approaches in literature. Xu et al. [3] proposed an API sequence based scanner for polymorphic malicious executable. This approach rests on an analysis based on the Windows API calling sequence that reflects the behavior of a piece of particular code. Although it could achieve good experiment results, the construction of the API calling sequences and the similarity measurement between the two sequences take too much computational time. Reddy et al. [4] presented an n-gram based computer virus detection, which combines several classifiers using Dempster Shafer Theory for better classification accuracy. But the training time is too much to apply to the antivirus applications. Tesauro et al. [5] developed a neural networks based method for computer virus recognition, which they deployed the neural network as a commercial product in IBM. Zhang et al. [6] proposed a Bayesian theory based method for unknown computer virus detection, which used the difference between the normal programs and suspicious programs to probably recognize unknown viruses. Wang et al. [7] proposed a support vector machines based approach for unknown virus detection. Zhang et al. [8] proposed a k-nearest neighbor algorithm based method for unknown virus detection. Chen et al. [9] presented a program behavior based method for unknown virus detection. Schultz et al. [10] proposed a data mining based approach for new virus detection. From the technical point of view, the approaches mentioned above are complex for two reasons. First, lots of malicious and benign codes as training dataset are difficult to collect. Second, they would consume lots of times when training the classifiers.

To improve the performance of the detector mentioned above and to effectively detect Windows PE viruses, a novel immune based approach for unknown Windows PE virus detection is proposed. Experiments were conducted and results show that this approach has better efficiency in the detection of known and unknown Windows PE viruses than the others.

In the following sections, we first describe the logical structure of Windows PE virus in section 2. Then we introduce the theory of our detection model which includes the detection process, the evolution of self and nonself, the antigen presenting and the generation of the antibody in section 3. Section 4 shows the implementation and experiment results. We state our conclusion in Section 5.

2 The Logical Structure of Windows PE Virus

PE (Portable Executable) is the native file format of Win32 and its specification is derived somewhat from the Unix COFF (Common Object File Format). The meaning of "portable executable" is that the file format is universal across Win32 platform: the PE loader of every Win32 platform recognizes and uses this file format even when Windows is running on CPU platforms other than Intel. Windows PE viruses take advantages of the PE file format to spread themselves among different Win32 platforms. Generally speaking, a Windows PE virus must include the following modules [11] to better infect other host programs, namely, the relocation module, the module of obtaining API address, the module of searching target files, the module of mapping file to the memory, the module of adding new section to infected files, and the module of returning to the target file. The logical structure of Windows PE virus is shown in Figure 1. We will briefly introduce them below.

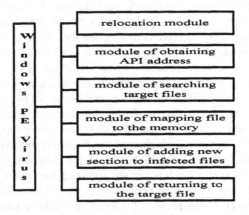

Fig. 1. The logical structure of Windows PE virus

2.1 The Relocation Module

Normal programs do not concern the location of variables or constants, because their locations in the memory were well calculated when compiled by the compiler program. Therefore, when programs are loaded into the memory, they do not need to relocate the position of variables or constants used in them. The variables or constants are directly used by their names. Similarly, the virus programs also use variables and constants. But the locations of virus variables or constants vary with the infected host programs, because of their attachment to different host programs resulting in different positions of the virus variables or constants when loaded in the memory with the host programs. Since these variables or constants do not have fixed addresses, the virus must rely on itself to relocate these addresses to normally access to the relevant resources when executed in the memory. Therefore, the Windows PE virus must have an inherent relocation module, which is usually at the beginning of the virus program with less code and little change, so as to be correctly executed in the Windows platform. In this study, we extract the relocation module as a gene from the virus to produce antibodies to detect unknown Windows PE virus.

2.2 The Module of Obtaining API Address

Windows programs generally run in Ring 3, the protection mode in the Windows operating system. The system API calls achieve through the dynamic link library in the Windows. Generally, normal programs have an import address table, inside which the actual addresses of API functions are. Thus, when being called by the program, the corresponding API functions addresses can be found in the import address table of the Windows PE file.

However, the Windows PE virus has only a code section, which does not include the import address table so as to reduce the virus source code. Unlike the normal programs, the Windows PE virus program can not directly obtain the address of API functions, and must firstly identify these addresses in dynamic link library. Therefore, the Windows PE virus must have such module that can obtain the addresses of Windows API functions called by the virus.

2.3 The Module of Searching Target Files

In order to spread themselves, a virus must have to continuously search target documents to implement its infection to expand its influence. Therefore, the Windows PE virus needs a target files searching module.

2.4 The Module of Mapping File to the Memory

Memory-mapping-file provides a group of independent functions that are the association of a file's contents with a portion of the virtual address space of a process. Processes read from and write to the file view using pointers, just as they would with dynamically allocated memory. The use of file mapping improves efficiency because the file resides on disk, but the file view resides in memory. In this way, the computer virus can quickly infect target files to reduce the possession of system resources. Therefore, the Windows PE virus generally has a memory-mapping-file module.

2.5 The Module of Adding New Section to Infected Files

The most effective way to infect target files for the Windows PE virus is to add a new section to host programs. While adding a new section to the target file, the virus must modify the start code in the place of AddressOfEntryPoint so as to firstly execute the virus code. Therefore, the Windows PE virus generally has the module of adding new section to infected files.

2.6 The Module of Returning to the Target File

In order to improve the viability, the virus should not destroy the infected target files. When infecting the target files, the virus should preserve the original value of AddressOfEntryPoint. After the execution, the virus should jump back to the original value of AddressOfEntryPoint to hand over control to the target files. Therefore, the Windows PE virus generally has the module of returning to the target file.

3 The Immune-Based Detection Theory

The main function of the immune system is how to distinguish between self and non-self [12], and thereafter protect self and kill nonself. Similarly, the main function of the computer virus detection system is how to discriminate viruses from benign programs. Given the similarity of the two systems, the computer virus detection system can draw inspirations from the immune system, so as to achieve better detection efficiency. We will elaborately introduce the immune-based approach below.

3.1 The Detection Process

The detection process of our approach consists of the following steps. Firstly, the relocation modules are extracted as virus genes from the viruses by antigen-presenting. Secondly, the qualified antibodies are generated from the virus genes through negative selection. Finally, the generated antibodies are used to detect the known and previously unknown viruses. The logic detection processes are shown in Figure 2.

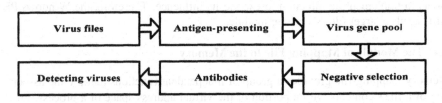

Fig. 2. The detection process

3.2 The Dynamic Evolution of Self and Nonself

In this study, *Self* is defined as the protected files, and *Nonself* suspicious files. Suppose AG is a question domain, that is, $AG = \bigcup_{i=1}^{\infty} H^i$, and H= (0,1,2,..., 9, A, B, C, D, E, F), a hexadecimal number set, i the positive integer. *Self* and *Nonself* satisfy the following conditions, respectively, that is, $Self \subset AG$, $Nonself \subset AG$, $Self \cup Nonself = AG$, $Self \cap Nonself = \varnothing$.

In the immune systems, the self and nonself are dynamic changing with the interaction between them. Similarly, the *self* and *nonself* in the computer immune systems change with the infection and the effect. In other words, a self becomes a nonself with the infection, and a nonself becomes a self with the repair. The dynamic evolutional equations of *Self* and *Nonself* are as follows.

$$Self(t) = \begin{cases} S_{initial}, t = 0 \\ Self(t-1) - Self_{del}(t) + Self_{new}(t), t \geq 1 \end{cases} \quad (1)$$

$$Self_{del}(t) = \{s \mid s \in Self(t-1) \wedge \exists y \in SA(t-1) \wedge <s, y> \in Match\} \quad (2)$$

$$Self_{new}(t) = \{s \mid s \in Nonself(t-1) \wedge \forall y \in SA(t-1) \wedge <s, y> \notin Match\} \quad (3)$$

$$Nonself(t) = \begin{cases} NS_{initial}, t = 0 \\ Nonself(t-1) - Nonself_{del}(t) + Nonself_{new}(t), t \geq 1 \end{cases} \tag{4}$$

$$Nonself_{del}(t) = Self_{new}(t) \tag{5}$$

$$Nonself_{new}(t) = Self_{del}(t) \tag{6}$$

where

$S_{initial}$ is the *Self* initial set that is composed of 500 normal Windows system files;

$Self_{del}$ is the *Nonself* set that has removed from the *Self* set;

$Self_{new}$ is the new generated *Self* set that are previously in the *Nonself* set, but are removed from it because of their non-matching with any antibodies;

$NS_{initial}$ is the *Nonself* initial set that are suspiciously infected by the viruses.

3.3 The Antigen-Presenting

The antigen-presenting is the process that extracts viruses' genes (virus relocation modules) from the suspicious files to form virus gene pool. The reasons why we choose relocation modules as virus genes are as follows. Firstly, the Windows PE virus relocation module is usually at the beginning of virus source code, and always small and little changed code easy to extract. Secondly, the other modules in the Windows PE virus such as the module of obtaining the API address, the module of searching target files and the module of memory-mapping file are also used in the normal programs. Thirdly, the module of adding a new section the infected files is extremely complex and difficult to analyze, though it is generally not found in the normal programs. The normally relocation module of the virus is shown in Figure 3. We extract the hex codes E8000000005B81EB2E1F4000 as the virus gene by anti-presenting.

.text: 00401F29	E8 00 00 00 00	call	$+5
.text: 00401F2E	loc_401F2E:		
.text: 00401F2E	5B	pop	ebx
.text: 00401F2F	81 EB 2E 1F 40 00	sub	ebx, offset loc_401F2E

Fig. 3. The relocation module of the virus

The virus gene pool through the antigen-presenting is defined as follows.

$$V = \{ v | v \in \bigcup_{i=8}^{32} H^i \wedge |v| = i \wedge v = Ap(x \in Nonself) \} \tag{7}$$

where

$Ap(x)$ is the antigen-presenting function;

v is the virus gene extracted from the virus relocation module, whose length is between eight and thirty-two hexadecimal codes.

3.4 The Generation of the Antibody

The acquired immune system that can protect against the specific viruses is generally acquired through vaccination to generate specific antibodies. The antibodies in this study are generated from the extraction of the vaccines in the virus gene pool, which are the virus genes obtained by antigen-presenting. Then, the detectors are generated from the antibodies to detect the viruses. For example, we will generate the detector E8000000005B from the virus gene pool. The detector set is defined as follows.

$$D = \{< d, affinity >| d \in \bigcup_{i=8}^{32} H^i, affinity \in N\} \tag{8}$$

where

d is the antibody;

affinity is the match between the antigen and the antibody.

3.5 The Detection of Windows PE Virus

After the detectors were generated, they can effectively detect Windows PE viruses. During the detection, the antigen whose affinity with the antibody is larger than the threshold value will be regarded as a virus. The dynamic evolutional equations of the antibodies and the detection of Windows PE viruses are as follows.

$$SA(t) = \begin{cases} \varnothing, t = 0 \\ SA(t-1) + SA_{new}(t), t \geq 1 \end{cases} \tag{9}$$

$$SA_{new}(t) = \{v | v \in D, \forall y \in Self, < v, y > \notin Match \wedge v.affinity \geq \beta\} \tag{10}$$

$$Match = \{< v, y >| v \in D, y \in AG, f_{match}(v.d, AP(y)) = 1\} \tag{11}$$

$$f_{match}(v, y) = \begin{cases} 1, f_{affinity}(v,y)/L_v \geq \alpha \\ 0, otherwise \end{cases} \tag{12}$$

$$f_{affinity}(v,y) = \max(x_1, x_2, ..., x_{|L_v - Ly|+1}) \tag{13}$$

$$x_i = \sum_{i=1}^{min(L_v, L_y)} \theta_{ij} \tag{14}$$

$$\theta_{ij} = \begin{cases} 1, v_i = y_{i+j-1}, 1 \leq i \leq |L_v - L_y|+1, 1 \leq j \leq L_v \\ 0, otherwise \end{cases} \tag{15}$$

where

SA is the specific antibody set;

SA_{new} is the new generated antibody set, whose affinity with self is greater than the threshold value β;

f_{match} is the matching function between antibody and antigen;

$f_{affinity}$ is the affinity function between antibody and antigen;

$Match$ is the set consisting of the antigens and the antibodies matched by the antigens;

θ_{ij} is the affinity value; if there is a matching between an antibody and an antigen, the value is 1, otherwise 0;

Lv is the vaccine length;
Ly is the antigen length.

4 Experiment and Results

The experiment was conducted in the computer virus and anti-virus laboratory, computer network and information security Institute of Sichuan University. Since there is no benchmark data set available for the detection of computer viruses unlike intrusion detection, the data sets including 100 viruses and 500 benign executables were collected from the website VX Heavens [13] and from system32 folder in Windows, respectively. The main goal of the experiment is to test the detection rate of known and unknown viruses and false-positive rate of the normal files. The experimental results are shown in Figure 4. Figure 4 shows that the detection rate of the Windows PE viruses is 97%, the omitting rate is 3%, and the false-positive rate (misidentification of legitimate programs as viruses) is only 3.6%. The good experimental result can own to the detectors generated from the relocation module that is the indispensable part of Windows PE viruses, which make them accurately detect Windows PE viruses with higher detection rate. The detectors can detect most of Windows PE viruses except the shelled and encrypted ones. Since the shelled and encrypted viruses were protected by the shell and the inner binary codes including the relocation part were disturbed with encryption, the detection of them will result in the omitting rate. Meanwhile, some legitimate system programs comprise the relocation module that in turn leads to false-positive rate.

In order to test the performance of the proposed approach, we conducted the related comparison experiments with the currently most mature antivirus technologies including the Kingsoft 2008, Panda 2008, KV 2008, Eset NOD32 and Kaspersky 7.0.

The comparison experiments results are shown in Figure 5 that the detection rate of our proposed approach is 97%, Eset NOD32 94%, Kaspersky 7.0 88%, Panda 2008 67%, Jiangmin KV2008 55%, and Kingsoft 2008 44%. Since most antivirus technologies are signature-based, they can only detect known computer viruses, and need to be updated frequently for its effectiveness. If their signature databases do not

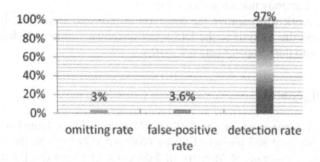

Fig. 4. The experiment results of our approach

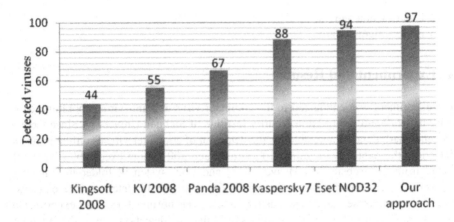

Fig. 5. The comparison experiments results

include a previously unknown virus signature, they cannot detect it. As a result, they have the higher detection rate of known viruses but lower detection rate of previously unknown viruses. Unlike them, our approach is non-signature-based technology, which can detect known and previously unknown viruses. The results indicate that our proposed approach has higher detection rate than the others, and efficiently testify the validity of our proposed approach.

5 Conclusions and Future Work

The Windows PE viruses have become an intriguing target of most virus writers, which leads to the continuously upgrade of the Windows PE viruses. At the same time, the currently antivirus is impossible to effectively detect unknown Windows PE viruses for most of them are signature-based. We draw inspirations from the immune system and the relocation module of the virus source code, and proposed the immune based approach for detection of the Windows PE viruses. The experimental results show that the proposed approach which is non-signature-based not only has a high detection rate, low false-positive rate and low omitting rate, but also its efficiency is better than the currently mature antivirus products.

The future work will improve the detection to take into account shelled information, and extend the analysis to the DLLs and unknown worms, which are presently the most threat to the computer network systems.

Acknowledgement

This work was sponsored by the National Natural Science Foundation of China (60573130), National 863 project of China (2006AA01Z435), and the New Century Excellent Expert Program of Ministry of Education of China (NCET-04-0870).The authors acknowledge the support of computer virus and antivirus Lab of Sichuan University and thank the VX Heavens!

References

1. Ford, R., Spafford, E.H.: Happy Birthday, Dear Viruses. Science 317, 210–211 (2007)
2. Balthrop, J., Forrest, S., Newman, M.E.J., et al.: Technological networks and the spread of computer viruses. Science 304, 527–529 (2004)
3. Xu, J.Y., Sung, A.H., Chavez, P.: Polymorphic malicious executable scanner by API sequence analysis. In: Fourth International Conference on Hybrid Intelligent Systems, pp. 378–383 (2004)
4. Reddy, D.K.S., Pujari, A.K.: N-gram analysis for computer virus detection. Journal in Computer Virology 2, 231–239 (2006)
5. Tesauro, G.J., Kephart, J.O., Sorkin, G.B.: Neural networks for computer virus recognition. IEEE Expert 11(4), 5–6 (1996)
6. Boyun, Z., Jianping, Y., Jingbo, G., Dingxing, Z.: Unknown Computer Virus Detection Based on Multi-naive Bayes Algorithm. Computer Engineering 32(10), 18–21 (2006)
7. Shuo, W., Ji-liu, Z., Bo, P.: Unknown virus detection based on API sequence and support vector machine. Journal of Computer Applications 27(8), 1942–1943 (2007)
8. Boyun, Z., Jianping, Y., Dingxing, Z., Jingbo, H.: Unknown Computer Virus Detection Based on K-Nearest Neighbor Algorithm. Computer Engineering and Applications 41(6), 7–10 (2005)
9. Yueling, C., Xiaozhu, J.: Computer Viruses Detection Method Based on Program Behavior. Journal of Qingdao University (Natural Science Edition) 19(2), 61–65 (2006)
10. Schultz, M.G., Eskin, E., Zadok, E.: Data Mining Methods for Detection of New Malicious Executables. In: IEEE Symposium on Security and Privacy (2001)
11. Guojpeng/CVC.GB.: The analysis of Win32 PE viruses (2003), http://www.hynubbs.cn/netstar/news_view.asp?id=61
12. Forrest, S., Perelson, A.S.: Self-nonself discrimination in a computer. In: IEEE Symposium on Security and Privacy, pp. 202–213 (1994)
13. VX Heavens, http://vx.netlux.org

Using Genetic Algorithms for Parameter Optimization in Building Predictive Data Mining Models

Ashish Sureka and Kishore Varma Indukuri

SETLabs, Infosys Technologies Ltd., Bangalore, India
Ashish_Sureka@infosys.com,
Kishore_Varma@infosys.com

Abstract. We present an application of genetic algorithms to search the space of model building parameters for optimizing the score function or accuracy of a predictive data mining model. The goal of predictive modeling is to build a classification or regression model that can accurately predict the value of a target column by observing the values of the input attributes. The process of finding an optimal algorithm and its control parameters for building a predictive model is a non-trivial process because of two reasons. The first reason is that the number of classification algorithms and its control parameters are very large. The second reason is that it can be quite time consuming to build a model for datasets containing a large number of records and attributes. These two reasons makes it impractical to enumerate through every algorithm and its possible control parameters for finding an optimal model. Genetic Algorithms are adaptive heuristic search algorithm and have been successfully applied to solve optimization problems in diverse domains. In this work, we formulate the problem of finding optimal predictive model building parameter as an optimization problem and examine the usefulness of genetic algorithms. We perform experiments on several datasets and report empirical results to show the applicability of genetic algorithms to the problem of finding optimal predictive model building parameters.

1 Introduction

Predictive Modeling is considered to be one of the most used data mining technology and has been applied to many engineering and scientific disciplines. The objective of predictive modeling is to a build a model from historical data assigning records into different classes or categories based on their attributes. A model is learned using the historical data and is then used to predict membership of new records. One of the fields in the historical data is designated as the target or class variable, and the other fields in the dataset are referred to as the independent variables (inputs or predictors).

There are several methods that fall under the group of classification-based predictive modeling algorithms.The range of classification methods include decision trees, neural networks, support-vector machines, bayes methods and nearest

C. Tang et al. (Eds.): ADMA 2008, LNAI 5139, pp. 260–271, 2008.

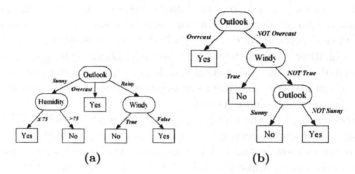

Fig. 1. (a) Decision Tree built using J48 learning scheme with the value of binary split control parameter set to false. (b) Decision Tree built using J48 learning scheme with the value of binary split control parameter set to true.

neighbor approach. Amongst the various classification methods, decision tree is arguably the most popular technique for predictive modeling. Many tree-building algorithms have been proposed in the literature and the various algorithms differ from each other in terms of their splitting criteria, pruning techniques, handling of missing values and continuous variables. Some of the algorithms used to build decision trees include ID3 [Qui86], C4.5, C5.0, SLIQ, CART (Classification and Regression Trees) and CHAID (Chi-square Automatic Interaction Detector). Each of these algorithms have several tuning parameters which can be varied and has an effect on the generated model. For example, the J48 algorithm, provided in the popular open source machine learning tool Weka [WF05], for generating an un-pruned or a pruned C4.5 decision tree has many tuning parameters. A user can set the value of a parameter called as binary splits to true or false. Similarly, the user has freedom to set values for other tuning parameters such as the usage of laplace option or sub-tree raising. The various algorithms to build predictive models combined with their respective tuning parameters results in a very large number of ways in which a model can be built. Applying different algorithms and their tuning parameters will result in a large number of potentially different models having potentially different predictive accuracy, precision and size.

Figures 1a and 1b illustrates two different models that we obtained by applying the J48 algorithm implemented in Weka. For the models shown in Figures 1a and 1b, the training data was the same and the values of all tuning parameters were same except for the parameter binary split. For the model in Figure 1a, the value of binary split parameter was set to false and for the model in Figure 1b, the value of binary split parameter was set to true. When we supplied same test data to both models, the accuracy results obtained were different.

There are several studies done in the past to compare various classification algorithms. A study was initiated by the European Commission under the Stat-Log project that compared many different classification algorithms on real-word problems [RKS95]. The authors used datasets from various domains such as medicine, finance, engineering etc and observed that the performance of an algorithms depends critically on the dataset [RKS95]. It is thus important to find an appropriate algorithm for a particular dataset. A study was done to review statistical tests for determining whether one classification algorithm is better than another on a particular learning task [Die98]. The author mentions that it is one of the most fundamental and difficult question in machine learning to answer which learning algorithm will produce more accurate classifiers for a particular dataset and domain [Die98].

The historical data or the input data used to build a model is called as the training set and in commercial data mining projects it is common to have the size of training dataset in the order of millions. The time required to build a predictive model (for example a decision tree model or a neural network model) increases with the increase in the number of training examples and the number of attributes in each record. For instance, depending on the computational resources, it can take several hours to build a predictive model from a training dataset that contains millions of records where each record contains several hundred attributes.

The process of building a predictive model is an iterative process where an analyst tries different mining methods and fine tunes their control parameters to build several models. The analyst then evaluates the various models obtained by comparing them on the basis of a user defined objective function. There are many important factors that need to be considered in deciding whether a learned model is appropriate to be deployed in an application. One of the parameter to judge the quality of a model is the classification error which signifies the accuracy of a model in assigning class labels to new classes. Other criteria can be the size of the model (for example the depth of a decision tree and the number of nodes in the tree) and the mis-detection rate for each of the target categories. Two models can have the same overall accuracy but may differ in their accuracy rates with respect to each individual categories or target classes. The appropriate model to select and deploy depends on the nature of the problem. All misclassification or errors may not be equally serious. For example, consider a situation in which a model is built for predicting presence of a heart disease in a patient based on his sugar level, age, gender, blood pressure etc. An error committed in diagnosing a patient as healthy when one is suffering from life-threatening heart disease (falsely classified as negative) is more serious than the opposite type of error where someone is diagnosed as suffering from a heart disease when one is in fact healthy (falsely classified as positive). If a choice has to be made between two models having the same overall error rate, then the one which has a low error rate for false negative decisions should be preferred to classify patients as ill or healthy. Thus distinguishing among error types is important and typically an analyst builds several models to decide which one is best suited.

There are thus two problems making it computationally expensive to find optimal predictive model building parameters. One problem is that the number of model building parameters are very large. The large number of parameters makes an exhaustive search infeasible. Other problem is that building a single

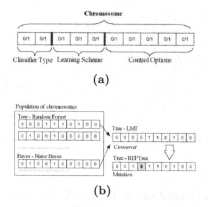

Fig. 2. (a) A binary string representation of predictive model building parameters. (b) An example of selection, crossover and mutation applied to a population of predictive model building parameters.

model itself can consume a substantial amount of time in cases where the dataset contains a huge number of records and attributes.

When enumeration over the entire space of solutions is not possible, heuristics like genetic algorithms and tabu search can be used to find a good solution which may not be the best solution by sacrificing completeness in return of efficiency. Metaheuristic search algorithms such as genetic algorithms have been applied successfully to a number of optimization problems in many engineering disciplines [Gol89], [HH04], [Mit98]. The work presented in this paper describes our design and experiences in applying genetic algorithms to search the space of predictive model building parameters. We present simulation results to show that genetic algorithms can serve as a useful technique to find a *good* predictive model in a *reasonable* amount of time.

2   Experimental Setup

Genetic algorithms are a rapidly growing area of artificial intelligence, inspired by Darwin's theory of evolution. It was invented by John Holland at University of Michigan in the 1960s and has been shown to work very well on some types of discrete combinatorial optimization problems. They are less susceptible to getting stuck at local optima than gradient search methods. Our problem requires searching through a huge number of possibilities in a search space whose structure is not well known and genetic algorithms have shown to perform well under such situations.

To carry out search by means of metaheuristic techniques such as genetic algorithms, several elements of the problem and search strategy must be defined: a model of the problem and a representation of possible solutions, transformation operators that are capable of changing an existing solution into an alternative solution and a strategy for searching the space of possible solutions using the

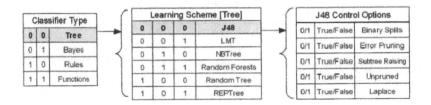

Classifier Type		
0	0	Tree
0	1	Bayes
1	0	Rules
1	1	Functions

Learning Scheme [Tree]			
0	0	0	J48
0	0	1	LMT
0	1	0	NBTree
0	1	1	Random Forests
1	0	0	Random Tree
1	0	1	REPTree

J48 Control Options		
0/1	True/False	Binary Splits
0/1	True/False	Error Pruning
0/1	True/False	Subtree Raising
0/1	True/False	Unpruned
0/1	True/False	Laplace

Fig. 3. An example mapping a ten bit chromosome into a predictive model building parameter

representation and transformation operators [Nil71]. We use genetic algorithms to explore the space of predictive model building parameters with the objective of finding a learning scheme and its control options that maximizes the overall accuracy of the classifier.

2.1   A Binary String Representation of Model Building Parameters

It is important to encode the solution and solution space in a format so that genetic algorithms can be applied. In this section, we present our design of transforming a model building parameter into a vector of binary variables in a form applicable to metaheuristic search. The classifier type, learning scheme and control options required to build a predictive model is represented as a candidate solution for the metaheuristic search and the objective is to efficiently explore the space of model building parameters and find a accuracy maximizing classifier. We represent candidate solutions as a binary string of $0's$ and $1's$. We set the size of a chromosome or a candidate solution to ten bits.

Figure 2a shows chromosomes in a GA population taking the form of bit strings. Chromosomes are divided into genes (single bits) that encode a particular element of the candidate solution. As shown in Figure 2a, the first two bits are used to represent a classifier type. We experiment with four classifier types: tree, bayes, rules and functions. Based on our encoding scheme, if the first two bits of a chromosome are 0 then it represents a tree classifier whereas if the first bit is 0 and the second bit is 1 then it represents a bayes classifier. Rules and function classifiers are represented by 10 and 11.

The next three bits are used to encode learning schemes within a classifier type. There are several learning schemes which fall under the category of tree based classifiers. Some of the decision tree inducing algorithms implemented in Weka are: J48, LMT, NBTree, Random Forests, Random Tree and REPTree [WF05]. Each of these tree building algorithms are represented by a unique string of three bits. The same logic follows for other classifier types. We prepared a list of algorithms implemented in Weka for each of the classifier types and assigned a unique string of three bits to each of them. The last five bits of the chromosomes represents tuning parameters for the various algorithms. For instance, some of the tuning parameters for the JRip algorithm algorithm includes setting the values for error rate, number of optimizations, value of minimal weights and whether to use pruning or not [Coh95]. Changing the values of these parameters can possibly result in different models resulting in different classification accuracies.

Due to limited space, it is not possible to provide a list of all learning schemes along with their tuning parameters and the values that they can take. Figure 3 illustrates how a ten bit chromosome is mapped to a predictive model building parameter. Figure 3 shows how a chromosome starting with 00 is translated to a tree based classifier and how the next three bits translates to a specific algorithm within a classifier type. For instance, a binary string of 0000010101 represents a J48 classifier [WF05], [Qui93] with binary splits, using sub-tree raising and laplace while setting the values of error-pruning and un-pruned to off.

2.2 Evaluation

The method used for computing solution fitness is a key component of genetic algorithms. Based on the fitness of the population, the algorithm stochastically selects individuals from the population to produce offspring via genetic operators like mutation and crossover.

In our experiments we use accuracy of a classifier as a measure of fitness. Accuracy is the percentage of correct predictions made by a predictive model over a data set. It measures how accurate a model's predictions are. There are other metrics such as precision, recall, F-measures, accuracy for each category to judge the performance of a classifier [JH00], [DJH00], [WF05]. The experiments performed in this work uses only the overall accuracy of a classifier as a measure of fitness.

2.3 Selection and Crossover

There are several selection criterion that can be employed and the intention behind all these selection criterion is to improve the overall quality of the population. Some of the selection criterion that have been used previously are proportionate selection, ranking selection and tournament selection [B94], [GD91]. The key point is that selection criterion should be such that good solutions are more likely to survive. In our experiments, we used the Best Chromosome selection criterion (retaining the fittest chromosome or configuration for next iteration) implemented in the JGAP (Java Genetic Algorithms Package)[1] tool.

In our experiments we apply the default crossover technique implemented in the JGAP (Java Genetic Algorithms Package tool. The default cross over rate is $\frac{populationsize}{2}$.

2.4 Mutation

The GA has a mutation probability, m, which dictates the frequency with which mutation occurs. For each string element in each string in the mating pool, the

---

[1] Homepage for JGAP: http://jgap.sourceforge.net/

GA checks to see if it should perform a mutation. If it should, it randomly changes the element value to a new one. In our representation of the binary strings, $1's$ are changed to $0's$ and $0's$ to $1's$. Mutation is performed after the crossover operation. In our simulations, we use the default values of $'m'$ implemented in JGAP (m is by default set to $\frac{1}{15}$).

Figure 2b is an example of selection, crossover and mutation applied to a population of predictive model building parameters. Two binary strings from a population of chromosomes are selected for performing crossover and mutation. The first chromosome encodes a Random Forest learning scheme and the second chromosome encodes Naive Bayes learning scheme. The two chromosomes are combined to produce an offspring that encodes a REPTree learning scheme. The shaded cell in the offspring chromosome represents the gene that was mutated.

3   Experimental Results

The experiments are carried out in 4 phases. The *first phase* is a sequential walk through all the algorithms with default control parameters. We measure the classification accuracies and the time taken by each of the algorithm. This phase is to show the accuracy and time variations for building a predictive model over a common dataset. In the first phase, the *control options field* is left unused. The *second phase* is a sequential walk through all the algorithms with various parameters and its values. In second phase, we iterate through the entire search space and test all the possible combinations (classifier types, algorithms as well as the control options). Our purpose was to check the accuracy variations across different classifier types (phase one) as well as the variations within the same classifier type and across different algorithms and control parameters within the same classifier type (phase two). The *third phase* is a default run of GA algorithms with the chromosome designed as discussed above. In this phase, the parameters of an algorithm can be changed by altering the *control options field* of the chromosome. The *fourth phase* involves some optimizations to speed up the GA algorithm by reducing the search space.

***Phase 1* : Execution times and accuracies across different classifier types.** In this phase, an iteration over each of the algorithm with their default parameters is performed and the execution time and accuracies are recorded. For example, the chromosome whose first 5 bits are 00000, represents a Tree classification algorithm: J48. All the chromosomes with the first 5 bits (MSB) represents J48 algorithm. We do not utilize he control options and use the default parameters. For example, the default parameters for J48 are: "-C 0.25 -M 2". This means that the *Pruning Confidence* is set as 0.25 and *minimum number of instances* as 2 respectively. The next classifier 00001 is RandomForest with default parameters as "-I 10 -K 0 -S 1". This means that the *number of trees* is set as 10, *number of features* is set as 0, *seed for random number generator* is set as 1 respectively.

Graph in Figure 4a shows that different classification models take different execution time and achieve different accuracies on a common dataset. Surprisingly, even the algorithms that are closely related may take completely different execution times and may result in completely different accuracies on a common dataset. For example, as shown in in Figure 4a, RandomTree and RandomForest results in varied execution time even though the accuracies are the same.

Phase 2 : **Execution times and accuracies across different classifier types and control options.** The maximum possible variations in parameters that can be tested in a particular Classification algorithm are 32 (as the number of bits in *control options field* is 5). For instance, the chromosome 0000000110 represents J48 Classification algorithm with parameters set as "-U -B -M 2". This means that in J48 algorithm, the flags *use unpruned tree* and *use binary splits only* are turned **ON** and parameter *set minimum number of instances per leaf* is set to 2 respectively. By altering the LSB of this chromosome, we get a new chromosome 0000000111. This chromosome represents the same J48 algorithm but with parameters "-S -R -N 3 -Q 1 -B -M 2 -A" which means that the flags *perform subtree raising* set to false, *use reduced error pruning* are turned **ON**, parameters *number of folds* is set to 3 and *seed for random data shuffling* is set to 1, flags *use binary splits only, minimum number of instances, laplace smoothing for predicted probabilities* is turned **ON** respectively. For our experiments, the Classification algorithms used are :

− Tree : J48, RandomForest, RandomTree, REPTree
− Bayes : NaiveBayes, NaiveBayesUpdateable
− Rules : ConjunctiveRule, JRip, NNge, OneR, PART
− Functions : MultilayerPerceptron, RBFNetwork, SimpleLogistic

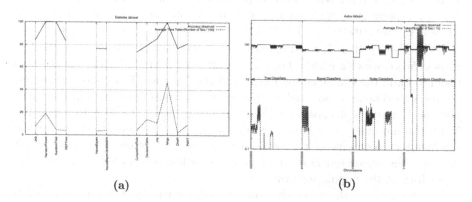

(a)   (b)

Fig. 4. (a) Execution times and accuracies across different classifier types, (b) Execution times and accuracies across different classifier types and control options

The maximum limit on number of algorithms in a particular category is 8. It may not always be possible to find all 8 algorithms for each of the category. The chromosomes corresponding to unassigned learning schemes will be rendered invalid and will be ignored during the GA execution.

To avoid chromosomes having null values in the sense that no classifier is assigned to it, we implemented a scheme that will make sure that none of the chromosome is left unassigned. All the values in different fields (like the classifier category, learning scheme and control options) are treated independently and assigned to existing classifiers in a cyclic fashion. This change increases the probability of trying more algorithms which otherwise would have been left out as invalid chromosome in default GA algorithm setup.

Figure 4b shows a sequential walk over each of the chromosome while recording their execution times and the prediction accuracies on the test dataset. Figure 4b shows variations in execution time and predictive accuracy across various classifiers. The variation is not only across different classifier types but also within different learning schemes within a classifier type. For example, as shown in Figure 4b, on an average Tree based classifier performs slightly better than Bayes based classifier in terms of the prediction accuracies. We also see a wide variation in prediction accuracies for Rule based classifiers (as compared to the other classifier types) for the specific Automobile dataset (obtained from UCI Machine Learning Repository).

In each of the categories (Tree Classifier, Bayes Classifier,etc.), we see that for some of the points the execution time taken tends to zero as we move from left to right. This is because we cache the results (accuracy and execution time) obtained during algorithm execution for later lookup. There are some classifiers which are mapped to multiple chromosomes (due to cyclic fashion used in assigning chromosomes to classifiers) and the classifier is only executed once (i.e., the first time) after which the cached results are reused.

Phase 3 : **GA Run with default parameters on two different datasets**
For our experiments, we used GA with its default Mutation probability and Cross over rate parameters (i.e. Mutation probability is $\frac{1}{15}$ and Cross over rate is $\frac{populationsize}{2}$). The Population Size parameter is varied from 2 to 20. The *Fitness Score*, which a Fitness Function returns can be a combination of the time taken to build the Classification model and the Accuracy it produces. However, for the experiments conducted in this work, a Fitness function which returns just the *Classifiers Accuracy* as *Fitness Score* is used. The Flag to retain the fittest chromosome over iterations is turned on i.e. GA is made to carry forward the fittest chromosome of an iteration to its next iteration. Parameter which indicates the maximum number of iterations allowed is varied from 20 to 50 depending on the population size.

In the Figure 5a, the x-axis denotes the target accuracy. The values on y-axis are in logarithmic scale and range from 1 to 15000. The y-axis is used to denote both the number of iterations and execution time. The figure shows results of one run of GA over anneal.ORIG dataset (obtained from UCI Machine Learning

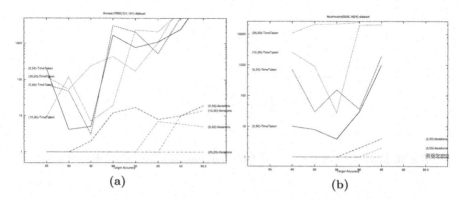

Fig. 5. (a) GA Run with default parameters on Anneal.ORIG dataset. (b) GA Run with default parameters on Mushroom dataset.

Repository) with 721 records in the training set and remaining 181 records in the testing set. The graph also shows the execution time and iterations for each of the combination of population size and maximum allowed iterations. For example, legend (2,50)-Iterations denotes the results for iterations in GA with population size set to 2 and maximum allowed iterations set to 50 It can be noted from the Figure 5a that, the execution time and iterations needed increase with the increase in target accuracy. It can also be noted that, the decrease in population size results in increase of the number of iterations needed to attain higher targets. As observed in the graph, when the population size is 20, GA achieves the target accuracy in single iteration except for a case where the target accuracy is 99.5. This happens because of two reasons. First being the population size 20 is quite high considering the small search space defined in our model. Second reason is that many classifiers yield high accuracies and hence finding one such solution with a high population size has high probability. However in a large scale implementation, where the search is of the much higher order, than the one used in this experiment, population size of 20 will be reasonable. We also performed similar experiments on a much larger dataset: Mushroom (obtained from UCI Machine Learning Repository) with 6506 records in training set and 1624 records in testing set . The results are plotted in Figure 5b. We see a similar pattern i.e. as the target increases the number of iterations required to achieve the desired accuracy also increases. However, this happens only after a threshold point (no increase is observed at 94 percent target accuracy). Also, as the population size increases we see a decrease in number of iterations required to achieve the target accuracy.

Phase 4 : **Optimized Search Space to make GA run faster** The 10-bit chromosome representation used so far, has some advantages and disadvantages. As the maximum limit on number of algorithms in a particular category is 8, we can accommodate more algorithms in all of the classifier categories in future. The advantage here is the ease in addition of more classifiers to a classifier category

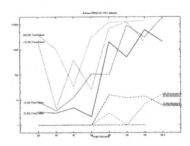

Fig. 6. Modified GA run with default parameters on Anneal.ORIG dataset

in future. However, the disadvantage in this strategy is the increase in search space. This phase has some optimizations to reduce the number of bits needed to represent the search space i.e. we try to reduce the chromosomes size. This in turn helps in speeding up the detection of the required predictive model. We do this by removing the boundaries among the 3 Fields in a chromosome. i.e. we dynamically count the total number of possible models[3] and assign them in a continuously manner to the entire range of chromosomes possible. The advantage of such an assignment is that, it reduces the search space by a factor of 2^k, if k is the number of bits saved by this continuous assignment. Figure 6 shows experiments on anneal.ORIG with the optimization as discussed in the previous paragraph.

There are several interesting possibilities for future research. We have done a preliminary investigation on the applicability of GAs. However, in this work the size of the search space (in terms of the number of algorithms and their control parameters) considered is small. More meaningful results and insights can be obtained by applying the approach with a much larger number of algorithms and parameters. Analyzing the effect of the search process and performance gains by tuning the various genetic algorithm parameters. We also plan to conduct further tests of the algorithms on other possibly more complex and large datasets. Another possibility is to add one more dimension to the search space. Along with the classifier types, learning scheme and control options, we plan to add the dimension of also finding the best subset of attributes or features from a dataset using search techniques [LS96], [VK93].

4   Conclusions

In this work, we apply genetic algorithms as an optimization tool for finding an accuracy maximizing predictive data mining model. The approach can be useful in situations where a user who may not be an expert in classification algorithms can find an optimal or near optimal predictive model from a space of a large number of possible models. The limitation of this approach is that genetic algorithm is a heuristic search techniques and is not guaranteed to find the optimal solution. No clean proof of convergence is known but our experiments show that the technique can be used to find good models in situations where it is computationally expensive to enumerate over all the possible models.

References

[B94]   Bck, T.: Selective pressure in evolutionary algorithms: A characterization of selection mechanisms. In: Proceedings of the first ieee conference on evolutionary computation. IEEE World Congress on Computational Intelligence (wcci) (1994)

[Coh95]   Cohen, W.W.: Fast effective rule induction. In: Proceedings 12th international conference on machine learning, Morgan kaufmann, San Francisco (1995)

[Die98]   Dieterich, T.G.: Approximate statistical tests for comparing supervised classification learning algorithms. Neural Computation 10(7), 899–7667 (1998)

[DJH00]   Hand, H.M.D.J., Smyth, P.: Principles of data mining. MIT Press, Cambridge (2000)

[GD91]   Goldberg, D.E., Deb, K.: A comparative analysis of selection scheme used in genetic algorithms. In: Rawlins, G. (ed.) Foundations of genetic algorithms. Morgan Kaufmann, San Mateo (1991)

[Gol89]   Goldberg, D.E.: Genetic algorithms in search, optimization, and machine learning, 1st edn. Addison-Wesley, Reading (1989)

[HH04]   Haupt, R.L., Haupt, S.E.: Practical genetic algorithms, 2nd edn. John Wiley and sons, Chichester (2004)

[JH00]   Kamber, M., Han, J.: Data mining: Concepts and techniques, 1st edn. Elsevier science and technology books, Amsterdam (2000) isbn: 1558604898

[LS96]   Liu, H., Setiono, R.: A probabilistic approach to feature selection - a filter solution. In: 13th international conference on machine learning (ICML), Bari, Italy, pp. 319–327 (1996)

[Mit98]   Mitchell, M.: An introduction to genetic algorithms. MIT Press, Cambridge (1998)

[Nil71]   Nilsson, N.J.: Problem-solving methods in artificial intelligence. McGraw-Hill companies, New York (1971)

[Qui86]   Quinlan, R.: Induction of decision trees. Machine learning 1, 81–106 (1986)

[Qui93]   Quinlan, R.: C4.5: Programs for machine learning. Morgan Kaufmann, San Mateo (1993)

[RKS95]   Feng, C., King, R., Shutherland, A.: Statlog: comparison of classification algorithms on large real-world problems. Applied artificial intelligence 9(3), 259–287 (1995)

[VK93]   Vafaie, H., De Jong, K.: Robust feature selection algorithms. In: Proceedings of the 5th IEEE International conference on tools for artificial intelligence, pp. 356–363. IEEE Press, Boston (1993)

[WF05]   Witten, I.H., Frank, E.: Data mining: Practical machine learning tools and techniques, 2nd edn. Morgan Kaufmann, San Francisco (2005)

Using Data Mining Methods to Predict Personally Identifiable Information in Emails

Liqiang Geng[1], Larry Korba[1], Xin Wang[2], Yunli Wang[1], Hongyu Liu[1],
and Yonghua You[1]

[1] Institute of Information Technology, National Research Council of Canada
Fredericton, New Brunswick, Canada
{liqiang.geng,larry.korba,yunli.wang,hongyu.liu,
yonghua.you}nrc-cnrc.gc.ca
[2] Department of Geomatics Engineering, University of Calgary, Calgary, Alberta, Canada
xcwang@ucalgary.ca

Abstract. Private information management and compliance are important issues nowadays for most of organizations. As a major communication tool for
organizations, email is one of the many potential sources for privacy leaks. Information extraction methods have been applied to detect private information in
text files. However, since email messages usually consist of low quality text, information extraction methods for private information detection may not achieve
good performance. In this paper, we address the problem of predicting the presence of private information in email using data mining and text mining methods. Two prediction models are proposed. The first model is based on
association rules that predict one type of private information based on other
types of private information identified in emails. The second model is based on
classification models that predict private information according to the content
of the emails. Experiments on the Enron email dataset show promising results.

1 Introduction

With the information explosion arising from marketing and other business requirements, today's organizations are facing increasing demands to assure privacy compliance with both internal and external policies, regulations, and laws. Externally,
corporations are required to comply with a variety of regulations depending on their
operational domains and sectors of business. Internally, good corporate practices
demand effective management, good decision making, clear accountability, effective
risk management, corporate integrity, etc. with respect to the collection, storage and
use of personally identifiable information (PII). Because of these increasing demands,
corporations are in need of automated tools that can assist in the monitoring of PII
data access in workflows, and in ensuring and demonstrating compliance with various
privacy requirements.

Email is one of the most important communication and information exchange tools
for modern organizations. It has greatly improved work efficiency of organizations.
However, with the increasing use of email, leaks and violations of the use of client PII
have become a serious issue that organizations are facing.

C. Tang et al. (Eds.): ADMA 2008, LNAI 5139, pp. 272–281, 2008.
© Springer-Verlag Berlin Heidelberg 2008

Two approaches can be used to ensure and to demonstrate privacy compliance for email. First, we can monitor the email content before the emails are sent out. Emails can be blocked if any violations have been detected according to policies and operational context. We call this approach *prevention*. The advantage of this approach is that the privacy violations can be prevented before an email is sent out. The disadvantage is that it may not be flexible enough. In real applications, there may be exceptions and emergencies which require immediate access to private information but which may not be allowed in normal process. The prevention approach may be a hindrance in these situations. In the second approach, which we called *audit*, we need software tools to find traces of the privacy leaks on an as-needed basis, or to report privacy violations on a regular basis. The advantage of this approach is that it provides the user great flexibility. The disadvantage is that it may work after the damage has been done.

The related work on detecting private information in emails is very limited. Armour et al. proposed an email compliance engine to detect privacy violations [3, 4]. This engine consists of two components: The entity extraction module which can identify private information such as names, phone numbers, social insurance numbers, student numbers, and addresses, and the privacy verification module which determines if the email should be blocked according to the type of private information detected, the recipients of the email, and the electronic policies or rules stored in a database. This method is aimed to prevent the private information leaks.

Carvalho and Cohen deal with private information leaks in email from another perspective [5]. They try to prevent the messages from accidentally being addressed to non-desired recipients. The approach does not detect private information in the emails directly. Instead, it predicts if an email is being sent to the wrong person based on the content of the email, the recipient, and the email history of the sender. They used an outlier detection method, which incorporates both content analysis and social network analysis.

It should be noted that private information discovery is different from privacy-preserving data mining [2, 6]. First, privacy-preserving data mining usually works on structured data, like databases, while private information discovery usually works on free text. Secondly, privacy-preserving data mining assumes that the location of the private information is known and uses this information as constraints for data mining process, while the aim of private information discovery is to identify the location and type of the private information. Thirdly, the information in databases for privacy-preserving data mining is more easily manageable than the free text used for private information discovery.

Our work on private information discovery is part of the Social Network Applied to Privacy (SNAP) project [8] underway within National Research Council of Canada. The project addresses the comprehensive issues in managing PII within organizations. The most important issues include identifying the PII in different kinds of documents stored in a computer and in network traffic, tracing user's access and entry of PII, and detecting the inappropriate access to or use of PII in workflow. The first step and the core of these functionalities is to identify the private information, such as email addresses, telephone numbers, addresses, social insurance numbers, etc.

Currently, PII detection algorithms have been implemented in SNAP to detect private information. For example, pattern matching and dictionary lookup [7] are used to identify the addresses, and Luhn algorithm [13] is used to identify credit card numbers. These algorithms can achieve high precision and recall for high quality documentations, but they may obtain poor performance for text of low quality, like email (i.e. text containing many acronyms, abbreviations, and misspellings). For example, a misspelling "Avenu" cannot be found in the dictionary of street types (we only store "Avenue" and "Ave" in the dictionary as the street type). Therefore, the algorithm will fail to identify the address containing "Avenu". Secondly, the information in the dictionary may evolve. If the dictionary cannot be updated in time, we will fail to detect the PII. For example, if new area codes have been added for the telephone numbers, they have to be updated in the dictionary to make sure that telephone numbers with the newly added area code can be identified. Thirdly, it is very easy for the sender of the email to circumvent the detection system by simply inserting some characters in the PII such that it is easy for human to comprehend, and yet difficult to detect with algorithms (an approach used in spam email messages). For example, the sentence "Tom's credit card number is 5*1*8*1*3*4*5*6*4*5*6*7*5*6*7*8" contains a credit card number, but most algorithms can not detect the pattern with "*" inserted.

2 Prediction Methods

In this paper, we address the problem of predicting PII in email using association rule mining and classification model mining. We do not intend to identify the detailed private information. Instead, we only predict if there is a private entity occurring in an email based on the subject and content of the email. This predicting model can be integrated with the existing information extraction-based private information detection algorithms in two ways, as shown in Figure 1. In Figure 1(a), we use the prediction model to improve the efficiency of the private information detection for the audit process. In practice, only a small portion of the emails contain private information. In this case, we can apply prediction model first to identify the emails that contain the private information with a high probability. Then we apply more time consuming detection algorithms to identify the detailed private information.

Figure 1(b) shows the second integration. It combines prediction models and the detection algorithms to improve the recall and precision of the detection system. In the case that the detection algorithm fails to identify private information and the prediction algorithm gives a positive prediction, we present the results to the user and the user must check the email manually.

In this paper, we consider four types of PII elements, *email addresses, telephone numbers, addresses,* and *money*. We employed two models for prediction, association rules and classification models. The association rules represent correlation between two itemsets [1]. In our case, we want to find the correlation among these four types of the PII elements and use the correlation to predict one type of PII elements based on other types of PII elements already detected or predicted in an email. The second model is based on the classification model. It predicts the private information based on the subject and content of the emails.

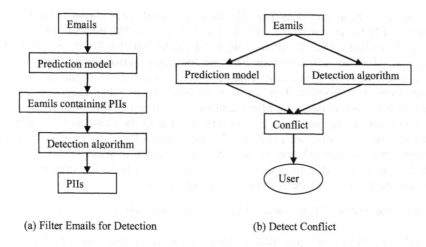

(a) Filter Emails for Detection   (b) Detect Conflict

Fig. 1. Integration of Prediction Model and the Detection Algorithms

2.1 Data Set

We worked on the Enron email dataset for our experiments. Enron was a U.S. corporation that conducted business in the energy sector from the 1980s until the early 2000s. With the rapid success of the business, Enron soon expanded their scope to include brokerage of a variety of commodities, including advertising time and network bandwidth. In 2001 the company collapsed due to accounting scandals. During the investigations that followed the collapse of the company, the Federal Energy Regulatory Commission made a large number of corporate email messages public. These emails have since been used as a useful source and benchmark for research in fields like link analysis, social network analysis, fraud detection, and textual analysis. There are different versions of the cleaned dataset. We chose the cleaned version from [12] to work on. The email dataset contains 252,759 messages from 151 employees distributed in around 3000 user defined folders. It is stored in a MySql database.

2.2 Using Association Rules to Predict Private Information

Association rule mining is a data mining approach which originated from the market basket problem. It discovers items that co-occur frequently within a data set. More formally, an association rule is defined in the following way [1]: Let $I = \{i_1, i_2, \ldots, i_m\}$ be a set of items. Let D be a set of transactions, where each transaction T is a set of items such that $T \subseteq I$. An association rule is an implication of the form $X \rightarrow Y$, where $X \subseteq I$, $Y \subseteq I$, and $X \cap Y = \Phi$. The rule $X \rightarrow Y$ holds for the dataset D with support s and confidence c if $s\%$ of transactions in D contain $X \cup Y$ and $c\%$ of transactions in D that contain X also contain Y. The confidence and support are measures that ensure the patterns found are statistically accurate and significant. For example, {milk, eggs} $\rightarrow$ {bread} is an association rule that says that when milk and eggs are purchased, bread is likely to be purchased as well.

In private information detection, we chose the emails sent during the period of January 1, 1999 to December 31, 2000 for our experiments. The number of the emails is 73,817. We first applied the privacy algorithm implemented in SNAP [8] to identify the private information in the emails. Then we constructed a two dimensional table, in which each row corresponds to an email and each column corresponds to a type of private elements. Therefore there are four attributes in the table, each representing *email address*, *phone number*, *address*, and *money*, respectively. If an email contains an *email address*, we put 1 to the cell corresponding to the email and the attribute *email address*. Otherwise, we put 0. We did the same for three other types of private elements. We then applied Apriori algorithm implemented in Weka [11] to mine association rules. We set support to 0.1% and confidence to 60%. The rules mined are shown in the following in the descending order of confidence.

EMAIL=true ADDRESS=true ==> PHONE=true   conf:(84%)

PHONE=true ADDRESS=true MONEY=true ==> EMAIL=true   conf:(82%)

EMAIL=true ADDRESS=true MONEY=true ==> PHONE=true   conf:(78%)

PHONE=true ADDRESS=true ==> EMAIL=true   conf:(73%)

PHONE=true MONEY=true ==> EMAIL=true   conf:(65%)

ADDRESS=true ==> PHONE=true   conf:(62%)

The first rule states that if an email contains an *email address* and an *address*, it will also contain a *telephone number* with the probability of 0.84 according to the dataset. In this case, if an *email address* and an *address* are detected in a new email, but the *phone number* is not detected. It may be worth a manual check into the email, because it is likely that the detection algorithm failed to find a phone number which occurs in the email.

Note that the experimental results may not be applied to other email dataset in different companies or sectors, because different companies may deal with different kinds of private information. However, the approach itself may be applied generally to different situations.

2.3 Using Classification Models to Predict Private Information

The classification problem is one of the major tasks in the area of data mining and machine learning. To address a classification problem, a classification model is built according to observed examples, which are represented in a two dimensional table. Each row in the table represents an object and each column represents an attribute. There is one attribute called the decision attribute, which represents the classes of the objects. All the other attributes are conditional attributes which serve as the condition for the classification. When a new example comes, its values for conditional attributes are inputted into the classification model. The model will classify the example into an appropriate class. The most well known classification systems include: Bayesian networks, neural networks, classification rules, and support vector machines [9].

We convert the private information prediction problem into a text classification problem. The conditional attributes are the words occurring in the emails, which we call features. The decision attribute is the attribute that indicates if there is a private element of some kind in the email. We first pre-process the email messages in the following way. We scan subjects and content of emails, remove stop words, and stem words using Porter algorithm [10]. After this processing, 5585 words are identified. Next, we select a subset of these words as features to train the classification model.

We use two methods to select the features for training. The first feature selection method that we use is based on the frequency of the words, and therefore is unsupervised. In this method, we choose the most frequent words as the features. Figure 2 shows the distribution of the words. The X-axis denotes the frequency threshold for pruning. The Y-axis denotes the number of words left after pruning. The distribution coincides with Zipf's law. For our experiments, we choose 100 for the frequency threshold and obtain 578 words as features. We use three representations: binary, frequency, and weighted, to construct the table. In the binary representation, if an email contains a word, we fill in the corresponding cell with 1, otherwise with 0. In the frequency representation, we record the frequency of a word occurring in the email. In the weighted frequency, we set the weight of the words in subject to 3, and weight of words in the content to 1. For example, if "trip" occurs once in subject and twice in content, its total importance value will be 5.

The second feature selection method is based on entropy and information gain, which is a supervised method. Our classification problem is a binary classification problem. If an email contains a piece of private element, we set the decision attribute $C = 1$, otherwise, we set $C = 0$. If a word w occurs in an email, we set condition attribute w to 1, otherwise it is set to 0. The entropy of the data is defined as

$$entropy\,(D) = -P(C = 0)\log_2 P(C = 0) - P(C = 1)\log_2 P(C = 1),$$

where $P(C = i) = $ *the number of the examples with class i / the number of all examples* denotes the probability of occurrences of class i. The entropy of data given a word w is defined as

$entropy(D \mid w) =$

$$- P(w = 0)(P(C = 0 \mid w = 0)\log_2 P(C = 0 \mid w = 0) + (P(C = 1 \mid w = 0)\log_2 P(C = 1 \mid w = 0))$$

$$- P(w = 1)(P(C = 0 \mid w = 1)\log_2 P(C = 0 \mid w = 1) + (P(C = 1 \mid w = 1)\log_2 P(C = 1 \mid w = 1))$$

where $P(w = 1) = $ *the number of the emails that contain word w / the number of all emails*, $P(w = 0) = $ *the number of the emails that do not contain word w / the number of all emails*. $P(C=0 \mid w= 0)$ denotes the conditional probability that an email does not contain private information given the word w does not occur in the email. With the same convention, it is straightforward to define $P(C= 1 \mid w= 0)$, $P(C= 0 \mid w= 1)$, $P(C= 1 \mid w= 1)$.

The information gain for word w is defined as

$$gain(w) = entropy(S) - entropy(S \mid w).$$

We chose the top 10% of words with the greatest information gain as features for training the classification models.

We chose C4.5 and SVM algorithms for the experiments. The C4.5 algorithm generates classification rules as classification models. It is an efficient algorithm and the

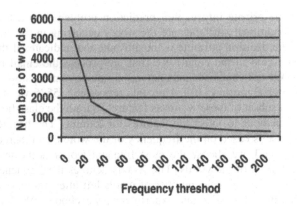

Fig. 2. Word distribution in terms of frequency

results offer easy comprehension. SVM is an optimization-based algorithm and is claimed to have good precision and recall on most datasets. We use the false positive rate (FPR) and false negative rate (FNR) to measure the performance of the classification modes. The false positive rate is defined as the ratio of the number of false positives to the number of all negatives. The false negative rate is defined as the ratio of the number of false negatives to the number of all positives. The reason that we use these two measures is due to the purpose of our task. In the case of the pre-detection, we do not want to miss any positive cases. Therefore, low false negative rate is desired. In the case of conflict detection, we do not want to provide too many false positive examples to increase the user's burden. Therefore, low false positive rate is desired.

We first did experiments for predicting *email addresses*. Table 1 shows the false positive rate. Table 2 shows the false negative rate.

Table 1. False positive rate for C4.5 and SVM

FPR	Binary	Frequency	Weighted	Information gain
C4.5	4.4%	3.8%	3.6%	3.0%
SVM	5.4%	1.8%	1.6%	3.2%

Table 2. False negative rate for C4.5 and SVM

FNR	Binary	Frequency	Weighted	Information gain
C4.5	55.3%	55.9%	54.9%	56.3%
SVM	44.4%	64.7%	61.0%	48.2%

From these two tables, we have several observations. First, the weighted representation always performs better than the frequency representation. Secondly, C4.5 is more insensitive to the representations than SVM is. Thirdly, the false negative rates are very high regardless of feature selection method. This is due to the fact that most of the examples are negative in terms of the private information. This makes our

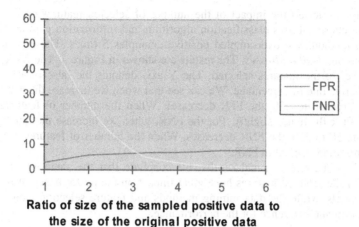

Fig. 3. Oversampling positive examples

classification problem an unbalanced one. To deal with this problem, we used an oversampling method to increase the number of the positive training examples. Figure 3 shows the false positive rate and false negative rate of the classification models learned from oversmapling.

The X-axis denotes the ratio of the size of the sampled positive data to the size of the original positive data. We can see that when the number of the positive samples for training increases, the false negative rate increases slightly, while the false positive rate decreases significantly. In this experimental setting, when we sample positive examples more than 5 times, there is no further improvement in either FPR or FNR.

We also did experiments for predicting *telephone number*, *addresses*, and *money*. We chose the C4.5 algorithm and the information gain feature selection method. We set the sampling ratio to 5. The experimental results are shown in Table 3.

Table 3. Oversampling for information gain feature selection

	Email	Telephone no.	Address	Money
FPR	7.9%	7.8%	1.9%	2.7%
FNR	1.5%	1.6%	0.4%	1.2%

We also experimented on the frequency selection method. The experimental results are shown in Table 4. We can see the information gain selection method produces smaller variances for FPR and FNR than frequency feature selection.

Table 4. Oversampling for frequency feature selection

	Email	Telephone no.	Address	Money
FPR	8.8%	3.2%	1.5%	1.1%
FNR	0.6%	11.7%	14.3%	16.9%

Finally, we tested the impact of the number of selected features on the performance. We chose C4.5 as classification algorithm and information gain as the feature selection method. We oversampled positive examples 5 times. The experiment was conducted on *email addresses*. The results are shown in Figure 4. The X-axis denotes the number of the features selected. The Y axis denotes the false positive rate and false negative rate in percentage. We can see that when we increase the number of the features from 50 to 250, the FPR decreases. When the number of features exceeds 250, the FPR fluctuates slightly. For the FNR, when we increase the number of features from 50 to 350, the FNR decreases. When the number of features exceeds 300, there is no improvement in FNR.

Based on the experimental results, we conclude that the sampling size and the number of the selected features have great impact on the performance of the classification models, while the data mining methods and feature selection methods do not show significant difference for the performance.

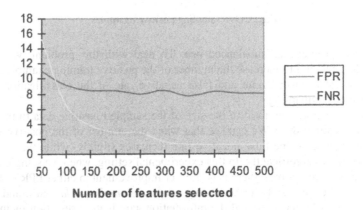

Number of features selected

Fig. 4. Number of selected features verses FPR and FNR

3   Conclusions and Future Work

In this paper we presented a data mining-based method to predict the presence of personally identifiable information in emails. We adopted association rule mining to predict private information according to other PII identified. We used classification models to predict the PII according to the content of the emails. Experimental results on the Enron data set show that our methods can achieve satisfactory false positive and false negative rates.

Currently, we only predict if there is a PII element of a certain type occurring in email. In the future, we may predict how many private elements of a certain type occur. We will also incorporate more information from the email to improve the performance of the system. For example, since different people have different wording habits, incorporating the user information may improve the prediction results. We can also utilize email thread information. For example, an email from A to B at time 0 requests some private information, and another email at time 1, in the same thread, from B to A may provide the private information. In this case, the content of the time

0 email may help predict private information in the time 1 email. Also, in the future, we will try to automatically determine the parameters in training the classification model, such as the number of the features and the size of the samples. Finally, we will do experiments to compare our method with the related methods for private information discovery.

References

[1] Agrawal, R., Srikant, R.: Fast Algorithms for Mining Association Rules. In: Proceedings of the 20th International Conference on Very Large Databases, Santiago, Chile, pp. 487–499 (1994)
[2] Agrawal, R., Srikant, R.: Privacy-Preserving Data Mining. In: Proceedings of the ACM SIGMOD Conference on Management of Data, Dallas, Texas, pp. 439–450 (2000)
[3] Armour, Q., Elazmeh, W., El-Kadri, N., Japkowicz, N., Matwin, S.: Privacy Compliance Enforcement in Email. In: Canadian Conference on AI, pp. 194–204 (2005)
[4] Boufaden, N., Elazmeh, W., Ma, Y., Matwin, S., El-Kadri, N., Japkowicz, N.: PEEP - An Information Extraction base approach for Privacy Protection in Email. In: CEAS (2005)
[5] Carvalho, V.R., Cohen, W.W.: Preventing Information Leaks in Email. In: SDM (2007)
[6] Evfimievski, A., Srikant, R., Agrawal, R., Gehrke, J.: Privacy Preserving Mining of Association Rules. In: Proceedings of 8th ACM SIGKDD International Conference on Knowledge Discovery and Data Mining (KDD) (2002)
[7] Han, H., Giles, C.L., Manavoglu, E., Zha, H., Zhang, Z., Fox, E.A.: Automatic Document Metadata Extraction Using Support Vector Machines. In: Proceedings of the 2003 Joint Conference o Digital Libraries (JDCL 2003), pp. 37–48 (2003)
[8] Korba, L., Song, R., Yee, G., Patrick, A., Buffett, S., Wang, Y., Geng, L.: Private Data Management in Collaborative Environments. In: Luo, Y. (ed.) CDVE 2007. LNCS, vol. 4674, pp. 88–96. Springer, Heidelberg (2007)
[9] Han, J., Kamber, M.: Data Mining: Concepts and Techniques. Micheline Kamber Publishers (2006)
[10] Jones, K.S., Willet, P.: Readings in Information Retrieval. Morgan Kaufmann, San Francisco (1997)
[11] Witten, I.H., Frank, E.: Data Mining: Practical Machine Learning Tools and Techniques, 2nd edn. Morgan Kaufmann, San Francisco (2005)
[12] http://www.isi.edu/~adibi/Enron/Enron.htm
[13] http://en.wikipedia.org/wiki/Luhn_algorithm

Iterative Reinforcement Cross-Domain Text Classification

Di Zhang, Gui-Rong Xue, and Yong Yu

Department of Computer Science and Engineering
Shanghai Jiao Tong University
No. 800 Dongchuan Road, Shanghai 200240, China
{aioria,grxue,yyu}@apex.sjtu.edu.cn

Abstract. Traditional text classification techniques are based on a basic assumption that the underlying distributions of training and test data should be identical. However, in many real world applications, this assumption is not often satisfied. Labeled training data are expensive, but there may be some labeled data available in a different but related domain from test data. Therefore, how to make use of labeled data from a different domain to supervise the classification becomes a crucial task. In this paper, we propose a novel algorithm for cross-domain text classification using reinforcement learning. In our algorithm, the training process is iteratively reinforced by making use of the relations between documents and words. Empirically, our method is an effective and scalable approach for text categorization when the training and test data are from different but related domains. The experimental results show that our algorithm can achieve better performance than several state-of-art classifiers.

1 Introduction

Text categorization is an important topic in data mining. Most traditional text categorization approaches rely on machine learning or statistical learning theories and techniques. Statistical learning makes an assumption that labeled training data should be drawn from the same underlying distribution as unlabeled test data. However, in many real application, this assumption often does not hold. For example, blog and news articles share some common topics, but their word usages differ a lot. As we know, there are quite amount of labeled news articles, but few labeled blog articles. As a consequence, we wonder if news articles can be used to supervise the classification on blog ones. Therefore, it raises an important issue how to classify documents across different domains, called *cross-domain learning* problem – an instance of *transfer learning* [1,2,3].

In this paper, a labeled training data set $\mathcal{D}_{\mathcal{L}}$ is given as well as an unlabeled test data set $\mathcal{D}_{\mathcal{U}}$. Here, $\mathcal{D}_{\mathcal{L}}$ and $\mathcal{D}_{\mathcal{U}}$ come from different albeit related domains. We call $\mathcal{D}_{\mathcal{U}}$ *in-domain* data set, and $\mathcal{D}_{\mathcal{L}}$ *out-of-domain* data set. And, our goal is to classify the unlabeled data in $\mathcal{D}_{\mathcal{U}}$ making use of the labeled data in $\mathcal{D}_{\mathcal{L}}$.

The basic idea of our work lies on statistical relational learning. Under the probabilistic text classification framework, the conditional probabilities (e.g.

C. Tang et al. (Eds.): ADMA 2008, LNAI 5139, pp. 282–293, 2008.

$p(c|d)$, $p(c|w)$, $p(w|d)$, etc.) are *local*, which means they will not change a lot when domain changes, where d denotes a document instance, w denotes a word and c denotes a class label. At another side, $p(c)$, $p(d)$ and $p(w)$ are *global*, which means they will change as domain changes. Most traditional classification algorithms minimize some criterion function under the global underlying distribution $p(d)$. Therefore, when labeled training data and unlabeled test data come from different domain, their global underlying distributions could be rather different from each other, and thus the learning algorithm might give poor performance on one distribution while training in another distribution. To address this problem, we design a classification algorithm depending on the global distributions very little. As discussed above, the local probabilities are often similar across related domains. Therefore, if we try to make use of the local information as much as possible to design a classification method, it is reasonable to believe that the cross-domain classification can be effective.

Empirically, the feature spaces (i.e. $p(w)$) among different domains vary a lot. Although related domains may share some common words, there are still quite amount of words only contained by one single domain. In order to enhance the training through local information provided by features, in our work, features are organized into several clusters, that each cluster collects similar words. The words are clustered based on the interrelationship between documents and words. After clustering the words, documents are classified based on the clustered features. Then, the document classification result will also boost the performance of word clustering using the interrelationship between documents and words. We design this process as an iterative reinforcement framework. In this framework, we iteratively perform document classification and word clustering, and show that the classification and clustering could co-boost each other's performance.

To evaluate our work, we conduct our experiments on three benchmark data sets. The experimental results show that, with the error rate-measure, our algorithm achieves significant improvement over the naive Bayes classifiers (NBCs), it also outperforms support vector machines (SVMs) and Transductive Support Vector Machines (TSVMs). In the experiments, we also discover that when the data size of training set varies, our algorithm still maintains a stable performance.

The contributions of our work are:

1. We claim that a good approach to solve the cross-domain text classification is to make use of the local information as much as possible, and consider the global information very little.
2. We relax the assumption of the traditional classification algorithms, and then design a framework to solve the cross-domain classification problem. Under our approach, the feature space and the categorization are updated based on the interrelationship between documents and words during iterative process.
3. The empirical results show that our framework improves the classification performance in the scenario of cross-domain learning.

The rest of the paper is organized as follows. In Section 2, we discuss the related works. We define the problem setting and present our iterative reinforcement categorization approach in Section 3. Experimental results together with the empirical analysis are presented in Section 4. Finally, we conclude the whole paper and give some future work in Section 5.

2   Related Work

In traditional classification, two techniques are mainly investigated: one is *supervised classification* [4,5] and the other is *semi-supervised classification* [6,7,8,9]. The difference between supervised and semi-supervised learning is the amount of labels they need. Both supervised and semi-supervised classification are based on the assumption that the distributions of the labeled and unlabeled data should be identical. However, when we address the issue of cross-domain categorization, the distributions of labeled and unlabeled data might be different, and thus the basic assumption of traditional classification learning is no longer satisfied well. As a consequence, traditional classification approaches may give poor performance.

In this paper, we address transfer learning across different domains. Transfer learning is a new however important topic in machine learning. Early works include [1,2,3]. A theoretical justification of transfer learning through multi-task learning was provided by Ben-David and Schuller [10]. [11] designed an ensemble-learning algorithm to solve transfer text classification problem. They assembled *predefined* classifiers based on training data, and calculated the *reliability score* for each classifiers. [12] denoted to cross-domain learning on neural network, while we focus on cross-domain text classification. [13] constructed a framework for learning *out-of-domain* texts based on *in-domain* data, even under the condition that labeled data is scarce.A statistical classifier was trained by using *Conditional Expectation Maximization*(CEM). [14] designed informative priors by estimate the covariance between words, and then apply these priors for classification. In order to work well, all the above approaches require some labeled data under the same distribution of test data. On the contrary, our framework can work without any labeled in-domain data.

Iterative reinforcement learning is used to solve our cross-domain classification. Iterative reinforcement learning has been widely applied in mining heterogeneous objects [15,16]. [15] proposed an reinforcement clustering algorithm, called ReCOM, which attempted to clustering heterogeneous objects by given inter-relationship among different types of objects and intra-relationships within one type. Similarly, IRC [16] classifies both web pages and queries simultaneously based on a bipartite graph which was modeled by the relationship between web pages and queries. In this paper, we model the bipartite graph as a document-word graph where the edge (or link) depicts the relation that document contains word. We apply iterative reinforcement link analysis method to the cross-domain categorization problem, and show the superior of our approach. The differences between their works and ours are: first, in their work, clustering (or classification) is conducted at both sides (query side and document side), while we do classification at the document side and clustering at the word side; second, they solve the heterogeneous object clustering (or classification) problem, while our problem is cross-domain text classification.

3   Cross-Domain Text Classification

In this section, we define the problem of classifying documents across different domains and then present our method to solve the problem.

3.1   Problem Formulation

Let $\mathcal{D}$ be the document sets that $\mathcal{D} = \mathcal{D}_\mathcal{L} \cup \mathcal{D}_\mathcal{U}$, where $\mathcal{D}_\mathcal{L}$ is the labeled (out-of-domain) data set and $\mathcal{D}_\mathcal{U}$ is the unlabeled (in-domain) data set. As assumed, the underlying distributions of $\mathcal{D}_\mathcal{L}$ and $\mathcal{D}_\mathcal{U}$ are different albeit related from each other. Our aim is to categorize $\mathcal{D}_\mathcal{U}$ as accurately as possible, by making use of the labeled data in $\mathcal{D}_\mathcal{L}$.

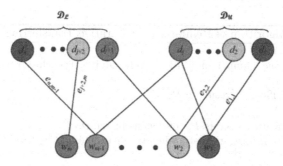

Fig. 1. Interrelations between Documents and Words

All the documents are represented by words which are denoted as $\mathcal{W} = \{w_1, w_2, \ldots, w_m\}$. As shown in Fig. 1, we define the edge e_{ij} as the interrelation between document $d_i \in \mathcal{D}$ and word $w_j \in \mathcal{W}$. Here, the interrelationship between a document and a word is whether a word is contained by a document, and the value of e_{ij} is set by the *term frequency* of w_j in d_i. If word w_j is not in this document, then let $e_{ij} = 0$.

For the document d_i, its feature vector is $E_{d_i} = [e_{i1}, \ldots, e_{im}]$, where m is the number of words. Similarly, the feature vector of word w_j is denoted as $E_{w_j} = [e_{1j}, e_{2j}, \ldots, e_{nj}]$, where n is the number of documents. We denote the feature vector set of documents in D as $E_\mathcal{D}$ and the feature vector set of $\mathcal{W}$ as $E_\mathcal{W}$.

3.2   Reinforcement Iterative Transferring Classification Algorithm

In this subsection, we present our novel framework, called *Reinforcement Iterative Transferring Classification* (RITC).

Our method is an iterative process. At the stage of initialization, we calculate the feature vectors $E_\mathcal{D}$ for document set $\mathcal{D}$. After that, iteration starts. One iteration is separated into two steps: the document classification step and the word clustering step. In the document classification step, we firstly classify the unlabeled data $\mathcal{D}_\mathcal{U}$ based on the training data $\mathcal{D}_\mathcal{L}$ using $E_\mathcal{D}$ as features. And then we update each word's feature vector E_{w_j} based on the document classification result. In the word clustering step, we cluster $\mathcal{W}$ into s (s is a parameter) clusters using $E_\mathcal{W}$ as features. Then, we update each document's feature vector E_{d_i} based on the word clustering result. We will describe the details of updating rule later.

As you will see later in the experiment part, the word clustering will enhance the classification performance, while document classification will also boost the effect of clustering on $\mathcal{W}$. Therefore, in this work, we iteratively repeat the word clustering and document classification steps, and let the clustering and classification co-boost each other. The iteration continues until the clustering and classification results converge.

The details of our algorithm are presented in **Algorithm 1.**

Algorithm 1. Algorithm of Reinforcement Iterative Transferring Classification

Input : $\mathcal{D}_\mathcal{L}$, $\mathcal{D}_\mathcal{U}$, $\mathcal{W}$
Parameters : s, the number of word clusters, and p, the cluster number of each document subset
Output : the classification result to $\mathcal{D}_\mathcal{U}$

1: Calculate the feature vectors $E_\mathcal{D}$ of document set $\mathcal{D}$.
2: Classify $\mathcal{D}_\mathcal{U}$ into k categories, according to the probability distribution of $\mathcal{D}_\mathcal{L}$ using $E_\mathcal{D}$ as features.
3: Update the words' feature vectors $E_\mathcal{W}$, with the parameter p (details in **Updating $\mathcal{W}$'s feature vectors**).
4: Cluster $\mathcal{W}$ into s clusters based on the newly $E_\mathcal{W}$.
5: Update documents' feature vectors $E_\mathcal{D}$ (details in **Updating $\mathcal{D}$'s feature vectors**)
6: Iterate step 2 to 5 until convergence.

In the above algorithm, note that p is not the class number of the documents but a parameter which we will use in Updating $\mathcal{W}$'s feature vectors session. In contrast, k is not a parameter but the class number of the documents, it is a constant.

Updating $\mathcal{W}$'s Feature Vectors. When we consider clustering on $\mathcal{W}$, a simple method is to use the $E_\mathcal{W}$ calculated using the interrelationship between each single document and each word, while the disadvantage of this method is obvious, that it could not utilize the information of classification on $\mathcal{D}_\mathcal{U}$. For the aim at obtaining more precise clustering on $\mathcal{W}$, we re-organize the feature vectors $E_\mathcal{W}$.

First we divide $\mathcal{D}$ into k subsets according to its current categories(here we merge $\mathcal{D}_{\mathcal{L}}$ and $\mathcal{D}_{\mathcal{U}}$ together); then clustering each subset into p clusters.Thus $\mathcal{D}$ are divided into:

$$\mathcal{D} = \mathcal{D}_{1_1}, \mathcal{D}_{1_2}, \ldots, \mathcal{D}_{1_p}, \ldots, , \ldots, \mathcal{D}_{k_1}, \mathcal{D}_{k_2}, \ldots, \mathcal{D}_{k_p}$$

At the beginning, $E_\mathcal{W}$ depicts the relations between m words and n documents; after this step,we have $k \times p$ clusters of documents instead of n documents. In order to depict the relations between m words and $k \times p$ sets of documents. We should re-calculate the feature vector of word j as following :

$$E_{w_j} = [SDC_{1_1}(j), SDC_{1_2}(j), \ldots SDC_{1_p}(j), \ldots, , \ldots,$$
$$SDC_{k_1}(j), SDC_{k_2}(j), \ldots, SDC_{k_p}(j)]$$

$$SDC_{u_v}(j) = \sum_{d_i \in \mathcal{D}_{u_v}} e_{ij} \quad (1 \leqq u \leqq k, 1 \leqq v \leqq p)$$

Updating $\mathcal{D}$'s feature vectors. The updating of documents' feature vectors is relatively simpler than $E_\mathcal{W}$. After step 4, clusters of words are generated as $\mathcal{WC} = \{wc_1, wc_2, \ldots, wc_s\}$. As we observed, each document consist of words , marked as $w_1, w_2, \ldots, w_j$. The feature vector of document i is:

$$E_{d_i} = [SWC_1(i), SWC_2(i), \ldots, SWC_s(i)]$$

there are s dimensions , corresponding to s word clusters. Thus for each SWC_u, we have

$$SWC_u(i) = \sum_{w_j \in \mathcal{WC}_u} e_{ij} \quad (1 \leqq u \leqq s)$$

3.3   Discussion

Before we analysis how our algorithm deals with the issue of private features between different domains, We define a binary boolean function.

$$f(w, D) = \begin{cases} 1 & \text{if feature } w \text{ appears in } D \text{ , here } D \text{ is a set of documents} \\ 0 & \text{otherwise} \end{cases}$$

Thus, in our problem, the features of documents could be separated into three subsets:

$$T_1 = \{w | f(w, D_U) \wedge f(w, D_L)\}$$
$$T_2 = \{w | \neg f(w, D_U) \wedge f(w, D_L)\}$$
$$T_3 = \{w | f(w, D_U) \wedge \neg f(w, D_L)\}$$

For cross-domain learning task, the set of T_2 and T_3 represent the difference of the two domain, which lead to unsatisfiable result for traditional classification. So we should try to shrink the T_2 and T_3's influence to the classification.

Though the underlying distribution of D_U and D_L are different, they share some features because they are related domains. For instance, $d_1 \in D_U$ contains features w_i which belongs to T_3; $d_2 \in D_S$ contains feature w_j which belongs to T_2; moreover, they share features $\{w_{k1}, w_{k2}, \ldots, w_{kn}\}$ which belong to T_1. In our algorithm RITC, d_1 and d_2 are likely to be assigned into the same document category after step 2 and then clustered into the same document clustering after step 3. As a result, w_i and w_j would be likely to be clustered into the same word cluster in step 4, because most documents that contain them are in the same document cluster. Now we can see that the bad influence of w_i and w_j has been eliminated. Therefor, features that share the similar meanings in T_2 and T_3 would be connected under the impact of T_1 through iteratively performing document classification and word clustering. As a common sense, the difference of distributions between labeled data and unlabeled data could not be too large. So the two domain must be related enough.

4   Experiments

In this section, we empirically evaluate our algorithm RITC. We compare the performance between traditional classifiers and our RITC algorithm on binary text classification. RITC is shown to be effective on solving cross-domain text classification.

4.1   Data Set

For evaluating the performance of our framework, several experiments are conducted on three data sets, 20 Newsgroups [17], SRAA [18] and Reuters-21578 [19]. Since these three data sets are not originally used for evaluating cross-domain classification, to fulfil the learning task, we split the data in the strategy as follows.

All these three data sets are organized by certain hierarchies. For instance, there are 7 top categories in the 20 Newsgroups, under which there are 20 subcategories. Since we conduct our experiments on binary text classification, we select two top categories and mark them as positive data and negative ones. Then, for each data set, we split it into two subsets according to its subcategories. For example, suppose A and B are two top categories which denotes positive and negative data respectively. A_1, A_2 are two subcategories under A; B_1, B_2 are two subcategories under B. We combine A_1 and B_1 to form the training set, the rest are used as the test set. After that, two data sets is generated. Since the training and test data are from different sub-categories, their domains can be considered as different. Meanwhile, since the positive data of training and test data come from the same top categories and also the negative data of training and test data come from the same top categories, they should be related.

Table 1 shows the details for all the data sets. We generate 5 cross-domain data sets from 20 Newsgroups. **auto vs aviation** and **real vs simulated** are

Table 1. The Composition of 10 Data Sets. There are too many subcategories in Reuters-21578, so we ignore composition details of last three data sets, which are from Reuters-21578.

Source	Data Set	Train/Test	Positive	Negative	#Instances
SRAA	auto vs aviation	train	sim-auto	sim-aviation	8,000
		test	real-auto	real-aviation	8,000
	real vs simulate	train	real-aviation	sim-aviation	8,000
		test	real-auto	sim-auto	8,000
20NG	rec vs talk	train	rec.autos rec.motorcycles	talk.politics.guns talk.politics.misc	3,669
		test	rec.sport.baseball rec.sport.hockey	talk.politics.mideast talk.religion.misc	3,561
	comp vs talk	train	comp.graphics comp.sys.mac.hardware comp.windows.x	talk.politics.mideast talk.religion.misc	4,482
		test	comp.os.ms-windows.misc comp.sys.ibm.pc.hardware	talk.politics.guns talk.politics.misc	3,652
	comp vs sci	train	comp.graphics comp.os.ms-windows.misc	sci.crypt sci.electronics	3,930
		test	comp.sys.ibm.pc.hardware comp.sys.mac.hardware comp.windows.x	sci.med sci.space	4,900
	comp vs rec	train	comp.graphics comp.sys.ibm.pc.hardware comp.sys.mac.hardware	rec.motorcycles rec.sport.hockey	4,904
		test	comp.os.ms-windows.misc comp.windows.x	rec.autos rec.sport.baseball	3,949
	sci vs talk	train	sci.electronics sci.med	talk.politics.misc talk.religion.misc	3,374
		test	sci.crypt sci.space	talk.politics.guns talk.politics.mideast	3,828
Reuters -21578	orgs vs places	train	orgs.*	places.*	1,078
		test	orgs.*	places.*	1,080
	people vs places	train	people.*	places.*	1,239
		test	people.*	places.*	1,210
	orgs vs people	train	orgs.*	people.*	1,016
		test	orgs.*	people.*	1,046

collected from SRAA. Since there are too many subcategories under Reuters-21578, we omit the details about the data sets, **orgs vs places**, **orgs vs people** and **places vs people**.

4.2 Comparison Methods

To show the advantage of our algorithm, we compare our *Reinforcement Iterative Transferring Classification* (RITC) to several existing algorithms. In the experiment, we select some state-of-art classifiers as baselines, such as Naive Bayes Classifier (NBC) [4], Support Vector Machines (SVM) [5] and Transductive Support Vector Machines (TSVM) [9].

4.3 Implementation Details

In the data preprocessing stage, we convert all the letters into lower-case, remove stop words, and stem all the words using Porter stemmer [20]. When selecting features, we use Document Frequency (DF) Thresholding [21]. Here we set the DF threshold to 3. To weighting the features, we use TF (for NBC) and TFIDF (for SVM) in training process.

To generate the baseline, we apply SVM^{light} as a tool to implement SVM [5] and TSVM [9]. Parameters are set to be default. While the algorithm of NBC is implemented by ourselves.

When implementing RITC, we use SVM as the basic classification algorithm; when cluster the objects, we use CLUTO [22] as the tool for clustering words and documents. The parameters of CLUTO is set to be default. The cluster numbers of words and documents (s and p) are both set to 32. These two parameters will be tuned empirically later.

4.4   Evaluation Metrics

The performance of the proposed methods was evaluated by test error rate. Let C be the function which maps from document d to its true class label $c = C(d)$, and F be the function which maps from document d to its prediction label $\hat{c} = F(d)$ given by the classifier. Test error rate is defined as

$$\epsilon = \frac{|\{d|d \in \mathcal{D}_\mathcal{U} \wedge C(d) \neq F(d)\}|}{|\mathcal{D}_\mathcal{U}|}$$

4.5   Experimental Results

Performance. Table 2 shows the comparative result between SVM, NBC, TSVM and our method RITC. The first column indicates the data sets. For instance, "A vs B", A and B represent the top categories. There are 10 data sets from three corpora which have been listed in Table 1. The first row indicate all the algorithms of classifications, the last one is our approach, Reinforcement Iterative Transferring Classification (RITC).

Since our algorithm is an iterative process, we should take the final results when it converges to a stable value. Empirical results show that the algorithm converges very fast, which will be shown later, and 5 iterations will be almost enough. Therefore, we take the number of iterations to be 5 in the experiments.

From the Table 2, we can see that the RITC makes significant improvement compared to SVM, while also be better than NBC. Generally, SVM should be more effective than NBC, however in the task of cross-domain classification, NBC is better than SVM. This implies that NBC is with better generality when the classification task crosses different domains.

Fig. 2 shows the influence of data size to different algorithms. The x-axis represents the size of training data. For instance , 0.4 means we randomly choose 40% of the original training data to form the new training set. Under these new sets, we compare the performance of our algorithm with SVM. From Figure 2,

Table 2. Test error rate for each classifier on each data set

Data Set	NBC	SVM	TSVM	RITC
real vs simulated	0.259	0.266	0.130	**0.054**
auto vs aviation	0.150	0.228	**0.102**	0.199
rec vs talk	0.235	0.233	0.040	**0.015**
comp vs talk	0.024	0.103	0.097	**0.017**
comp vs sci	0.207	0.317	0.183	**0.066**
comp vs rec	0.072	0.165	0.098	**0.029**
sci vs talk	0.226	0.226	0.108	**0.045**
orgs vs places	0.377	0.454	0.436	**0.334**
people vs places	0.216	0.266	0.231	**0.208**
orgs vs people	0.289	0.297	0.297	**0.248**

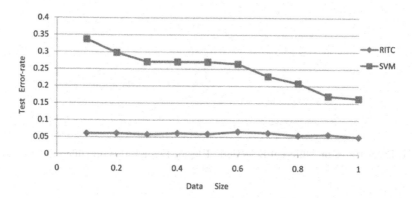

Fig. 2. Test error rate curve on different data sizes on the `simulated vs real` data set

we can see that the size of training data strongly affects the performances of SVM algorithm. In contrast, our algorithm hold a stable error-rate though the size of training set varies a lot.

Convergence. Since RITC is an iterative method, it is important to show the convergence issue to it. Fig. 3 gives more details about convergence. The x-axis represents the times of iterations, y-axis denotes the error-rate. As shown in the figure, error-rates are decrease after every iteration. All curves come to perfectly convergence. The error-rates achieve a fixed value after 5 or 6 iterations, and thus we set the number of iteration to 5 in the experiments.

Parameter Tuning. In Algorithm 1, there are two parameters: one is the number of document clusters p in *Step 3*; the other is the number of word clusters s in *Step 4*. We perform the parameter tuning on the **real vs simulated** data set. The error-rates derived from varied ps are plotted in Fig. 4. From the Fig. 4, we set p to 32, since the algorithm performs best when $p = 32$. Likewise, we set $s = 32$ according to Fig. 5.

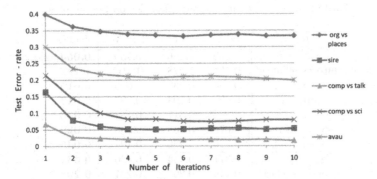

Fig. 3. Test error rate curve on different data size of `simulated vs real` data set

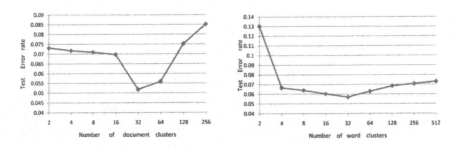

Fig. 4. Error Rates on Different Selection of p

Fig. 5. Error Rates on Different Selection of s

5   Conclusion and Future Work

In this paper, we proposed an iterative reinforcement transferring classification algorithm to categorize documents across different domains. This algorithm utilizes relationships between documents and words. We consider these relationships as feature vectors for both words and documents, and then we classify documents and cluster words simultaneously. Classification and clustering co-boost each other, and the iterative process converges very well. Experiment shows that our approach RITC can significantly improve cross-domain classification performance against traditional supervised and semi-supervised classfication algorithms.

For future work, we would like to extend this algorithm to other learning tasks. For instance, we could aim to classify web categories based on the relationship between web pages and their hyperlinks. We wonder whether our algorithm is effective in these other learning tasks.

References

1. Mitchell, T.M.: 6. In: Machine Learning, p. 179. McGraw Hill, New York (1997)
2. Schmidhuber, J.: On learning how to learn learning strategies. Technical Report FKI-198-94, Fakultat fur Informatik (1994)

3. Caruana, R.: Multitask learning. Machine Learning 28(1), 41–75 (1997)
4. Lewis, D.D.: Representation and learning in information retrieval. Ph.D thesis, Amherst, MA, USA (1992)
5. Boser, B.E., Guyon, I., Vapnik, V.: A training algorithm for optimal margin classifiers. In: Proceedings of the Fifth Annual Workshop on Computational Learning Theory (1992)
6. Zhu, X.: Semi-supervised learning literature survey. Technical Report 1530, University of Wisconsin–Madison (2006)
7. Blum, A., Mitchell, T.: Combining labeled and unlabeled data with co-training. In: Proceedings of the Eleventh Annual Conference on Computational Learning Theory (1998)
8. Nigam, K., McCallum, A.K., Thrun, S., Mitchell, T.: Text classification from labeled and unlabeled documents using em. Machine Learning 39, 103–134 (2000)
9. Joachims, T.: Transductive inference for text classification using support vector machines. In: Proceedings of Sixteenth International Conference on Machine Learning (1999)
10. Ben-David, S., Schuller, R.: Exploiting task relatedness for multiple task learning. In: Proceedings of the Sixteenth Annual Conference on Learning Theory (2003)
11. Bennett, P.N., Dumais, S.T., Horvitz, E.: Inductive transfer for text classification using generalized reliability indicators. In: Proceedings of ICML 2003 Workshop on The Continuum from Labeled and Unlabeled Data (2003)
12. Swarup, S., Ray, S.R.: Cross-domain knowledge transfer using structured representations. In: Proceedings of the Twenty-First National Conference on Artificial Intelligence (2006)
13. DauméIII, H., Marcu, D.: Domain adaptation for statistical classifiers. Journal of Artificial Intelligence Research 26, 101–126 (2006)
14. Raina, R., Ng, A.Y., Koller, D.: Constructing informative priors using transfer learning. In: Proceedings of Twenty-Third International Conference on Machine Learning (2006)
15. Wang, J., Zeng, H., Chen, Z., Lu, H., Tao, L., Ma, W.: ReCoM: reinforcement clustering of multi-type interrelated data objects. In: Proceedings of the 26th annual international ACM SIGIR conference on Research and development in information retrieval, pp. 274–281 (2003)
16. Xue, G., Shen, D., Yang, Q., Zeng, H., Chen, Z., Yu, Y., Xi, W., Ma, W.: IRC: An Iterative Reinforcement Categorization Algorithm for Interrelated Web Objects. In: ICDM 2004: Proceedings of the 4th IEEE International Conference on Data Mining, pp. 273–280 (2004)
17. Lang, K.: Newsweeder: Learning to filter netnews. In: Proceedings of the Twelfth International Conference on Machine Learning (1995)
18. McCallum, A.K.: Simulated/real/aviation/auto usenet data, http://www.cs.umass.edu/~mccallum/code-data.html
19. Lewis, D.D.: Reuters-21578 test collection, http://www.daviddlewis.com/
20. Porter, M.F.: An algorithm for suffix stripping. Program 14(3), 130–137 (1980)
21. Yang, Y., Pedersen, J.O.: A comparative study on feature selection in text categorization. In: Proceedings of Fourteenth International Conference on Machine Learning (1997)
22. Karypis, G.: Cluto – software for clustering high-dimensional datasets, http://glaros.dtc.umn.edu/gkhome/views/cluto

Extracting Decision Rules from Sigmoid Kernel*

Quanzhong Liu, Yang Zhang**, and Zhengguo Hu

College of Information Engineering, Northwest A&F University, P.R. China, 712100
liuqzhong@nwsuaf.edu.cn,
zhangyang@nwsuaf.edu.cn,
zghu@sina.com

Abstract. Sigmoid kernel is widely applied in neural networks for classification tasks. SVM classifier, which is applied with sigmoid kernel, has excellent classification accuracy. However, as sigmoid kernel has complicated structure, it is generally difficult for human expert to interpret and understand how the sigmoid kernel makes its classification decision. As decision rule classifier is understandable to human expert, in this paper, we present our InterSIG algorithm, which mines decision rules from the classification hyper-plane which is constructed by SVM with sigmoid kernel. InterSIG expands sigmoid kernel into its Maclaurin series, and then mines classification rules which make great contribution to classification from the classification hyper-plane. Experiment results show that InterSIG classifier is more understandable to human experts without jeopardizing the accuracy than the original SVM with sigmoid kernel. Furthermore, compared with 3 association classifiers, CMAR, CBA, CPAR and C4.5, a decision tree classifier, InterSIG classifier is very encouraging over the 9 datasets.

1 Introduction

Support Vector Machines (SVMs) are state-of-the art data mining technique which have proven performance in many applications [1], such as credit scoring [2], bioinformatics, medical diagnosis, and so on. The sigmoid kernel, which originates from neural networks, is applied broadly in non-linear SVM [3].

SVM [4] has excellent classification performance. However, in many applications, not only high classification accuracy, but also an understandable classifier is desired. For example, for medical diagnosis, it is great helpful for human experts to understand how the system makes its decisions, so as to be confident of its predictions. For credit scoring, when credit has been denied to a customer, the financial institution should provide specific reasons why the application was rejected; indefinite and vague reasons for denial are illegal [5]. However, the classification model of non-linear SVM is a black box, which is difficult for human

---

* This work is supported by Talent Fund of Northwest A&F University (01140402, 01140406) and Young Cadreman Supporting Program of Northwest A&F University (01140301).
** Corresponding author.

C. Tang et al. (Eds.): ADMA 2008, LNAI 5139, pp. 294–304, 2008.

experts to understand and interpret. Hence, several approaches for extracting rules from SVM classification model have been proposed by research community, including extracting IF-THEN rules [6][7][8], extracting decision trees [9][10], and extracting association rules [11].

Mining association rules for building associative classifier has been extensively studied in data mining community, with a lot of successful associative classifiers being proposed, such as CMAR [12], CBA [13], CPAR[14], etc. They have excellent classification performance and understandable classification model.

In order to interpret the classification model of SVM with sigmoid kernel into decision rules, so as to make its classification model understandable, in this paper, we present our InterSIG (Interpreting SIGmoid) algorithm. InterSIG expands sigmoid kernel into its Maclaurin series, and then mines decision rules which make great contribution to classification from the classification hyper-plane constructed by SVM. The experiment results show that the rules extracted by our algorithm are understandable to human experts. Furthermore, compared with SVM with the original sigmoid kernel, CMAR[12], CBA[13], CPAR[14], and C4.5[15], InterSIG classifier is very competitive over the 9 datasets.

This paper is organized as follows: we expand sigmoid kernel into its Maclaurin series for extracting classification rules in section 2. Section 3 presents the method to calculate the weight of the classification rules. Section 4 explains how to extract classification rules from classification hyper-plane which is constructed by SVM with sigmoid kernel. Experiment results are described in section 5. Finally, we conclude our paper and present our future work in section 6.

2   Sigmoid Kernel

Suppose $U \in R^n$, $V \in R^n$, $\rho \in R$, $\zeta \in R$, sigmoid kernel is defined as:

$$K(U, V) = \tanh(\rho\langle U, V\rangle + \zeta) \tag{1}$$

Here, ρ and ζ are hyper-parameters of sigmoid kernel.

In this paper, we focus on classification tasks when sample data only have discrete attributes. Numerical attributes could be discretized into discrete attributes. For a discrete attribute A, if there are $|A|$ possible values for this attribute, then we can use $|A|$ Boolean literals to represent this attribute, with each Boolean literal representing the occurrence or non-occurrence of the corresponding attribute value.

After pre-processing in the above way, the input space of sample data becomes $\{0, 1\}^n$.

We consider the function $\tanh(x)$, and rewrite it into the following formula:

$$\tanh(x) = \frac{e^x - e^{-x}}{e^x + e^{-x}} = \frac{1 - e^{-2x}}{1 + e^{-2x}} = \frac{2}{1 + e^{-2x}} - 1 \tag{2}$$

Suppose:

$$f(x) = (1 + e^{-2x})^{-1} \tag{3}$$

According to Maclaurin series of elementary functions:

$$(1+x)^{-1} = 1 - x + x^2 + \cdots + (-1)^n x^n + \cdots, \qquad |x| < 1 \qquad (4)$$

formula (3) could be expanded into the following series:

$$f(x) = \sum_{i=0}^{n}(-1)^i(e^{-2x})^i = 1 - e^{-2x} + (e^{-2x})^2 + \cdots + (-1)^n(e^{-2x})^n$$

$$= 1 - e^{-2x} + e^{-4x} - e^{-6x} + e^{-8x} + \cdots$$

$$+ (-1)^n(e^{-2nx}), \qquad |e^{-2x}| < 1 \qquad (5)$$

The prerequisite for the above formula is $|e^{-2x}| < 1$. For sigmoid kernel, if we select reasonable values for hyper-parameter ρ and ζ, the prerequisite $|e^{-2x}| < 1$ could be satisfied.

We expand $(-1)^n(e^{-2nx})$ in formula (5) into Maclaurin series:

$$-e^{-2x} = - \left[1 + \frac{(-2)^1}{1!}x + \frac{(-2)^2}{2!}x^2 + \frac{(-2)^3}{3!}x^3 + \frac{(-2)^4}{4!}x^4 + \cdots \right.$$

$$\left. + \frac{(-2)^n}{n!}x^n + o(n) \right]$$

$$e^{-4x} = \left[1 + \frac{(-4)^1}{1!}x + \frac{(-4)^2}{2!}x^2 + \frac{(-4)^3}{3!}x^3 + \frac{(-4)^4}{4!}x^4 + \cdots \right.$$

$$\left. + \frac{(-4)^n}{n!}x^n + o(n) \right]$$

$$\cdots \cdots$$

$$(-1)^n e^{-2nx} = (-1)^n \left[1 + \frac{(-2n)^1}{1!}x + \frac{(-2n)^2}{2!}x^2 + \frac{(-2n)^3}{3!}x^3 + \frac{(-2n)^4}{4!}x^4 + \cdots \right.$$

$$\left. + \frac{(-2n)^n}{n!}x^n + o(n) \right] \qquad (6)$$

By combining corresponding terms of formula (6), we have:

$$f(x) = \left(\frac{1}{1!}\sum_{t=1}^{n}(-1)^t(-2t) \right)x + \left(\frac{1}{2!}\sum_{t=1}^{n}(-1)^t(-2t)^2 \right)x^2 +$$

$$\left(\frac{1}{3!}\sum_{t=1}^{n}(-1)^t(-2t)^3 \right)x^3 + \cdots + \left(\frac{1}{n!}\sum_{t=1}^{n}(-1)^t(-2t)^n \right)x^n +$$

$$\sum_{t=0}^{n}(-1)^t + o(n) \qquad (7)$$

According to formula (2), (3) and (7), we get:

$$\tanh(x) = 2f(x) - 1$$

$$= \left(\frac{2}{1!}\sum_{t=1}^{n}(-1)^t(-2t)\right)x + \left(\frac{2}{2!}\sum_{t=1}^{n}(-1)^t(-2t)^2\right)x^2 +$$

$$\left(\frac{2}{3!}\sum_{t=1}^{n}(-1)^t(-2t)^3\right)x^3 + \cdots + \left(\frac{2}{n!}\sum_{t=1}^{n}(-1)^t(-2t)^n\right)x^n +$$

$$2\sum_{t=0}^{n}(-1)^t - 1 + o(n), \qquad\qquad |e^{-2x}| < 1 \qquad (8)$$

We set $\zeta = 0$ and $\rho > 0$ in our experiment, then, $|e^{-2(\rho\langle U,V\rangle)+\zeta}| = |e^{-2(\rho\langle U,V\rangle)}| < 1$ holds. Following formula (5) and formula (8), the sigmoid kernel could be represented as:

$$K(U,V) = \tanh(\rho\langle U,V\rangle + \zeta) = \tanh(\rho\langle U,V\rangle)$$

$$= \left(\frac{2}{1!}\sum_{t=1}^{n}\left((-1)^t(-2t)\right)\right)\rho\langle U,V\rangle$$

$$+ \left(\frac{2}{2!}\sum_{t=1}^{n}\left((-1)^t(-2t)^2\right)\right)\rho^2\langle U,V\rangle^2 + \cdots$$

$$+ \left(\frac{2}{n!}\sum_{t=1}^{n}\left((-1)^t(-2t)^n\right)\right)\rho^n\langle U,V\rangle^n + 2\sum_{t=0}^{n}(-1)^t - 1$$

$$+ o(n) \qquad\qquad (9)$$

Here, $\langle,\rangle$ represents the inner product between two vectors.

Let's consider the term $I_p = X_{j_1}X_{j_2}\ldots X_{j_p}, (1 \le j_1 < j_2 < \cdots < j_p \le n)$. The length of I_p is p. The coefficient of I_p in formula (9) could be represented as:

$$\sum_{k=p}^{\infty}\left(\frac{2}{k!}\sum_{t=1}^{n}(-1)^t(-2t)^k\right)\rho^k h(k,p) \qquad (10)$$

Here, $h(z,p)$ represents the sum of the coefficients of terms with length p in the expansion of $\langle U,V\rangle^z (z \in N)$. $h(z,p)$ could be calculated by:

$$\begin{cases} h(z,1) = 1 \\ h(z,p) = p^z - \sum_{k=1}^{p-1}\binom{p}{k}h(z,k) & p \le z \\ h(z,p) = 0 & p > z \end{cases} \qquad (11)$$

The detailed proof of the above formula is omitted here for lacking of space.

3   Weight of the Classification Rules

A dataset with d samples could be represented as $\{\vec{X_i}, y_i\}, i = 1, 2, \ldots, d$, with $\vec{X_i} \in \{0,1\}^m$, representing a sample data, and $y_i \in \{+1, -1\}$, representing the class label of this sample. For a testing sample X, the classification function learned by non-linear SVM with sigmoid kernel could be represented as:

$$F(X) = \text{sgn}\left(b + \sum_{i=1}^{d} \alpha_i y_i K(\overrightarrow{X_i}, X)\right) \qquad (12)$$

Here, $\alpha_i (1 \leq i \leq d)$ and b are knowledge learned by SVM; sgn() represents the sign function. Let's consider the following function:

$$g(X) = b + \sum_{i=1}^{d} \alpha_i y_i K(\overrightarrow{X_i}, X) \qquad (13)$$

Suppose $\lambda_i = \alpha_i y_i K(\overrightarrow{X_i}, X)$, and $K(\overrightarrow{X_i}, X)$ is expanded by formula (9). Then, for λ_i, the contribution of dimension $X_{j_1} (1 \leq j_1 \leq m)$ to classification could be represented as:

$$\frac{\partial \lambda_i}{\partial X_{j_1}} = \alpha_i y_i (\overrightarrow{X_i})_{j_1} \sum_{k=1}^{\infty} \left(\frac{2}{k!} \sum_{t=1}^{n} (-1)^t (-2t)^k \right) \rho^k h(k, 1) \qquad (14)$$

Here, we borrow terminology from the research of mining association rules. If we look the dimension X_{j_1} as an item, then formula (14) could be looked as the classification weight of 1-itemset $\{X_{j_1}\}$ in λ_i.

Following the above discussion, for 2-itemset $\{X_{j_1}, X_{j_2}\}$, $(1 \leq j_1 < j_2 \leq m)$ in λ_i, the classification weight could be represented as:

$$\frac{\partial \lambda_i}{\partial (X_{j_1} X_{j_2})} = \alpha_i y_i (\overrightarrow{X_i})_{j_1} (\overrightarrow{X_i})_{j_2} \sum_{k=2}^{\infty} \left(\frac{2}{k!} \sum_{t=1}^{n} (-1)^t (-2t)^k \right) \rho^k h(k, 2) \qquad (15)$$

Therefore, for p-itemset $\{X_{j_1}, X_{j_2}, \ldots, X_{j_p}\}, (1 \leq j_1 < j_2 < \ldots < j_p \leq m)$ in λ_i, the classification weight is:

$$\frac{\partial \lambda_i}{\partial (X_{j_1} X_{j_2} \cdots X_{j_p})} = \alpha_i y_i (\overrightarrow{X_i})_{j_1} (\overrightarrow{X_i})_{j_2} \cdots (\overrightarrow{X_i})_{j_p}$$
$$\sum_{k=p}^{\infty} \left(\frac{2}{k!} \sum_{t=1}^{n} (-1)^t (-2t)^k \right) \rho^k h(k, p) \qquad (16)$$

Following the above discussion, for an itemset I_p with length p, the contribution of I_p to classification could be represented as:

$$\frac{\partial g(x)}{\partial (X_{j_1} X_{j_2} \cdots X_{j_p})} = \sum_{i=1}^{d} \alpha_i y_i (\overrightarrow{X_i})_{j_1} (\overrightarrow{X_i})_{j_2} \cdots (\overrightarrow{X_i})_{j_p}$$
$$\sum_{k=p}^{\infty} \left(\frac{2}{k!} \sum_{t=1}^{n} (-1)^t (-2t)^k \right) \rho^k h(k, p) \qquad (17)$$

So, the classification function of InterSIG could be represented as:

$$F(X) = \operatorname{sgn}(b + \sum_{1 \le i \le m} \alpha_i y_i + (X_{j_1}) \sum_{1 \le j_1 \le m} \frac{\partial g(X)}{\partial(X_{j_1})}$$

$$+ (X_{j_1} X_{j_2}) \sum_{1 \le j_1 < j_2 \le m} \frac{\partial g(X)}{\partial(X_{j_1} X_{j_2})} + \cdots$$

$$(X_{j_1} X_{j_2} \cdots X_{j_n}) \sum_{1 \le j_1 < j_2 < \cdots < j_n \le m} \frac{\partial g(X)}{\partial(X_{j_1} X_{j_2} \cdots X_{j_n})}$$

$$+ \cdots) \tag{18}$$

Theoretically, in formula (18), $n \le m$. However, we set $n \le 4$ in our experiment, and this is explained in next section.

4   Extracting Rules from Sigmoid Kernel

Our InterSIG classifier is working in the following steps:

1. Constructing classification hyper-plane from training data by SVM with sigmoid kernel.
2. Extracting decision rules from the classification hyper-plane.
3. Classifying testing data by these decision rules.

In the classification model learned by SVM, positive support vectors are the support vectors which satisfy $y_i = +1$, and negative support vectors are the support vectors which satisfy $y_i = -1$. Here, we write SV_P and SV_N for the set of positive support vectors and the set of negative support vectors, respectively.

Theoretically, we need to mine itemsets with length up to m. However, according to the theory of Occam's razor [16], we should emphasize the contribution to classification made by short itemsets, reducing the contribution made by long itemsets, so as to ensure the good classification accuracy of sigmoid kernel. Therefore, we only need mine out itemsets with reasonable length. Hence, we mine itemsets with length up to $MaxLiteral$, a user defined parameter. We simply set $MaxLitral = 4$ in our experiment, as our pilot experiments show that this is a good value.

Let's write $WEIGHT(r)$ for the weight of rule r, rules which satisfy $WEIGHT(r) \le MinWeight$ are filtered, as they made little contribution to classification. Here, $MinWeight$ is a user defined parameter.

After rule filtering in the above way, we still could get a big size of rule set. In order to further reduce the size of rule set, we sort the classification rules descendingly according to $WEIGHT(r)$, and only top $Lambda$ percent of the rules in the list are moved into the final rules set. Here, $Lambda$ is also a user defined parameter. It is shown in our pilot experiments that a good value of $MinWeight$ is $0.001 \times b$, and $Lambda$ is 50. Here b is the parameter learned by SVM.

Algorithm 1. Extracting Rules from sigmoid kernel

Input:　The set of positive support vectors, SV_p,
　　　　　The set of negative support vectors, SV_n,
　　　　　Minimal rule weight, $MinWeight$,
　　　　　Maximum literal, $MaxLiteral$,
　　　　　Threshold $Lambda$,

Output: Rule set

1: Mining 1-itemset classification rule set $R_{1,P}$ and $R_{1,N}$ from SV_p and SV_n respectively, following formula(17);

$$R_{1,P} = \{r|WEIGHT(r) \geq MinWeight\}$$
$$R_{1,N} = \{r|WEIGHT(r) \geq MinWeight\}$$

2: $R_{all} = \phi, n = 2$;

3: Mining n-itemset classification rule set $R_{n,P}$ and $R_{n,N}$ from SV_p and SV_n respectively, following formula(17);

$$R_{n,P} = \{rr'|r \in R_{n-1,P} \wedge r' \in R_{1,P} \wedge WEIGHT(rr') \geq MinWeight\}$$
$$R_{n,N} = \{rr'|r \in R_{n-1,N} \wedge r' \in R_{1,N} \wedge WEIGHT(rr') \geq MinWeight\}$$

4: $R_{all} = R_{all} \cup R_{n,N} \cup R_{n,P}$;

5: If $n = MaxLiteral$ goto 6 else $n = n + 1$ goto 3;

6: Sort rules in R_{all} descendingly according to weight of rules, and move top $Lambda$ percent of the rules in the list into R'_{all};

7: Output R'_{all}

Following the above discussion, Algorithm 1 shows our algorithm for extracting rules from sigmoid kernel. In step 1, 1-length rules are mined out from classification hyper-plane. In step 2, 3 and 4, rules with length up to $MaxLiteral$, are mined out. In step 6, we sort the classification rules descendingly according to $WEIGHT(r)$, and only top $Lambda$ percent of the rules in the list are moved into the final classification rules set R'_{all}.

5　Experiment Result

5.1　Classification Performance

In order to validate classification performance of InterSIG classifier, we test 9 datasets from UCI[1] machine learning repository. In this section, we report our experimental results by comparing the classification accuracy of InterSIG against associative classifiers CMAR [12], CBA [13], CPAR [14] and decision tree classifier C4.5 [15]. We selected 9 datasets for experiments because their classification performance on these datasets is available in the literature for comparison.

10-fold cross validation was performed on each dataset and the average results on the 10 folds are reported here as final result. This experiment setting is widely used by the research community.

---

[1] URL: http://www.ics.uci.edu/~mlearn/MLRepository.html

Table 1. Comparing InterSIG with CMAR, CBA, CPAR, C4.5

datasets	SVM	CMAR	CBA	CPAR	C4.5	InterSIG
Austral	85.5	86.1	84.9	86.2	84.7	84.8
Cleve	82.6	82.2	82.8	81.5	78.2	81.2
Crx	85.5	84.9	84.7	85.7	84.9	85.7
German	70	74.9	73.4	73.4	72.3	70.7
Hepatic	79.2	80.5	81.8	79.4	80.6	85.8
Heart	83.7	82.2	81.9	82.6	80.8	83.3
Hypo	98.2	98.4	98.9	98.1	99.2	98.2
Sonar	84.7	79.4	77.5	79.3	70.2	87.5
Sick	96.8	97.5	97	96.8	98.5	96.8
Average	85.1	85.1	84.8	84.8	83.3	**86.0**

Our experiment is made on a PC with Pentium 4, 3.0GHZ CPU and 512MB memory. The algorithms were implemented in Java, and the LIBSVM[2] software package was used for SVM learning.

In our experiment, we set hyper-parameter of sigmoid kernel $\rho = 0.01$ and $\zeta = 0$.

Table 1 compares the classification accuracy of InterSIG with CMAR [12], CBA [13], CPAR [14], C4.5 [15], and SVM with sigmoid kernel on 9 UCI datasets. In table 1, column 1 lists the name of the datasets. Column 2 gives the classification accuracy of SVM with sigmoid kernel. Column 3, 4, 5 and 6 represents the classification accuracy of CMAR, CBA, CPAR and C4.5 respectively. These results are copied from [12], [13], [14] and [15]. The last column gives the classification accuracy of InterSIG. The row at the bottom of table 1 gives the average accuracy on the 9 datasets.

From table 1, we could observe that InterSIG classifier achieves better classification accuracy than other classifiers in datasets Crx, Hepatic and Sonar. Compared with other classifiers, the average accuracy of InterSIG classifier over the 9 datasets has been improved, InterSIG classifier is very competitive.

5.2   Interpreting Rules

Here, we take the *heart* dataset for example to explain the rules extracted by our InterSIG algorithm. There are 13 attributes in the original *heart* dataset. There is only one possible value for attribute *RestBP*, *Cholesterol*, *BloodSugar*, and *ECG*. These attributes are ignored, as they can make no contribution to classification. Table 2 gives the detailed information for discretizing the *heart* dataset. In table 2, column 1 lists the name of the original attributes; column 2 gives the detailed data for discretizing the corresponding attribute; column 3 lists the attributes after discretizing.

Averagely, we could obtain 1325.2 rules for *heart* dataset by 10-fold cross validation. Due to space limitation, we only list 8 rules, which are chosen from

---

[2] URL: http://www.csie.ntu.edu.tw/~cjlin/

Table 2. Discretizing the attributes of the *heart* dataset

Attribute	Discretization	Boolean Attribute
Age	(-INF, 54.5)	A_1
	[54.5,+INF)	A_2
Sex	(-INF, 0.5)	A_3
	[0.5,+INF)	A_4
ChestPain	(-INF, 3.5)	A_5
	[3.5,+INF)	A_6
MaxHeartRate	(-INF, 147.5)	A_7
	[147.5,+INF)	A_8
Angina	(-INF, 0.5)	A_9
	[0.5,+INF)	A_{10}
OldPeak	(-INF, 1.7)	A_{11}
	[1.7,+INF)	A_{12}
STSlope	(-INF, 1.5)	A_{13}
	[1.5,+INF)	A_{14}
Vessels	(-INF, 0.5)	A_{15}
	[0.5,+INF)	A_{16}
Thal	(-INF, 4.5)	A_{17}
	[4.5,+INF)	A_{18}

Table 3. Classification rules for *breast* dataset

Rule	Weight	Class Label
A_2	7.9546	*presence*
A_5	-22.3990	*Absence*
$A_2 \wedge A_3$	3.6554	*presence*
$A_1 \wedge A_5$	15.9691	*presence*
$A_3 \wedge A_{10} \wedge A_{14}$	3.8970	*presence*
$A_4 \wedge A_6 \wedge A_{12}$	5.9536	*presence*
$A_6 \wedge A_8 \wedge A_{15} \wedge A_{17}$	6.7497	*presence*
$A_4 \wedge A_8 \wedge A_{16} \wedge A_{18}$	-6.1872	*Absence*
......		

the final rule set randomly, in table 3. In this table, column 1 lists the rules extracted by our InterSIG algorithm; column 2 gives the weight of the rules; and column 3 gives the class label suggested by the corresponding rule.

Let's write r for a rule, and t for a testing sample. Rule r could suggest the *presence* class if r matches t and $WEIGHT(r) > 0$; and r could suggest the *Absence* class if r matches t and $WEIGHT(r) < 0$.

Take the rule $A_1 \wedge A_5$ for example, it could be understood as: If $Age \in (-INF, 54.5)$ and $ChestPain \in (-INF, 3.5)$, then class label is *presence*, with rule weight 15.9691.

Following above discussion, it is obvious that the rules extracted by our algorithm are understandable to human experts. On the one hand, human experts can use these rules to understand why a certain testing sample is classified into a certain class. On the other hand, human experts could embody their individual domain knowledge into the classification system by modifying these rules, with the hope that their domain knowledge could help to further improve the classification accuracy of the system.

6   Conclusion and Future Work

The complex structure of sigmoid kernel makes it difficult to be understood. In this paper, we expand it into its Maclaurin series, and extract classification rules from the classification hyper-plane which is constructed by SVM with sigmoid kernel, so as to construct InterSIG decision rule classifier. Experiment results on 9 UCI datasets show that InterSIG classifier is more understandable to human experts without jeopardizing the accuracy than the original SVM with sigmoid kernel. Furthermore, compared with association classifier CMAR, CBA, CPAR and decision tree classifier C4.5, InterSIG classifier is very competitive.

For non-understandable sigmoid kernel, we construct decision rule classifier InterSIG, which can help human experts to understand sigmoid kernel better.

In the future, we will try to study better algorithm for rule selection, so as to further reduce the size of the rule set while keeping its classification accuracy.

References

1. Cristianini, N., Shawe-Taylor, J.: An introduction to Support Vector Machines and Other Kernel-Based Learning Methods. Cambridge University Press, New York (2000)
2. Baesens, B., Van Gestel, T., Viaene, S., Stepanova, M., Suykens, J., Vanthienen, J.: Benchmarking State-of-the-art classification algorithms for credit scoring. Journal of the Operational Research Society 54(6), 627–635 (2003)
3. Lin, H.T., Lin, C.J.: A study on sigmoid kernels for SVM and the training of non-PSD kernels by SMO-type methods. Technical Report, Neural Computation. Department of Computer Science and Information Engineering, National Taiwan,Taipei (2003)
4. Shawe-Taylor, J., Cristianini, N.: Kernel Methods for Pattern Analysis. Cambridge University Press, Cambridge (2004)
5. Martens, D., Baesens, B., Van Gestel, T., Vanthienen, J.: Comprehensible Credit Scoring Models Using Rule Extraction from Support Vector Machines. European journal of operational research 183(3), 1466–1476 (2007)
6. Zhang, Y., Su, H., Jia, T., Chu, J.: Rule extraction from trained support vector machines. In: Ho, T.-B., Cheung, D., Liu, H. (eds.) PAKDD 2005. LNCS (LNAI), vol. 3518, pp. 61–70. Springer, Heidelberg (2005)
7. Nunez, H., Angulo, C., Catala, A.: Rule-extraction from support vector machines. In: Proc. European Symposium on Artificial Neural Networks, pp. 107–112 (2002)
8. Fung, G., Sandilya, S., Bharat Rao, R.: Rule extraction from linear support vector machines. In: Proceeding of the eleventh ACM SIGKDD international conference on Knowledge discovery and data mining, pp. 32–40 (2005)

9. Barakat, N., Diederich, J.: Eclectic rule-extraction from support vector machines. International Journal of Computational Intelligence 2(1) (2005)
10. Barakat, N., Diederich, J.: Learning-based Rule-Extraction from Support Vector Machines. In: The 14th International Conference on Computer Theory and applications, ICCTA 2004 (2004)
11. Zhang, Y., Li, Z.H., Tang, Y., Cui, K.B.: DRC-BK: Mining Classification Rules with Help of SVM. In: Dai, H., Srikant, R., Zhang, C. (eds.) PAKDD 2004. LNCS (LNAI), vol. 3056, pp. 191–195. Springer, Heidelberg (2004)
12. Li, W., Han, J., Pei, J.: CMAR: Accurate and Efficient Classification Based on Multiple Class Association Rules. In: IEEE International Conference on Data Ming, pp. 369–376 (2001)
13. Liu, B., Hsu, W., Ma, Y.: Integrating Classification and Association Rule Mining. In: Pro. the 4th International Conference on Knowledge Discovery and Data Mining (KDD 1998), pp. 80–86 (1998)
14. Yin, X., Han, J.: CPAR: Classification Based on Predictive Association Rules. In: Proc. 2003 SIAM Int'I Conf. Data Ming (SDM 2003) (2003)
15. Quinlan, J.R.: C4.5:Programs for Machine Learning. Morgan Kaufmann, San Francisco (1993)
16. Mitchell, T.M.: Machine Learning. McGraw-Hill Press, New York (1997)

DMGrid: A Data Mining System
Based on Grid Computing*

Yi Wang, Liutong Xu,
Guanhui Geng, Xiangang Zhao, and Nan Du

Beijing Key Laboratory of Intelligent Telecommunications Software and Multimedia,
Beijing University of Posts and Telecommunications, Beijing
{wangyi.tseg,gengguanhui,zhaoxiangang}@gmail.com,
{xliutong,dunan}@bupt.edu.cn

Abstract. Researchers in the field of data mining now confront a common problem that data mining tasks are time-consuming in that these tasks have to process large-scale datasets. Grid computing focuses on integrating distributed, heterogeneous and idle computers from the Internet to be a service system with high performance. Thus, it is possible to take advantage of grid computing to provide high performance computation capability to effectively reduce task durations. Here, we have successfully developed DMGrid, a grid handling data mining applications. In DMGrid, it not only considers efficient parallel computing as a crucial aspect, but also takes into account dynamic resource configuration. Unlike many existing data mining grids, DMGrid also provides an engine to execute the algorithm flow specified in an application. Moreover, it offers application execution monitoring. At last, we perform experiments and design two applications: Customer Churning Analysis and Customer Value Analysis through which the feasibility of DMGrid is validated.

1 Introduction

The technique of data mining concentrates on obtaining valuable information from large scale datasets, leading to a problem that data mining tasks are time-consuming. According to our experience, on a single computing node, such a task costs several hours on medium scale datasets, but even several days on large scale ones, like telecom datasets. The difficulty of low efficiency can be addressed by parallel computing with high performance, so grid computing is a good candidate. Grid computing has the capability of integrating those idle computers to be a high performance system, where every computing node undertakes some parts of computation work.

In the light of those advantages of grid computing, a data mining grid called DMGrid has been specially created to handle data mining applications. In DMGrid, data mining algorithms run in parallel on distributed computing nodes

---

* This work is supported by the National Natural Science Foundation of China under Grant 60402011 and National Eleven Five-Year Scientific and Technical Support Plans under Grant 2006BAH03B05.

C. Tang et al. (Eds.): ADMA 2008, LNAI 5139, pp. 305–316, 2008.

in order to reduce execution time effectively. In addition, DMGrid is different from those common computing platforms because it provides friendly user manipulation interfaces: dynamic resource configuration and application execution monitoring. When a function can be fulfilled with more than one algorithm, the former allows users to select one of them according to their requirements. By the later, it is convenient for users to monitor the execution progress of data mining applications.

In most cases, a practical application consists of not a single algorithm but several ones collaborating with each other. In DMGrid, such a requirement has been seriously taken into account so that Algorithm Flow Engine is involved in DMGrid to schedule the execution sequence of algorithms in an application.

In the end, two experimental applications: Customer Churning Analysis and Customer Value Analysis, have also been designed to validate the feasibility of DMGrid.

The rest of the paper is organized as follows: Section 2 reviews related work. Section 3 introduces the architecture of DMGrid and a typical process procedure and section 4 its implementation. Section 5 gives experimental analysis, including performance analysis, job scheduling analysis and failure analysis. Section 6 displays two representative applications: Customer Churning Analysis and Customer Value Analysis. Section 7 concludes.

2   Related Work

Since I. Foster proposes the grid conception which concentrates on integrating a mass of idle computing resources into a supercomputer to provide various services to scientific domains, grid techniques have been a hot topic in the parallel computing environment[1].

The Kensington data mining system provides a distributed knowledge discovery environment and it allows the execution of data mining tasks on remote servers with support of Enterprise JavaBean[2]. The algorithm development and mining system (ADaM) is an agent-based data mining framework, which comprises a mining engine and a daemon-controlled database[3]. THE KNOWLEDGE GRID is a middleware for implementation of knowledge discovery services in a wide range of high performance distributed applications[4][5].

The technique of data mining grid is gradually integrated with web service. Wu-Shan Jiang puts forward a service-oriented architecture abstracting mining algorithms and distributed datasets as web services[6]. Ping Chen introduces a data mining metadata service into grid environment[7]. Peter Brezany proposes a service based architecture for distributed and high-performance data mining in computational grid environment[8]. María S. Pérez also focuses on architecture design for distributed data mining [9]. Grid-VirtuE is a layered architecture for grid virtual enterprises[10].

It is true that parallel computing, distributed datasets and dynamic resource configuration are fully considered in those systems discussed above, but as a practical system, it should further offer friendly user interfaces, such as monitoring working progress, which are neglected by many systems. What's more, a practical application involves the execution of an algorithm flow, not a single algorithm. Therefore many discussed above belong to not data mining systems but just computing platforms. In [11], Ramos Ruy proposes a distributed data mining system HARVARD that allows users to specify the workflow of the sub-tasks composing the whole knowledge discovery process[11].

CIShell is an "empty shell" that supports easy integration of new datasets and algorithms by algorithm developers and easy usage of algorithms by algorithm users. Its plug-and-play architecture supports the integration and utilization of diverse modeling, visualization interfaces, scheduler[12][13].

3   DMGrid Architecture

As discussed above, data mining applications encounter four challenges: (1) a practical application involves several algorithms composed of an algorithm flow; (2) data mining tasks are time-consuming; (3) datasets are distributed; (4) users have requirements to monitor data mining applications. Thus, in DMGrid, we define four corresponding roles: scheduler, worker, dataset provider and progress monitor.

3.1   DMGrid Architecture

Fig. 1 shows the whole architecture.

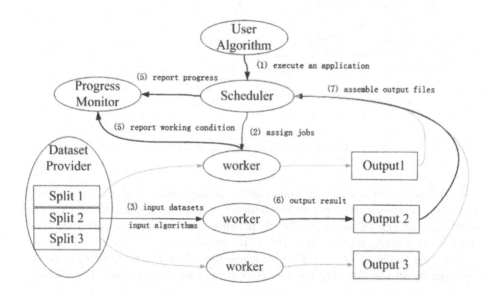

Fig. 1. The collaboration overview

Algorithm Flow Engine as a scheduler has the following duties: (1) It receives data mining applications from users. (2) It manages algorithm execution sequences. For example, when algorithm A's output is algorithm B's input, B has to wait until A is completed. (3) It assembles running results of workers and stores intermediary results of the algorithm flow. After a whole application is accomplished, it returns ultimate results to users.

Every computing node acts as a worker who receives instructions from Algorithm Flow Engine, processes some part of a dataset from dataset providers and takes on some part of computation. When computing nodes are running, they have obligations to report their processing progress to Progress Monitor. After they have accomplished their tasks respectively, workers will submit results to Algorithm Flow Engine to be assembled.

Dataset providers store original datasets to be mined and algorithms to be executed.

Progress Monitor is responsible to monitor Algorithm Flow Engine as well as every computing node and then informs users of their progress information.

3.2 A Typical Process Procedure

Fig. 2 shows a typical process procedure of a data mining application on DMGrid.

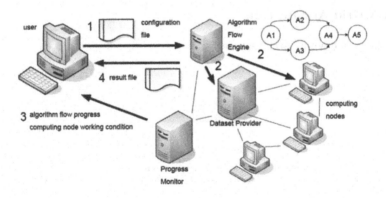

Fig. 2. A typical process procedure

1. Before a user want to submit a data mining application, he/she can select required algorithms, specify the number of computing node to execute an algorithm, set the requirement of CPU performance, etc. All the information is recorded in a configuration file in the XML format.

Here, we display a configuration example file where there are 5 steps in all (see Fig. 3). In the first step the user selects the algorithm kmeans, specifies at

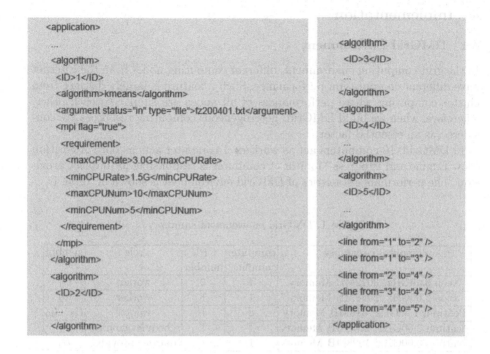

Fig. 3. A fraction of the sample file

the best 10 computing nodes to execute it and also requires that CPU frequency must be between 1.5G Hz and 3.0G Hz. We omit detail information of the other 4 steps for brevity.

2. When receiving the configuration file, Algorithm Flow Engine checks existing resources in the grid to judge whether to execute the application. For instance, if there are not enough available computing nodes, Algorithm Flow Engine returns a message to the user and tells him/her that his/her requirements fail to be satisfied.

Once all the requirements of the user can be fulfilled, Algorithm Flow Engine will execute the algorithm flow according to the sequence specified in the file. In our example of Fig. 3, Algorithm 1 runs first. Algorithm 2 and 3 have to wait until Algorithm 1 is completed because Algorithm 1's output files are Algorithm 2 and 3's input ones. Similarly, Algorithm 4 can not run until both Algorithm 2 and 3 finish. Algorithm 5 will run in the end and its result is the one of the whole application.

3. During the execution of an application, the user observes not only the progress of Algorithm Flow Engine but also the working condition of every worker.

4. As the application has been accomplished, Algorithm Flow Engine has the responsibility to transfer the result to the user.

4   Implementation

4.1   DMGrid Environment

In the grid-computing environment, different computing nodes from the Internet have different computation performance. Such a feature is largely distinct from cluster computing where performances of all nodes are similar to each other. Therefore, when we build DMGrid, heterogeneous computing resources are considered as an essential factor.

In DMGrid, 10 computers act as workers. 1 computer acts as both Algorithm Flow Engine and Progress Monitor. 1 computer is responsible for dataset provision. The performance statistics of DMGrid environment is shown in Table 1.

Table 1. DMGrid environment summary

computer capability	computer number	CPU number	role	symbol
Xeon 3.40GHz; 3072MB Memory	1	2	worker	C_1
Xeon 3.00GHz; 2048MB Memory	1	1	worker	C_2
Pentium 1.50GHz; 512MB Memory	8	1	worker	$C_3\sim C_{10}$
Pentium 3.00GHz; 2048MB Memory	1	1	scheduler,monitor	S_1
Pentium 3.00GHz; 1028MB Memory	1	1	dataset provider	D_1

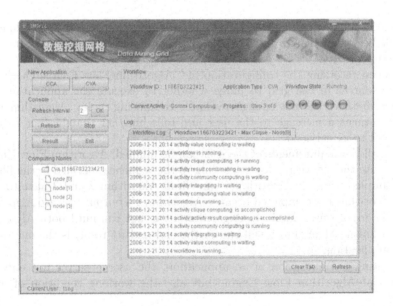

Fig. 4. User interface of DMGrid

4.2   Critical Techniques

Here, we rest on workflow engine proposed in [14] and Gmpi in [15] as Algorithm Flow Engine and a computing platform respectively. Gmpi provides MPI interfaces under grid environment, so those parallel algorithms under traditional cluster environment are easy to be ported to grid environment. Moreover, both techniques provide working progress report, so we just develop a monitor receiving reports from Algorithm Flow Engine and computing nodes. In addition, we depend on Network File System to transfer datasets to computing nodes.

4.3   User Interface

A GUI client is shown in Fig. 4. The upper right part shows the progress of Algorithm Flow Engine, the lower left part displays computing nodes and the lower right part records the detailed information of the working progress of Algorithm Flow Engine and computing nodes.

5   Experimental Evaluation

In DMGrid, a job means a certain amount of calculation assigned to a single worker when DMGrid is executing a parallel algorithm. A parallel algorithm detecting all maximum cliques in the network (Peamc) is employed to validate the performance of DMGrid[16]. In [16], Peamc has been validated to be effective under the cluster environment. Test datasets are call pairs from a telecom operator where one record is a call pair and then a call graph consists of nodes representing callers or callees and edges representing communications between them. Peamc is used to discover all maximum cliques from such a huge network in a parallel way.

5.1   Load Test of a Computing Node

In many cases, more than one job will run in a single computing node. Such a situation will lead to CPU slice schedule among these algorithms and make their efficiency declined. Due to heterogeneous computing resources in the grid environment, computing nodes with different performance result to different load-dealing performance. Here, we select workers C_1, C_2, C_3, three nodes with performance distinction, to perform load experiments. In order to test these workers, the dataset amount a job processes is in inverse proportion to job numbers. For example, if there is 1 job , it processes 1000000 records while if there are 10 jobs, each processes 100000 ones. As shown in Fig. 5 (a), the load of more jobs leads to longer complete time in all three testers, but C_1 is fastest and C_3 is slowest.

5.2   Load Balance among Computing Nodes

From the conclusion in the first experiment, if we execute a parallel algorithm and assign identical loads on computing nodes with different performance, low performance ones run more slowly than those with high performance and eventually the duration of the whole parallel algorithm lasts long. Such an assignment strategy is not suitable for grid environment. Here, we adopt a simple but unbalanced strategy according to CPU frequency, that is, high performance nodes take on more work while low ones undertake less. All computing nodes (from C_1 to C_{10})are included in this experiment. The results are shown in Fig. 5 (b). Here, a job processes about 50000 records averagely.

5.3 Dataset Transfer Duration

An experiment is designed that a dataset provider transfers distinct amounts of a dataset to different performance workers, and we check whether or not their corresponding transfer duration will be distinct. Here, the transfers of 7 datasets containing records from 150000 to 600000 are tested on C_1, C_2, C_3 whose results are shown in Fig. 5 (c).

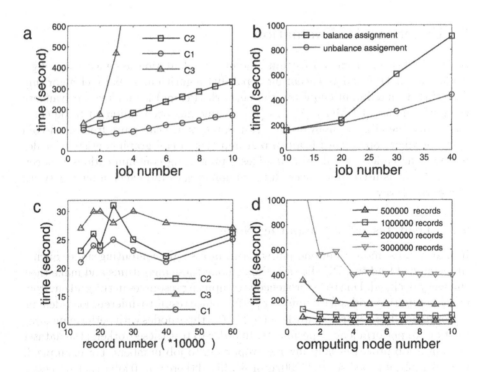

Fig. 5. Experiment results

5.4 Overall Parallel Performance

Here, in order to test overall parallel performance of DMGrid, we execute Peamc on different dataset volumes and different worker numbers, depending on unbalanced load strategy. All computing nodes are included in the experiment and one job exactly runs in only one node. Their results are shown in Fig. 5 (d).

5.5   Computing Node Failure

This experiment explores which conditions a computing node will refuse to work in. We discover that a worker collapses mainly as a result of available memory exhaustion. For workers from C_3 to C_{10}, they will collapse if more than 20 jobs are assigned while C_1 or C_2 has the capability of undertaking more than 100 jobs.

5.6   Scheduler Failure

From this experiment, if we submit more than 40 applications in a minute to Algorithm Flow Engine, that is, the scheduler, it will collapse.

6   Two Representative Applications

In order to validate the utility of our architecture and its demo system, we design two applications: one is called "Customer Churning Analysis" that is used to analyze those churning customers from a large-scale customer dataset in the telecom field. The other is "Customer Value Analysis" whose goal is to discover those most profitable customers.

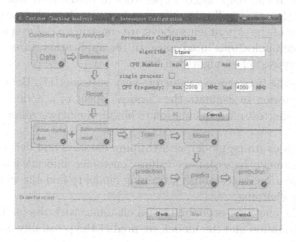

Fig. 6. The configuration interface of Customer Churning Analysis (Client version)

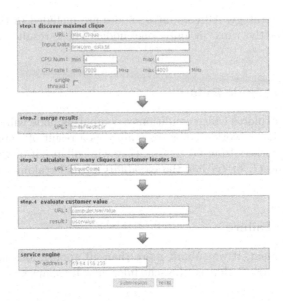

Fig. 7. The configuration interface of Customer Value Analysis (Web browser version). The 2nd step is a subsidiary algorithm to combine result fractions generated from several computing nodes into one result file.

6.1   Customer Churning Analysis

The goal of this application is to analyze churning customers from large customer datasets. It can help telecom operators to predictively discover churning customers and then they will take measures to maintain such customers in time. In the same way of the experiments above, we construct a call graph from records of customer communications in advance. In the application, three algorithms as follows are composed of an algorithm flow:

1. Calculate the betweenness value of every customer[17]. Betweenness is regarded as a criterion to evaluate the "bridge" effect of a node in the network and we rest on shortest path calculation to obtain the betweenness value of some node.

2. Establish a churning model with training datasets and betweenness value. Combining customer betweenness values, customer information and history churning information, we establish a training model to find out which customers are likely to be churning.

3. Predict the churning probability of a customer with the model. According to current information and the model, we predict the possibility a customer will become churning.

Here, the first algorithm is a time-consuming task, so in the configuration file we may set the first algorithm to run on more than one computing node. The other two algorithms only execute in a single computing node. The execution sequence of three algorithm is linear, that is, the first algorithm's output is the second algorithm's input while the second algorithm's output is the third algorithm's input.

The goals of the second and third algorithms are to establish a model and to make predictions with the model. Lots of techniques, such as Decision Tree, Bayesian Classification, Rule-Based Classification [18], can accomplish such two goals. However, it is users that decide which one to be selected and our system is so flexible as to provide multi-algorithms to satisfy users' requirements.

6.2 Customer Value Analysis

Similar to the first application, this application is used to find out those profitable customers. Three algorithms are composed of the application.

1. Discover maximal cliques[16]. Its basic idea has been discussed above and in reality, a clique usually represents a group of persons with close connections. The step focuses on discovering those groups.

2. Calculate how many cliques a customer locates in. This step makes statistics of how many groups a customer locates in and a higher quantity means the higher activeness of a customer.

3. Evaluate customer values. We combine activeness value with other customer information to evaluate their overall values.

The execution sequence of three algorithm is linear too.

We obtain value scores of 95675 customers from 800K records in the way. The proportion of customers whose scores are between 0 and 20 is 73%, the proportion from 21 to 40 is 26.6%, the proportion from 41 to 60 is 3%, the proportion from 61 to 80 is 0.5% and the proportion from 81 to 100 is 0.3%. The higher scores corresponds to more profitable customers. As we see, a mass of customers are just "ordinary customers" while 287 customers may be "profitable customers".

7   Conclusions

We have successfully achieved a grid serving data mining applications. It has the following properties: (1) it allows users to configure an application dynamically. (2) it offers Algorithm Flow Engine to manage the algorithm execution sequence in an application. (3) Users can monitor the working progress of DMGrid.

We also perform experiments on DMGrid, including loading analysis, data transfer analysis and overview parallel performance analysis. In addition, two representative applications are also designed. Through them, the feasibility, effectiveness and high efficiency of DMGrid are validated.

In the future, we will improve Algorithm Flow Engine to be capable of processing more applications submitted in a short duration. Due to our limited conditions, DMGrid involves only 12 computers. What DMGrid behaviors are under the condition more computers participate in it is another question we will address.

References

1. Foster, I., Kesselman, C.: The Grid: Blueprint for a New Computing Infrastructure, 2nd edn.
2. Chattratichat, J., Darlington, J., Guo, Y., Hedvall, S., Köler, M., Syed, J.: An architecture for distributed enterprise data mining. In: HPCN Europe 1999: Proceedings of the 7th International Conference on High-Performance Computing and Networking, pp. 573–582 (1999)
3. Hinke, T.H., Novotny, J.: Data mining on nasa's information power grid. hpdc 292, 292 (2000)
4. Cannataro, M., Talia, D.: The knowledge grid. Communications of the ACM 46, 89–93 (2003)
5. Cannataro, M., Pugliese, A., Talia, D., Trunfil, P.: Distributed data mining on grids: Service, tools, and applications. IEEE transactions on system, man, and cybernetics-part B:cybernetic 34(6), 2451–2465 (2004)
6. Jiang, W., Yu, J.: Distributed data mining on the grid. Proceedings of 2005 International Conference on Machine Learning and Cybernetics 4, 2010–2014 (2005)
7. Chen, P., Wang, B., Xu, L., Wu, B., Zhou, G.: The design of data mining web service architecture based on jdm in grid environment. In: International Symposium on Pervasive Computing and Applications, pp. 684–689 (2006)
8. Brezany, P., Janciak, I., Woehrer, A., Tjoa, A.M.: Gridminer: A framework for knowledge discovery on the grid – from a vision to design and implementation. In: Cracow Grid Workshop (2004)
9. Pérez, M.S., Sánchez, A., Robles, V., Herrero, P., Peña, J.M.: Design and implementation of a data mining grid-aware architecture. Future Generation Computer Systems 23, 42–47 (2007)
10. Alessandro, D., Amihai, M.: Virtue a formal model of virtual enterprises for information markets. J. Intell. Inf. Syst. 30(1), 33–53 (2008)
11. Ramos, R., Camacho, R., Souto, P.: A commodity platform for distributed data mining – the harvard system. In: Perner, P. (ed.) ICDM 2006. LNCS (LNAI), vol. 4065, pp. 49–61. Springer, Heidelberg (2006)
12. http://cishell.org
13. http://nwb.slis.indiana.edu
14. Zheng, Y.E., Ma, H., Zhang, L.: A temporal logic based grid workflow model and scheduling scheme. In: Proceedings of the sixth International Conference on Grid and Cooperative Computing, pp. 338–345 (2007)
15. Zhang, L., Ma, H., Jiang, Y., Zheng, Y.E.: Gmpi: A grid based mpi framework and its implementation. Journal of Huazhong University of Science and Technology (Nature Science) 35 (sup. II), 16–19 (2007)
16. Du, N., Wu, B., Wang, B.: A parallel algorithm for enumerating all maximal cliques in complex network. In: Proceedings of the 6th International Conference on Data Mining Workshop, pp. 320–324 (2006)
17. Chen, P., Wang, Y., Wu, B.: Betweenness research in telecom society network. The Journal of Dynamics of Continuous, Discrete and Impulsive Systems (DCDIS)
18. Han, J., Kamber, M.: Data Mining: Concepts and Techniques, 2nd edn

S-SimRank: Combining Content and Link Information to Cluster Papers Effectively and Efficiently

Yuanzhe Cai[1,2], Pei Li[1,2], Hongyan Liu[3], Jun He[1,2], and Xiaoyong Du[1,2]

[1] Key Labs of Data Engineering and Knowledge Engineering, Ministry of Education, China
[2] Department of Computer Science, Renmin University of China, China
{yzcai,lp,hejun,duyong}@ruc.edu.cn
[3] Department of Management Science and Engineering, Tsinghua University, China
liuhy@sem.tsinghua.edu.cn

Abstract. Both Content analysis and link analysis have its advantages in measuring relationships among documents. In this paper, we propose a new method to combine these two methods to compute the similarity of research papers so that we can do clustering of these papers more accurately. In order to improve the efficiency of similarity calculation, we develop a strategy to deal with the relationship graph separately without affecting the accuracy. We also design an approach to assign different weights to different links to the papers, which can enhance the accuracy of similarity calculation. The experimental results conducted on ACM Data Set show that our new algorithm, *S-SimRank,* outperforms other algorithms.

1 Introduction

Nowadays, with more and more papers are published, we find that it is difficult to cluster all possible papers in one field. In past several decades, researcheres have proposed many methods to calculate the similarity among documents by content analysis, such as Vector Space Model [1], Boolean model, etc. However, these methods may not be available for automatically recommending bibliographies.

Table 1. Professor Jeffrey D. Ullman's publication about universal relation assumption

Author	Paper	Classify
Jeffrey D. U.	A simplified universal relation assumption and its properties	Theory
	SYSTEM/U: a database based on the universal relation assumption	System
	On Kent's 'Consequences of assuming a universal relation'	Theory
	The revenge of the JD	Theory

Table 1 lists a series of papers about universal relation assumption which are written by Professor Jeffrey D. Ullman. We can clearly find that research on universal relation assumption is a long process: Firstly, researchers propose a new theory of assumption. Next, they develop a new system called SYSTEM/U, based on universal

C. Tang et al. (Eds.): ADMA 2008, LNAI 5139, pp. 317–329, 2008.

relation assumption. Thirdly, they find new problems of this assumption and improve their theory. Clearly, if we only calculate the similarity between two documents by analyzing document contents, the similarity between "A simplified universal relation assumption and its properties" and "SYSTEM/U: a database system based on the universal relation assumption" is very small. Because the former one is a paper about theory but the later one is about system. Obviously, words used in papers about theory are much different from words used in the papers about system. However, these two papers should be similar because they are all in the same theory system.

Further thinking about the above-mentioned problem, we discover that these papers have the same author, Professor Ullman. In addition, these papers are all published on SIGMOD, a top conference in database area. Can we use author and conference information to solve this problem? If two papers are written by the same author, these two papers are more similar. In the same way, the similarity of two papers is higher, if they are published on the same conference. [2] [3] [4] introduces the way to calculate the similarity by paper link analysis. In these methods, we can discover more implicit relationship between documents. However, a new problem appears.

Table 2. Professor Gautam Das's research area

Author	Research Area
Gautam Das	Ranking and Top-k Queries
	Data Mining
	Sampling and Approximate Queries

From Table 2 we see that Professor Gautam Das published many papers in database areas on conferences such as ICDE, VLDB, and SIGMOD. Because these papers are written by the same author and published on the same conferences, we can't distinguish these papers which are in area of top-k queries, area of data mining and area of sampling respectively by only considering link analysis.

A natural way to solve "implicit relevance" and "topic default" is to combine content similarity with link analysis. In this aim, we propose a new algorithm, *S-SimRank*, to improve the calculation of similarity. Our algorithm has a strong relationship to SimRank [2]. However, SimRank algorithm contains three disadvantages to measure documents similarity. Firstly, this algorithm doesn't consider term frequency in documents. Secondly, because SimRank is concerned with global similarity calculation, it spends lots of time in calculating the similarity between two terms which have weak or no relationship. Thirdly, although each part of links has a different degree of importance, SimRank does not set weight for different parts of link. Based on these observations, we propose a new algorithm, *S-SimRank*. The main contributions of this work are as follows:

- Term frequency is considered in *S-SimRank* to calculate similarity between documents, which improves the accuracy of similarity between papers.
- *S-SimRank* leaves out unnecessary similarity calculations so that *S-SimRank* is much more efficient than SimRank.

● We propose a method to set weights for different kinds of links, which dramatically improves the similarity calculation accuracy between documents.

The rest of this paper is organized as follows: Section 2 presents related works. In section 3, we introduce our algorithm, *S-SimRank* (means *Star SimRank*), to find related papers. Section 4 shows the experimental result. Finally, we present the conclusion in Section 5.

2 Related Work

Currently, there are mainly three kinds of methods to measure the similarity between documents: content analysis, link analysis and hierarchical domain structure analysis.

Content analysis includes two models: Vector Space Model and Boolean model. In Vector Space Model [1], each document is represented as a vector of terms. And relevance is measured by the similarity (e.g. cosine of angle) between each vector.

The similarity between documents can be calculated by analyzing links between documents. Some works focus on analysis of citation between documents. The analysis of citation graph aims to find related papers using citing relationship among them. The most common measures are based on co-citation [5] and co-coupling [6]. Co-citation means if two papers are often cited together by others, they may discuss related topics. Similarly, co-coupling means if two papers cite many papers in common, they may focus on the similar topic. In [7], Amsler proposed to fuse bibliographic co-citation and co-coupling measures to determine the similarity between documents. Some recent works, [8] further leveraged citation and provided a good mechanism to discover more implicitly similar objects. [9] demonstrated that citation and term could be integrated effectively into VSM. [10] [11] [12] [13] combined both citation and term to calculate the similarity between two documents. [14] proposed an algorithm to take two different features, content and citation, into account simultaneously and let them reinforce each other to get better performance. Some other works focus on the analysis of documents' out-links. [3] analyzed the DBLP data set and discovered that if two papers have the same author, these two documents are much more similar and if two papers are published on the same conference, they also have the similar topic. In addition, [3] also designed an effective algorithm to cluster the relative papers by documents link analysis.

Some other works focus on hierarchical domain structure analysis. [15] and [16] calculate the similarity by analysis of path length and nearest-common ancestor of two documents. [15] proposed that hierarchical domain structure analysis, compared with traditional similarity measures, matches human intuition better.

3 S-SimRank

In this section, we will first introduce a method using content information to calculate document similarity. Then, we will give an effective and efficient algorithm, *S-SimRank*, to compute similarity by considering both content and links. Finally, we propose a method to calculate weights for different links so that accuracy can be improved.

3.1 Content-Based Similarity Calculation

The relationship between the paper and its content can be considered as links between the paper and words in content. [2] presented that two objects are similar if they are linked with similar objects, and the similarity between two objects x and y is defined as the average similarity between objects linked with x and those with y. Thus, if two documents link with many same words, these two documents are much more similar. Furthermore, if two words are in the same document, these two words may be in the same topic. However, method proposed in [2] does not consider word frequency in documents. Thus, it gets wrong similarity result between documents in some cases.

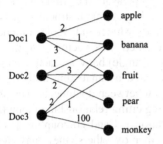

Table 3. Documents' similarity matrix (C=0.8)

	Doc1	Doc2	Doc3
Doc1	1.000	0.497	0.497
Doc2	0.497	1.000	0.497
Doc3	0.497	0.497	1.000

Fig. 1. Relationship between documents and words

For example, consider document-word graph shown in Figure 1, nodes on the left hand represent document doc1, doc2, and doc3, while nodes on the right hand represent words occurred in each documents. Apparently, Doc1 contains three words, apple which appears 2 times, banana 1 time and fruit 3 times, analogously to Doc2 and Doc3. Similarity result between documents calculated by SimRank[2] is shown at Table 3. Because [3] neglects word frequency in each document, similarity of Doc1 and Doc2 is equal to similarity of Doc2 and Doc3. Clearly, that is not right.

The inspiration comes from people random walks at a graph [17] [18]. When a person stand at node "Doc1" in Figure 1, probability of this person walking to word "banana" is $1/(2+3+1)$, the probability to "apple" is $2/(2+3+1)$ and to word "fruit" is $3/(2+3+1)$. In addition, when a person stand at the node "banana", the probability of this people walks to Doc1 is $1/(1+1+2)$, to Doc2 is $1/(1+1+2)$ and to Doc3 is $2/(1+1+2)$. After we iterate this computation for several times, the similarity has been distributed at each node in the graph.

Following this motivation, we have the following formula to calculate similarity between object a and b, i.e., $s(a,b)$:

$$s(a,b) = \begin{cases} 1 & \text{if } a=b \\ d\sum_{i=1}^{|O(a)|}\sum_{j=1}^{|O(b)|} \dfrac{tf(O_i(a))}{\sum_{k=1}^{|O(a)|} tf(O_k(a))} \dfrac{tf(O_j(b))}{\sum_{k=1}^{|O(b)|} tf(O_k(a))} s(O_i(a),O_j(b)) & \text{otherwise} \end{cases} \quad (1)$$

Decay factor d is a constant between 0 and 1. If a is a document, $tf\,(O_i(a))$ is the frequency of the ith word occurred in a. If a is a word, $tf\,(O_i(a))$ is the frequency of this word a in document $O_i(a)$. $O(a)$ describes the set of objects linking to a, and $O_i(a)$ is the ith object linking to a. The same thing holds for $tf\,(O_j(b))$, $O(b)$ and $O_j(b)$. Similarity matrix recalculated by formula (1) is shown in Table 4.

Table 4. Similarity matrix calculated by formula (1) (d=0.8)

	Doc1	Doc2	Doc3
Doc1	1.000	0.498	0.231
Doc2	0.498	1.000	0.231
Doc3	0.231	0.231	1.000

In Table 4, similarity between Doc1 and Doc2 is much higher than similarity between Doc1 and Doc3. In addition, similarity between Doc1 and Doc3 is equal to similarity between Doc2 and Doc3. Clearly, this result matches well with human intuition for these documents.

3.2 *S-SimRank* Algorithm Introduction

Before we talk about *S-SimRank* algorithm, we will discuss our model for document similarity calculation. This model is illustrated by Figure 2.

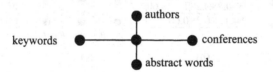

Fig. 2. Documents similarity model

We calculate similarity between two papers by considering four aspects: keywords and abstract words, authors and conference.

3.2.1 Problems of SimRank

When we calculated SimRank algorithm for Figure 2, we discover that the SimRank result matrix is a sparse matrix which contains a great number of zeroes, so it consumes a large amount of calculation for unnecessary similarity calculation in the graph. For example, when we calculate similarities between 1000 papers by SimRank algorithm, result matrix has nearly 64000000 values, while only about 100000 of them in the matrix will affect documents similarity calculation. However, others in the matrix remain 0 during the whole process of running the algorithm.

For example, we calculate similarity matrix for Figure 3 by SimRank algorithm and similarity result matrix is shown at Table 5. In this table, we can discover that similarity between node set A and node set B are equal to 0 and similarity between node set B and node set C are also equal to 0. However, SimRank has to calculate similarity between these unnecessary nodes.

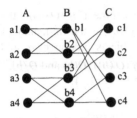

Fig. 3. Documents similarity model

Table 5. Similarity matrix, $d=0.8$

	a1	a2	a3	a4	b1	b2	b3	b4	c1	c2	c3	c4
a1	1	0.55	0.25	0.25	0	0	0	0	0.40	0.40	0.40	0.40
a2	0.55	1	0.25	0.25	0	0	0	0	0.40	0.40	0.40	0.40
a3	0.25	0.25	1	0.55	0	0	0	0	0.40	0.40	0.40	0.40
a4	0.25	0.25	0.55	1	0	0	0	0	0.40	0.40	0.40	0.40
b1	0	0	0	0	1	0.36	0.26	0.36	0	0	0	0
b2	0	0	0	0	0.36	1	0.36	0.26	0	0	0	0
b3	0	0	0	0	0.26	0.36	1	0.36	0	0	0	0
b4	0	0	0	0	0.36	0.26	0.36	1	0	0	0	0
c1	0.40	0.40	0.40	0.40	0	0	0	0	1	0.55	0.25	0.25
c2	0.40	0.40	0.40	0.40	0	0	0	0	0.55	1	0.25	0.25
c3	0.40	0.40	0.40	0.40	0	0	0	0	0.25	0.25	1	0.55
c4	0.40	0.40	0.40	0.40	0	0	0	0	0.25	0.25	0.55	1

3.2.2 *S-SimRank* Method

One intuitive method comes from Bipartite SimRank algorithm. We try to extend bipartite SimRank algorithm to calculate similarity. For example, we calculate the similarity between nodes in node set A by considering their links to node set B ($A \leftarrow B$, for simplicity), then $B \leftarrow C$ and iterate for several times. However, some new problems occur.

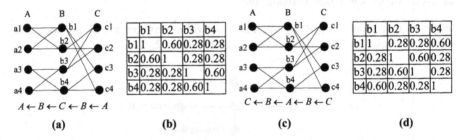

Fig. 4. Different ways to calculate nodes similarity, $d = 0.8$

As shown in Figure 4 (a) and (c), we try two different orders to calculate nodes similarity. Result matrix of similarity of node set B are shown at (b) and (d) respectively. Surprisingly, they are different. Clearly, these similarity matrixes are not equal to the result of SimRank, and they don't match our observation either because result should be like $s(b1,b2) = s(b1,b4) = s(b3,b4) = s(b2,b3)$.

The reason is that by SimRank method, in the $(k+1)^{th}$ iteration, the similarity between node a_i and node b_j is computed based on similarity scores of all of a_i and b_j's neighbors in the kth iteration. Therefore, it is unrelated to order of calculation. However, when we calculate similarity among nodes in node set B, we only consider one side of these nodes, not considering both sides simultaneously. For example, when we compute by the order of , in formula (1), we will calculate node set B's similarity by node set C, and then compute node set B's similarity by node set A for one iteration. Because each time the similarity will multiplied decay factor d, the influence of node set C to node set B is much stronger than the influence of node set A to node set B. Thus, we get false result that similarity of node set B is order-dependent. In sum, when we compute the node set B' similarity, we need to take both node set A and node set C into consideration equally.

We extend this observation to star shape graph (we call it star graph). In a star graph, we should calculate similarity of center node set by considering all node sets around them, which leads to our new algorithm, *S-SimRank*, described as follows.

Definition 1. An *n*-star graph SG is a graph consisting of one set C of center nodes, and (n-1) sets of side nodes. Let S_i be the ith set of side nodes, and $S=\{S_1, S_2, ..., S_{n-1}\}$. Each set S_i of side nodes only have relationship with center nodes, which is represented by edge between them in the graph.

For example, Figure 3 shows a 3-star graph. In this graph, $B=\{b1, b2, b3, b4\}$ is the set of center nodes, $A=\{a1, a2, a3, a4\}$ and $C=\{c1, c2, c3, c4\}$ are two sets of side nodes. There are edges between A and B, and between C and B. There is no edge between A and C.

Obviously, this *n*-star graph can be divided into (n-1) bipartite graphs, and each bipartite graph consists of a set of center nodes and a set of side nodes. In the bipartite graph C–S_x shown in Figure 5(b), C and S_x are node sets. To model the random walk after landing on a node, a probability distribution matrix should be given, which we call transfer matrix.

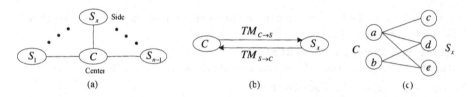

(a)   (b)   (c)

Fig. 5. n-Star Model and C–S_x bipartite model

Definition 2. The transfer matrix $TM_{C \to S_x}$ of a bipartite graph C–S_x in an *n*-star graph SG consists of $|C|$ vectors, where $|C|$ is the number of nodes in C. Each vector describes the probability of a node in C to each node in S_k, with elements nonnegative and added up to 1.

For the bipartite graph shown in Figure 4(c), we can get a transfer matrix

$$TM_{C \to S_x} = \begin{bmatrix} 1/3 & 1/3 & 1/3 \\ 0 & 1/2 & 1/2 \end{bmatrix}$$

from node set C to node set S_x. It shows that for node a, it has the probability of 1/3 to node c, and the same probability to node d and e.

In *S-SimRank*, Each iteration can be divided into two steps: (1) compute the transferred similarity in one bipartite graph; (2) make each bipartite graph reasonably weighted. In step (1), we set $s(c,d)$ as the similarity between node c and d. $s(c,d)$ has relationship with node a and b, because c and d connect to them. The transfer matrix $TM_{C \to S_x}$ plays a great role in describing this relationship.

Let $Sim_{kx}(C)$ donate the kth iterative similarity matrix ($|C|\times|C|$) of C by bipartite graph $C-S_x$, $Sim_k(Sx)$ (x=1, 2, , n-1) donate the kth iterative similarity matrix of S_x, and let $Sim_k(C \rightarrow Sx)$ donate the computing process of getting $Sim_{kx}(C)$ according to transfer matrix $TM_{C \rightarrow S_x}$. Constant d is a decay factor, showing that along with iteration, the influence transferred from other nodes becomes weak. As discussed above, for $a_i, a_j \in S_x$, c_i, c_j in node set C, we can write iteration equations for $Sim_{k+1}(C \rightarrow S_x)$:

$$s_{k+1}(a_i, a_j) = d \cdot \sum_{l=1}^{|S_x|} \sum_{p=1}^{|S_x|} (TM_{C \rightarrow S_x})_{il} \cdot (TM_{C \rightarrow S_x})_{jp} \cdot Sim_k(a_i, a_j) \tag{2}$$

And for $Sim_{k+1}(S_x \rightarrow C)$:

$$s_{k+1}(c_i, c_j) = d \cdot \sum_{l=1}^{|C|} \sum_{p=1}^{|C|} (TM_{S_x \rightarrow C})_{il} \cdot (TM_{S_x \rightarrow C})_{jp} \cdot Sim_k(c_i, c_j) \tag{3}$$

For $a_i = a_j$, $s_k(a_i, a_j) = 1$, and analogously for $s_k(c_i, c_j)$. When $k = 0$, $s_0(a_i, a_j)$ is a initial similarity matrix. Following our motivation, if $a_i = a_j$ then $s_0(a_i, a_j)$ should be 1, otherwise 0. Therefore, $Sim_0(S)$ can be initialized to be a identity matrix, and analogously for $Sim_0(C)$.

Based on these definitions and notations given above, the main steps of our Unweighted *S-SimRank* approach can be shown as follows.

Algorithm Unweighted S-SimRank
Input: decay factor d, transfer matrix $TM_{C \rightarrow S_x}$, $TM_{S_x \rightarrow C}$, $1 \leq x \leq n-1$, tolerant factor $\mathcal{E}$.
Output: similarity matrix $Sim(C)$.

$k \leftarrow 0$
$Sim_0(C) \leftarrow$ identity matrix
for each $S_x \in S$ (x=1,2, ...,n-1)
$\quad Sim_0(S_x) \leftarrow$ identity matrix
while (max($Sim_{k+1}(C) - Sim_k(C)$) > $\mathcal{E}$)
$\quad$ **for each** $S_x \in S$
$\quad\quad$ compute $Sim_k(C \rightarrow S_x)$
$\quad\quad$ compute $Sim_k(S_x \rightarrow C)$ getting $Sim_{kx}(C)$
$$Sim_{k+1}(C) = \frac{1}{n-1} \sum_{x=1}^{n-1} Sim_{kx}(C)$$
$\quad k = k+1$
return $Sim_{k+1}(C)$

Unweighted *S-SimRank* tries to get similarity matrix from each bipartite graph, and gain mean value as iterative result of center node set. Also the newly changed similarity matrix of center node set will influence the similarity matrix of each side node sets. Obviously, in Unweighted *S-SimRank*, the status of every bipartite graph is equal. By adequately weighted, the bipartite graph with higher score will play a greater role than lower ones. Weighted *S-SimRank* will be discussed in Section 3.3.

Let us analyze the time and space complexity for this method of computing *S-SimRank*. Let d_1 be the average number of nodes in the node sets and n is the number of node set. The space required is simply $O(nd_1^2)$ to store the results R_k. Let d_2 be the average of $|O(a)||O(b)|$ over all node pairs (a, b), and k the iteration number. The time required is $O(knd_1^2d_2)$, since for each iteration, the similarity score of every node-pair (d_1^2 of these) is updated with values from its in-neighbor pairs (d_2 of these on average). As it corresponds roughly to the square of the average in-degree, d_2 is likely to be a constant with respect to d_1 for many domains.

3.3 Weighted *S-SimRank*

[19] shows that in web page, words in different parts have the different importance. For example, the words in title are much more important than the words in contents.

Thus, in *n*-Star Model SG_n, we define Weighted *S-SimRank* formula as follows:

$$Sim_{k+1}(C) = \sum_{x=1}^{n-1} Sim_{kx}(C) \cdot w_x \qquad where \quad \sum_{x=1}^{n-1} w_x = 1 \qquad (4)$$

However, how to learn weight value is a challenging problem. Some classification algorithm [20] such as Bayes algorithm, Decision Tree, and Neural Network learn the math model by training data and then evaluate the model by test data. In the same way, we can also get the weight values from training data and then use the learned weight values to calculate other data.

We use each factor's influence degree to decide the importance of the factor. In our model, we calculate documents similarity by each factor, cluster these documents and then compare the result with the standard documents category (final result). We use formula (5) to calculate weight of each factor.

$$accuracy(S_x) = \frac{right(S_x)}{count(paper)}$$

$$w_x = accuracy(S_x) \Big/ \sum_{x=1}^{n-1} accuracy(S_x) \qquad (5)$$

In formula (5), $right(S_x)$ means the number of correctly classified documents only considering factor S_x, and $count(paper)$ is the total number of papers, $|C|$.

4 Experiment and Evaluation

4.1 Experiment Setup

In this section we report experiments to examine the efficiency and effectiveness of *S-SimRank*. The dataset includes 14000 papers downloaded from ACM [21]. We want to focus our analysis on these computer science papers and group them into clusters so that each cluster of papers is in a certain research area. We remove conferences and journals that are not well known. As a result, there are 90 conferences or journals left. We select 1077 most productive authors, each having at least 3 publications. We choose 132063 most frequent words stems from abstracts of these papers, excluding 46 most frequent words which are removed as stop words. There are four types of objects to calculate documents similarity: 1077 authors, 90 conferences or journals, and 15342 keywords and 132063 word stems in abstracts.

We take PAM [20], a *k*-medoids clustering approach, to cluster papers based on similarities calculated by our method. We randomly select the initial centroids for 50 times when do clustering and choose the most accurate result. All our experiments are running on a PC with a 1.86G Intel Core 2 Processor, 2GB memory, under windows XP Professional environment. All of our programs are written in java. Every experiment is performed at least 3 times, except the case when the number of papers is above 600 for SimRank.

We generate 6 datasets which include 100, 200, 400, 600, 800, 1000 papers from the paper set respectively for the performance evaluation experiments, among which the first and the last datasets are used for accuracy test. All of the 100 papers come from three areas, Information Systems, Computing Milieux, and Software. All of the 1000 papers are from three areas, Hardware, Software, and Information Systems.

4.2 Experiment Results

In the first set of experiments, we want to compare the accuracy among SimRank, Vector Space Model, *S-SimRank* and Weighted *S-SimRank*. At the beginning, We study the weight from 100 documents. The weight value of each factor is shown at Table 6. In Figure 6, we draw an accuracy contrast diagram for each algorithm for datasets including 100 and 1000 papers respectively. In these experiments, VSM performs worst among these algorithms, because it only considers the documents content. Weighted *S-SimRank* has the better result than Unweighed *S-SimRank*, because the importance of each factor is different.

Table 6. Learning weights from 100 papers

Training set : 100 Papers	Key Words	Authors	Sources	Abstracts
Weight(W)	0.227	0.218	0.256	0.299

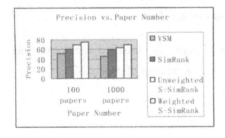

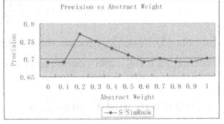

Fig. 6. Precision vs. Paper Number   **Fig.7.** Precision vs. Weight

In the second set of experiments, we want to test whether or not our method is an effective way to determine the weight. Figure 7 illustrates cluster precision for the different abstract weights. Between 0.2 and 0.3, we gain the highest precision of the clustering. The weight of abstract based on formula (5) is 0.299, which is very close to our experiments

We use the formula 6 to evaluation the convergence performance.

$$Dv(k) = \max_{i=1, j=1}^{|C|,|C|} \left(\left| s_k(c_i, c_j) - s(c_i, c_j) \right| \right) \qquad c_i, c_j \in C \qquad (6)$$

In formula (6), k is the iteration number. Dv (Different value) means maximal change value of the similarity for the k-iteration to convergence value. Figure 8 describes the convergence performance of each algorithm, which shows that SimRank is the best. Because SimRank will calculate all of the nodes in graph in each iteration, it needs less iteration times than *S-SimRank* to converge. In addition, we discover that with the increase of the number of nodes in the graph, the speed of convergence improves. However, since in each iteration SimRank need to do much more computation than *S-SimRank*, the time spent for each iteration differs a lot, which is shown in Table 7.

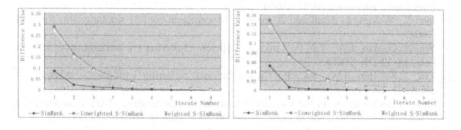

(a) Convergence for 100 papers   (b) Convergence for 1000 papers

Fig. 8. Convergence

Table 7. Performance on each iteration

Paper# Algo.Time(s)	200	400	600	800	1000
VSM	0.463	1.76	4.199	6.853	10.034
SimRank	789.128	2448.039	6791.292	12807.081	21754.430
S-SimRank	*33.297*	*163.528*	*454.490*	*886.492*	*1463.465*

After these algorithms have iterated for ten times, we get the average value of time used for each iteration. In Table 7, it can be seen that average time consumed in one iteration for SimRank is about 20 times more than that of *S-SimRank*.

In sum, we can see that *S-SimRank* is the most competitive method, since it reaches higher accuracy, and is more efficient than SimRank.

5 Conclusion

In this paper we propose an effective and efficient approach, *S-SimRank*, to group related papers. We take term frequency into consideration when calculating the similarity between documents. Besides this kind of content information, we also consider information linked to each paper, such as keywords, abstract words, authors and conferences. Using the star shape linked information, we improve existing algorithm, SimRank, to neglect unnecessary computations by decomposing the graph. In the meantime, we also assign different weights to each link. Experiment results show *S-SimRank* achieves high efficiency and accuracy in clustering related papers.

Acknowledgments. This work was supported in part by the National Natural Science Foundation of China under Grant No. 70471006, 70621061, 60496325 and 60573092; the 985 Project of Renmin University under Grant No. 21357232.

References

1. Salton, G., Wong, A., Yang, C.S.: A vector space model for information retrieval. In: Communications of the ACM (1975)
2. Jeh, G., Widom, J.: SimRank: A measure of structural-context similarity. In: SIGKDD (2002)
3. Yin, X.X., Han, J.W., Yu., P.: Linkclus: Efficient clustering via heterogeneous semantic links. In: VLDB (2006)
4. Yin, X.X., Han, J.W., Yu., P.: Cross-relational clustering with user's guidance. In: SIGKDD (2005)
5. Small, H.: Co-citation in the scientific literature: A new measure of the relationship between two documents. Journal of the American Society for Information Science (1973)
6. Kessler, M.M.: Bibliographic coupling between scientific papers. American Documentation (1963)
7. Amsler, R.: Applications of citation-based automatic classification. Linguistic Research Center (1972)
8. Xue, G.R., Zeng, H.J., Chen, Z., Ma, W.Y., Yu, Y.: Similarity Spreading: A New Algorithm for Similarity Calculation of Interrelated Objects. In: WWW (2004)
9. Salton, G.: Associative document retrieval techniques using bibliographic information. Journal of the ACM (1963)
10. Wen, J.R., Nie, J.Y., Zhang, H.J.: Clustering user queries of a search engine. In: WWW (2001)
11. Bharat, K., Henzinger, M.: Improved Algorithms for Topic Distillation in a Hyperlinked Environment. In: SIGIR (1998)
12. Chakrabarti, S.: Automatic Resource Compilation by Analyzing Hyperlink Structure and Associated Text. In: WWW (1998)
13. Chakrabarti, S., Dom, B.E., Kumar, S.R., Raghavan, P., Rajagopalan, S., Tomkins, A.D.: Mining the Web's link structure. Computer 32(8) (1999)
14. Huang, S., Xue, G.R., Zhang, B.Y., Chen, Z., Yu, Y., Ma, W.Y.: TSSP: A Reinforcement Algorithm to Find Related Papers. In: WI (2004)
15. Ganesan, P., Molina, H.G., Widom, J.: Exploiting hierarchical domain structure to compute similarity. In: ACM Transactions on Information Systems (2003)
16. Maguitman, A.G., Menczer, F., Roinestad, H.: Algorithmic Detection of Semantic Similarity. In: WWW (2005)

17. Lov´asz, L.: Random Walks on Graphs: A Survey, 2nd edn., pp. 1–46. Bolyai Society Mathematical Studies (1993)
18. Tong, H.H., Faloutsos, C., Pan, J.Y.: Fast RandomWalk with Restart and Its Applications. In: Perner, P. (ed.) ICDM 2006. LNCS (LNAI), vol. 4065. Springer, Heidelberg (2006)
19. Song, R., Liu, H., Wen, H.F., Ma, J.R.,, W.Y.: Learning Block Importance Models for Web Pages. In: WWW (2004)
20. Han, J.W., Kamber, M.: Data Mining Concepts and Techniques. Morgan Kaufmann Publishers, San Francisco (2001)
21. ACM dataset, http://portal.acm.org/portal.cfm

Open Domain Recommendation: Social Networks and Collaborative Filtering

Sarah K. Tyler and Yi Zhang

University of California, Santa Cruz

Abstract. Commercial enterprises employ data mining techniques to recommend products to their customers. Most of the prior research is usually focused on a specific domain such as movies or books, and recommendation algorithms using similarities between users and/or similarities between products usually performs reasonably well. However, when the domain isn't as specific, recommendation becomes much more difficult, because the data could be too sparse to find similar users or similar products based on purchasing history alone. To solve this problem, we propose using social network data, along with rating history to enhance product recommendations. This paper exploits the state of art collaborative filtering algorithm and social net based recommendation algorithm for the task of open domain recommendation. We show that when a social network can be applied, it is a strong indicator of user preference for product recommendations. However, the high precision is achieved at the cost of recall. Although the sparseness of the data may suggest that the social network is not always applicable, we present a solution to utilize the network in these cases.

1 Introduction

Recommendation systems use information from both users and products to predict which products a given user might prefer. Many **Collaborative filtering** techniques have been proposed to recommend products to a user using information from other users with similar tastes and preferences.

However, prior research work on recommender systems are usually limited to a specific domain, such as movie recommendation with either the MovieLens or Netflix data. While the number of movies in general may be large, the number of new movies produced each year is relatively small, and the number of blockbusters seen by large audiences is even smaller. For most of the similar user pairs, there are often some movies seen by both of them, and for most similar movie pairs, there are often a lot of over lap of viewers. If two users have both rated the same subset of movies, one can aggregate the information to see where their similarities and differences lie; if they share similar genre tastes, favorite actors or other aspects in common. If the number of movies they have both rated is relatively small, it is harder to determine the underlying causes that makes the ratings either similar or dissimilar with respect to each other. In these contexts, additional information could be helpful. Similarly, the problem exists for product

C. Tang et al. (Eds.): ADMA 2008, LNAI 5139, pp. 330–341, 2008.

pairs. In close domain recommendation, especially the widely studied movie recommendation scenario, one can usually achieve a reasonable degree of accuracy, because this problem does not dominate the average performance. However, this becomes a serious problem in open domain recommender systems.

To solve this problem, especially for open domain recommender systems, we exploit additional contextual information, the social and trust networks, for recommendation. If the user has selected a group of friends or identify a group of people he/she trusts, we assume they share some interests in common. While a user may add anyone to their social network, there is an implicit assumption of kinship: work acquaintance might share a professional interest while social friends may share hobbies. While the connection between any two individuals may be tenuous, a large group of connections can potentially bias the recommendation system in the right direction. Our goal is to combine these multiple types of information to enhance prediction when a small number of training ratings per product hamper the accuracy of traditional methods.

This paper compared several representative recommendation techniques on a open domain recommendation task. We found that the trust network method worked the best in terms of precision, but was applicable in a limited context thus having low recall. The regularized Singular Value Decomposition method, a collaborative filtering technique, on the other hand, fell victim to the perceptivity of the data. Being a more complex model, it did not have sufficient data to learn the hidden representations and was not able to outperform a simple baseline.

2   Related Work

Typically recommendation filtering uses collaborative filtering. The idea is to find similar individuals, and similar products, in order to make the best recommendation. For example, memory based heuristics, and model based approaches have been used in collaborative filtering tasks [1] [2] [8] [10] [17]. The drawback to these approaches is that they require significant amounts of data per user and per product.

Content based approaches such as latent semantic indexing[7], also help improve recommendation[15], but face scaling issues. As new items are introduced, they may have additional, never before seen features. This is especially true when the context includes natural language such as product description terms, where, according to Zipf's law we can expect to see new words, regardless of how large our training set is.

The notion of using trust networks is not new, both with implicit and explicit networks. Referral Chains use word co-occurrences to build an informal network and uses the network to enhance web search[9]. Yet the question seems to be how to apply it since social connections are not necessarily the same as trusted connections, and may be tenuous at best [14].

TidalTrust is a recommendation technique that allows users to specify a degree of trust for each person in the network [5][6]. The trust is then accumulated over neighbors of varying distance to create a ranked list approach. The top ranked items are then presented to the user, and are the only ones used in the evaluation.

Other recommendation work involving social networks has focused on the user profiles. Liu et al.[12] harvested profile pages on Friendster, Orkut and MySpace, using the user supplied interests to create Interest Maps to form taste cliques for product recommendation. Their work, however, focused on the profiles and not the connections between users.

The trust network approach has been discussed in conjunction with the same data set we use. Massa et al.[13] showed the potential power of trust networks, and argued for a way of propagating trust over all users. Leskovec et al. [11] also did a study of information cascades, which is typically studied in the blog domain. In their study, users could select who to share a product with. As a result, Leskovec et al. were able to see how the social network influenced the cascade of products in a recommendation environment.

3   Methods

To see how existing recommendation techniques perform on an open domain recommendation task, we looked at three types of methods. The first approach is a base line weighted average that had no personalization. The second approach made predictions based on the social network. Lastly, a collaborative filtering approach commonly used for product recommendation in the movie domain was applied.

3.1   Baseline

In order to determine whether personalized recommendation will help, we first needed a baseline which predicts each product rating independent of the users and sans personalization. The baseline predicts a product's rating by taking the average rating for the given product in the training set. This is a common approach when the number of ratings per product and per user are small. In these instances there is not enough data to model the hidden variables and more complex models can not be trained well. In our case users review on average 2 products, and products have on average 2.4 ratings.

One added benefit of this approach is that it is very fast and simple, as there are no hidden features to estimate. This method also has two drawbacks. First, the predicted rating can easily be skewed by a single review when the training data is sparse. Second, some individuals have a predisposition to rate products either high or low and this model does not account for individual user's rating bias. This algorithm assumes a user's rating of a product i is the average rating of that particular product. The approach is detailed in Equation 1.

$$r_i = \frac{1}{n_i} \Sigma_u r_{iu} \tag{1}$$

Where r_{ui} is user u's ratings of product i. n_i is the number of users that have a non missing rating for product i, $n_i = ||\{ \text{ Number of users where } r_{iu} \text{ is defined}\}||$.

3.2 TidalTrust

We used TidalTrust as our social network recommendation system since it provides a way of propagating trust as Massa et al.[13] called for. TidalTrust utilizes the extended trust network for users by creating a trust flow metric. If two users do not trust each other directly, the amount of trust between them is the product of the trust along each part of the path. In cases where there is more than one path, only the path with the highest trust score is used. When a prediction is needed for a specific user and product, the trust network is explored to find other users who rated the same product. If a member of the trust network has rated the item, their opinion is weighted according to their distance from the initial user, and by how much trust is exhibited along the path between the two users. This method only needs to walk the trust graph to make a prediction which can be very fast. Most users trust a very small fraction of the overall user set. The approach is outlined in Equation 2.

$$r_{iu_1} = \frac{\Sigma_{u_2 \in S} t_{u_1 u_2} r_{iu_2}}{\Sigma_{u_2 \in S} t_{u_1 u_2}} \tag{2}$$

Where $t_{u_1 u_2}$ is the trust of u_1 to u_2 and r_{iu_2} is the rating of product i by user u_2. In our dataset, each trust instance had the same weight. The t_{u_1,u_2} term was constant and dropped out of the equation. The predicted rating in this instance is the average of the rating in the trust network. Used in this manner, TidalTrust is similar in effect to the baseline.

3.3 Singular Value Decomposition

For our collaborative filtering approach we used singular value decomposition [1]. We first create a sparse user-product rating matrix. Each user is represented as a vector of products where the index into the vector indicates a given product's rating. Each product is represented as a vector of users where the index into the vector indicates a given user's rating of the product. The singular value decomposition technique is then used to find the hidden representation of users and products in a low dimensional space. Finally a new user-product rating matrix without missing entries is reconstructed using the learned low dimensional representation.

Singular value decomposition[3] is one of the effective collaborative filtering techniques that works well on the well know Netflix data set, which contains 100 Million explicit movie ratings from about 1 Million Netflix customers over a long period of time (1998-2005). It scales well, and is capable of learning the hidden factors that account for individual's uniqueness and rating patterns. It performs much better than Pearson Correlation and Netflix's own system.

In our case, the singular value decomposition will likely be less effective because of how simultaneously diverse and sparse our data is. When dimensionality of the user vectors is high, each user begins to look equally far away from the

---

[1] We acquired our implementation of Singular Value Decomposition from Timely Development[3] which they used for the Netflix Prize and distribute freely[16].

rest. For our data, we varied the number of hidden features. Since the size of our data is limited, it would be difficult to learn many features, however our diverse domain indicates more features would be necessary.

4 Data

The data set used was collected from Epinions.com[4] in January of 2008. Epinions.com is a commercial site that allows users to rate products, give reviews, and share their opinions with other users. Each user can also specify which other users he or she trust. Collecting these individual trust instances creates a directed graph of trust.

One of the advantages of Epinions compared to other review sites is that users can rate any kind of item they wish, from mattresses to restaurants. While a benefit to the epinions.com user base, this increases the size of the product space on which to make predictions. As a result, the number of hidden features required to make an accurate prediction in this domain is likely greater than the number needed in domains where there is more consistency between products.

Second, the same feature value may have very different effects on two different products. For example, a $100 laptop may seem like a steal, but a $100 pack of gum is likely over priced. Here the same feature value for price influences the recommendation in two different ways even for the same user.

The data sample itself consists of 85,139 user-product ratings, each on a scale of 1-5. The average user-product rating was 4.02 with a standard deviation of

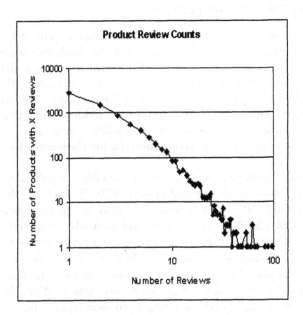

Fig. 1. The graph of the number of products in the test set with N reviews in the training set. Not shown here is the number of the 7428 products with zero reviews.

1.14. There are 35,137 unique products and 41,696 unique users. This means each user has an average of two reviews, and each product has on average 2.4 ratings. Compared with commonly used recommendation data sets, which usually have hundreds of ratings per user and tens of thousands of ratings per product, it is much harder to do well on this data set. Figure 1 shows the that data follows an approximately Zipf law curve.

In the initial TidalTrust paper, users could specify the degree to which they trusted another user. In our data set, however, all we can see is whether or not a user trusts another user. There is no notion of why a user is trusting another user, or how much trust between exists between the users. In this setting we are forced to assume uniform trust in our implementation.

5   Evaluation

In order to evaluate the different models, we need to establish some objectives. In the first case we wanted to see how closely the model conforms to ground truth and we use Mean Square Error as the objective. However, finding the ground truth value is not the primary goal of recommender systems. When creating a recommender system the primary task is to ensure that the item recommended is desirable to the user. Items that are unrelated and not recommended are less important. Therefore, in the second case, we examine whether the highly rated products are desirable to the end users.

The ratings follow a roughly Gaussian distribution, with a center of 4.02. Therefore, to achieve the first objective we used mean squared error (MSE) which follows naturally from the distribution. For the second objective we used several different methods. The first was a precision recall curve, which describes the precisions of recommended items at different "desirable" (or user preference) thresholds. For example, if the "desirable" threshold is 4, we assume a user who rated the product with a 4 or a 5 liked the given product, but a user who rated it with a 1, 2 or 3 did not. In recommender systems, precision is usually more important than recall, so our discussion often centers on precision.

Often users will only look at the first couple of items. To measure how well our models would perform in this environment, we also include macro averages Precision@K and AverageRating@K. It turns out in our environment the number of reviews per product is often low, following a long tail distribution. For example, half of the products that exist in our testing set, do not exist in the training set. Half of those that do, only occur once in the training set. The number of ratings per user follows a similar distribution. Since a small percentage of our products have more than one rating, we often let K=1 for our macro averages.

We also looked at an aggregate Precision@K that was independent of users, where all user-product pairs are ordered according to rating and the precision is calculated for the top K product-user ratings. For this evaluation, we selected only two thresholds for "desirable" when computing these measures. The first, 4.0 reflects the average rating users tend towards. Using the average tends to lead to very good results for all models, so we also choose a threshold of 4.5. Since users are bound by integer ratings, only products that received a 5/5 were deemed interesting. The models needed to make a prediction that rounded to 5.

Our original 20% split of our 80/20 partitioning consisted of 14,873 test cases. However, only 7,445 test instances contained a product or user also in the 80% partition used for testing. For our evaluations we used this subset of users.

5.1 Baseline

For our first objective, we calculated an MSE of 1.36. The F-measure for the baseline in Figure 2 exhibits a knee at 3.5. This is partially due to the fact that the average measurement calculated in the baseline can be skewed by either a very strong or very negative rating. The closer the threshold for "desirable" is to the maximum value or minimum value, the less likely it is for the average rating to recover from a strongly dissenting rating, especially when half of the data that occurs in the test set occurs less than twice. This is also reflective in the sharp downtick of precision, recall and F-measure around 4.5.

Coincidentally, the average rating is 4.02 with a standard deviation of 1.14. The high precision, recall and F-measure for the "desirable" threshold of less than 3 are inflated since the data is so strongly skewed.

The AverageRating@K for $k = 1$ was 4.0 and the AveragePrecision@K for $k = 1$ item was 0.84 and 0.59 for the 4.0 and 4.5 thresholds of "desirability" respectively. This demonstrates that the baseline is reasonably accurate in predicting whether an item is in the top half of all items, but is not as accurate at predicting the very top rated items.

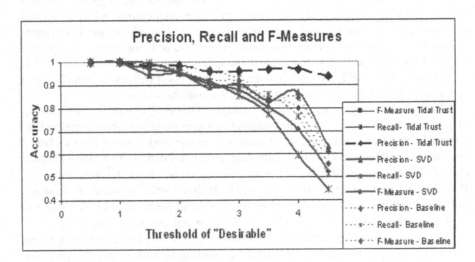

Fig. 2. A Graph of the overall precision, recall and F-measure for the each model. The recall and F-measure for Tidal Trust was less than 0.015 at all thresholds.

5.2   TidalTrust

The TidalTrust MSE was extremely low, 0.52, less than half of the MSE for the baseline although we only calculated the MSE in products where prediction was possible. Along similar lines, precision was very high as shown in Figure 2. Recall, however, was less than 0.008 for all "desirable" thresholds. This was an artifact of how few instances could be rated with TidalTrust. While TidalTrust was able to make strong predictions, it was only able to make a prediction in 75 of the 7,445 test cases, or 1% of the time. It appears that if a product was rated by someone in the given trust network, the two users often agree both in polarity and in magnitude of the rating. However, most of the time two users in a given trust network do not rate the same product. In our data set, a given trust network generally may only have one item that exists in common with more than one user. Still, this approach shows promise.

The strong MSE metric in general, along with the precision curve show that trust networks do have a positive effect on rating prediction, but more work needs to be done to harness that power.

The baseline, when run over the 75 instances that could be predicted using TidalTrust, had a MSE of 0.49, very close and on the surface slightly better than the MSE of TidalTrust. However, in those 75 instances, TidalTrust exactly agreed with the true rating value in 59 instances. In contrast, the baseline was within 0.25 of the true rating in only 32 instances. If we increase the window to 0.5 the baseline was within the true value in 38 instances. When the trust network could make a prediction, it seems to be more accurate than the baseline at finding the exact rating.

In fact, TidalTrust so closely matched the predicted value, that it was only off from the actual value by more than 1 in three of the seventy five instances. When it was off, however, the difference was significant. In one instance TidalTrust's predicted rating was off by 4 from the true rating, and in another it was off by 3. In contrast, the greatest the baseline was off on these 75 instances was 2.2, however there were 10 instances where the baseline was off by more than 1 and less than 2 to the true rating. If you treat the three instances of magnitude greater than 2 as outliers from both the baseline and TidalTrust, the MSE of TidalTrust is 0.23 where the MSE of the baseline is still 0.48. While in general MSE may not be an appropriate measure for recommendation accuracy, the measure does support that Tidal Trust, on average, beats the baseline.

Figure 3 and 4 offer a different perspective on the same phenomenon with the Precision@K metric. Here, items are ranked according to their predicted rating, independent of users. We see that the precision values are near 1 for all values of K. In environments were precision far outweighs recall, such as product recommendation, there is a clear advantage for Tidal Trust.

AverageRating@K for $k = 1$ was 4.1. The average precision rating for the top 1 item per users are also reflective of the same nature, 96.7 and 93.4 for the 4.0 and 4.5 thresholds respectively. This shows that Social Network information consistently influences product recommendations when they can be applied.

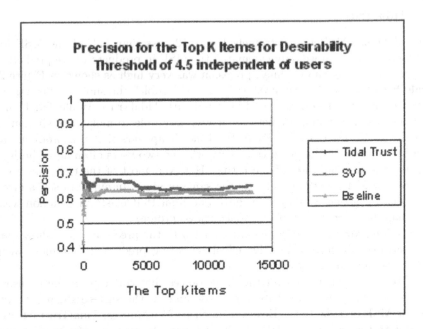

Fig. 3. A graph of the baseline precision, recall and F-measure for different thresholds of "desirable". The Knee around 3-3.5 occurs before the average product rating.

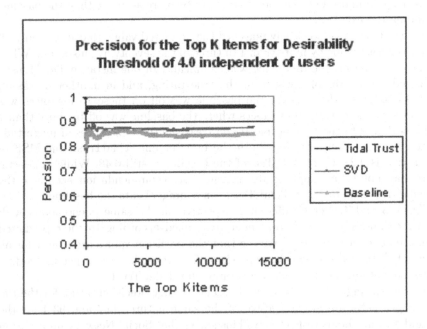

Fig. 4. A graph of the baseline precision, recall and F-measure for different thresholds of "desirable". The Knee around 3-3.5 occurs before the average product rating.

5.3   Singular Value Decomposition

The final approach used was collaborative filtering in the form of singular value decomposition.

In this case the MSE dropped considerably to 1.5, just above the baseline. This is indicative of two things. The data itself is so sparse that the hidden features cannot be trained well, and that collaborative filtering may require much more data than is available.

The precision and recall curves are similar to the curves in Figure 2, and are nearly identical to the baseline. We see, however that Percision is slightly higher than the baseline by Figures 3 and 4 according to the Precision@K metric.

In terms of the macro average, Precision@K for k of 1, SVD scores 86.2 62.7 for thresholds of 4.0 and 4.5 respectively. Like the baseline, the SVD model is more accurate when it predicts a product is in the top 50

Netflix Data. It is worth noting that Singular Value Decomposition is the collaborative filtering technique that is often used in the movie domain because it is able to distill the movies and users into smaller feature vectors where better inferences can be drawn over them. The MSE on a sample of Netflix data was 0.77, half the MSE of the Epinions.com data. This is also better than most reported MSE for Netflix, but only slightly better and could be due to the sampling bias.

The key difference between Netflix and Epinions is the amount of reviews per user and product. In a random sample of approximately 4589 Netflix users, each user has made an average of 27.9 reviews and each product had an average of 15.4 reviews. This additional information provides more certainty when learning the hidden features.

Our Epinions.com data is simultaneously very sparse, making it difficult to learn hidden features, and very vast, making a greater number of hidden features necessary. This makes sense since we have, on average, 2.4 ratings per product and many products have 1 rating. Learning multiple hidden features is difficult with the limited amount of data.

6   Conclusions

It is clear that the dimensionality requirements of Singular Value Decomposition makes the model complexity too high in the epinions.com context. Although Singular value decomposition outperforms the baseline, it does not outperform it by much. This indicates it was unable to adequately learn the hidden features and improve recommendation accuracy.

The trust network proved to be very useful in the limited number of times it could be applied. It's accuracy was higher than the baseline for both evaluation objectives. Even without considering the possible outliers, the trust network preformed very well. It seems when a product is reviewed by your trust network, your opinion of it will be closer to that of your network, rather than the entire user base. Unfortunately, it could rarely be applied, limiting it's utility. In our sample it was only able to make a prediction less than 1% of the time. If the social network information could be applied in more cases, the accuracy of the recommendation would surely increase.

7   Future Work

The social network aspect of the data shows great promise for improving recommendation, but the current system is not capable of capitalizing on it. If one can bootstrap the trust network, they may see a significant improvement.

While a specific product may not be common in a trust network, the trust network may share general interests, which then influences what products they would like to purchase. Thus the trust network's relative opinions of similar products may be useful for rating prediction. For example, a Single Lens Reflex (SLR) is a type of advanced lens for digital cameras. For the average user, the additional cost may be prohibitive for them to purchase a camera with such a lens, but to an amateur photographer, the lens may be worthwhile. It is likely that our amateur photographer has friends, colleagues or acquaintances with whom he or she shares his or her interests. If these acquaintances are in the social network of our amateur photographer, they may rate similar products with SLR lenses. Therefore, other products with similar features may have an average rating in the social network that is close to our amateur photographers' true rating for the given product. This can help us estimate the rating for a new, unseen product from the explicit network in the same way that collaborative filtering is often applied for the implicit network.

We propose using the products' contextual features to find similar products. The social network recommendation for each product can be weighted according to the similarity of the desired product in addition to the trust distance between the user and the network. This approximate rating can be used in cases where the predicted rating cannot be established directly. It is our belief that this method will show continued improvement over collaborative filtering in this general domain.

References

1. Breese, J.S., Heckerman, D., Kadie, C.: Empirical analysis of predictive algorithms for collaborative filtering. Technical report, Microsoft Research, One Microsoft Way, Redmond, WA 98052 (1998)
2. Delgado, J., Ishii, N.: Memory-based weightedmajority prediction for recommender systems. In: ACM SIGIR 1999 Workshop on Recommender Systems (1999)
3. T. Development. Timely development singular value decomposition inplementation (visited on January 20, 2008) (2008),
   http://www.timelydevelopment.com/Demos/NetflixPrize.htm
4. Epinions.com (Crawled between January 11th and January 19th, 2008) (2008),
   http://www.epinions.com
5. Golbeck, J.: Personalizing applications through integration of inferred trust values in semantic web-based social networks. In: Proceedings of Semantic Network Analysis Workshop (2005)

6. Golbeck, J.: Generating predictive movie recommendations from trust in social networks. In: Proceedings of the Fourth International Conference on Trust Management (2006)

7. Hofmann, T.: Latent semantic models for collaborative filtering. ACM Trans. Inf. Syst. 22(1), 89–115 (2004)

8. Jin, R., Chai, J.Y., Si, L.: An automatic weighting scheme for collaborative filtering. In: SIGIR 2004: Proceedings of the 27th annual international ACM SIGIR conference on Research and development in information retrieval, pp. 337–344. ACM Press, New York (2004)

9. Kautz, H., Selman, B., Shah, M.: Referral web: combining social networks and collaborative filtering. Commun. ACM 40(3), 63–65 (1997)

10. Konstan, J.A., Miller, B.N., Maltz, D., Herlocker, J.L., Gordon, L.R., Riedl, J.: GroupLens: Applying collaborative filtering to Usenet news. Communications of the ACM 40(3), 77–87 (1997)

11. Leskovec, J., Singh, A., Klienberg, J.: Patterns of influence in a recommendation network. In: Ng, W.-K., Kitsuregawa, M., Li, J., Chang, K. (eds.) PAKDD 2006. LNCS (LNAI), vol. 3918, pp. 380–389. Springer, Heidelberg (2006)

12. Liu, H., Maes, P.: Interestmap: Harvesting social network profiles for recommendation. In: Beyond Personalization (2005)

13. Massa, P., Bhattacharjee, B.: Using trust in recommender systems: An experimental analysis. In: Jensen, C., Poslad, S., Dimitrakos, T. (eds.) iTrust 2004. LNCS, vol. 2995, pp. 221–235. Springer, Heidelberg (2004)

14. McDonald, D.W.: Recommending collaboration with social networks: a comparative evaluation. In: Proceedings of the SIGCHI conference on Human factors in computing systems (2003)

15. Melville, P., Mooney, R.J., Nagarajan, R.: Content-boosted collaborative filtering for improved recommendations. In: Proceedings of the Eighteenth National Conference on Artificial Intelligence (AAAI 2002), Edmonton, Canada (2002)

16. Netflix. Netflix prize (visited on November 30, 2006) (2006), http://www.netflixprize.com

17. Zhang, S., Wang, W., Ford, J., Makedon, F., Pearlman, J.: Using singular value decomposition approximation for collaborative filtering. In: CEC 2005: Proceedings of the Seventh IEEE International Conference on E-Commerce Technology, Washington, DC, USA, pp. 257–264. IEEE Computer Society, Los Alamitos (2005)

An Effective Approach for Identifying Evolving Three-Dimensional Structural Motifs in Protein Folding Data*

Hui Yang and Lin Han

Department of Computer Science
San Francisco State University, San Francisco, CA 94132, USA
huiyang@cs.sfsu.edu, lhan@sfsu.edu

Abstract. Molecular Dynamics-based simulations have been employed to study the protein folding process, in which a protein acquires its functional three-dimensional structure. This has resulted in a large number of protein folding trajectories. As a result, it becomes increasingly important to analyze such data to facilitate a deeper understanding of the protein folding mechanism. In this paper, we focus on identifying important 3D structural motifs in the folding data. We have proposed a multi-step algorithm that is not only computationally efficient but also captures the evolving nature of the folding process. Empirical evaluation demonstrates that such motifs are effective at characterizing a protein's structural evolution in its folding process. We also show that such motifs can be utilized to address important folding issues such as detecting important folding events, and structurally characterizing a folding pathway.

1 Introduction

Understanding the protein folding mechanism–the process in which a protein acquires its functional 3D native structure (or conformation)–remains one of the most challenging problems in computational biology and molecular biology. To facilitate this understanding, Molecular Dynamics (MD) based computer simulations have often been utilized. Empowered with high performance computing (e.g., distributed and parallel computing) and large-capacity storage devices, such simulations can study the folding process in atomistic details with femtosecond resolution [6,11]. This has led to the accumulation of a huge number of folding trajectories, each corresponding to a time series of 3D conformations of the protein under study. Accordingly, effectively managing and analyzing such data has become increasingly important.

Several approaches have been proposed for protein folding data analysis [3,4,9,10]. However, they are greatly limited since a folding trajectory is often abstracted to a series of points. Each point corresponds to one 3D conformation

---

* This work was partially supported by a Microsoft e-science grant. Correspondence should be addressed to Hui Yang.

C. Tang et al. (Eds.): ADMA 2008, LNAI 5139, pp. 342–354, 2008.

and consists of one or more scalars to measure the global properties of this conformation. Examples of such measurements include radius of gyration, contact order [12], and SASA (Solvent Accessible Surface Area) [4]. Such an abstraction prevents one from detecting important structural changes (e.g., the formation of an α-helix) caused by interactions among amino acids (or atoms) in the folding process, not to say capturing the the evolving nature of such changes. The acquisition of such information is critical to a detailed understanding of the folding process. In this article, we present a spatio-temporal approach to achieving this.

Unlike existing methods, this approach focuses on both the temporal and spatial aspects of folding trajectories. It considers each conformation as it should be, i.e., a spatial structure consisting of a collection of interacting entities. Depending on the chosen granularity, such entities can either be individual amino acids or atoms. We adopt the former in this article. Our approach takes two main stages. The first stage discovers important structural motifs along a folding trajectory, and the second stage characterizes the evolving nature of such motifs and their interactions over time. This article will focus on the first stage.

It is challenging to characterize structural motifs in the folding data due to the following reasons: First, one cannot simply adopt the same definitions for well-known motifs such as regular secondary structures including α-helices and β-sheets, as they are defined w.r.t. native protein conformations and do not take into account the dynamic nature of the folding process. Second, it is important to extract both local and non-local motifs, where the former capture the interactions among amino acids close to each other on the primary sequence (e.g., the amino acids in positions of i and $i + 4$), and the latter the interactions among amino acids that are distant from each other on the primary sequence. Finally, it is computationally expensive to directly work in the 3D space due to the complexity of the subgraph isomorphism problem [5].

To address such challenges, we have proposed a 3-step algorithm to identify important structural motifs in the protein folding data. The first step converts each 3D protein conformation to a 2D contact map and then extracts all the maximal 2D patterns in this contact map. Such 2D patterns can capture both local and non-local interaction among amino acids. For each of these non-local patterns, the second step identifies its corresponding 3D substructure(s), and then characterizes their geometric properties (e.g., an α-helix) by applying the commonly used DSSP vocabulary [7]. The above 2D and 3D patterns are clustered into groups respectively based on pattern similarity. Finally, the results from the previous two steps are combined to derive structural motifs.

After structural motifs are identified, the next stage studies how such motifs evolve and interact with each other. We utilize the spatio-temporal association mining framework proposed earlier [16] to accomplish this goal. This framework is designed to analyze spatio-temporal data produced in several scientific domains. It proposes different types of Spatial Object Association Patterns (SOAP) and SOAP episodes to capture the interaction among objects. The focus of this article is on the first stage–the 3-step algorithm for identifying significant 3D structural motifs in folding trajectories. Please also note that the studies reported in this article is a continuation of one of our earlier studies [15]. However, this earlier work primarily focuses on 2D non-local patterns in contact maps. It also attempted to identify the relationships between such patterns and their corresponding 3D counterparts. This was, however, done manually using a small sample, and thus highly inaccurate. This aspect will be further discussed in Sections 2.4 and 3.3.

A variety of evaluations were conducted to demonstrate the effectiveness of these identified structural motifs. We utilized two folding datasets and a collection of native protein structures for this purpose. (See Section 3.3.)

In summary, we have made the following main contributions in this work: First, we propose an effective approach to identifying 3D structural motifs in protein folding trajectories. This approach is computationally efficient as it begins with identifying non-local patterns in 2D contact maps. It then utilizes such 2D patterns as anchors to identify 3D substructures. Second, the proposed approach naturally considers the evolving nature of the protein folding process. Finally, a variety of evaluation demonstrates the effectiveness of such motifs and their applications in addressing important biological problems.

2   Algorithm

Problem Statement. Given a set of folding trajectories of a protein of interest, our main goal is to design an automated procedure identifying meaningful 3D structural motifs in such trajectories.

We next describe this procedure, which consists of 3 main steps as shown in Fig. 1. We will first describe the input data–protein folding trajectories, and then proceed to explain the procedure in detail. We will also discuss the main motivation behind each step.

Input : Protein folding trajectories
Output: A set of 3D structural motifs
Algorithm:
Step 1. Extract and classify 2D maximal non-local patterns.
    1.1 Transform a trajectory from a series of 3D conformations to a series of 2D contact maps.
    1.2 Identify the maximal 2D non-local patterns.
    1.3 Cluster the 2D non-local patterns into groups based on geometric similarity.
Step 2. Identify and classify the 3D substructures based on the 2D non-local patterns.
    2.1 Recognize local structures in each conformation on the trajectory.
    2.2 Construct 3D substructures based on 2D non-local patterns
    2.3 Cluster all the 3D substructures into different groups based on mutual similarity.
Step 3. Generate 3D structural motifs.

Fig. 1. Algorithm: the main steps for identifying 3D motifs in protein folding data

2.1   Protein Folding Trajectories

The output of MD-based simulations is a collection of *protein folding trajectories*, each of which is a time series of 3D conformations of the protein under study. Such conformations are usually sampled regularly (e.g., every 200fs) during a simulation. In this article, we also refer to a conformation as a *frame*. Each

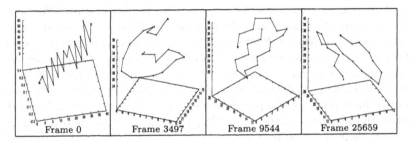

Fig. 2. Sample frames (with backbone shown) on a trajectory of the small protein Beta3S

frame is often described by a PDB file–a format introduced by the Protein Data Bank programs. This file records the 3D coordinates of all the atoms in a protein. Fig. 2 illustrates 4 frames along a folding trajectory of a small protein Beta3S.

2.2 Step 1: Contact Map Generation and Maximal Non-local Pattern Identification

This step first transforms a folding trajectory from a series of 3D conformations to a series of 2D contact maps. It then extracts all the maximal 2D non-local patterns in these contact maps. Finally, such 2D patterns are categorized into different groups. This procedure was first proposed and discussed in details by Yang *et al.* [14,15]. We include a brief description here (1) to make this algorithm self-contained; and (2) to discuss why we believe this step is important to the identification of 3D motifs in protein folding data.

Transform a Folding Trajectory from 3D to 2D. Contact map is being utilized to achieve this transformation. When generating contact maps, we consider the Euclidean distances between α-carbons (C_α) of each amino acid. Two C_αs are in contact if their distance is within a distance threshold δ (e.g. 8.5Å). Thus, for a protein of N residues, its *contact map* is an $N \times N$ binary matrix, where the cell at (i, j) is 1 if the ith and j^{th} C_αs are in contact, 0 otherwise. Since contact maps are symmetric across the diagonal, we only consider the bits below the diagonal. We also ignore the C_α pairs whose distance in the primary sequence is ≤ 2, as they are in contact by default.

The rationale behind the above transformation is twofold: first, the use of contact maps can significantly reduce the computational complexity; second, contact maps are effective at preserving potential interactions among residues in the folding context [17].

Identify Maximal Two-Dimensional Non-Local Patterns. Every bit in a contact map has eight neighbor bits. For an edge position, we assume its out-of-boundary positions contain 0s. In a contact map, a non-local pattern is a collection of bit-1 positions, where for each 1, at least one of its neighbors is 1. Correspondingly, a *maximal non-local pattern*, also referred to as a *2D pattern*, to be a non-local pattern p where every neighbor bit not in p is 0. We apply a simple region growth algorithm to identify all the 2D patterns in each contact map in a folding trajectory. Each identified 2D pattern is then represented as a feature vector that characterizes its geometric properties, for instance, shape and the number of in-contact C_α pairs. (See [14] for details of this vector.)

Note that such 2D patterns can capture the potential interactions among residues without prescribing a priori interacting patterns (e.g., an α-helix). Furthermore, the involved residues in a 2D pattern are not necessarily near each other w.r.t. their positions on the backbone, as long as their 3D Euclidian distance is within the contact threshold δ, thereby the name *non-local patterns*. It is due to such properties that we believe these 2D patterns can effectively facilitate the identification of 3D structural motifs in the next step.

Cluster Maximal Two-Dimensional Non-Local Patterns. The 2D patterns extracted above are then partitioned into approximately equivalent groups, each of which consists of 2D patterns exhibiting similar geometric properties. This is achieved by running a k-means based clustering algorithm [8], where k is the number of clusters that will be produced. To determine an optimal value of k an entropy-based method is used. Please see [14] for more details. Finally, we characterize each of these 2D clusters by its centroid, which will be utilized to characterize the 3D structural motifs identified later.

2.3 Step 2. Identify and Classify 3D Non-local Substructures Based on 2D Non-local Patterns

Extract 3D Local Substructures in Each Frame. Unlike recognizing 3D local substructures in native protein structures, where one mainly focuses on recognizing regular substructures (e.g., α-helices) and their spatial topology, one needs to take into account the dynamics in the folding process. Since both experimental and computational studies have demonstrated that many (small) proteins often fold hierarchically: first forming local substructures, then secondary structures, and finally their native structures [2], we hypothesize that the folding process might produce many local substructures, which form the building blocks of regular substructures. Therefore, we can utilize DSSP [7], a commonly used program identifying secondary structural elements, to identify 3D local substructures.

DSSP classifies such structural elements into eight categories: **H**, α-helix; **E**, β-strand; **G**, 3_{10} helix, a helix with backbone-backbone hydrogen bonds between positions i and $i+3$; **I**, π helix, a helix with backbone-backbone hydrogen bonds between positions i and $i+5$; **B**, bridge, a single residue β-strand; **T**, a hydrogen bonded turn; **S**, bend; and **C**, any residue that does not belong to any of the previous seven groups.

We apply the DSSP method to each 3D frame in a trajectory and extract all the local 3D substructures. Each substructure is then represented as a vector

$< trjID, frmID, Type, R\_list >$, where $trjID$ and $frmID$ identify the trajectory and frame that contain this substructure, $type$ is one of the above eight DSSP types, and R_list identifies the residues involved this substructure.

Construct 3D Substructures Based on 2D Non-Local Patterns. For each 2D non-local pattern identified in *Step 1*, this step constructs its corresponding 3D non-local substructure, which comprises all the 3D local structures that belong to this 2D pattern. A 3D local substructure belongs to a 2D non-local pattern if its R_list shares one or more residues with this 2D pattern. Examples of 3D non-local substructures include $ETEG$, SSH and ST.

Cluster 3D Non-Local Substructures. The goal here is to identify similar 3D non-local substructures and put them into the same group. One key issue is to define a distance function that properly measures the similarity between two 3D substructures–S_1 and S_2. Based on our observation, we have designed the following function for this purpose:

$$dist(S_1, S_2) = \omega_1 \times (isContinuous(S_1) = isContinuous(S_2)?1 : 0$$
$$+ \omega_2 \times (isMaxGap(S_1, \Delta) = isMaxGap(S_2, \Delta))?1 : 0$$
$$+ \omega_3 \times EditDistance(list_{ss}(S_1), list_{ss}(S_2)) \qquad (1)$$

where $isContinuous(S)$ indicates whether the residues of S cover a continuous segment in the primary sequence, $isMaxGap(S, \Delta)$ indicates whether the distance on the primary sequence between two neighboring residues of S is $\geq \Delta$, a user-specified parameter, and $list_{SS}(S)$ returns the list of 3D local substructures (or DSSP elements) of S. ω_1, ω_2 and ω_3 are user-specified weights. In general, ω_3 should be larger than the other two to emphasize the structural difference. For instance, we set them to 1, 1 and 7.5 respectively in our evaluation. Using this distance function, we apply a k-means clustering algorithm to identify groups of similar 3D substructures. An entropy-based method is adopted to determine the "optimal" value of k–the number of clusters. We next use such clusters of 3D substructures together with the clusters of 2D patterns to construct different 3D structural motifs for a protein folding dataset.

2.4 Step 3. Generate Three-Dimensional Structural Motifs

For the 3D substructures in each cluster, we further partition them into sub-clusters. In each sub-cluster, the corresponding 2D patterns will all belong to the same 2D cluster. Let $C_{i,j}$ be a sub-cluster as a result of combining the ith 3D cluster and the jth 2D cluster, we can then characterize $C_{i,j}$ by its centroid, which corresponds to a structure that shares similar 3D properties with substructures in the ith 3D cluster, and similar 2D properties with patterns in the jth 2D cluster. Such a centroid is regarded as a structural motif. For a given dataset, let N_2 and N_3 be the number of 2D and 3D clusters identified respectively, our algorithm will identify a total of $N_2 \times N_3$ structural motifs. Fig. 3 presents several examples of such structural motifs.

3   Evaluation

We have conducted a variety of studies, both qualitatively and quantitatively, to evaluate the the 3D motifs identified by the proposed algorithm. We report the main results in this section.

3.1   Evaluation Datasets and Parametric Setting

Evaluation Datasets: We applied the proposed algorithm to three datasets: BBA5, Beta3S, and Native. The first two are folding datasets and Native consists of 1544 native structures. See Table 1 for further details.

Parametric Setting: To evaluate the impact of different values of δ–the contact distance threshold (see Section 2.2) on the quality of the 3D motifs, we varied its value from $5.5\mathring{A}$ to $8.5\mathring{A}$ at an $1.0\mathring{A}$ interval, i.e., $\delta \in \{5.5\mathring{A}, 6.5\mathring{A}, 7.5\mathring{A}, 8.5\mathring{A}\}$. Among these four values, we observed that $5.5\mathring{A}$ tends to be too restricted such that it could only capture a limited number of non-local 2D or 3D patterns. In contrast, $8.5\mathring{A}$ tends to be too relaxed that it rendered many redundant 3D motifs. We hence will focus on discussing the results from $\delta = 6.5\mathring{A}$ and $7.5\mathring{A}$.

We also examined the impact from different weighting schemes in $dist(S_1, S_2)$ (Formula (1) in Section 2.3). Specifically, we have set $(\omega_1, \omega_2, \omega_3)$ to $(1, 1, 1)$ and $(1, 1, 7.5)$. The former weighs the three contributing factors of $dist(S_1, S_2)$ equally; whereas the latter weighs the third factor–the list of 3D local substructures–much more significantly than the other two. We noticed that the latter often led to high-quality clustering results of 3D non-local substructures. This makes sense as it stresses on the inherent structural difference between two 3D non-local substructure. For instance, a substructure of SH (an α-helix) should be considered significantly different from another structure of SE (a β-strand), regardless of the state of these other two factors in the distance function. For this reason, we thus will report results from the second weighting schema.

3.2   Qualitative Evaluation of the Identified 3D Motifs

Table 2 summarizes the main results obtained over the two folding datasets–BBA5 and Beta3S, corresponding to the three main steps in the proposed algorithm

Table 1. Evaluation datasets: BBA5 and Beta3S are MD simulation data, produced by the *folding@home* research group; and Native is constructed by randomly selecting 1544 proteins from SCOP (http://scop.mrc-lmb.cam.ac.uk/scop/)

Name	#(frames/proteins)	Rem.
BBA5	2 trajs.: T_1–192 frames; T_2–150 frames	PDB ID: BBA5; Primary sequence: 23 residues; Designed protein; Native structure: Residues 1-10 form a β hairpin, and 11-23 an α-helix
Beta3S	2 trajs.: T_1: 25,664 frames; T_2: 30,075 frames	Name: GSGS or Beta3s; Primary sequence: 20 residues; Designed protein; Native structure: three stranded anti-parallel β-sheets with turns at 6-7 and 14-15
Native	1,544 proteins	All α proteins: 180; All β proteins: 245; α/β proteins: 192; $\alpha + \beta$ proteins: 275; others: 84; unclassified: 568

Table 2. Main results from the two folding datasets BBA5 and Beta3S, where δ is the distance threshold for contact map generation

Dataset	δ	#(non-local patterns)	#(2D Clusters)	#(3D Clusters)	#(3D Motifs)
BBA5	6.5Å	796	9	13	117
BBA5	7.5Å	1,054	11	20	220
Beta3S	6.5Å	62,980	10	11	110
Beta3S	7.5Å	69,695	10	13	130

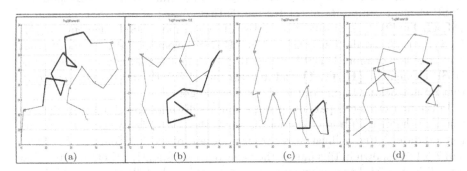

Fig. 3. 3D motif examples, which are highlighted on the backbone: (a) a motif identified for BBA5, consisting of one helical substructures **H**; and involving 11 residues, among which 15 pairs are in contact (≤ 6.5Å); (b) a motif identified for Beta3S, consisting of one hydrogen bonded turn and two β-strands **TEE**; (c) a motif identified for BBA5, consisting of two local substructures **ST**; and involving 7 residues, among which 6 pairs are in contact of ≤ 6.5Å; and (d) a motif identified in the BBA5 dataset. It consists of two local substructures **TT**; and involves 7 residues, among which 8 pairs are in contact of ≤ 7.5Å.

(Fig. 1). At first glance of Table 2, it may seem counterintuitive that our algorithm produced fewer motifs in Beta3S than in BBA5, since the former rendered significantly more non-local patterns than the latter. This can be explained by the relatively simpler native structure of Beta3S (Table 1). Compared to BBA5 that contains both an α-helix and a β-hairpin, Beta3S exhibits only one type of local secondary structures– a three-stranded anti-parallel β-sheet. If one considers the folding process of a protein as the process of finding a path to its native structure, based on the analysis of BBA5 and Beta3S, *it seems that a protein tends to follow a structurally "economic" path.* In other words, the simpler the destination structure is, the less diverse the non-local substructures are. This explains why Beta3S in general has fewer motifs than BBA5, even though the Beta3S dataset is far larger than BBA5 in volume.

As discussed in Section 2.3, the 3D motifs identified by the proposed algorithm should be able to cover not only well-defined substructures such as α-helices and β-strands, but also evolving (or intermediate) substructures. Such substructures can either be local or non-local. This is supported by the resulted 3D motifs in both BBA5 and Beta3S datasets. As shown in Fig. 3, Fig. 3(a) represents an α-helical structure, Fig. 3(b) a β-strand, whereas Figs. 3 (c-d) present two motifs corresponding to intermediate substructures. Note that the motifs can be local (Figs. 3(a-c)) or non-local (Fig. 3(d)).

3.3   Cross-Comparison of Three-Dimensional Motifs

To gain more insights into the identified motifs, we conducted two types of cross-comparison. For the convenience of conducting such comparison, all the identified motifs are organized into 6 coarser categories according to their corresponding DSSP element composition: (1) 1α: motifs that consist of one DSSP element in $\{H, G, I\}$; (2) $2_+\alpha$: motifs that consist of two or more DSSP elements in $\{H, G, I\}$; (3) 1β: motifs that consist of one **E** DSSP element; (4) $2_+\beta$: motifs that consist of two or more **E** DSSP element; (5) $\alpha\beta$: motifs that consist at least one DSSP element in $\{H, G, I\}$ and at least one **E** DSSP; and (6) *Other*: motifs that do not belong to any of the above five categories.

In the first cross-comparison, given a contact distance threshold (δ) value, we compare the distribution of the motifs w.r.t. the above six categories across all three datasets. Fig. 4 illustrates the distribution of motifs identified $\delta = 6.5\text{\AA}$ and $7.5\text{\AA}$. As shown in this figure, the value of δ only slightly affects the distribution. Take $\delta = 7.5\text{\AA}$ as one example, each dataset has the following distribution [1]: **BBA5**–*Other* (49%), 1α(30%), $2_+\beta$ (15%), 1β (3%), $\alpha\beta$ (3%), and $2_+\alpha$ (0%); **Beta3S**–1β (37.9%), *Other* (32%), $2_+\beta$ (30%), 1α(0.1%), $2_+\alpha$ (0%), and $\alpha\beta$ (0%); and **Native**–$2_+\beta$ (45%), $2_+\alpha$ (20%), $\alpha\beta$ (35%), 1α(0%), 1β (0%), and *Other* (0%). Combining these numbers and Fig. 4, one can observe the following: first, the two folding datasets have a large portion of *Other* motifs, whereas the Native has zero. This is because that the *Other* motifs correspond to intermediate substructures that can only appear in folding data; second, unlike the Native dataset, whose motifs consist of at least two DSSP structural elements, many of motifs in the two folding datasets only consist of one helical or β DSSP element. Again, this reflects the evolving nature of the folding process; and finally, the motif distribution of BBA5 and Beta3S further supports an earlier observation that a protein tends to select a structurally "economic" path to reach the destination structure, as one can observe that the dominant motifs are remarkably consistent with the secondary structural composition in their native conformations. These observations have demonstrated that the effectiveness of the proposed algorithm.

For the second cross-comparison, the main goal is to show whether 2D non-local patterns as discussed in Section 2.2 are sufficient to characterize a folding trajectory. Given a contact distance threshold (δ) value, we first identify one 2D cluster from each of the three datasets, such that the centroids of these three 2D clusters are approximately similar to each other. We next examine the distribution of the motifs associated with each of these 2D clusters w.r.t. the above six motif categories. Fig. 5 shows the motif distribution associated with two sets of similar 2D clusters. One can clearly observe that the motif distributions of similar 2D clusters from different datasets are significantly different from each

---

[1] The percentages below have had their decimal parts rounded up to the 1% position.

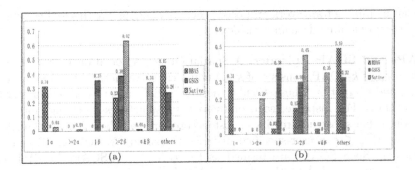

Fig. 4. A comparison of the 3D motif distribution in the three datasets. The 3D motifs are consolidated into six categories as shown on the X-axis. The Y-axis indicates the percentages of 3D motifs in each category w.r.t. the entire set of 3D motifs identified in a dataset. (a) contact distance threshold (δ) = 6.5Å; and (b) contact distance threshold (δ) = 7.5Å.

other. This indicates that using 2D non-local patterns to characterize the folding data can be misleading; it is thereby necessary and important to identify motifs in three-dimensional structural space.

3.4 Using Three-Dimensional Motifs to Analyze Folding Trajectories

In this section, we demonstrate that the identified 3D motifs can be utilized to effectively address important biological issues. To do this, we employ a spatio-temporal

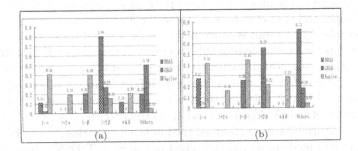

Fig. 5. A comparison regarding the distribution of 3D motifs within three similar 2D clusters, drawn from the three datasets respectively. The 3D motifs are consolidated into six categories as shown on the X-axis. The y-axis indicates the ratio of each 3D category: (a) the distribution of 3D motifs in 2D clusters whose 2D patterns on average involve 7 − 8 residues, among which 6 pairs are within a distance of 6.5Å, and the 1-bits form a 150° angle; and (b) the distribution of 3D motifs in 2D clusters whose 2D patterns on average involve 10 − 12 residues, among which 15 pairs are within a distance of 7.5Å, and the 1-bits form a 160° angle.

association mining framework proposed previously [13,16]. We this earlier work in the context of folding data analysis next.

SOAPs and SOAP Episodes. A Spatial Object Association Pattern of size k, denoted as k-SOAP, consists of k 3D non-local substructures labeled by their corresponding motifs. These k substructures satisfy a set of specified spatial relationships. For instance, each of these k substructures is a neighbor of at least one other substructure. Two substructures are neighbors if their Hausdorff distance [1] is $\leq \epsilon$, a user-specified distance threshold. We set ϵ to 10Å in our evaluation. Such SOAPs are termed as $(minLink = 1)$-SOAPs in [16]. Let $M = \{m_1, m_2, \ldots, m_r\}$ be the r motifs identified by the proposed algorithm in a folding dataset, an example of $(minLink = 1)$-SOAPs could be (m_1, m_1, m_2), which says that there exist three non-local 3D substructures, labeled as motifs m_1, m_1 and m_2 respectively, such that each of them is a neighbor of one or more of the remaining two substructures. A SOAP is said to be frequent if it is contained in $\geq minSupp$ frames in a folding trajectory. We set $minSupp$ to 5.

We next construct SOAP episodes to characterize the evolving nature of a folding trajectory. A SOAP episode is defined as follows: $E = (p, F_b, F_e)$, where p is a SOAP, F_b and F_e identify a maximum sequence of continuous frames where p was present. Note that for a given p, it can be created more than once in a trajectory, and thus can have more than one episode.

Main Results. It has been suggested that α-helices and β-turns commonly form on the timescale of about 100 ns and 1 μs, respectively [11], i.e., the former is formed more rapidly than the latter. We utilized SOAP episodes to check whether this is the case in the two BBA5 folding trajectories. The answer is inconclusive. In one trajectory, α-helices were formed as early as in the 68th frame, far before the first appearance of β-turns in the 153th frame. However, it is the opposite in the other trajectory: the first appearance of β-turns was in the 20th frame, and that of α-helices was in the 39th frame.

Another interesting result is concerned with the Beta3S trajectories. We have observed the presence of α-helical substructures in the middle of both trajectories. Specifically, α-helical substructures were present in frames 8837-9813 in the trajectory of 25644 frames, and in frames 16867-18220 in the other trajectory.

We also used SOAP episodes to identify the temporal associations among different types of motifs. Especially, what motifs preceded the formation of an α-helix or a β-turn? We have observed the following scenarios in both BBA5 and Beta3S: (1) intermediate motifs composed of the **S** or **T** DSSP elements often preceded the formation of an α-helical motif, and the frequency of **S** or **T** was approximately equal; and (2) the motifs that preceded a β-strand or turn on the other hand were often those composed of only the **S** element. That is, a bend was formed before a β-strand or turn was formed for both BBA5 and Beta3S.

The final set of results characterize the structural evolution that involve a set of residues of interest. For the small protein BBA5, we are interested in identifying the evolving paths of the following two sets of residues: 1-10, and 11-23. The former is expected to form a β hairpin, and the latter an α-helix

Table 3. The evolving paths of the BBA5 and Beta3S proteins. These paths were constructed based on SOAP episodes. Each path is represented as a sequence of 3D motifs, where a motif is described by its corresponding set of DSSP elements. See Section 2.3 for the meaning of each symbol. A vertical bar between two motifs means that they alternated between each other.

Protein	Residues	Native	Traj.	Evolving Path
BBA5	1-10	β turn	T_1	S→ EES → SS → EES → EET
			T_2	EEH → EET → EE → EET → EES →EEG → EET → EES
BBA5	11-23	α-helix	T_1	T → G → H → HS → SH
			T_2	T → G → small H → large H
Beta3S	1-15	β turn	T_1	SS → ESS → ETE → SS → SET|SSE → ESE
			T_2	SS → SES|ESE → SST|STT → TSS
Beta3S	8-20	β turn	T_1	SS → SET → ESE
			T_2	SS → SES → ESE|SES → TTS|TSS

(See Table 1). For Beta3S, we are interested in the evolving paths of the following two sets of residues: 1-15 and 8-20. Both are expected to form a β-turn. We identify such evolving paths by combining the relevant SOAP episodes discussed above. See Table 3 for detailed information on such paths. One can observe that different trajectories took different paths attempting to reach the same structure. However, not every path leads to the expected structure. One should also notice the similarity among different paths. To generalize such observations would require more folding trajectories, but this SOAP episode-based approach is applicable to any number of folding trajectories.

4 Conclusions

In this article, we have described an effective approach for identifying three-dimensional non-local structural motifs in protein folding trajectories. The proposed approach takes three major steps by first transforming a protein folding trajectory from 3D space to 2D. Extensive empirical studies were conducted to evaluate the quality of such motifs. These studies show that the motifs generated by the proposed algorithm can well capture the dynamic nature of the folding process. We have also utilized such motifs to address important issues related to protein folding. The findings further demonstrate the effectiveness of the proposed method and the potential power of the identified motifs.

References

1. Atallah, M.J.: A linear time algorithm for the hausdorff distance between convex polygons. Information Processing Letters 17, 207–209 (1983)
2. Baldwin, R.L., Rose, G.D.: Is protein folding hierarchical? local structure and peptide folding. Trends in Biochemical Sciences 24(1), 26–33 (1999)
3. Berrar, D., Stahl, F., et al.: Towards data warehousing and mining of protein unfolding simulation data. J. of clin. monit. & comp. 19(4-5), 307–317 (2005)
4. Ferreira, P.G., Silva, C.G., et al.: A closer look on protein unfolding simulations through hierarchical clustering. In: Proceedings of CIBCB (2007)

5. Garey, M.R., Johnson, D.S.: Computers and Intractability: A Guide to the Theory of NP-Completeness (1979)
6. Germain, R.S., et al.: Blue matter on blue gene/l: massively parallel computation for biomolecular simulation. In: Proc.of the 3rd IEEE/ACM/IFIP int'l conf. on HW/SW codesign & sys. syn., pp. 207–212 (2005)
7. Kabsch, W., Sander, C.: Dictionary of protein secondary structures. Biopolymers 22, 2577–2637 (1983)
8. MacQueen, J.: Some methods for classification and analysis of multivariate observation. In: Proc. of the 5th Berkeley Symposium on Math. Stat. and Prob., vol. 1, pp. 281–297 (1967)
9. Parida, L., Zhou, R.: Combinatorial pattern discovery approach for the folding trajectory analysis of a beta-hairpin. PLoS Comput. Biol. 1 (June 2005)
10. Russel, D., Guibas, L.: Exploring protein folding trajectories using geometric spanners. In: Pacific Symposium on Biocomputing, pp. 40–51 (2005)
11. Snow, C.D., Nguyen, H., et al.: Absolute comparison of simulated and experimental protein-folding dynamics. Nature 420, 102–106 (2002)
12. Snow, C.D., Sorin, E.J., et al.: How well can simulation predict protein folding kinetics and thermodynamics? Ann. Rev. Biophys. BioMol. Struct. 34, 43–69 (2005)
13. Yang, H., Parthasarathy, S., et al.: Towards association based spatio-temporal reasoning. In: Proc. the 19th IJCAI Workshop on Spatio-temporal Reasoning (2005)
14. Yang, H., Marsolo, K., et al.: Discovering spatial relationships between approximately equivalent patterns. In: BIOKDD, pp. 62–71 (2004)
15. Yang, H., Parthasarathy, S., Ucar, D.: A spatio-temporal mining approach towards summarizing and analyzing protein folding trajectories. J. of A.M.B. 2 (2007)
16. Yang, H., Parthasarathy, S., Mehta, S.: A generalized framework for mining spatio-temporal patterns in scientific data. In: Proceeding of ACM SIGKDD, pp. 716–721 (2005)
17. Zagrovic, B., Snow, C.D., et al.: In simulation of folding of a small alpha-helical protein in atomistic detail using worldwide distributed computing. J. Mol. Biol. (2002)

Texture Image Retrieval Based on Contourlet Transform and Active Perceptual Similarity Learning[*]

Huaijing Qu[1,2], Yuhua Peng[1], Honglin Wan[1], and Min Han[1]

[1] School of Information Science and Engineering, Shandong University,
Jinan, Shandong, People's Republic of China
[2] School of Information & Electric Engineering, Shandong Jianzhu University,
Jinan, Shandong, People's Republic of China
huaijqu@sdu.edu.cn, pyuhua@sdu.edu.cn

Abstract. This paper proposes a new texture image retrieval scheme based on contourlet transform and support vector machines (SVMs). In the scheme, the energies and the generalized Gaussian distribution (GGD) parameters are used to represent the contourlet subband features. Using the representations, a two-run SVM retrieval algorithm which employs an one-class SVM followed by a two-class SVM is proposed to carry out the perceptual similarity measurement. For the query image, the one-class SVM is used to obtain the effective initial training set with positive and negative samples. Using these initial samples, the two-class SVM is applied to refine on the image classification subject to the user's relevance feedback. Compared with existing texture image retrieval methods, the proposed retrieval scheme is demonstrated respectively to be effective on the VisTex database of 640 texture images and the Brodatz database of 1760 texture images. Experimental results have shown that the proposed retrieval scheme can attain 99.38% and 98.07% of the average rates respectively for the two databases.

Keywords: Contourlet transform, generalized Gaussian distribution, support vector machine, relevance feedback, texture image retrieval.

1 Introduction

With the explosive growth in the volume of digital image databases, content-based image retrieval (CBIR) has recently become one of the most effective accessing tools [1]. Usually, texture features play an important role in describing the content of visual images. Moreover, texture is also a key component of human visual perception. Therefore, texture is one of efficient and effective models used in CBIR systems [2].

The research and development of texture image retrieval system in the past decades can be reviewed by the works around finding good visual features or defining robust similarity measurements. The methods of texture feature extraction can be classified

---

[*] This project is sponsored by SRF for ROCS, SEM (2004.176.4) and NSF SD Province (Z2004G01) of China.

C. Tang et al. (Eds.): ADMA 2008, LNAI 5139, pp. 355–366, 2008.

into statistical methods, model-based methods and signal processing methods [3]. Among these methods, the signal processing methods have advantages in the characterization of the directional and scale features of textures. They include the use of discrete wavelet transform, Gabor wavelets and complex wavelets. However, these methods suffer from the limitation of directional information or heavy computational complexity. Thus, contourlet transform, which can provide a different number of directions at each scale and has less computational complexity, has recently received an increasing attention [4], [5].

On the other hand, developing good similarity measurements which match the texture features and reflect human perception is an important and challenging task [1]. The traditional similarity measurement schemes adopt the distance metrics [6]. An alternative method is to consider jointly the two problems of feature extraction and similarity measurement [7]. However, two issues of how to represent high level concepts using low level computable features and how to measure the similarity to reflect the subjectivity of human perception [8], need to be further explored to obtain satisfactory CBIR performance.

To address these issues, the relevance feedback technique as a powerful tool has been widely used in CBIR [8]. However, this technique has some limitations, such as requiring much iteration to meet user's expectation; previous feedback results being not retained in the system; the weighting method being heuristic and lacking of optimal justification [9].

The recent results have shown that support vector machines (SVMs) provide an efficient methodology to construct automatic and adaptive learning algorithm to update the weights for CBIR by using the relevance feedback technique [9]. Typically, one-class SVM or two-class SVM has been found wide applications in the retrievals of texture images [10], [9]. However, the image retrieval performance based on one-class SVM is unsatisfactory due to the lack of the help of negative sample information, and for two-class SVM, the selection of the training sample is very challenging [11].

This paper proposes a new retrieval scheme by seeking the synergy of the contourlet transform and SVMs. That is, based on energy and the generalized Gaussian distribution (GGD) parameters of contourlet subbands of the texture images, a two-run SVM retrieval algorithm is adopted. First, according to the extracted feature set, one-class SVM is used for obtaining the initial training set with positive and negative samples and providing the initial retrieval results for a subsequent two-class SVM for refined classification. The classification process of the two-class SVM keeps going on subject to the user's relevance feedback. The proposed retrieval scheme has several advantages over existing texture image retrieval schemes. First of all, the GGD parameters provide richer information and improve the retrieval accuracy. Second, the one-class SVM provide good negative and positive training samples required by the two-class SVM. As a result, this scheme can significantly improve texture image retrieval performance compared with the method of using one-class or two-class SVM alone. Experimental results have demonstrated the improvements made by the proposed texture image retrieval scheme.

2 Background

2.1 Contourlet Transform

The contourlet transform, developed by Do and Vetterli [4], is a true 2-D sparse expansion method. It starts from the discrete-domain by using 2-D non-separable filter banks, and then converges to a continuous-domain expansion in a multiresolution analysis framework. Usually, it outperforms the wavelet transform in capturing the directional information of natural images [4].

The contourlet transform has the pyramid directional filter bank structure. It consists of a Laplacian pyramid (LP) followed by a directional filter bank (DFB). At first, the LP decomposes the input image into a lowpass version and multiple scale bandpass versions. Then, the DFB decomposes each scale bandpass version into different numbers of directional subbands. Typically, for an $N \times N$ bandpass image and an L-level DFB, the first half of the 2^L directional subbands is $N/2^{L-1} \times N/2$ in size, while the other half is $N/2 \times N/2^{L-1}$ in size.

2.2 One-Class SVM and Two-Class SVM

Recently, SVM has emerged as a very successful texture classification method [13]. In our work, one-class and regular two-class SVM are used in the texture image retrieval. We adopt the LIBSVM algorithm (available at: http://www.csie.ntu.edu.tw/~cjlin/libsvm) where one-class SVM uses the Scholkopf et al.'s method [14] and two-class SVM uses the Vapnik's method [12].

2.2.1 One-Class SVM (OCSVM)

The one-class SVM, proposed by Scholkopf et al. [14], is used to estimate the support of a high-dimensional distribution and to predict the relevant (positive) and the non-relevant (negative) images in CBIR. To be more specific, we consider training vectors $X_i \in R^n$, $i = 1, \cdots, l$ without any class information, where l is the number of training samples, and n is the dimension of a training vector. In order to separate the training samples from the origin, One-class SVM solves the following primal problem

$$\min_{\mathsf{W}, \xi, \rho} \frac{1}{2} \|\mathsf{W}\|^2 + \frac{1}{vl} \sum_{i=1}^{l} \xi_i - \rho \tag{1}$$

$$\text{Subject to } \xi_i \geq 0 \text{ and } \mathsf{W}^T \Phi(x_i) \geq \rho - \xi_i, i = 1, \cdots, l$$

where ξ_i denotes the slack variables indicating how far the outliers deviated from the surface of the hyperplane, and ρ denotes threshold. $\Phi(\cdot)$ is a kernel map which transforms the training samples of the input space into a high-dimensional inner product space. The parameter $v \in (0,1]$ controls the tradeoff between training error and model complexity.

The above optimization problem can be transformed into its dual optimization problem by using the Lagrangian approach [15] as follows

$$\overline{\alpha} = \arg\max_{\alpha}\left\{-\frac{1}{2}\sum_{i=1}^{l}\sum_{j=1}^{l}\alpha_i\alpha_j K(x_i,x_j)\right\}$$

(2)

Subject to $0 \le \alpha_i \le \frac{1}{vl}, i = 1,\cdots,l$ and $\sum_{i=1}^{l}\alpha_i = 1$

where $K(x_i,x_j) = \Phi(x_i)^T\Phi(x_j)$ is the Mercer kernel [12]. Accordingly, the decision function can be described as

$$f_1(x) = \text{sgn}(\overline{W}^T\Phi(x) - \overline{\rho}) = \text{sgn}\left(\sum_{i=1}^{l}\overline{\alpha}_i K(x_i,x) - \overline{\rho}\right)$$

(3)

Where $\overline{W} = \sum_{i=1}^{l}\overline{\alpha}_i\Phi(x_i)$, $\overline{\rho} = \sum_{i=1}^{l}\overline{\alpha}_i K(x_i,x_i)$, and x is a new sample point.

In texture image retrieval, the retrieved images can be ranked by following the decreasing values of decision function

$$f_2(x) = \sum_{i=1}^{l}\overline{\alpha}_i K(x_i,x) - \overline{\rho}$$

(4)

The images with higher values are more similar to the query image.

2.2.2 Two-Class (Binary Case) SVM (BCSVM)

The regular two-class SVM, developed by Vapnik [12], solves a classification problem by finding a maximum margin hyperplane. Assume that the training data set with l samples is represented by $(x_i, y_i), i = 1,\cdots,l$ where $x_i \in R^n$ is an $n-$ dimensional input vector and $y_i \in \{\pm 1\}$ is an output label. The classification hyperplane is denoted as $W^T\Phi(x) + b = 0$. Therefore, the regular two-class SVM solves the following primal problem

$$\min_{W,b,\xi}\frac{1}{2}\|W\|^2 + C\sum_{i=1}^{l}\xi_i$$

(5)

Subject to $\xi_i \ge 0$ and $y_i\left(W^T\Phi(x_i) + b\right) \ge 1 - \xi_i, i = 1\cdots l$.

where ξ_i is the i-th slack variable that represents the margin errors for the non-separable training samples; C is the penalty of training error and controls the tradeoff between model complexity and training error in order to achieve good generalization performance; b is a parameter to control the bias; and $\Phi(\cdot)$ is a nonlinear map from the input data space to the high-dimensional inner product space.

The above optimization problem can be transformed into its dual problem as follows

$$\overline{\alpha} = \arg\max_{\alpha}\left\{\sum_{i=1}^{l}\alpha_i - \frac{1}{2}\sum_{i=1}^{l}\sum_{j=1}^{l}\alpha_i\alpha_j y_i y_j K(\mathbf{x}_i,\mathbf{x}_j)\right\}$$

(6)

Subject to $0 \le \alpha_i \le C, i = 1,\cdots,l$ and $\sum_{i=1}^{l}\alpha_i y_i = 0$

where $K(\mathbf{x}_i,\mathbf{x}_j) = \Phi^T(\mathbf{x}_i)\Phi(\mathbf{x}_j)$ is a Mercer kernel. The decision function of classification then is of the form

$$f_1(\mathbf{x}) = \mathrm{sgn}(\overline{\mathbf{W}}^T\Phi(\mathbf{x})+\overline{b}) = \mathrm{sgn}\left(\sum_{i=1}^{l}\overline{\alpha}_i y_i K(\mathbf{x}_i,\mathbf{x})+\overline{b}\right)$$

(7)

In (7), $\overline{\mathbf{W}} = \sum_{i=1}^{l}\overline{\alpha}_i y_i \Phi(\mathbf{x}_i)$, $\overline{b} = -\frac{1}{2}\overline{\mathbf{W}}(\Phi(\mathbf{x}_m)+\Phi(\mathbf{x}_n))$, where $\mathbf{x}_m$ and $\mathbf{x}_n$ are support vectors, $\overline{\alpha}_m > 0, \overline{\alpha}_n > 0$, $y_m = 1, y_n = -1$, and $\mathbf{x}$ is a new sample.

In texture image retrieval, the retrieved images can be ranked by following the decreasing values of decision function

$$f_2(\mathbf{x}) = \sum_{i=1}^{l}\overline{\alpha}_i y_i K(\mathbf{x}_i,\mathbf{x})+\overline{b}$$

(8)

The images with higher values are more similar to the query image.

3 Contourlet-Based Texture Image Retrieval

3.1 Texture Feature Selection and Similarity Measurement

In the contourlet-based texture image retrieval system, the extracted features are chosen as the subband energies given by $f_1 = [\mu_1\ \sigma_1\ \mu_2\ \sigma_2 \cdots \mu_m\ \sigma_m]$ with

$$\mu_k = \frac{1}{MN}\sum_{i=1}^{M}\sum_{j=1}^{N}|C_k(i,j)|$$

(9)

$$\sigma_k = \left[\frac{1}{MN}\sum_{i=1}^{M}\sum_{j=1}^{N}(|C_k(i,j)|-m_k)^2\right]^{1/2}$$

(10)

where $C_k(i, j)$ is the k-th contourlet subband coefficient of an image, $M \times N$ is the size of the k-th subband, m is the number of total subbands, and m_k is the mean value of the k-th subband coefficients. For the energy features, the similarity is measured by using a normalized Euclidean distance.

Here we choose GGD parameters of contourlet subband coefficients in addition to the subband energies. We have estimated the GGD parameters using an improved maximum likelihood method, see [5], [16]. The GGD feature representations are given by $f_2 = [\sigma_1^2 \ \beta_1 \ \sigma_2^2 \ \beta_2 \cdots \sigma_n^2 \ \beta_n]$, where the variance σ_k^2 and the shape parameter β_k are from the k-th of n contourlet detail subbands of an image. To measure the similarity, we employ the Kullback-Leibler distance (KLD) [7], [16].

3.2 Standard Texture Image Databases

In our studies, we consider two standard texture image databases which are also used by other literatures, in order to make a fair comparison.

Database D1. It consists of 40 texture images representing 40 texture classes. The images in the database are obtained from the VisTex database [7]. These images are of 512×512 pixels. In our studies, only grey-scale levels of the images (computed from the luminance components) are used. Each image is divided into sixteen nonoverlapping subimages, thus we have a test database of 640 texture images.

Database D2. It is referred to as Brodatz database [17] consisting of 110 different texture images. The Brodatz database includes inhomogenous and large-scale texture images. Thus, it is a good and challenging platform for CBIR performance analysis. In database D2, each texture image is of 512×512 pixels with 256 grey-scale level image, and it is decomposed of sixteen nonoverlapping subimages of 128×128 pixels, thus we totally have 1760 texture images.

3.3 Retrieval Performance and Comparisons

In our following work, only the texture database D1 is adopted. In retrieval experiments, a query texture image is any one of 640 images. According to the extracted features and corresponding similarity measurements, the distances between the query image and any image from the database are computed and then ranked in increasing order and the closest top 16 images are then retrieved. Thereby, the average retrieval rate of database D1 can be computed.

Table 1 shows the retrieval performance and the comparisons, where the comparisons of retrieval performances are made with the conventional wavelet pyramid transform (DWT) with three decomposition levels using the Daubechies' filter db4 [7], [18]. In the experiments based on contourlet transform, LP and DFB adopt PKVA filters [4], and LP decomposition uses three levels and corresponding DFB uses 8, 4, 4 directional decompositions from the finest scale to the coarser ones. It is shown that the use of the GGD feature representations and the KLD outperforms the traditional approach which uses the subband energy representations and the normalized Euclidean distance. Moreover, the retrieval

Table 1. Average retrieval rate (%) of 40 classes of texture images of database D1

Type of decomposition	Methods	
	Energy	GGD
DWT [7]	64.83	76.57
Contourlet	69.51	78.09

performance of thecontourlet-based CBIR is superior to the one of the wavelet-based CBIR.

4 Texture Image Retrieval by a Two-Run SVM Retrieval Algorithm

4.1 Two-Run SVM Retrieval Algorithm

The two-run SVM is formed by an one-class SVM and a two-class SVM. For any query image, two initial relevant (positive) and two initial non-relevant (negative) samples are respectively obtained by using a traditional retrieval method. Then, the two positive samples are used as the training samples for an one-class SVM. The classification results of the one-class SVM are fed to a two-class SVM. Finally, the satisfactory retrieval results are obtained through the classification of the two-class SVM. The detailed retrieval steps for a query image are described as follows.

Step 1. Sample Initialization
To save the retrieval time, two initial relevant and two non-relevant samples are chosen by a traditional texture image retrieval method where only the mean of the absolute values of the contourlet subband coefficients (see (9)) is used as feature, and the normalized Euclidean distance is used to perform the similarity measurement. For each query image, the top two similar images are taken as the initial positive samples, and the top two dissimilar images are taken as the initial negative samples.

Step 2. Feature Extraction and Normalization
Assume that there are N texture images in the database (either D1 or D2). Then, the feature set can be represented as $F = [F_1, \cdots, F_N]$, where $F_i = [f_{i,1}, \cdots, f_{i,M}]^T$, $i = 1, \cdots, N$ denotes the feature vector of each texture image and M is the length of the vector F_i. In the proposed retrieval algorithm, the feature set F_i of each image in the database consists of contourlet-based subband energies and GGD parameters of contourlet detail subband coefficients.

In order for each individual feature component to receive equal emphasis while avoiding the numerical difficulties in the retrieval process, we normalize the entries of the feature set F_i to the range of $[0,1]$ for every image. The normalization is done by replacing the feature components and feature vector respectively with

$$f'_{i,m} = \frac{f_{i,m} - f_{i\min}}{f_{i\max} - f_{i\min}}, \quad F'_i = \left[f'_{i,1}, \cdots, f'_{i,M}\right]^T, i = 1, \cdots, N \quad m = 1, \cdots, M$$

where $f_{i\min}$ and $f_{i\max}$ denote the minimum and maximum values in the feature vector F_i. Then the normalized feature set can be represented as $F' = [F'_1, \cdots, F'_N]$.

Step 3. One-Class SVM for Coarse Retrieval
For any query image, two texture images of the same class are first extracted by using the query examples resulting from step1, and the corresponding feature vectors $F'_q = [F'_{qi}, i = 1, 2]$ are obtained from the feature set F'. At the same time, the feature vectors of the other images in database are extracted, which are denoted as $F'_C = [F'_{Ci}, i = 1, 2, \cdots, N - 2]$. Then, an OCSVM takes F'_q as the training samples to obtain the decision function $f_O(x)$ (see (4)). And then, OCSVM takes F'_C as the testing samples to test. The images retrieved by the OCSVM are ordered on the basis of their decreasing values of $f_O(F'_{Ci})$, $i = 1, \cdots, N - 2$. Finally, the top 14 ranked images are output to user. By using this method, we can also obtain the retrieval rate of each query image.

Step 4. Relevance Feedback
The user classifies the 14 images into relevant ones or non-relevant ones. If they all belong to the same class as that of the two query examples, the retrieval process using the query image ends and its retrieval rate is 100%. Otherwise, the two query samples and their relevant images in 14 images are labeled as "+1" referring to the positive instances, and their non-relevant images are labeled as "-1" referring to the negative instances.

Step 5. Two-Class SVM for Refined Retrieval
The BCSVM takes the feature vectors of the positive and negative instances of Step4 as the training samples to obtain the decision function $f_B(x)$ (see (8)). Then, the BCSVM takes remaining parts of F'_C as the testing samples to test. The retrieved images are ranked in terms of the decreasing values of $f_B(F'_{Ci})$. Like Step3, only the top 14 similar images are output to user. In the ranking calculation, the retrieval rate of each query image is obtained as well.

Step 6. The Retrieval Refinement Using Relevance Feedback
If the previous retrieval results do not meet the user's expectation, Step4 and Step5 are repeated for new feedback results.

4.2 Retrieval Performance of the Two-Run SVM Retrieval Algorithm

4.2.1 Average Retrieval Accuracy by Using Energy Features and Comparisons
We consider applying the two-run SVM retrieval algorithm respectively in a wavelet-based CBIR system and in a contourlet-based CBIR system. For a fair comparison to

the retrieval results of using the traditional similarity measurements as described in Section 3.3, all the feature representations in the two system are chosen as the same as the subband energies as given in Section 3.1.

First, experiments on the texture images of database D1 are conducted. In our experiments, four iterations of the relevance feedbacks are performed in the BCSVM, and the Gaussian radial basis kernel function used in the SVM is taken as $K(x,y) = \exp\left(-\|x - y\|^2 / (2\sigma^2)\right)$, where σ is the width of the Gaussian function. For each iteration of BCSVM classification, the scaling on the training and testing samples is conducted. The main advantage of scaling is to select a proper value for the kernel parameter. The average retrieval rates (%) are shown in Table 2. Comparing with Table1, we can conclude that the two-run SVM retrieval algorithm obviously outperforms the schemes of using traditional similarity measurements for both CBIR systems, and contourlet-based method is superior to wavelet-based approach. Moreover, the proposed schemes can be stable within three or four iterations for BCSVM classification. It is practically important as pointed in [19] because the traditional relevance feedback scheme usually requires many numbers of iterations to improve retrieval performance [9]. The same conclusions can be drawn on the image database D2, as shown in Table 3. Therefore, the proposed two-run SVM retrieval algorithm provides an effective means to the texture image retrieval.

Table 2. Retrieval performance comparisons of DWT and contourlet transform by using energy features and the proposed retrieval scheme in database D1

Type of decomposition	OCSVM	BCSVM iterations			
		1	2	3	4
DWT	72.34	85.47	87.97	90.63	91.41
Contourlet	79.53	94.06	95.00	96.41	96.56

Table 3. Retrieval performance comparisons of DWT and contourlet transform by using energy features and the proposed retrieval scheme in database D2

Type of decomposition	OCSVM	BCSVM iterations			
		1	2	3	4
DWT	68.98	82.05	84.43	86.48	86.93
Contourlet	73.81	87.10	89.38	90.57	90.85

4.2.2 Retrieval Effectiveness and Retrieval Time

In the experiments, we consider the contourlet-based CBIR over database D1 and D2. The feature representations take both the subband energy features and the GGD model parameters of detail subbands. The obtained average retrieval rates are reported in the Table 4. The data in the table clearly show that the CBIR system using the GGD feature representations and the two-run SVM retrieval algorithm significantly improves the performance of the texture image retrieval. Comparison with the data in Table 3 and Table 4 also demonstrates that the proposed two-run SVM retrieval algorithm preserves the capability of SVM to efficiently exploit information from the additional features with increasing the number of good texture features [13].

Moreover, the results in the table also show that the proposed retrieval algorithm can rapidly stable within two or three iterations for BCSVM classification. For given two query samples (from Step 1 in Section 4.1), the retrieval CPU times for given feature sets of database D1 and D2 are respectively listed in the last column of Table 4 (the experiments are done on a Pentium IV computer with 2.40 GHz). This merit is desirable in practice. It takes the advantage of using two-run SVM where the one-class SVM provides the complementary sample information to the two-class SVM.

Table 4. Retrieval effectiveness and retrieval times of the proposed retrieval scheme

Database	OCSVM	BCSVM iterations				Total time (s)
		1	2	3	4	
D1	90.31	98.12	99.06	99.22	99.38	0.59
D2	87.95	95.85	97.05	97.78	98.07	3.54

4.2.3 Comparisons of Retrieval Performances

Lastly, we compare the performance of the two-run SVM retrieval algorithm with that of the retrieval algorithm of using the OCSVM or the BCSVM alone, in order to show the efficiency of the proposed retrieval scheme in the active perceptual similarity learning. We perform the relevance feedback scheme of the OCSVM and BCSVM respectively over D1 and D2. The retrieval algorithms are similar to those described in Section 4.1. For the OCSVM algorithm, only positive samples are exploited in each feedback. For the BCSVM algorithm, two positive and two negative samples are used in the first classification, which are obtained in terms of Step 1 in Section 4.1. The obtained average retrieval rates are summarized in Table 5. From Table 4 and Table 5, we can see that the proposed two-run SVM retrieval algorithm outperforms the OCSVM algorithm and the BCSVM algorithm. This can be explained like this. The OCSVM algorithm lacks of the support of negative sample information and the BCSVM algorithm requires good initial samples. In the case of small samples, the representation of the negative sample class is much poorer due to its much more complex distribution. Therefore, for the BCSVM algorithm, the small number of labeled samples can not effectively classify the positive and negative sample classes.

Table 5. Comparisons of different schemes in average retrieval rate (%)

Database	Methods	Iterations				
		1	2	3	4	5
D1	OCSVM	90.31	97.81	98.59	98.59	98.59
	BCSVM	12.50	90.63	98.28	98.59	98.91
D2	OCSVM	87.95	93.92	95.40	95.74	96.42
	BCSVM	12.50	88.12	95.85	96.53	97.33

5 Conclusions

We have presented a texture image retrieval scheme based on contourlet transform and active perception similarity learning. In the scheme, the GGD parameters of detail subbands together with subband energies are used as representations of the texture features. Since the contourlet transform can better capture directional information of texture image than the wavelet transforms, the proposed feature representations are more sufficient to distinguish different textures, and in turn to improve the retrieval accuracy. To further improve the retrieval performance in both the accuracy and the retrieval speed in the present of small samples, a two-run SVM retrieval algorithm is proposed to carry out the relevance feedback retrieving. In the two-run SVM scheme, the one-class SVM with a relatively small number of one class training samples is first applied to obtain the effective initial training set for the followed two-class SVM which is used for classification and refined retrieval subject to the user's relevance feedback. The GGD feature representation and the two-run SVM retrieval algorithm give rise to the proposed CBIR scheme. The effectiveness of the proposed CBIR scheme has been examined through experiments on the standard texture database D1 and D2. The experimental results show that the proposed CBIR scheme improves significantly the retrieval performance. Therefore, the proposed scheme provides a robust and efficient means for texture image retrieval.

References

1. Smeulders, A.W.M., Worring, M., Santini, S., Gupta, A., Jain, R.: Content-based image retrieval at the end of the early years. IEEE Trans. Pattern Anal. Mach. Intell. 22(12), 1349–1380 (2000)
2. Smith, J.R., Chang, S.–F.: Automated binary texture feature sets for image retrieval. In: Proc. ICASSP 1996, Atlanta, GA (1996)
3. Randen, T., Husoy, J.H.: Filtering for texture classification: A comparative study. IEEE Transactions on Pattern Analysis and Machine Intelligence 21(4), 291–310 (1999)
4. Do, M.N., Vetterli, M.: The contourlet transform: an efficient directional multiresolution image representation. IEEE Transactions on Image Processing 14(12), 2091–2106 (2005)
5. Qu, H., Peng, Y., Sun, W.: Texture Image Retrieval Based on Contourlet Coefficient Modeling with Generalized Gaussian Distribution. In: Kang, L., Liu, Y., Zeng, S. (eds.) ISICA 2007. LNCS, vol. 4683, pp. 493–502. Springer, Heidelberg (2007)
6. Kokare, M., Chatterji, B.N., Biswas, P.K.: Comparison of similarity metrics for texture image retrieval. In: Proceedings of IEEE Conference on Convergent Technologies for Asia-Pacific Region, vol. 2, pp. 571–575 (2003)

7. Do, M.N., Vetterli, M.: Wavelet-based texture retrieval using generalized Gaussian density and Kullback-Leibler distance. IEEE Transactions on Image Processing 11(2), 146–158 (2002)
8. Rui, Y., Huang, T.S., Ortega, M., Mehrotra, S.: Relevance feedback: a power tool for interactive content-based image retrieval. IEEE Transactions on Circuits and Video Technology 8(5), 644–655 (1998)
9. Tian, Q., Hong, P., Huang, T.S.: Update relevant image weights for content-based image retrieval using support vector machines. In: Proceedings of IEEE International Conference on Multimedia and Expo., Hilton New York & Towers, New York, vol. 2, pp. 1199–1202 (2000)
10. Chen, Y., Zhou, X.S., Huang, T.S.: One-class SVM for learning in image retrieval. In: Proceedings of IEEE International Conference on Image Processing, Thessaloniki, Greece, vol. 1, pp. 34–37 (2001)
11. Vasconcelos, N., Lippman, A.: A probabilistic architecture for content-based image retrieval. In: Proceedings of IEEE Conference on Computer Vision and Pattern Recognition, Hilton Head Island, SC, USA, vol. 1, pp. 216–221 (2000)
12. Vapnik, V.: Statistical Learning Theory. Wiley, New York (1998)
13. Li, S., Kwok, J.T., Zhu, H., Wang, Y.: Texture classification using the support vector machines. Pattern Recognition 36, 2883–2893 (2003)
14. Scholkopf, B., Platt, J.C., Shawe-Taylor, J., Smola, A.J., Williamson, R.C.: Estimating the support of a high-dimensional distribution. Neural Computation 13(7), 1443–1471 (2001)
15. Fletcher, R.: Practical Methods of Optimization, 2nd edn. John Wiley & Sons, New York (1987)
16. Qu, H., Wu, Y., Peng, Y.: Contourlet Coefficient Modeling with Generalized Gaussian Distribution and Application. In: Proceeding of International Conference on Audio, Language and Image Processing, Shanghai, China (to appear, 2008)
17. Brodatz, P.: Texture: A Photograph Album for Artists and Designers. Dover, New York (1966)
18. Daubechies, I.: Ten lectures on wavelet. SIAM, Philadelphia (1992)
19. Korfhage, R.R.: Information storage and Retrieval. John Wiley & Sons, New York (1997)

A Temporal Dominant Relationship Analysis Method [*]

Jing Yang [1], Yuanxi Wu [1], Cuiping Li [2], Hong Chen [2], and Bo Qu[1]

[1] Information School, Renmin University of China
Beijing 100872, China
{jingyang,yuanbao,qubo}@ruc.edu.cn
[2] Key Lab of Data Engineering and Knowledge Engineering of MOE
Beijing 100872, China
{licuiping,chong}@ruc.edu.cn

Abstract. Recent research on skyline queries has attracted much interest in the database and data mining community. The concept of dominant relationship analysis has commonly used in the context of skyline computation, due to its importance in many applications. Current methods have only considered so-called min/max hard attributes like price and quality which a user wants to minimize or maximize. However, objects can also have temporal attribute which can be used to represent relevant constraints on the query results. In this paper, we introduce novel skyline query types taking into account not only min/max hard attributes but also temporal attribute and the relationships between these different attribute types. We find the interrelated connection between the time-evolving attributes and the dominant relationship. Based on this discovery, we define the novel dominant relationship based on temporal aggregation and use it to analyze the problem of positioning a product in a competitive market while the time frame is required. We propose a new and efficient method to process temporal aggregation dominant relationship queries using corner transformation. Our experimental evaluation using a real dataset and various synthetic datasets demonstrates that the new query types are indeed meaningful and the proposed algorithms are efficient and scalable.

1 Introduction

Recently, the concept of dominance has attracted much interest in the skyline context in relation to answering preference queries. Dominant relationship is commonly used in the computation of skyline which has attracted considerable attention by the database community [1,2,3,4,5]. This problem can be seen as a special class of Pareto preference queries [6]. Efficient skyline querying methodologies have been studied extensively [8,9,10,11,12]. Because it is the basis of many applications, e.g., multi-criteria decision making [4], rank-aware query, user-preference queries [6] and micro-economic analysis [7]. In this paper, we propose extending the concept for business analysis based on temporal aggregation using corner transformation.

[*] This research is partly supported by the National Science Foundation of China (60673138, 60603046), Key Program of Science Technology Research of MOE (106006), and Program for New Century Excellent Talents in University.

C. Tang et al. (Eds.): ADMA 2008, LNAI 5139, pp. 367–378, 2008.
© Springer-Verlag Berlin Heidelberg 2008

Given an N-dimensional dataset S, let $D = \{D_1,...,D_N\}$ be the set of dimensions. Let p and q be two data points in S. We then denote the values of p and q on dimension D_i as p_i and q_i.

Definition 1 (Dominate, p < q). For each of the dimension D_i, we define an order $\prec D_i$. We say that p is better than q in dimension D_i (denoted as $p_i < q_i$) if p_i comes before q_i based on $\prec D_i$ or conversely, q_i is worse than p_i (also denoted as $q_i < p_i$). If p_i and q_i are equals, we denote them as $p_i = q_i$.

This paper points out that a product dominates a customer if the product is no worse than the requirement of a customer in all attribute, it means that the product definitely satisfies all the requirements of the customer. When the customer needs to purchase this kind of product, he will prefer to choose this one. Given any product, the numbers of dominated customers can be used as measurements to gauge how good the positioning of the product is in the market. Obviously, it is best to dominate as many customers as possible. Therefore, Li et al. [7] propose to extend the concept of dominance and three types of queries called LOQ, SAQ, CDQ for dominant relationship analysis from a microeconomic perspective. These queries have practical significance that allow us to find an interesting market position in the product attribute space which can dominate more customers while remaining profitable. Current methods have only considered so-called min/max hard attributes like price and quality which a user wants to minimize or maximize. However, objects can also have temporal attribute which can be used to represent relevant constraints on the query results, which was however, not mentioned in [7].

Table 1. The scenario of seven customers who book the hotels

Objects(Customer)	Time Period (Startdate~Enddate)	Hotels(Price , Quality)
a	Jan. 2nd ~ Jan. 8th	A (1 , 2)
b	Jan. 4th ~ Jan. 5th	B (2 , 3)
c	Jan. 1st ~ Jan. 5th	C (3 , 5)
d	Jan. 4th ~ Jan. 8th	D (4 , 7)
e	Jan. 1st ~ Jan. 2nd	E (5 , 3)

Example 1. Consider the six customers listed in Table 1. They all selected a hotel during different time periods. If we compare these hotels based on the price and quality attributes as shown in Figure 1(b), then we can see that hotel A is the only one skyline point among the six hotels. This is because all other hotels are dominated by the hotel A in terms of quality and price.

From a customer's perspective, the skyline of a set of hotels is useful when selecting a hotel to stay since it is obvious that the hotel A will always be a better choice when compared to B, C, D, E and F if he/she wants to trade-off quality for price.

However, whether a hotel is popular (or comfortable to customers) is not only determined by its min/max hard attributes such as price and star numbers (quality),

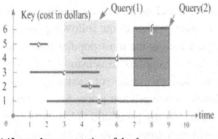
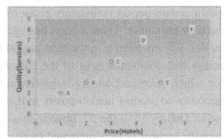

(a)Interval representation of the 6 customers
in temporal dimension x

(b) Location of hotels preferred by the 6 customers
in min/max dimensions quality and price

Fig. 1. Temporal and Min/Max dimensions quality and price

sometimes it is affected by the its soft attributes such as human environment, service, public praise in certain period. When the firstly considered attribute by a customer is time-evolving attribute, he/she will choose a more popular hotel in the expectant period. The occupation rate of the hotel may vary from time to time. In this paper, we propose a novel skyline query type taking into account not only min/max hard attributes but also temporal attribute.

Answering such preference queries [4] is one reason why skyline computation has emerged as a hot research topic. Besides quality and price, however, temporal attribute is also an important aspect that affects customer decision. In Fig. 1, although the hotels *B, C, D, E and F* are not in skyline result related to hard attributes, their managers also want to know how many customers they dominate in certain period, from which the manager can know the business position of their hotels in the local area. Generally speaking, in one period the more customers the hotel dominates, the more popular it is in the market. Going back to our running example, we suppose that C is the most popular hotel, because it is chosen by the most customers from January 1st to the 5th on Figure 1(a). If the customer c is attending a conference in this period, he/she might consider staying in the hotel C although it is not in the skyline result in term of hard attributes such as price and quality.

Note that unlike the quality and price attributes in which "good" and "better" are defined right from the start, the preferred values for temporal attributes can be determined only with respect to some given reference date. To distinguish these two types of attributes, we will call attributes such as *quality* and *price **min/max** **hard** attributes and attributes such as Jan. 2nd and Jan. 5th **temporal attributes**. Temporal has received considerable attention due to the large number of applications that require efficient query of data with time-evolving attributes. While previous research on skyline queries has investigated the perspective of a customer who wants to find a good trade-off between hotel price and quality, minimizing the price for a given quality, our research is motivated by the hotel management point of view. The objective of a hotel manager is to maximize the price (and consequently, the profit) for a given quality within certain period constraints given by the price and quality of competing hotels and their proximity. Thus, a hotel manager may want to answer the following type of queries: For my hotel q in the time period $[x, y]$, which is the most popular price and quality that dominates most of the customers in the min/max dimensions. It means that which price and quality is preferred by the largest number of customers? The purpose is to product market position: If my hotel service product prices \$5, and push out on January 1st to the 3th, how many customers will my product dominant? In this case, the number of the dominated customers will vary from day to day, the more the number of the dominated customers, the more competitive the service product p of the hotel .we call p the *most popular dominator of q* and denoted as *count* (q). Which hotel q is profitable according to that constraint while having the largest *sum* (q), i.e. has the largest number of temporal aggregation between all the hotels or their service products?

This corresponds to the second query in the earlier example. Inspired by the above motivating applications, we call this new family of query types considering the relationship between min/max hard and temporal attributes *temporal dominant relationship analysis* and propose a novel algorithm *temporal aggregation dominant queries* (TADQs) . In order to process these TADQs efficiently, this paper explores temporal aggregation query into the dominant relationship analyze.

The efficient process of temporal aggregations present a number of unique challenges not found in the case of non-temporal aggregation. One challenge is temporal grouping, a process in which we must group aggregate results by time. In this case, the above discussion can change into this problem. For example, a hotel department that preserves the following information about service products booked by its customers: (1) the starting/ending date of each reservation, and (2) its cost (in dollars). Figure 1 illustrates the interval representation of 6 customers, where the key of each interval (i.e. its projection on the vertical axis) denotes its cost, while the horizontal projection corresponds to its duration or following the common terminology in the literature, its lifespan. For example, the lifespan of a is the interval [2, 8]. A data is alive during its lifespan, and dead outside it. Let us assume that the granularity of date is one day. A hotel manager may want to answer the following types of queries:

1) Given a key range qk and an interval qt, please retrieve the total number of data intervals that are alive during qt with keys in range qk. This kind of query is called *temporal count query*. For example, **Query 1** in Figure 1(a) (light shaded rectangle) represents the query "return the number of customers in period $qt= [3, 6]$". It can be answered by counting the number of intervals intersecting the query rectangle (i.e., in our example the result is 4).

Query 2. Figure 1(a) (dark shaded rectangle) represents the query "return the number of customers in period $qt= [7, 9]$, with costs in $qk= [2, 6]$". The result is 2.

2) Assuming that each data interval is associated with a *weight*□retrieves the sum of the weights of the qualifying records. This kind of query is called the *temporal sum query*, which, For instance, if the database also stores the number of persons involved in each reservation (i.e., it is possible to have tourisms with more than two customers, but they leave only one record), then a temporal sum query returns the total number of persons in all the records of reservation that qualify *qk* and *qt*.

Clearly, computing these aggregate results is significantly more intricate than aggregation without the additional time dimension.

The remainder of the paper is organized as follows. The query processing strategies for temporal aggregation dominant relationship analysis using corner transformation is described in Section 2. The performance analysis is reported in Section 3.

2 The Transform-Based Temporal Aggregation Method of Dominance Analyse

In this section, we introduce the transform-based temporal aggregation processing method proposed in this paper. The method first transforms data objects with extent on time dimension into points without extents using corner transformation [13], and then, performs aggregation. Based on the temporal aggregation results, we can conclude the dominance analysis.

2.1 Transformation

In this section, we first introduce how to transform a data object with extents into a point without extents using corner transformation. Corner transformation transforms the MBR (minimum bound rectangle) of a data object in the n-dimensional original space into a point in the 2n-dimensional transformed space. In corner transformation, the coordinates of a point in the 2n-dimensional space are determined by the minimum and maximum values of the MBR on each of the n axes in the original space [13]. For example, a one-dimensional object whose minimum and maximum values on the x-axis are lx and rx, respectively, is transformed into the point (lx, rx) in the two-dimensional transformed space.

A query that finds data objects overlapping with a given region in the original space is transformed into a query that finds point objects contained in a certain region in the transformed space [13].

Figure 2 shows relationships between a point and regions in the transformed space. Here, objects overlapping with the region r in the original space (Figure 2(a)) are transformed into points in the regions A, B, C, or D in the transformed space (Figure 2(b)).

Using these characteristics, the original space temporal aggregate that compute over all tuples whose valid intervals overlap with the interval r can be processed by the operation that aggregates points in the union of the transformed space regions A, B, C, and D, which constitutes the shaded part in Figure 2(b).

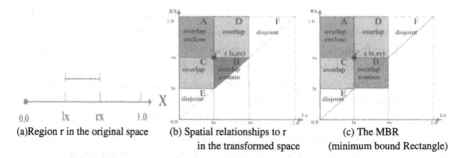

(a)Region r in the original space

(b) Spatial relationships to r in the transformed space

(c) The MBR (minimum bound Rectangle)

Fig. 2. Transformed space regions having various spatial relationships with the query region r in the original space. Here, r̀ is the transformed point of r [13].

Example 2 Using this method, if we first ignore the cost dimension (we will discuss how to process this kind of non-time dimension later), the interval representation of 6 customers in Figure 1 (as Figure 3(a)) can be transformed into the 6 red points in Figure 3(b). Similarly, the query region of Query 1 can be transformed into the blue point in Figure 3(b). It can be found that, to answer Query 1, we only need to count the number of red points in the shaded region of Figure 3(b).

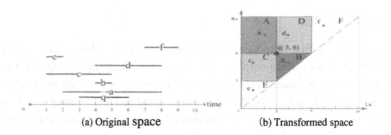

(a) Original space

(b) Transformed space

Fig. 3. Objects in the original and transformed space

2.2 Aggregation

Now, the problem is how to aggregate those points in the shaded part. Since there is no point under the diagonal, the aggregation of the shaded part in Figure 2(b) is equal to that of the regular MBR whose left-bottom corner and right-up corner are (0.0, lx) and (rx, 1.0) respectively (as shown in Figure 2(c)). It becomes a typical range query problem in data cube philosophy. A range query applies an aggregation operation over all selected cells of an OLAP data cube where the selection is specified by providing ranges of values for numeric dimensions [14].

Much research has gone into efficiently range query processing. Let D = {1, 2, 3..., d} denote the set of dimensions, where each dimension corresponds to a functional attribute. We will represent the d-dimensional data cube by a d-dimensional array A of size $n_1 \times n_2 \times ... \times n_d$. Where $n_j >= 2, j \in D$. We assume an array has a starting index 0. For convenience, we will call each array element a cell.

We will describe all range queries with respect to array A. The problem of computing a range-sum query in a D-dimensional data cube can be formulated as follows:

$$Sum\ (l_1{:}h_1, ..., l_d{:}h_d) = \sum_{i1=l1}^{h1} ... \sum_{id=ld}^{hd} A[i_1,...,i_d].$$

Similarly, a range-count query in a D-dimensional data cube can be formulated as Count $(l_1{:}h_1,..., l_d{:}h_d)$.

In this paper, we adopt the method proposed in [14] to process a range query. The essential idea is to pre-compute some auxiliary information that is used to answer ad hoc queries at run-time. By maintaining auxiliary information which is of the same size as the data cube, all range queries for a given cube can be answered in constant time, irrespective of the size of the sub-cube circumscribed by a query. Response to a range query requires access to some cells of the auxiliary information.

Let P be a d-dimensional array of size $N = n_1 \times n_2 \times ... \times n_d$ (which has the same size as A). P will be used to store various pre-computed (Pre-Count or Pre-Sum in our example) of A. we will pre-computed, for all $0 \leq x_j < n_j$ and $j \in D$,

$$P[x_1, x_2, ..., x_d] = Sum(0{:}x_1, 0{:}x_2, ..., 0{:}x_d) = \sum_{i1=0}^{x1} \sum_{i2=0}^{x2} ... \sum_{id=0}^{xd} A[i_1, i_2, ..., i_d]. \quad (1)$$

For example, Table 2 (a) shows a 2-dimensional array A of size 6×3. Table 2 (b) shows of its corresponding Pre-Sum array P whose size is same as array A. P is used to store various pre-computed prefix-sums of A. Each cell

$$P[x, y] = Sum\ (0{:}x, 0{:}y) = \sum_{i=0}^{x} \sum_{j=0}^{y} A[i, j].$$

Table 2. The original array A and its prefix-sum array P

(a)Index	0	1	2	3	4	5
0	3	5	1	2	2	3
1	7	3	2	6	8	2
2	2	4	2	3	3	5
(b)Index	0	1	2	3	4	5
0	3	8	9	11	13	16
1	10	18	21	29	39	44
2	12	24	29	40	53	63

For example, the value of cell P (1, 1) is the sum of A (0, 0), A (0, 1), A (1, 0), A (1, 1), i.e. 18. The value of cell P (0, 3) is the sum of A (0, 0), A (0, 1), A (0, 2), A (0, 3), i.e. 11. Having the auxiliary information (Pre-Sum array P in our example), any range query of A can be computed from up to 2^d appropriate elements of P according the following theorem proposed in [14].

Theorem 1. For all $j \in D$, let $S(j) = \begin{cases} 1, & if & x_j = h_j, \\ -1, & if & x_j = l_j - 1 \end{cases}$ Then, for all $j \in D$

$$Sum\ (l_1:h_1,...,l_d:h_d) = \sum_{\forall x_j \in \{l_j-1, h_j\}} \left\{ \left(\prod_{i=1}^{d} s(i) \right) * p[x_1, x_2,...x_d] \right\} \tag{2}$$

The theorem above provides how any range-sum of A can be computed from up to 2^d appropriate elements of P. The left hand side of Equation 2 specifies a range-sum of A, The right hand side of Equation 2 consists of 2^d additive terms, each is from an element of P with a sign "+" or "-" defined by product of all s(i)'s. For notational convenience, let $P[x_1, x_2, ..., x_d] = 0$ if $x_j = -1$ for some $j \in D$.

For example, when d=2, the range-sum $Sum(l_1:h_1,l_2:h_2)$ can be obtained in three computation steps as $P[h_1,h_2]$ - $P[h_1,l_2-1]$ - $P[l_1-1,h_2]$ + $P[l_1-1,l_2-1]$. For instance in Table 2, the range-sum $Sum(1:2, 2:3)$ (red region in Table 2) can be derived from P[2, 3] - P[0, 3] - P[2, 1] + P[0, 1] = 40 - 11 - 24 + 8 = 13.

2.3 Pre-computation

The basic method to pre-compute a prefix array P needs d phases, where d is the dimension number. During the first phase, one-dimensional prefix aggregation of A along dimension 1 for all elements of A is performed and the result is stored in P (denoted P_1). During the i-th phase, for all $2 \le i \le d$, one-dimensional prefix-aggregation of P_{i-1}(the output from previous phase) along dimension i is performed and the result is stored back to P (denoted P_i). Note that only one copy of P is needed because the same array is reused during each phase of pre-computation.

For example, in order to compute the prefix sum array in Table 2(b) for the original array A in Table 2(a), we need first perform one-dimension prefix-sum along the horizontal axis, and then perform one-dimension prefix-sum along the vertical axis.

The basic algorithm is somewhat naïve in that it needs to scan the original array d times to compute the prefix aggregation along d dimensions.

In this Section, we present a more efficient method which will scan the original array only once. We impose an arbitrary order for the dimensions as $d_1, ..., d_n$. We also impose a lexicographical order on the cells of A such that p is ordered before q if and only if there exists an i such that $p_i < q_i$ and for all $j<i$, $p_j=q_j$.

We observe that the prefix aggregation of a cell can be obtained by utilizing the aggregations of its children in different subspaces. Intuitively, we can compute the prefix array in a divide-and-conquer and bottom-up manner. For each cell p, since it can be the child of other cell in any dimension, we need compute for it $p_1, p_2, ..., p_n$. Here, p_i represents the prefix aggregation in subspace $d_i...d_n$. In order to compute the aggregates for all cells, we can search the cell enumeration tree in a depth-first manner according to a user-specified dimension order. Hereafter, except for specifically mentioned, we will use the same assuming for the dimension order.

The pseudo code of the prefix aggregation computation algorithm is shown in Algorithm 1. It is inspired by the BUC algorithm proposed by Bayer and Ramakrishnan [15]. It recursively partitions objects in a depth-first manner so that objects prefixed by the same cell are grouped together at the time of computation for the cell's prefix aggregation. The partitioning is performed on different dimensions at each level of the recursion so that different groupings can be formed.

After initialization, the main algorithm calls Enumerate () for the smallest cell [0, 0... 0]. The function Enumerate () will then implement depth first search and perform recursive computation of prefix aggregation for each cell on the enumerating tree.

For each dimension D between dim and numDims-1, the input data set is partitioned on dimension D (Line 4). Line 5 iterates through the partitions for each distinct value in a descending order. The partition becomes the input data set in the next recursive call to Enumerate (), which compute the prefix aggregation on the partition for dimensions D+1 to numDims-1.

Note that the descending order is very important in computing the prefix aggregation. This order guarantees when a cell is processing, all its children's prefix information has already been known.

Now, we look at the procedure PrefixCompute() in the second line of function Enumerate(). Given the input cell, PrefixCompute's task is to compute the prefix aggregation of cells in all subspaces. The algorithm proceeds from the last dimension to the first dimension. For each dimension d, the prefix aggregation of the cell in subspace $d_i...d_n$ is computed and stored in PreAgg[d].

Algorithm 1: Enumerate(C, n)

  Input: C: A set of points.

   N: The total number of dimensions.

  Output: A prefix array.

  Method: let cell=[0,…,0] and Call Enumerate(cell, C, 1);

  Function Enumerate (cell, input, dim)

  5.   **for** i=cardinality[D] to 1 **do**
  6.   part=point partition for value xi of D
  7.   let cell[D]=i
  8.   Enumerate(cell, part, D+1)

  Algorithm 2: PrefixCompute (cell, PreAgg, dim)

  1. Initialize temp to be the value of cell;
  2. **for** i=dim to 1 do

  Input: cell: the cell to be processed.

  input: the partition.

  dim: the starting dimension for this iteration.

  1. **if** dim==N+1 do
  2.   PrefixCompute(cell, PreAgg, dim-1)
  3. **for** D=dim to N do
  4.   partition input on dimension D
  3.   **if** cell[i]<cardinality[i]do
  4.   tempcell=child(cell,i)
  5.   //compute index of tempcell in subspace $d_i…d_n$
  6.   temp += PreAgg[i][index];
  7.   //compute index of cell in subspace $d_i…d_n$
  8.   PreAgg[i][index] = temp;

2.4 Top-k Dominating Search

Up to now, we discussed how to process the temporal count or sum query with an interval qt. Based on the results of prefix aggregation computation (count in Example 3) in the transformed space, we can do the dominance analysis. This part presents an eager approach for evaluating one of the dominance queries called top-k dominating query based on above mentioned temporal aggregation, which traverses the cell enumeration tree in a depth-first manner and computes each prefix array P (count q), for example when customer wants to query top-k dominating hotels with the k-largest *count* (q) owns a product service which is comparable to many other hotels.

Algorithm 3 shows the pseudo code of the Counting-Guided Temporal Aggregation Dominance Query Algorithm (TADQ), which directs search by counting upper bound scores of examined non-leaf entries of the cell enumeration tree. A max-heap H is employed for organizing the array to be visited in descending order of their scores. W is a min-heap for managing the top-k dominating points as the algorithm progresses, while γ is the k-th score in W (used for pruning). First, the upper bound scores μ(q) of the cell enumeration tree root entries are computed in batch (using the **Enumerate** algorithm) and these are inserted into the max-heap H. While the score μ(p) of H's top entry e is higher than γ (implying that points with scores higher than γ may be indexed under e), the top entry is deheaped, and the node Z pointed by e is visited. If Z is a non-leaf node, its entries are enheaped, after **Enumerate** is called to compute their upper score bounds. If Z is a leaf node, the scores of the points in it are computed in batch and the top-k set W (also) is updated, if applicable.

Algorithm3: Temporal Aggregation Dominance Query (TADQ)

Algorithm TADQ (Tree R, Integer k)

```
1: H:=new max-heap; W:=new min-heap;
2: γ :=0; .                           // the k-th highest score found so far
3: Enumerate(R.root,{e⁻ | e ∈R.root});
4: for all entries e ∈ R.root do
5:     enheap(H, <e, μ(e⁻)>);
6: while |H| > 0 and H's top entry's score > γ  do
7:     e:=deheap(H);
8:     read the child node Z pointed by e;
9:     if Z is non-leaf then
10:        Enumerate (R.root,{ec⁻ | ec∈Z});
11:        for all entries ec∈ Z do
12:            enheap(H, <ec, μ(ec⁻)>);
13:    else                            // Z is a leaf
14:        Enumerate (R.root,{p | p∈Z});
15:        update W and γ , using <p, μ(p)>, p ∈Z
16: report W as the result;
```

3 Experimental Results

We experimented that the algorithms are in high availability to evaluate the efficiency and effectiveness of our method, we conducted extensive experiments. We implemented all algorithms using Microsoft Visual C++ V6.0, and conducted the experiments on a DELL PC with Pentium 4 CPU 2.40GHz, main memory size 256MB, disk 40GB, running Microsoft Windows XP Professional Edition. We conducted experiments on both synthetic and real life datasets. However, due to space limitation, we will only report results on synthetic datasets here. Results from real life datasets mirror the result of the synthetic datasets closely. The default value of data size is 100,000.

We use two experiments to evaluate our algorithm TADQ. We evaluate it with the datasets different in sizes, dimensions and distribution which can be defined to three kinds (correlated, independent and anti-correlated).

The first experiment is shown as the Figure 4(a), which explores the running time of our method for each type of data distribution with increasing dimensionality. Clearly, we can obtain comparable running time on all three datasets. Among the three distributions, correlated data gives the best effect as many attributes in the same

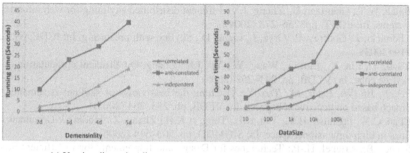

(a) Varying dimensionality   (b)Varying number of points

Fig. 4. Query Performance for TADQ

tuple are related which accelerating our methods. Independent dataset is the second in the terms of the running time. There is no relationship between the attributes in the same tuple. This means that some attributes may have the high value, but the others in the same tuple may not have the high value. So when we compute the dominate relationship between two tuples, the dominate relationship between the corresponsive attributes of two tuples has no meaning on that of another couples of the two tuples.

Anti-correlated data sets have the longest running time. The reason is that when some attributes of a tuple have the high value, the other must have the low value. This means that this tuple can't be dominated by other tuples because it has the high values on some attributes, at the same time it can't dominate other points too because the other attributes of it have the low value. The result is that we have a large result sets with small dominate count for each point in it, which means we need more time to compute it .

Figure 4(b) is about the second experiment, it shows how running time of our method TADQ scales up as the number of points goes up. We can see that running time gets longer as the number of points increase. At the same time, the correlated data sets perfect best, the following is the independent data sets, and the last is the anti-correlated data sets.

References

1. Ramsak, F., Kossmann, D., Rost, S.: Shooting stars in the sky: An online algorithm for skyline queries. In: VLDB (2002)
2. Papadias, D., Tao, Y., Fu, G., Seeger, B.: An optimal and progressive algorithm for skyline queries. In: SIGMOD (2003)
3. Tan, K., et al.: Efficient progressive skyline computation. In: VLDB (2001)
4. Kossmann, D., Borzsonyi, S., Stocker, K.: The skyline operator. In: ICDE (2001)
5. Lin, W.W.X., Yuan, Y., Lu, H.: Stabbing the sky: efficient skyline computation over sliding windows. In: ICDE (2005)
6. Kieling, W.: Foundations of preferences in database systems. In: VLDB, pp. 311–322 (2002)
7. Li, C., Ooi, B.C., Tung, A.K.H., Wang, S.: DADA: A data cube for dominant relationship analysis. In: SIGMOD, pp. 659–670 (2006)

8. Balke, W.T., Guentzer, U., Zheng, J.X.: Efficient distributed skylining for web information systems. In: EDBT, pp. 256–273 (2004)
9. Chomicki, J., Godfrey, P., Gryz, J., Liang, D.: Skyline with presorting. In: ICDE, pp. 717–719 (2003)
10. Yuan, Y., Lin, X., Liu, Q., Wang, W., Yu, J.X., Zhang, Q.: Efficient computation of the skyline cube. In: VLDB, pp. 241–252 (2005)
11. Pei, J., Jin, W., Ester, M., Tao, Y.: Catching the best views of skyline: A semantic approach based on decisive subspaces. In: VLDB, pp. 253–264 (2005)
12. Chan, C.Y., Jagadish, H.V., Tan, K.L., Tung, A.K.H., Zhang, Z.: Finding k-Dominant skylines in high dimensional space. In: SIGMOD, pp. 503–514 (2006)
13. Seeger, B., Kriegel, H.-P.: Techniques for Design and Implementation of Efficient Spatial Access Methods. In: Proc. the 14th Int'l Conf. on Very Large Data Bases, Los Angeles, California, August 1988, pp. 360–371 (1988)
14. Ho, C.-T., Agrawal, R., Megiddo, N., Srikant, R.: Range queries in olap data cubes. In: SIGMOD Conference, pp. 73–88 (1997)
15. Beyer, K.S., Ramakrishnan, R.: Bottom-up computation of sparse and iceberg cubes. In: SIGMOD 1999, Proceedings ACM SIGMOD International Conference on Management of Data, Philadelphia, Pennsylvania, USA, June 1-3, 1999, pp. 359–370 (1999)

Leakage-Aware Energy Efficient Scheduling for Fixed-Priority Tasks with Preemption Thresholds

XiaoChuan He and Yan Jia

Institute of Network Technology and Information Security
School of Computer Science
National University of Defense Technology
Changsha, China 410073

Abstract. Dynamic Voltage Scaling (DVS), which adjusts the clock speed and supply voltage dynamically, is an effective technique in reducing the energy consumption of embedded real-time systems. However, most existing DVS algorithms focus on reducing the energy consumption of CPU only, ignoring their negative impacts on task scheduling and system wide energy consumption. In this paper, we address one of such side effects, an increase in task preemptions due to DVS. We present energy-efficient Fixed-priority with preemption threshold (EE-FPPT) scheduling algorithm to solve this problem. First, we propose an appropriate schedulability analysis, based on response time analysis, for supporting energy-efficient FPPT scheduling in hard real-time systems. Second, we prove that a task set achieves the minimal energy consumptions under Maximal Preemption Threshold Assignment (MPTA).

1 Introduction

Low power utilization has become one of the key challenges to the designer of battery-powered embedded real-time computing systems. Dynamic Voltage Scaling (DVS), which adjusts the supply voltage and its corresponding clock frequency dynamically, is one of the most effective low-power design technique for embedded real-time systems. Since the energy consumption of CMOS circuits has a quadratic dependency on the supply voltage, lowering the supply voltage is one of the most effective ways of reducing the energy consumption.

With a recent growth in the portable and mobile embedded device market, where a low-power consumption is an important design requirement, several commercial variable voltage microprocessors were developed. Targeting these microprocessors, many DVS algorithms have been proposed or developed, especially for hard real-time systems [1,2]. Since lowering the supply voltage also decreases the maximum achievable clock speed [3], various DVS algorithms for hard real-time systems have the goal of reducing supply voltage dynamically to the lowest possible level while satisfying the tasks'timing constraints.

Each DVS algorithm is known to be quite effective in reducing the energy/ power consumption of a target system [1,2,4]. However, the existing DVS

C. Tang et al. (Eds.): ADMA 2008, LNAI 5139, pp. 379–390, 2008.
© Springer-Verlag Berlin Heidelberg 2008

algorithms mainly focus on reducing energy consumption of CPU only, ignoring their negative impacts on system-wide energy consumption. For example, when the tasks'execution times are increased due to a lowered clock speed, the patterns of device usage and memory traffic may be changed, potentially increasing the energy consumption in system buses, I/O devices and memory chips. In particular, when a lower-priority task's execution time is extended with a lowered clock speed, it may be preempted more often by higher-priority tasks. According to the experiments reported in [5], the number of task preemptions can grow up to 500% under dynamic voltage scaling over non-DVS executions.

The increase in the number of task preemptions can negatively impact on the system energy consumption in several ways. First, the preemption overhead may increase the energy consumption in memory subsystems. In multi-tasking real-time systems, when a task is preempted by a higher priority task, the memory blocks used by the preempted task are displaced from the cache by the memory blocks used by the preempting higher priority task. Later, when the preempted task resumes its execution, a considerable amount of time is consumed to reload the previously displaced memory blocks into the cache. When preemptions are frequent due to the lengthened task execution time, cache-related preemption costs can take a significant portion of processor time and energy consumption in memory subsystems [6]. In addition, since the voltage scaling is performed usually at each context switching point, such frequent preemptions may degrade not only the system energy efficiency but also the system utilization when the voltage scaling overhead is not negligible as shown in [7].

Second, the lengthened task lifetime may increase the energy consumption in system devices [8]. Since the execution of a preempted task should be delayed while a preempting task is running, its lifetime - the time interval between its activation and completion - is lengthened. If we assume that the system devices are active (i.e., powered up) during the lifetime of the task (that use the system devices), the increased lifetime of the task may also increase the energy consumption in the system devices. Furthermore, as the number of simultaneously activated tasks increases, the number of active system devices is likely to increase, consuming more energy. In addition, since the code and data sections of the activated tasks should be kept in memory, the amount of active memory may increase, thus increasing the leakage power in memory subsystems.

Fixed-priority preemptive (FPP) scheduling algorithms [9] and fixed-priority non-preemptive (FPNP) scheduling algorithms [10] are two important classes of real-time scheduling algorithms. To obtain the benefits of both FPP and FPNP algorithms, there are several other algorithms trying to fill the gap between them. The fixed-priority with preemption threshold (FPPT) scheduling algorithm [11] is one of them. Under FPPT, each task has a pair of priorities: regular priority and preemption threshold, where the preemption threshold of a task is higher than or equal to its regular priority. The preemption threshold represents the tasks running-time preemption priority level. It prevents the preemption of the task from other tasks, unless the preempting tasks priority is higher than the preemption threshold of the current running task. Saksena and Wang have shown that task sets scheduled with FPPT can have significant schedulability improvements over task set using fixed priorities [11]. The regular priority of a task can be predefined or obtained by algorithms [9,10], but the preemption threshold is usually calculated during a schedulability analysis [12,13]. All preemption thresholds of a task set form a preemption threshold assignment or assignment for simplification. If an assignment can make each task schedulable by FPPT, the assignment is called valid.

This paper extends the current work on FPPT in [12] by importing a energy-efficient scheme in FPPT scheduling. Efficient schedulability analysis, which combine the variable voltage processor model, DVS mechanisms and the scheduling algorithm into consideration, is needed to guarantee the timeliness requirement. In this paper, an algorithm to analyze the schedulability of energy efficient FPPT (EE-FPPT) scheduling is provided. In order to reduce the total energy consumption of systems, another algorithm to calculate the optimal preemption threshold assignment for maximal energy saving is also presented.

2   Computational Model

This study deals with the fixed priority preemptive scheduling of tasks in a real-time systems with hard constraints, i.e., systems in which the respect of time constraints is mandatory. The activities of the system are modeled by periodic tasks. The model of the system is defined by a task set T of cardinality n, $T = \{\tau_1, \tau_2, ..., \tau_n\}$. The j_{th} job of task τ_i is denoted as $J_{i,j}$. The index, j, for jobs of a task is started from zero. A periodic task τ_i is characterized by a 4-tuple (C_i, T_i, D_i, f_i) where each request of τ_i, called instance, has an execution requirement of C_i, and a deadline D_i. T_i time units separate two consecutive instances of τ_i (hence T_i is the period of the task). Each task τ_i is assigned with different clock frequency f_i from a presumed clock frequency set of cardinality m, $\Phi = \{FLK^1, FLK^2, ..., FLK^m\}$, where $FLK^1 < FLK^2 < ... < FLK^m$. These respective clock frequency for tasks are assumed to have being already calculated by certain DVS-related algorithms [1,2,4].

Note that C_i is the worst-case execution cycles (WCEC) of the task τ_i, so the worst-case execution time (WCET) of the task τ_i is C_i/f_i, which represented by C_i. The system is said schedulable if each instance finishes before its deadline.

Each task is associated with a deadline D_i, that D_i may be arbitrarily large. This means that many instances of the same task can be active (in the ready queue) at the same time. We assume that the scheduler handles tasks with the same priorities using a FIFO rule. Hence an early instance of a task has priority over a later, and must be completed before the later instance is allowed to start.

We further assume that the total utilization of all tasks, U, is strictly less than 1. This will later be shown to be a necessary condition for the analysis.

We assume that (a) the tasks are independent, i.e., there is no blocking due to shared resource, (b) tasks do not suspend themselves, except at the end of their execution, and (c) the overheads due to context switching, etc., are negligible (i.e., assumed to be zero).

We also associate with each task τ_i a unique priority $\pi_i \in \{1, 2, ..., n\}$ such that contention for resources is resolved in favor of the job with the highest priority that is ready to run.

Hereafter, we use the notion $\mathcal{T} = \{\tau_i = (C_i, D_i, T_i, f_i) | i = 1, 2, ..., n\}$ to denote the set of n tasks composing our real-time workload. We will use the tuple $(\mathcal{T}, \Pi)$ to denote the workload $\mathcal{T}$ along with some priority assignment Π.

3   Schedulability Analysis for EE-FPPT

In this section, we will discuss the schedulability analysis for FPPT considering the dynamic voltage scaling mechanism described in Section 1. The schedulability analysis method for EE-FPPT is proposed by extending the algorithm proposed in [12,14].

We consider the model in a system with a memory hierarchy in the following, where the system is equipped with an on-chip instruction and data cache and that the main external memory has a constant access latency. To accurately model the WCET in systems with memory hierarchies, the effect of frequency scaling must be described exactly. The WCEC C_i of a task τ_i can be split into two portions. The first portion C_i^{pc} captures the ideal number of cycles required to execute the task assuming perfect caches. In other words, C_i^{pc} does not scale with frequency. The second portion, C_i^{cm}, counts the total number of instruction and data cache misses for the task τ_i. Obviously, C_i^{cm} scales with frequency and depends on the memory access latency. If a system without caches is considered, C_i^{pc} would count the total number of cycles used for non-memory operations while C_i^{cm} would count the total number of memory references. Thus, the WCEC C_i of a task τ_i can be expressed as follows:

$$C_i = C_i^{pc} + C_i^{cm} \cdot N_m \tag{1}$$

where N_m is the number of cycles required to access the memory, which depends on the latency of the memory L and the frequency of the processor f_i. In general, N_m can be represented by $L \cdot f_i$. In practical real-time applications, C_i^{pc} and C_i^{cm} can be identified statistically by program profiling or other techniques, and L can be measured by some physical instrument too, Thus, the WCEC C_i of a task τ_i should be the function of the frequency of the processor f_i in static time analysis [15,16] of a task, denoted as:

$$C_i = C_i^{pc} + C_i^{cm} \cdot L \cdot f_i \tag{2}$$

then the WCET C_i of a task τ_i can be written as:

$$C_i = C_i^{pc}/f_i + C_i^{cm} \cdot L \tag{3}$$

With above considerations, the calculation of a task τ_i response time under EE-FPPT can be conducted through the following equations.

$$B_i = \max_{\tau_j \in \mathcal{T}} \{C_j^{pc}/f_j + C_j^{cm} \cdot L | \pi_i > \pi_j \wedge \pi_i \leq \gamma_j\} \tag{4}$$

$$L_i = B_i + \sum_{\forall j, \pi_j \geq \pi_i} \lceil \frac{L_i}{T_j} \rceil \cdot (C_j^{pc}/f_j + C_j^{cm} \cdot L) \tag{5}$$

$$S_i^k = B_i + k \cdot (C_i^{pc}/f_i + C_i^{cm} \cdot L) + \\ \sum_{\forall j, \pi_j > \pi_i} \left(1 + \lfloor \frac{S_i^k}{T_j} \rfloor \right) \cdot (C_j^{pc}/f_j + C_j^{cm} \cdot L) \tag{6}$$

$$F_i^k = S_i^k + (C_i^{pc}/f_i + C_i^{cm} \cdot L) + \\ \sum_{\forall j, \pi_j > \gamma_i} \left(\lceil \frac{F_i^k}{T_j} \rceil - \left(1 + \lfloor \frac{S_i^k}{T_j} \rfloor \right) \right) \cdot (C_j^{pc}/f_j + C_j^{cm} \cdot L) \tag{7}$$

$$R_i = {}^{max}_{k=0,1,2,\ldots,\lfloor \frac{L_i}{T_j} \rfloor} (F_i^k - k \cdot T_i) \tag{8}$$

4 Preemption Threshold Assignment for Minimal Energy Consumption

In this paper, the optimal preemption threshold assignment is the assignment that can minimize the power consumption of task set. A description of the method to find out the optimal preemption threshold assignment regarding the analysis described earlier is given in this section. The regular priority assignment of a task set is assumed predefined, which can be conducted by algorithms [10].

In this section we assume that the priority of each task in T has been already assigned. We would like to find a preemption threshold assignment Γ that is feasible and make the power consumption minimal. A preemption threshold assignment Γ is *feasible* if and only if the system is schedulable according to the conditions presented earlier in section 3. Hereafter, the set of all feasible preemption threshold assignments for the task set T will be denoted by $\mathcal{G}(T, \Pi)$. A particular feasible assignment of special interest is defined below:

Definition 1. (Identity Preemption Threshold Assignment, IPTA) *We define the identity preemption threshold assignment, $\Gamma^I \in \mathcal{G}(T, \Pi)$, as the preemption threshold assignment where all tasks have been assigned preemption thresholds that are equal to the tasks' priority (i.e. $\gamma_i = \pi_i$ for all $i \in [1, n]$.*

Since the tasks priorities and parameters are preassigned according to some scheduling algorithm (e.g. RM, DM, EDF, etc), so the identity assignment is always known. Moreover, $\mathcal{G}(T, \Pi)$ is never empty since it will at least contain the identity assignment.

Given two preemption threshold assignments, $\Gamma, \Gamma' \in \mathcal{G}(T, \Pi)$, we say that Γ is larger than Γ', and denote it by $\Gamma \succ \Gamma'$, if and only if all member preemption thresholds of Γ are equal to or greater than the corresponding preemption thresholds of Γ' (i.e. $\forall i, \gamma_i \geq \gamma_i'$). The largest of all preemption threshold assignments is of particular interest and is defined as follows:

Definition 2. (Maximal Preemption Threshold Assignment, MPTA) *We define the maximal preemption threshold assignment, denoted by $\Gamma^{max} = (\gamma_1^{max}, \gamma_2^{max}, ..., \gamma_n^{max}) \in \mathcal{G}(T, \Pi)$, as the largest preemption threshold assignment in $\mathcal{G}(T, \Pi)$. That is, $\Gamma^{max} \succ \Gamma'$ for all $\Gamma \in \mathcal{G}(T, \Pi)$.*

The MPTA was presented in [12] firstly, then was analyzed by Chen et al.[17], and was shown to always find the maximal preemption threshold assignment if one exists [17]. Since in our case we always start with a feasible assignment, namely the identity assignment (IPTA), the maximal preemption threshold assignment always exists (in the worst-case being equal to the identity assignment) and will always be found.

We now present the main theorem for this section. In proving this theorem, we will denote the total power consumption of a task set T and a particular preemption threshold assignment Γ by $E_{total}(T, \Gamma, \Pi)$.

Theorem 1. *Given two real-time systems (T, Γ, Π) and (T, Γ', Π) with preemption thresholds assignments Γ and Γ' in $\mathcal{G}(T)$ such that $\Gamma \succ \Gamma'$. The power consumption $E_{total}(T, \Gamma', \Pi)$ can be no smaller than $E_{total}(T, \Gamma, \Pi)$.*

Proof. Without loss of generality, let us assume that $\gamma_k = \gamma'_k$ for all $k = 1, 2, ..., i-1, i+1, ..., n$ and let $\gamma'_i < \gamma_i$ for some arbitrary $i \in (1, 2, ..., n)$. It should be clear that $\Gamma \succ \Gamma'$ according to our definition.

When the preemption threshold of τ_i changes from γ_i to γ'_i, the worst-case response time of any task τ_k with $\pi_k > \gamma'_i$ will not change. The worst-case response time of a task τ_k with $\gamma'_i > \pi_k > \pi_i$ will also stay the same. Furthermore, any task τ_k with priority $\gamma'_i < \pi_k \le \gamma_i$ will have no worse worst-case response time with γ'_i than with γ_i, and will make another interference in the normal execution of task τ_i, which would further squeeze the τ_i's computation time of its own. In the course of schedulability test of task set T (equation 4, 5, 6, 7, 8), task τ_i is associated with a clock frequency f_i, which represents the processor speed when task τ_i is scheduled to run, faster processor speed for task τ_i would reduce the execution requirement of task τ_i, but resulting in more power consumption of task τ_i. If the decrease on γ_i (just like mentioned above) make the task τ_i itself unschedulable, increasing the processor speed for task τ_i from f_i to f'_i ($f'_i > f_i, f'_i \in \Phi$) would be the only way to oppose its effect and remake task τ_i schedulable again.

When the processor speed of task τ_i changes from f_i to f''_i ($f''_i < f_i, f''_i \in \Phi$), τ_i's computation time of its own will be relaxed, and then the worst-case response time of task τ_i will increased by $C_i^{pc}(1/f''_i - 1/f_i)$, if $R_i + C_i^{pc}(1/f''_i - 1/f_i) \le D_i$, then the slowdown of clock frequency for task τ_i would be feasible and thus lead to power saving. For any task τ_k with priority $\pi_k < \pi_i$, the increment $C_i^{pc}(1/f''_i - 1/f_i)$ on τ_i's computation time will contribute more interference time to their worst-case response time. Now let $\tau_j \in T$ be the task belonging to the task subset with priority $\pi_k < \pi_i$, where τ_j's worst-case response time is closest to its deadline D_j. if the increment mentioned above make τ_j unschedulable, the preemption threshold γ_j of τ_j can be promoted to recover τ_j's schedulability if $\gamma_j < \gamma_j^{max}$. For any task τ_k with priority $\pi_i < \pi_k < \gamma_i$, this increment maybe make the blocking time of τ_k rise. From equation 4 we know that the blocking time for task τ_k is essentially a upper boundary which is almost impossible to attain, and make little difference in the worst-case response time of task τ_k in most of the situations, based on the theorem2 in [17].   □

Corollary 1. *The MPTA finds the preemption threshold assignment with the smallest possible total power consumptions.*

Proof. Theorem 3 in [13] shows that the MPTA finds the maximal preemption threshold assignment Γ^{max} with the essential property that $\Gamma^{max} \succ \Gamma$ for all $\Gamma \in \mathcal{G}(\mathcal{T})$. Combining this with theorem 1 proves this corollary. □

Given the real-time system $(\mathcal{T}, \Pi, \Gamma^I)$, how this minimal possible total power consumptions under MPTA can be produced practically? Algorithm 1 in the following accomplishes this goal efficiently.

Input: $(\mathcal{T}, \Pi, \Phi, \Gamma^I)$
Output: $[f_1^{opt}, f_2^{opt}, ..., f_n^{opt}]$
1 $\Gamma \leftarrow \Gamma^I$ /* initialize preemption threshold to identity assignment */
2 sort $\mathcal{T}$ by descending priority order
3 **for** $(i = 1; i \leq n; i \neq n)$ **do**
4   **while** $((\text{schedulable} = \textit{True})$ and $(f_i \neq FLK^1))$ **do**
5   **if** $(f_i = FLK^k)$ **then**
6 $f_i \leftarrow FLK^{k-1}$
7   **end**
8   **for** $(j = 1; j \leq \pi_i - 1; j \neq \pi_i - 1)$ **do**
9 $\textit{schedulable} \leftarrow$ False
10   **while** $((\text{schedulable} = \textit{False})$ and $(\gamma_j \leq n))$ **do**
11 $\textit{schedulable} = \text{SchedulabilityTest}(\tau_j)$
12   **if** $(\text{schedulable} = \textit{False})$ **then**
13 $\gamma_j \leftarrow \gamma_j + 1$
14   **end**
15   **end**
16   **if** $(\gamma_j \leq n)$ **then**
17 $\textit{schedulable} \leftarrow$ True
18   **end**
19   **else**
20 $f_i \leftarrow FLK^k$;
21   **end**
22   **end**
23   **for** $(k = \pi_i + 1; k \leq \gamma_i; j \neq \gamma_i)$ **do**
24 $\textit{schedulable} = \text{SchedulabilityTest}(\tau_k)$
25   **if** $(\text{schedulable} = \textit{False})$ **then**
26 $f_i \leftarrow FLK^k$;
27   **end**
28   **end**
29   **end**
30 **end**

Algorithm 1. FindMaxEnergySaving

The algorithm *FindMaxEnergySaving* examines the task set $\mathcal{T}$ from the task with highest regular priority to the task with lowest regular priority, when τ_i is considered, the processor speed for τ_i is relaxed tentatively, then other tasks's schedulability whose worst-case response time can be affected are checked, these tasks include any task τ_k with priority $\pi_k < \pi_i$ and any other task τ'_k with priority $\pi_i < \pi_k \le \gamma_i$. If some task's schedulability is compromised, the preemption threshold of the task would be promoted to regain its schedulability. If the preemption threshold of the task can be promoted already, thus the slowdown of τ_i would be infeasible.

5   Case Studies and Simulations

Section 4 showed that EE-FPPT will always render the controlled task preemptions and thus reduced energy consumptions that will maintain the schedulability of the workload. We now evaluate the impact of EE-FPPT on energy saving in two ways. First, we use EE-FPPT to schedule a real workload developed for controlling an Unmaned Aviation Vehicle (UAV). Second, we use randomly-generated workloads to examine broad trends across a range of design points.

Our experiments were accomplished on the Transmeta's Crusoe processor, which utilize the LongRun2 technology. LongRun2 technology is a suite of advanced power management, leakage control and process compensation technologies that can diminish the negative effects of increasing leakage power and process variations in advanced nanoscale designs, software could adjust Mhz and voltage to most efficient power level.

5.1   Paparazzi Benchmark

The Paparazzi project of Brisset and Drouin [18] targets a cheap fixed-wing autonomous UAV executing a predefined mission. Nemer et al. [19] used the Paparazzi project to develop a real-time benchmark called PapaBench. Papabench is composed of two workloads with tasks for controlling the servo system, and handling navigation and stabilization. In this section we used EE-FPPT to schedule and optimize the autopilot controller (MCU0) tasks from PapaBench listed in Table 2with their worst-case execution cycles (WCEC).

For this evaluation, we assume that the task precedence relationships and utilization are unknown and hence assume that a fully-preemptive scheduling approach is required.

The lowest possible maximum processor speed for each task was computed using the *lpps/RMS* algorithm by Youngsoo et al. [20]. This DVS-related technique make the number of task preemption rise by 95.8% (on the worst-case condition), then the application of EE-FPPT scheduling scheme put a curb on this phenomenon, and make the the number of task preemption merely rise by 30.9% (under MPTA). This holds for the utilization levels examined (32% to 93%). Indeed, EE-FPPT with the MPTA provides us with a simple systematic method that can be applied directly to any real-time system independent of the fixed-priority assignment policy used.

Table 1. The real-time tasks composing the Fly-By-Wire benchmark

Task	Name	Frequency	WCEC
τ_1	manage_radio_orders	40Hz	17,191
τ_2	stabilization	20Hz	13,579
τ_3	send_data_to_servo	20Hz	5,640
τ_4	receive_GPS_data	4Hz	1,813
τ_5	navigation	4Hz	1,676
τ_6	altitude_control	4Hz	1,897
τ_7	climb_control	4Hz	1,697
τ_8	reporting_task	10Hz	3,154

5.2   Generic Real-Time Workloads

We next investigate workload characteristics that affect the limitation of task preemptions and energy saving optimality level attainable through EE-FPPT. We now simulate and analyze randomly generated systems of tasks to better understand EE-FPPT.

To cover a wide range of design points, 20,000 real-time task sets with 10 tasks each were randomly generated. These were created so 1000 have a utilization of 50%, 1000 have 52% utilization, and so on up to 90%. For each group of task sets who hold the same utilization, those were created so 20 have a C_i^{pc}/C_i of 50%, 20 have 51%, and so on up to 100%. Task periods have a normal distribution with a mean, $\bar{T}$, of 100 time units and a standard deviation, σ_T, of 15%, 45%, and 75%, respectively. Moreover, task deadlines were set equal to their respective periods (for simplicity, though not necessary). Tasks' WCETs were set to incur the required overall system utilization. Tasks' associated processor clock frequencies were calculated by *lpps/RMS* algorithm [20]. All 20,000 real-time task sets generated were schedulable with a fully preemptive policy.

We first investigate the effect of the limited task preemption on the DVS-used real-time task sets using EE-FPPT. Using the MPTAA, the number of task preemptions required by each system was computed. The average normalized number of preemptions were then plotted as a function of the overall system utilization. The results are shown in figures 1(a) and 1(b).

We then investigate the effect of the system utilization on the minimal power consumption achieved by EE-FPPT. Using the MPTA, the minimal power consumption produced by each system was computed and normalized to the power consumption required by the fully-preemptive version of the system. The average normalized power consumptions were then plotted as a function of the overall system utilization and the standard deviation in the task periods. The results are shown in figures 2(a).

At low utilizations the systems power requirements might be less than 30% of those of a fully preemptive system. However, at higher utilization levels, the variation in the tasksperiods increasingly affects the savings attainable. With $\sigma_T = 15\%$ the savings are only slightly dependent on the utilization level. On

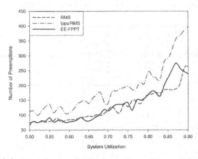 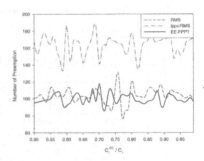

(a) Number of Preemption rise with system utilization for EE-FPPT, but decline compared with some DVS-related methods

(b) Number of Preemption fluctuate with the increment of processor-intensive instructions's percent, on the condition that system utilization = 0.67

Fig. 1. Experiment results for limited preemption of EE-FPPT

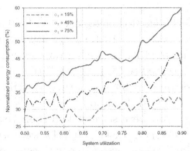 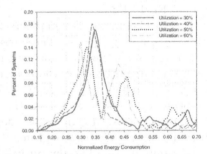

(a) Power consumption produced for EE-FPPT rises with both task period variability and system utilization

(b) EE-FPPT dramatically accomplishes the energy savings, even for high-utilization systems

Fig. 2. Experiment results for power saving of EE-FPPT

the other hand, as the standard deviation of the periods increases, the savings attainable decrease significantly at higher utilizations. This can be attributed to the fact that for systems with large variations in their periods it is much harder to maintain the systems schedulability while minimizing preemptions. For example, if a system contains two tasks that have a large difference in frequencies, it is difficult, if not impossible, to limit the higher frequency task from preempting the slower while maintaining system schedulability. This becomes very apparent at high-utilization system where there is much less slack time.

Another interesting property is the distribution of the 20,000 systems among the different normalized power consumption levels. Figure 2(b) show this distribution for the overall system utilization levels of 30%, 40%, 50%, and 60%, respectively. As can be seen, the workloads scheduled with the fixed-priority schemes depend on the system utilization level to some extent.

6   Conclusions

We have discussed the possible side effects of a DVS algorithm on the system energy consumption, and investigated using preemption threshold scheduling to reduce the number of task preemptions while keeping the energy efficiencies of the existing DVS algorithms. Two major contributions have been presented. First, response time analysis for EE-FPPT with a given priority assignment has been described. Second, an efficient algorithm that assigns the optimal preemption threshold configuration has been presented to maximize the energy savings of a task set. Our experimental results show that EE-FPPT under MPTA can accomplish the least number of preemption, minimal power consumption as the same time keep the schedulability of task set.

References

1. Kim, W., Kim, J., Min, S.L.: A dynamic voltage scaling algorithm for dynamic-priority hard real-time systems using slack time analysis. In: Paris, F. (ed.) Design, Automation and Test in Europe Conference and Exposition, pp. 788–794. IEEE Computer Society, Los Alamitos (2002)
2. Kim, W., Kim, J., Min, S.L.: Dynamic voltage scaling algorithm for fixed-priority real-time systems using work-demand analysis. In: Roh, I.V., Hyung (eds.) ISLPED, Seoul, Korea, pp. 396–401. ACM, New York (2003)
3. Sakurai, T., Newton, A.R.: Alpha-power law mosfet model and its applications to cmos inverterdelay and other formulas. IEEE Journal of Solid-State Circuits 25(2), 584–594 (1990)
4. Padmanabhan Pillai, K.G.S.: Real-time dynamic voltage scaling for low-power embedded operating systems. In: 18th ACM Symposium on Operating System Principles, Chateau Lake Louise, Banff, Alberta, Canada, vol. 35, pp. 89–102. ACM, New York (2001)
5. Kim, W., Shin, D., Yun, H.S., Kim, J., Min, S.L.: Performance comparison of dynamic voltage scaling algorithms for hard real-time systems. In: 8th IEEE Real Time Technology and Applications Symposium, San Jose, CA, USA, pp. 219–228. IEEE Computer Society, Los Alamitos (2002)
6. Lee, S., Min, S.L., Kim, C.-S., Lee, C.-G., Lee, M.: Cache-conscious limited preemptive scheduling. Real-Time Systems 17(2-3), 257–282 (1999)
7. Saewong, S., Rajkumar, R.: Practical voltage-scaling for fixed-priority rt-systems. In: 9th IEEE Real-Time and Embedded Technology and Applications Symposium, Toronto, Canada, p. 106. IEEE Computer Society, Los Alamitos (2003)
8. Vishnu Swaminathan, K.C.: Pruning-based, energy-optimal, deterministic i/o device scheduling for hard real-time systems. ACM Transactions on Embeded Computing Systems 4(1), 141–167 (2005)
9. Liu, C.L., Layland, J.W.: Scheduling algorithms for multiprogramming in a hard-real-time environment. Journal of the ACM 20(1), 46–61 (1973)
10. George, L., Nicolas Rivierre, M.S.: Preemptive and non-preemptive real-time uniprocessor scheduling. Technical Report RR-2966, INRIA, France (1996)

11. Manas Saksena, Y.W.: Scalable real-time system design using preemption thresholds. In: 21st IEEE Real-Time Systems Symposium, pp. 25–34 (2000)
12. Wang, Y., Saksena, M.: Scheduling fixed-priority tasks with preemption threshold. In: 6th International Workshop on Real-Time Computing and Applications Symposium, Hong Kong, China, pp. 328–335. IEEE Computer Society, Los Alamitos (1999)
13. Chen, J., Ashif Harji, P.B.: Solution space for fixed-priority with preemption threshold. In: 11th IEEE Real Time and Embedded Technology and Applications Symposium (RTAS 2005), San Francisco, CA, USA, pp. 385–394. IEEE Computer Society Press, Los Alamitos (2005)
14. Regehr, J.: Scheduling tasks with mixed preemption relations for robustness to timing faults. In: IEEE Real-Time Systems Symposium, pp. 315–326 (2002)
15. Muller, F.: Timing analysis for instruction caches. Real-Time Systems 18(2/3), 217–247 (2000)
16. Park, C.Y.: Predicting program execution times by analyzing static and dynamic program paths. Real-Time Systems 5(1), 31–62 (1993)
17. Chen, J.: Extensions to Fixed Priority with PreemptionThreshold and Reservation-Based Schedulin. Ph.D thesis, University of Waterloo (2005)
18. University, E.: The paparazzi project (2007)
19. Nemer, F., Cassé, H., Sainrat, P., Bahsoun, J.P., De Michiel, M.: Papabench: a free real-time benchmark. In: Mueller, F. (ed.) 6th Intl. Workshop on Worst-Case Execution Time (WCET) Analysis, Germany, Internationales Begegnungs- und Forschungszentrum fuer Informatik (IBFI), Schloss Dagstuhl, Germany. Dagstuhl Seminar Proceedings, vol. 06902 (2006)
20. Shin, Y., Choi, K., Sakurai, T.: Power optimization of real-time embedded systems on variable speed processors. In: Sentovich, E. (ed.) 2000 IEEE/ACM International Conference on Computer-Aided Design, San Jose, California, USA, IEEE, Los Alamitos (2000)

Learning and Inferences of the Bayesian Network with Maximum Likelihood Parameters*

JiaDong Zhang, Kun Yue, and WeiYi Liu

Department of Computer Science and Engineering,
School of Information Science and Engineering, Yunnan University,
Kunming, 650091, P.R. China
jiadongzhang@yahoo.cn

Abstract. In real applications established on Bayesian networks (BNs), it is necessary to make inference for arbitrary evidence even it is not contained in existing conditional probability tables (CPTs). Aiming at this problem, in this paper, we discuss the learning and inferences of the BN with maximum likelihood parameters that replace the CPTs. We focus on the learning of the maximum likelihood parameters and give the corresponding methods for 2 kinds of BN inferences: forward inferences and backward inferences. Furthermore, we give the approximate inference method of BNs with maximum likelihood hypotheses. Preliminary experiments show the feasibility of our proposed methods.

Keywords: Bayesian network, Inference, Maximum likelihood hypothesis, Support vector machine, Sigmoid.

1 Introduction

In real applications, it is necessary to make probabilistic inference for a set of query variables according to some observed evidence. Fortunately, the Bayesian network is a powerful uncertain knowledge representation and reasoning tool, which is widely studied and applied [1], [2], [3].

The basic task for BN inferences is to compute the posterior probability distribution for a set of query variables by search result, given some observed evidence. For example, in Fig. 1, we can deduce the probability distribution for *cholesterol standards* of somebody whose *age* is 60. However, some queries are often submitted on arbitrary evidence values. For example, if we know John is 65 years old, how to deduce the probability distribution for his *cholesterol standards*? One the other hand, if we know his *cholesterol standard* is 160, how to deduce the probability distribution for his *age*? These 2 questions are said to be the forward inference and the backward inference with a BN respectively.

The ordinary inference with the BN by search cannot answer the above 2 questions, since there is no data about patients of 65 years old and 160 *cholesterol standard* in the existing CPTs. For the forward inference, we discussed the

* This work was supported by the National Natural Science Foundation of China (No. 60763007) and the Cultivation Project for Backbone Teachers of Yunnan University.

C. Tang et al. (Eds.): ADMA 2008, LNAI 5139, pp. 391–399, 2008.

A	P(A)
a_1=60	0.3
a_2=70	0.2
a_3=80	0.3
a_4=90	0.2

A · C

P(C|A)	a_1=60	...	a_4=90	a'=65
c_1=150	2/3	...	0	$h_{c1}(a')$
c_2=170	1/3	...	0	$h_{c2}(a')$
c_3=190	0	...	1	$h_{c3}(a')$

Fig. 1. The BN with the maximum likelihood hypothesis for a'

A	P(A)
a_1=60	0.3
a_2=70	0.2
a_3=80	0.3
a_4=90	0.2

A · C

P(C|A)	A=a
c_1=150	$h_{c1}(a)$
c_2=170	$h_{c2}(a)$
c_3=190	$h_{c3}(a)$

Fig. 2. The BN with maximum likelihood hypotheses

inference method via learning maximum likelihood hypotheses (i.e., the column corresponding to $a' = 65$ in Fig. 1) from data to compute posterior probability distributions for arbitrary evidence values [4]. A *maximum likelihood hypothesis* is an hypothesis that maximizes the probability of appearance of original samples [5].

In order to compute posterior probability distributions for arbitrary evidence values, the method given in [4] needs concern original samples to find the maximum likelihood hypothesis during inferences. Actually, the probabilistic inference in a BN generally just applies the conditional probability parameters instead of concerning the original samples. In addition, the scales of CPTs are often large and difficult to be maintained when the size of sample data is great. Thus, in this paper, we look upon the maximum likelihood parameters as the component of a BN replacing the conventional CPTs. We are to mainly discuss the learning method for parameters of maximum likelihood hypotheses when a BN is constructed from data [6]. The desired BN corresponding to Fig. 1 is shown in Fig. 2. Therefore, we concentrate on how to obtain the BN like Fig. 2, on which the forward inference can be made accordingly.

Following, as for the backward inference, we are to give the method based on the Bayes formula and linear interpolation for parameters of maximum likelihood hypotheses.

To sum up, centered on learning the parameters of maximum likelihood hypotheses, the forward and backward inferences can be addressed.

Fortunately, support vector machine (SVM) is a new machine learning method based on the structural risk minimization principle from statistical learning theory [7]. SVMs are learning systems that use a hypothesis space of linear functions in a high dimensional feature space and SVMs are quite suitable for the learning on small sample [8]. Furthermore, by training the parameters of an additional sigmoid function, the SVM outputs can be mapped into probabilities [9].

Based on the SVM, the maximum likelihood hypothesis with non-probabilistic outputs can be obtained by using the samples to train the SVM, and the non-probabilistic outputs of the SVM can be mapped into the probabilities via fitting a sigmoid for according with the requirement of BNs.

Further, since exact inference in large and connected networks is difficult [1], we are to give a improved Gibbs sampling algorithm for approximate probabilistic inference of BNs with maximum likelihood hypotheses.

Generally, the main contributions of this paper can be summarized as follows:

- We give the method to learn the BN with maximum likelihood parameters to replace the conventional CPTs. Therefore, the BN can be applied to the inferences even the given evidence is not contained in the CPTs.
- Based on BN with maximum likelihood parameters, we give the methods for forward inference and backward inference respectively.

2   Bayesian Networks with Maximum Likelihood Hypothesis

In this section, we focus on the learning of the maximum likelihood parameters and give the corresponding methods for 2 kinds of BN inferences: forward inferences and backward inferences.

2.1   Maximum Likelihood Hypothesis Based on the SVM and Sigmoid

It is known that SVM classification is to construct an optimal hyperplane, with the maximal marginal of separation between 2 classes [8]. By introducing the kernel function, SVMs can handle non-linear feature spaces and carry out the training considering combinations of more than one feature [8].

The unthresholded output of the standard 2-*classes* (i.e., *class* $\in \{-1, 1\}$) SVM [7] is

$$f(x) = \sum_{i=1}^{n} y_i \alpha_i k(x_i, x) + b, \tag{1}$$

where n is the number of sample and $k(x_i, x)$ is a kernel function.

Obviously, the output f is not a probability, where $f = f(x)$. To map the SVM outputs into probabilities, we adopt the method that applies a parametric model to fit the posterior $P(y = 1|f)$ (i.e., $P(class|input)$) directly. And the parameters of the model should be adapted to give the best probability outputs. The probability $P(y = 1|f)$ should be monotonic in f, since the SVM is trained to separate most or all of positive examples from negative examples. Moreover $P(y = 1|f)$ should lie between 0 and 1. Bayes' rule suggests using a parametric form of a sigmoid [9]:

$$P(y = 1|f) = \frac{1}{1 + \exp(\beta f + \gamma)}. \tag{2}$$

This means that if the maximum likelihood hypothesis $h = P(y = 1|f)$ has been obtained (i.e., parameters α, β and γ have been obtained), the posterior probability distribution $P(y|f(x))$ for query variable y can be easily computed, given arbitrary evidence values x by the following method. First the non- probabilistic output $f(x)$ of the SVM can be computed based on equation (1). Then the non-probabilistic output of the SVM can be mapped into the probability $P(y = 1|f(x))$ based on equation (2).

Note that it is known SVM and sigmoid need be trained and be fitted respectively for obtaining parameters α, β and γ. The methods for learning relevant parameters of the maximum likelihood hypothesis will be introduced in Subsection 2.2 and Subsection 2.3 respectively.

2.2 Training the SVM for Obtaining Parameters α

Here we are to train the SVM for obtaining the parameters α.

In a BN, each node corresponds to a variable, denoted as y, and the set of parents of y is denoted as x. Through extracting the values of variables x and y from the original samples for constructing the BN, the training set, denoted as $\{(x_i, y_i)\}$, can be easily obtained for the node. Then the parameters α can be solved by the conventional methods [7]:

$$\begin{cases} \min_{\alpha} \frac{1}{2} \sum_{i=1}^{n} \sum_{j=1}^{n} y_i y_j \alpha_i \alpha_j k(x_i, x_j) - \sum_{i=1}^{n} \alpha_i \\ s.t. \sum_{i=1}^{n} y_i \alpha_i = 0 \\ \quad 0 \le \alpha_i \le c, \ i = 1, \cdots, n \end{cases} \tag{3}$$

where $k(x_i, x)$ is a kernel function.

2.3 Fitting the Sigmoid for Obtaining Parameters β and γ

The parameters β and γ can be fitted based on maximum likelihood estimation from a training set $\{(f_i, t_i)\}$, which is defined based on the training set $\{(x_i, y_i)\}$ as follows:

- In Subsection 2.2, we obtain the parameters α, so f_i can be obtained based on the following equation:
$$f_i = f(x_i). \tag{4}$$

- t_i, which is the target probability, can be obtained based on the following equation:
$$t_i = \frac{y_i + 1}{2}. \tag{5}$$

Consequently, the sigmoid can be fitted by the following method.

The parameters β and γ are found by minimizing the negative log likelihood of the training set $\{(f_i, t_i)\}$, which is a cross-entropy error function [9]:

$$\min_{\beta, \gamma} - \sum_{i=1}^{n} t_i \log(p_i) + (1 - t_i) \log(1 - p_i), \tag{6}$$

where

$$p_i = \frac{1}{1 + \exp(\beta f_i + \gamma)}.$$

However, based on equations (4) and (5), two issues arise in the optimization problem (6): a biased estimate of the distribution of f out of the training set $\{(x_i, y_i)\}$ and over-fitting this set. Cross-validation method is applied for forming an unbiased training set of the output of the SVM f_i. On the other hand, to avoid over-fitting this set, the equation (5) is replaced by the following equation [9]:

$$t_i = \begin{cases} \frac{N_+ + 1}{N_+ + 2} & y_i = 1 \\ \frac{1}{N_- + 2} & y_i = -1 \end{cases} \tag{7}$$

where N_+ and N_- denote the number of positive examples (i.e., $y_i = 1$) and negative examples (i.e., $y_i = -1$) in the training set $\{(x_i, y_i)\}$ respectively.

Till now, based on the BN structure and the maximum likelihood parameters, the forward inference can be done for arbitrary evidence values.

2.4 Backward Inference of the BN with Maximum Likelihood Hypotheses

The definitions of x and y are the same as those in Subsection 2.2. According to the arbitrary evidence value y' of y, the posterior probability distribution $P(x|y')$, namely backward inference, can be obtained by the following method.

First, the backward inference $P(x|y')$ can be transformed into the forward inference $P(y'|x)$ by the Bayes formula:

$$P(x|y') = \frac{P(y'|x)P(x)}{P(y')}. \tag{8}$$

In equation (8), $P(y'|x)$ can be obtained by linear interpolation for parameters of maximum likelihood hypotheses, $P(x)$ can be obtained directly by maximum likelihood hypotheses, and $P(y')$ is merely a scale factor that can be ignored during computation.

Suppose $y_i \le y' \le y_j$ and $y_i \ne y_j$, $P(y'|x)$ can be obtained by the following linear interpolation equation [10]:

$$P(y'|x) = \frac{y' - y_i}{y_j - y_i} P(y_i|x) + \frac{y_j - y'}{y_j - y_i} P(y_j|x), \tag{9}$$

where y_i and y_j are two adjacent state values of the variable y, and $P(y_i|x)$ and $P(y_j|x)$ can be obtained directly by maximum likelihood hypotheses.

Thus, the backward inference of the BN with maximum likelihood hypotheses can be solved by the following method. First, the backward inference can be transformed into the forward inference based on equation (8). Then linear interpolation for parameters of maximum likelihood hypotheses is applied for computing corresponding posterior probability distributions by equation (9). The details are interpreted by the following example.

Example 1. Assume the maximum likelihood hypotheses $h_{c_1}(a)$, $h_{c_2}(a)$ and $h_{c_3}(a)$ have been obtained in Figure 2, considering computing posterior probability distribution $P(A|c' = 160)$:

Step1. According to equation (8),

$$P(a_1|c' = 160) = \frac{P(c' = 160|a_1)P(a_1)}{P(c' = 160)} = 0.3kP(c' = 160|a_1),$$

where $P(a_1) = 0.3$ and $k = 1/P(c' = 160)$.

Step2. According to equation (9),

$$\begin{aligned}
P(c' = 160|a_1) &= \tfrac{c'-c_1}{c_2-c_1}P(c_1|a_1) + \tfrac{c_2-c'}{c_2-c_1}P(c_2|a_1) \\
&= 0.5h_{c_1}(a_1) + 0.5h_{c_2}(a_1) \\
&= 0.5(1/3 + 2/3) = 0.5.
\end{aligned}$$

Therefore, we have $P(a_1|c' = 160) = 0.15k$. Analogously, we have $P(a_2|c' = 160) = 0.1k$, $P(a_3|c' = 160) = 0.05k$ and $P(a_4|c' = 160) = 0$. After normalization, we can obtain $P(a_1|c' = 160) = 1/2$, $P(a_2|c' = 160) = 1/3$, $P(a_3|c' = 160) = 1/6$ and $P(a_4|c' = 160) = 0$.

By virtue of the above basic ideas of forward and backward inferences, following we give an algorithm for approximate inferences on a BN with maximum likelihood parameters.

3   Approximate Inference of Bayesian Networks with Maximum Likelihood Hypothesis

The intractability of exact inference of interval probability is obvious. Based on the property of Markov blankets, we consider adopting Gibbs sampling algorithm [2] for approximate inference with the BN. A Markov blanket $MB(x)$ [1] of a node x in a BN is any subset $S(x \notin S)$ of nodes for which x is independent of $U - S - x$ given S, where U is a finite set of nodes. We extend the Gibbs-sampling probabilistic algorithm to the BN with maximum likelihood hypotheses in Algorithm 1, which also has been proved to be convergent [4].

Algorithm 1. Approximate inference in Bayesian networks with maximum likelihood hypotheses

Input:

   BN: a Bayesian network with maximum likelihood hypotheses

   $\overrightarrow{Z}$: the nonevidence nodes in BN

   $\overrightarrow{E}$: the evidence nodes in BN

   x: the query variable

   $\overrightarrow{e}$: the set of values of the evidence nodes $\overrightarrow{E}$

   n: the total number of samples to be generated

Output: The estimates of $P(x|e)$.

Variables:

   $\overrightarrow{z}$: the set of values of the nonevidence nodes $\overrightarrow{Z}$

   $N_x(x_i)(i = 1, \cdots, n)$: a vector of counts over probabilities of x_i, where $x_i(i = 1, \cdots, n)$ is the value of x.

Step1. Initialization:

$\vec{z} \leftarrow$ random values;

$\vec{e} \leftarrow$ evidence values of $\vec{E}$;

$N_x(x_i) \leftarrow 0 \ (i = 1, \cdots, n)$

Step2. For $i \leftarrow 1$ to n do

(1) Compute the probability values $P(x_i|MB(x))$ of x in the next state where $MB(x)$ is the set of the current values in the Markov blanket of x. $P(x_i|MB(x))$ can be obtained based on the maximum likelihood hypotheses.

(2) Generate a random number r, where r is uniformly distributed over $(0,1)$, we determine the values of x:

$$
x = \begin{cases}
x_1 & r \leq P(x_1|MB(x)) \\
x_2 & P(x_1|MB(x)) < r \leq P(x_1|MB(x)) + P(x_2|MB(x)) \\
\vdots & \vdots
\end{cases}
$$

(3) Count:

If $x = x_i$ then $N_x(x_i) \leftarrow N_x(x_i) + 1$

Step3. Estimate $P(x|e)$:

$P(x_i|e) \leftarrow N_x(x_i)/n$.

Note that here Algorithm 1 is different from have been shown in [4], since the computation of $P(x_i|MB(x))$ in Setp2 is independent of CPTs, which is obtained based on maximum likelihood hypotheses and linear interpolation for parameters of maximum likelihood hypotheses.

4   Experimental Results

To verify the feasibility of our proposed methods in this paper, we tested their accuracy and effectiveness for learning maximum likelihood hypotheses. Let us consider the database concerning *America Cleveland heart disease diagnosis* downloaded from UCI machine learning repository [11]. In order to focus on the idea of our proposed method, we only consider the 4-attributes of *age*, *resting blood pressure* (mm Hg), *serum cholesterol* (mg/dl) and *diagnosis* of *heart disease* (the predicted attribute), which are denoted as variables A, B, C and D respectively.

By the existing method to construct BNs from sample data [6], we can obtain the structure of the BN G shown in Fig. 3, in which $D = \{0,1\}$ represents absence and presence of heart disease in the patient respectively.

Based on the structure of Fig. 3, we first computed CPTs for the 4-attributes using the BN learning tool - PowerConstructor [6]. Then we learned maximum likelihood hypotheses h_B, h_C and h_D based on our proposed method. Finally, the posterior probability distributions corresponding to CPTs can be obtained. Consequently, errors were obtained by the absolute values of the posterior probability distributions learned by our proposed method minus the corresponding conditional probabilities computed by PowerConstructor.

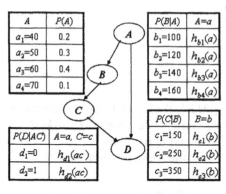

Table 1. Errors on the maximum likelihood hypothesis H_D

age(A)	serum cholesterol(C)	Error
40	150	0.2495
40	250	0.1627
40	350	0.0352
40	450	0.0005
50	150	0.0776
⋮	⋮	⋮
70	150	0.0495
70	250	0.1066
70	350	0.0630
70	450	0.0005

Fig. 3. The structure of the Bayesian network G

We specifically considered 16 different combinational states of *Age* and *serum cholesterol* (mg/dl) for *diagnosis*. Errors are given in Table 1. Then, the general maximum, minimal and average errors are 0.2495, 0.0005 and 0.0871 respectively.

From above results of the accuracy tests, we can conclude that our proposed method is effective and accurate to a great extent, and thus can be applied into corresponding inferences in disease diagnosis.

5   Conclusion and Future Work

In this paper, we focus on the learning of the maximum likelihood parameters and give the corresponding methods for 2 kinds of BN inferences: forward inferences and backward inferences. Furthermore, we give the approximate inference method of BNs with maximum likelihood hypotheses. Preliminary experiments show the feasibility of our proposed methods. Our methods also raise some other interesting research issues. For example, the method to learn the maximum likelihood hypotheses uses based on their inverse functions instead of linear interpolation can be further studied.

References

1. Pearl, J.: Probabilistic reasoning in intelligent systems: network of plausible inference. Morgen Kaufmann publishers, Inc., San Mates (1998)
2. Heckerman, D., Wellman, M.P.: Bayesian networks. Communication of the ACM 38(3), 27–30 (1995)
3. Russel, S.J., Norving, P.: Artificial intelligence - a modern approach. Pearson Education Inc., Prentice-Hall (2002)
4. Liu, W.Y., Yue, K., Zhang, J.D.: Augmenting Learning Function to Bayesian Network Inferences with Maximum Likelihood Parameters. Expert Systems with Applications: An International Journal, ESWA 41(2) (to appear, 2008)

5. Mitchell, T.M.: Machine Learning. McGraw-Hill Companies, Inc, New York (1997)
6. Cheng, J., Greiner, R., Kelly, J., Bell, D., Liu, W.: Learning Bayesian network from data: an information-theory based approach. Artificial Intelligence 137(2), 43–90 (2002)
7. Vapnik, V.: Statistical learning theory. John Wiley and Sons, Inc., Chichester (1998)
8. Burges, C.J.C.: A tutorial on support vector machines for pattern recognition. Data Mining and Knowledge Discovery 2(2), 121–167 (1998)
9. Platt, J.C.: Probabilistic Outputs for Support Vector Machines and Comparisons to Regularized Likelihood Methods. In: Advances in Large Margin Classifiers (1999)
10. Bergh, J., Lofstrom, J.: Interpolation Spaces an Introduction. Springer, Inc., Heidelberg (1976)
11. http://www.ics.uci.edu/~mlearn/MLRepository.html (2007)

TARtool: A Temporal Dataset Generator for Market Basket Analysis

Asem Omari, Regina Langer, and Stefan Conrad

Heinrich-Heine University Duesseldorf
Institute of Computer Science
Databases and Information Systems
Duesseldorf, Germany
{omari,conrad}@cs.uni-duesseldorf.de,
Regina.Langer@uni-duesseldorf.de

Abstract. The problem of finding a suitable dataset to test different data mining algorithms and techniques and specifically association rule mining for Market Basket Analysis is a big challenge. A lot of dataset generators have been implemented in order to overcome this problem. ARtool is a tool that generates synthetic datasets and runs association rule mining for Market Basket Analysis. But the lack of datasets that include timestamps of the transactions to facilitate the analysis of Market Basket data taking into account temporal aspects is notable. In this paper, we present the TARtool. The TARtool is a data mining and generation tool based on the ARtool. TARtool is able to generate datasets with timestamps for both retail and e-commerce environments taking into account general customer buying habits in such environments. We implemented the generator to produce datasets with different format to ease the process of mining such datasets in other data mining tools. An advanced GUI is also provided. The experimental results showed that our tool overcomes other tools in efficiency, usability, functionality, and quality of generated data.

1 Introduction

Data mining is the process of finding interesting information from large databases. An important field of research in data mining is Market Basket Analysis. The authors in [1] list the most challenging problems in data mining research. One of that problems is mining sequence data and time series data. Temporal data mining [2] is the process of mining databases that have time granularities. The goal is to find patterns which repeat over time and their periods, or finding the repeating patterns of a time-related database as well as the interval which corresponds to the pattern period [3]. The work presented in [4] studies the problem of association rules that exist in certain time intervals and thus display regular cyclic variations over time.

Association rule mining is the main task to perform Market Basket Analysis. The purpose of association rule mining is to describe strong relationships

C. Tang et al. (Eds.): ADMA 2008, LNAI 5139, pp. 400–410, 2008.

between objects or items of the transactions by means of implication rules of the form $X \Rightarrow Y$, where X and Y are sets of items and have no items in common. Given a database of transactions D where each transaction $T \in D$ is a set of items, $X \Rightarrow Y$ denotes that whenever a transaction T contains X then there is a probability that it contains Y too. The rule $X \Rightarrow Y$ holds in the transactions set T with confidence c if $c\%$ of transactions in T that contain X also contain Y. The rule has support s in T if $s\%$ of all transactions in T contains both X and Y. Association rule mining is finding all association rules that have support and confidence values greater than or equal a user-specified minimum support ($minsup$), and minimum confidence ($minconf$) respectively. Recently, researchers aim not only finding relationships between different items in the market basket, but also finding an answer to important questions with temporal dimensions such as:

- Are there any relationships between items and specific days of the week?
- Which temporal dependencies exist between distinct items?
- Which seasonal distances exist between the purchase of the same item?
- How does the selling behavior of a set of products change over time?

Because of the increasing importance of temporal data mining as an interesting field of research, researchers look for datasets that have temporal attributes to test, develop, or improve their algorithms for temporal data mining. Those algorithms may also be of interest in many other topics of research that imply a temporal aspect such as weather data, or stock market data. Unfortunately, the availability of temporal data for downloading from the web is very low, especially when we talk about temporal Market Basket data. This unavailability of suitable datasets leads to the conclusion, that we need to generate Market Basket datasets with timestamps to test, and develop data mining algorithms taking into account temporal granularities. This paper is structured as follows: in section 2 we investigate the problem of the availability of datasets for Market Basket Analysis, we also make a comparison between real world and synthetic datasets. Then, in section 3, we discuss some well-known dataset generators and the available software solutions. The detailed description of TARtool is presented in section 4. We evaluate our tool in section 5. Finally, in section 6, we summarize our paper and present some ideas for future work.

2   Datasets for Market Basket Analysis

Since Market Basket Analysis is an important tool for improved marketing, many software solutions are available for this purpose. Business tools like *Microsoft SQL Server 2005*, or *IBM DB2 Data Warehouse* focus on the analysis of relational business data. Software tools which are available for free download like ARMiner [5], ARtool [6], or WEKA [7], are more dedicated to research. They do not only analyze data but also give additional information on the effectiveness of algorithms performed. So, in order to generate data to be used by those tools, we have to investigate which kinds of datasets can be generated.

2.1 Datasets for Association Rule Mining

A normal transaction consists of a transaction-id and a list of items in every row or sentence. Sometimes, the items are represented as boolean values 0 if the item is not bought, or 1 if the item is bought. But the commonly used format for Market Basket data is that of numeric values for items without any other information:

```
1 3 5 9 11 20 31 45 49
3 7 11 12 15 20 43...
```

This format has to be converted in order to be used by ARMiner and ARtool, since those tools can only evaluate binary data. ARMiner and ARtool have a special converter for that purpose which have to be performed before analyzing the data. WEKA needs a special ASCII-Data format (*.arff) for data analysis containing information about the attributes and a boolean representation of the items. Since there is no unique format for input-data, it is impossible to evaluate the same dataset in one format with different tools. In this paper, we present a dataset generator that is able to generate datasets that are readable by ARMiner, ARtool, WEKA and other data mining tools. Additionally, the generator has the ability to produce large Market Basket datasets with timestamps to simulate transactions in both retail and e-commerce environments.

2.2 Real World versus Synthetic Datasets

In the beginning of data mining research, generated data was mostly used to test or develop algorithms for Market Basket Analysis. Meanwhile, there are both generated and real world datasets available for download which can be found on data mining related websites. But both types of data suffer from disadvantages. Real world datasets can be influenced or made unusable by:

- Uncomplete or missing attributes
- Seasonal influences like religious occasions
- Marketing for special products
- Good or bad weather
- Location e.g. in or outside the town.

Therefore, some researchers prefer generated datasets. But they also have some drawbacks such as:

- The quality of the data depends on the generator used
- They do not really reflect customers purchasing habits
- Algorithms performances differ when performed on generated data

The study in [8] compares five well-known association rule algorithms using three real-world datasets and an artificial dataset from IBM Almaden. The authors showed that algorithms (APRIORI, FP-Growth, Closet, Charm and Magnum-Opus) do not have the same effectiveness on generated data as they have on real world data. Hahsler et al. showed in [9] visually the differences between simulated data and supermarket data. They found that support and confidence of itemsets with a small support are higher in supermarket data than in generated data.

3   Dataset Generators and Software Solutions

There are many software solutions for data mining, and specifically Market Basket Analysis. The following tools belong to the well-known data mining and generation software solutions.

3.1   The IBM Generator

In the literature, a lot of researchers use the IBM generator [10] provided by the Almaden Research Center to run their experiments and test their algorithms. This generator is no longer provided by IBM, and other implementations written in C/C++, which are available for download, produce compile errors when executed.

3.2   An E-Commerce Generator

The dataset generator developed by Groblschegg [11] produces datasets for an e-commerce Market Basket. It depends on Ehrenberg's *Repeat-Buying-Theory* [12], which refers to seasonal customer habits. Ehrenberg used for his studies the so-called *consumer panels* to derive information on the intervals consumer used to purchase certain products. The generator of Groblschegg uses these intervals to generate Market Basket data by producing purchasing timestamps for each product and customer on a time axis. This time axis is cut by the intervals into transactions for every customer. The generator produces timestamps for the transactions as decimal numbers between 0 and 1, which are not really suitable for temporal data mining, because they cannot be mapped to attributes like specific day of a week, or hour of a day.

3.3   ARMiner

ARMiner [5] is a tool for data mining from the University of Boston, Massachusetts. As mentioned before, it can analyze binary sequential datasets by performing different algorithms. It finds frequent itemsets, and association rules depending on the specified minimum support and confidence values. Effectiveness of algorithms can be benchmarked by execution time and required passes over the dataset. Datasets and algorithms can be added dynamically. Furthermore, there is a test data generator available. The software is executed in the command line. There is no GUI. It is written in Java and can be maintained as necessary.

3.4   The ARtool Generator

ARtool [6] is an enhancement of ARMiner, with nearly the same capability. It is now executed by using a GUI. A few functions can only be executed in the command line. It has some more algorithms implemented, but it can only analyze the same binary datasets as ARMiner. ARtool has also a test data generator.

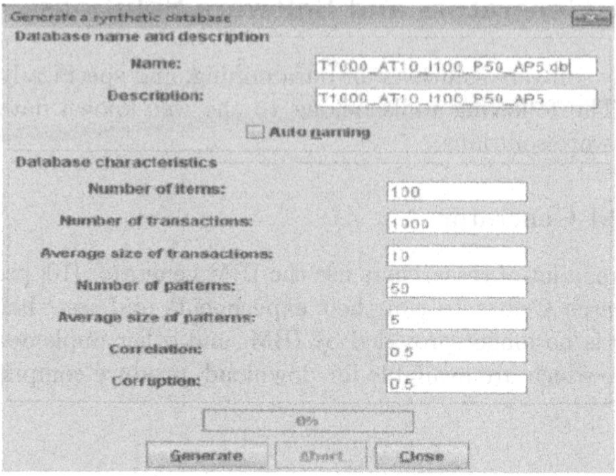

Fig. 1. ARtool GUI

The ARtool Generator is a Java implementation of the IBM Generator. It uses the parameters and variables described by Agrawal et al. in [10] to generate Market Basket data. The parameters, which are entered in a panel of the GUI (see Fig. 1), are as follows:

- Name and description of the dataset produced
- Number of items
- Number of transactions
- Average size of transactions
- Number of patterns
- Average size of pattern
- Correlation level
- Corruption level

Defaults are provided and a progress bar shows the generation process. The output is, as mentioned, a sequential binary dataset with a header containing dataset name, description, the generated item names $C_1, ..., C_n$, the number of transactions and items, and consecutively the transactions. To read this format, it has to be converted by a conversion tool provided by ARtool. The conversion tool can only be executed in the command line, not in the GUI.

3.5 WEKA

WEKA [7] is a tool designed for evaluating special ASCII-Datasets and relational data. It gives information on the effectiveness of algorithms and can visualize results. In general, it has much more functionality than ARMiner or ARtool, but it has no dataset generator available.

From previous, we can say that there is no tool designed for the purpose of temporal data mining. Furthermore, there is no algorithm in any tool on-hand, that can generate dataset with timestamp functionality. What we need is

a dataset generator to generate temporal Market Basket data to ease the process
of Market Basket Analysis.

4   Enhancements for ARtool

As a result, we can say that ARtool synthetic dataset generator is the mostly
referred to and used generator. TARtool is an enhancement to the ARtool. TAR-
tool includes the following enhancements:

- Generate datasets for retail and e-commerce environments
- Generate a timestamp for each transaction
- Generate dataset that are readable by ARtool, WEKA, and other data min-
  ing tools
- The possibility to mine those temporal datasets with algorithms provided in
  both tools and other data mining tools

All these features can be entered as parameters in the GUI. An example is
provided in Fig. 2. New parameters to enter are:

- Check box for dataset generation with timestamps
- Startdate and enddate for the timestamps of the generated dataset
- Buttons to choose between dataset generation for retail or e-commerce
  environment
- Up to two daily peaks per day with more transactions in a specific time
- Check box for generation of additional datasets with same values readable
  by WEKA and other data mining tools (.arff format)

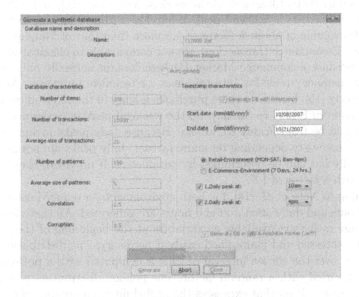

Fig. 2. TARtool GUI

The output provided when generating a dataset with timestamp has ASCII-format with the dataset extension ".dat". An example output file looks like this:

```
1193987598500 (Fri Nov 02 08:13:18 CET 2007) 2 7 8 9 10
1193988231400 (Fri Nov 02 08:24:51 CET 2007) 4 5 8 9
1193988790000 (Fri Nov 02 08:29:10 CET 2007) 2 4 7 8 9
```

This ASCII-file can be selected in TARtool as a database to be mined. The output consists of a timestamp as a 4-byte long value, containing the seconds since 1/1/1970 (the first column in the sample dataset above). This value is provided by the Java-Classes *Date* and *Gregorian Calendar* and can therefore easily be implemented in other software to handle the timestamp for analysis. Additionally, there is a readable version of the timestamp provided to see what timestamps have been generated, followed by the numerical product lists, which are generated according to the algorithm described by Agrawal et al. [10].

4.1 Timestamp Generation

The timestamp generation depends on the startdate and enddate provided in the chosen environment (i.e. retail or e-commerce). When retail environment is selected, the timestamps will be generated weekly from Monday to Saturday from 8am to 8pm. Sundays and holidays are omitted. On the other hand, If e-commerce is selected, timestamp generation will be consecutive 7 days a week, 24 hours a day. In a supermarket, there are no uniformly distributed purchases, but there are hours with a big sales volume, and hours with less. To simulate this distribution, an algorithm was implemented to achieve a rather realistic sales volume over all hours of the day. Based on the *Retail Market Basket Data Set* provided by Brijs [13] as well as the work of Neto et al. [14], and Vallamsetty et al. [15], there exists a weekend-peak of purchases from Thursday to Saturday with a sales volume of about a factor of 1.5 more than that of Monday through Wednesday. E-commerce transactions are not comparable to classical supermarket data, because e-commerce Market Baskets contain normally only few purchases, for instance, items for entertainment, or technical purchases. According to Vallamsetty [15], buyers do these purchases mainly in the after-office-hours or at weekends from Friday to Sunday. So the weekend peak in e-commerce transactions should be from Friday to Sunday. Because daily peaks in supermarkets and e-commerce vary depending on many factors, daily peaks are not generated automatically but can be determined by parameters. If provided, they will also be rated with a factor of 1.5.

According to Neto et al. [14], for both environments, a reduced sales volume at night hours and daily start and end hours are generated. All these factors for sales volume rating are available as variables at the beginning of the TARtool and can be accessed and maintained easily if necessary. The distribution of the transactions over the chosen interval of time is computed with a poisson distribution and varied with a random factor. The poisson distribution is a discrete probability distribution that expresses the probability of a number of events occurring in a fixed period of time if these events occur with a known average rate

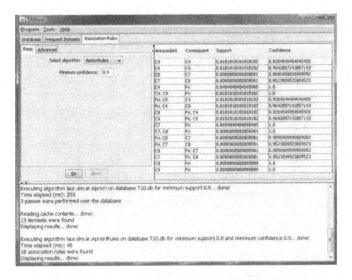

Fig. 3. An example of generated association rules

and independently of the time since the last event. The generated ASCII-file can be selected in TARtool for analysis like the binary datasets. To evaluate the timestamps, the attributes week day and hour of the day from the timestamp are chosen and given as items to the association rule algorithms. An example of generated association rules can be seen in Fig. 3.

5 Evaluation

To evaluate and test the efficiency of our tool, we generated a .dat-file and two related WEKA-readable .arff-files. They have the WEKA-special .arff-Format with definitions for the attributes and boolean values for the items. The first WEKA-readable dataset is named *.arff. It contains boolean values 0 and 1 for each item of the related .dat-file. The second file is named *q.arff and contains the values ? and 1 for the items. Because WEKA will find a lot of association rules within the first kind of dataset, the second one is generated to omit rules like: *IF A AND NOT B ⇒ C.*

In Fig. 4 the *q.arff-file opened in WEKA, which was generated for a retail environment with two peaks per day, is provided. The distribution of the number of transactions per hour of the day can be seen in the visualization on the right-hand side. The first peak is at 10 am and the second peak is at 5 pm. Those two peaks have been chosen in that specific time intervals in order to simulate real retail environment which, normally, have such peaks in those time points according to Vallamsetty [15]. Then, the *q.arff-file is mined in WEKA and the related *.dat-file is mined in TARtool using the APRIORI-algorithm, which is implemented in both tools. An example of the comparison of the frequent

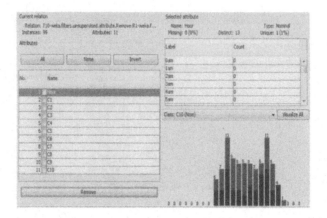

Fig. 4. Opening of an *.arff-file in WEKA

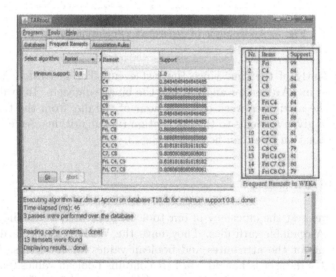

Fig. 5. A Comparison of frequent itemsets in TARtool and WEKA for the same generated dataset

itemsets is given in Fig. 5. The comparison shows a very high degree of similarity of frequent itemsets under both TARtool and WEKA when mining the same generated dataset. The amount of time and space for generating binary datasets and ASCII-files in the enhanced generator depends extensively on the parameters and the output chosen. The generation of binary datasets, i.e. those datasets without timestamps, needs much more time but less space than the ASCII-files. The generation of the *.dat-file is ten times faster than producing the .db-file but needs twice as much space. Table 1 presents some costs of generation for datasets with 100 items executed on a desktop with Pentium D Dual Core 2*1.6 GHz

Table 1. Generation costs for binary and ASCII files

# of Transactions	.db Dataset Millisec.	KB	.dat Dataset Millisec.	KB
1,000	359	50	157	72
10,000	3,046	436	391	729
100,000	298,91	4,340	3,031	7,342
1,000,000	298,672	418,26	297,65	73,671
10,000,000	Not executed	...	331,875	742,164

processor, 2048 MB RAM under Windows Vista. The generation of the binary file with 10,000,000 transactions was not executed due to the large amount of time it would have needed. But it was generated as a .dat-file.

6   Summary and Future Work

In this paper, we developed the TARtool which is a tool based on the ARtool. TARtool has the capability to generate datasets with timestamps for both retail and e-commerce environments, taking into account general customer buying habits in such environments. We also implemented the generator to produce datasets with ARFF format to ease the process of mining such datasets in other data mining tools. An advanced GUI is also provided. The experimental results showed that our tool overcomes other tools in efficiency, usability, functionality, and quality of generated data. As a future work we plan to do the following:

- Enhance our tool to be able to generate biographic information of customers such as customer gender, age, and address. Because for e-commerce environments, such information are normally presented in a web-portal, where customers have to register for purchasing.
- Make it possible to determine detailed attributes of the timestamps being generated by the TARtool (now only day and hour are chosen automatically).
- Build visualization tools in order to ease the process of reading and analyzing the generated/mined data.
- Find a real world dataset and generate a dataset that simulates that real world dataset in order to compare the quality of generated dataset with the real one.
- We also plan to develop the process of data generation by building a graph in which nodes represent customers. The customers have different relationships between each other such as friendship and neighborhood. Through those relationships, the customers influence each other in the decision of buying some product. In that way, we can model the purchasing process much more realistically.

References

1. Yang, Q., Wu, X.: 10 Challenging Problems in Data Mining Research. International Journal of Information Technology and Decision Making 5, 597–604 (2006)
2. Antunes, C., Oliveira, A.: Temporal Data Mining: An Overview. In: Proceedings of the Workshop on Temporal Data Mining, of Knowledge Discovery and Data Mining (KDD 2001), San Francisco, USA (2001)
3. Lin, W., Orgun, M.A., Williams, G.: An Overview of Temporal Data Mining. In: Proceedings of the 1st Australian Data Mining Workshop, Canberra, Australia, pp. 83–90. University of Technology, Sydney (2002)
4. Ozden, B., Ramaswamy, S., Silberschatz, A.: Cyclic Association Rules. In: ICDE 1998: Proceedings of the Fourteenth International Conference on Data Engineering, Washington, DC, USA, pp. 412–421. IEEE Computer Society, Los Alamitos (1998)
5. Cristofor, L.: ARMiner Project, University of Massachusetts, Boston (last called in 15.09.2007), http://www.cs.umb.edu/~laur/ARMiner/
6. Cristofor, L.: ARtool Project, University of Massachusetts, Boston (last called in 15.09.2007), http://www.cs.umb.edu/~laur/ARtool/
7. Witten, I.H., Frank, E.: Data Mining: Practical Machine Learning Tools and Techniques. Morgan Kaufmann Publishers, San Francisco (2005)
8. Zheng, Z., Kohavi, R., Mason, L.: Real World Performance of Association Rule Algorithms. In: Provost, F., Srikant, R. (eds.) Proceedings of the Seventh ACM SIGKDD International Conference on Knowledge Discovery and Data Mining, pp. 401–406 (2001)
9. Hahsler, M., Hornik, K.: New Probabilistic Interest Measures for Association Rules. Intelligent Data Analysis, vol. 11, pp. 437–455 (2007)
10. Agrawal, R., Srikant, R.: Fast Algorithms for Mining Association Rules. In: Proceedings of the 20th VLDB Conference, Santiago, Chile, pp. 487–499 (1994)
11. Groblschegg, M.: Developing a Testdata Generator for Market Basket Analysis for E-commerce Applications. Vienna University of Economics and Business Administration, Vienna, Austria (2003)
12. Ehrenberg, A.: Repeat-Buying: Facts, Theory and Applications. Charles Griffin & Company Ltd., London (1988)
13. Brijs, T.: Retail Market Basket Data Set, University of Limburg, Belgium (last called in 12.9.2007), http://fimi.cs.helsinki.fi/dat/retail.pdf
14. Neto, H., Almeida, J., Rocha, L., Meira, W., Guerra, P., Almeida, V.: A Characterization of Broadband User Behaviour and Their E-Business Activities. ACM SIGMETRICS Performance Evaluation Review, Special Issue: E-Commerce, vol. 32, pp. 3–13 (2004)
15. Vallamsetty, U., Kant, K., Mohapatra, P.: Characterization of E-commerce Traffic. In: Proceedings International Workshop on Advanced Issues of E-Commerce and Web Based Information Systems, pp. 137–147. IEEE Computer Society, Los Alamitos (2002)

Dimensionality Reduction for Classification[*]
Comparison of Techniques and Dimension Choice

Frank Plastria[1], Steven De Bruyne[2], and Emilio Carrizosa[3]

[1] Vrije Universiteit Brussel
Frank.Plastria@vub.ac.be
[2] Vrije Universiteit Brussel
Steven.De.Bruyne@vub.ac.be
[3] Universidad de Sevilla
ecarrizosa@us.es

Abstract. We investigate the effects of dimensionality reduction using different techniques and different dimensions on six two-class data sets with numerical attributes as pre-processing for two classification algorithms. Besides reducing the dimensionality with the use of principal components and linear discriminants, we also introduce four new techniques. After this dimensionality reduction two algorithms are applied. The first algorithm takes advantage of the reduced dimensionality itself while the second one directly exploits the dimensional ranking. We observe that neither a single superior dimensionality reduction technique nor a straightforward way to select the optimal dimension can be identified. On the other hand we show that a good choice of technique and dimension can have a major impact on the classification power, generating classifiers that can rival industry standards. We conclude that dimensionality reduction should not only be used for visualisation or as pre-processing on very high dimensional data, but also as a general pre-processing technique on numerical data to raise the classification power. The difficult choice of both the dimensionality reduction technique and the reduced dimension however, should be directly based on the effects on the classification power.

1 Introduction

Dimensionality reduction of the feature space has long been used in data mining. So is principal component analysis, first introduced in [3], often used as a pre-processing step for problems with an extreme high dimensionality. Linear discriminant analysis, first introduced in [2], on the other hand, while sharing many properties, is used to solve the problem immediately by reducing the dimensionality of the feature space to one. The optimal number of dimensions for principal component analysis has been investigated many times [6], but with the goal of finding the number of non-trivial components. We on the other hand use another criterion, namely maximization of the 10-fold cross validation results of

[*] Partially supported by the research project OZR1372 of the Vrije Universiteit Brussel.

C. Tang et al. (Eds.): ADMA 2008, LNAI 5139, pp. 411–418, 2008.
© Springer-Verlag Berlin Heidelberg 2008

the classifiers yielded by the algorithms. The optima for both these criteria do not necessarily coincide.

We start by defining the different techniques we use. Some of them are standard techniques while others are new. Later we compare them to see which one delivers superior results.

To evaluate the effect of the dimensionality reduction, we use two-class data sets on which we apply two classification algorithms. The first one is an algorithm that normally functions in the original feature space and we are interested to see if the reduction of the dimensionality can have positive effects nonetheless. The second algorithm is a new algorithm that directly uses the properties of the new feature space introduced by the transformation and reduction of the dimensionality.

A full overview of each possible combination of dimensionality reduction technique, dimension choice and algorithm is presented and analysed.

2   Dimensionality Reduction Techniques

The reduction of the dimension of the attribute vector is executed in three steps. First, we compute a square transformation matrix of dimension the number of attributes. Second, the attribute vectors are transformed by multiplying them with this matrix. Finally, the actual reduction consists of keeping a fixed number of the most discriminating new attributes (features).

Several techniques to compute an effective transformation matrix are evaluated. Principal components and linear discriminants are selected as standard solutions. The principal components orientate the data so that the variance is maximized firstly along the first axis, secondly along the second axis etc. Principal components ignore the existence of multiple classes. Linear discriminants however take into account the existence of multiple groups by trying to find orientations that favour a high spread of the total data while avoiding those yielding a high spread within the different homogenous groups. These two techniques are complemented by four new ones. The first one, which we named principal separation, is by idea similar to linear discriminants but looks for orientations in which pairs of instances of different classes lie far apart. The three final approaches exploit the fact that only two groups exist and that a straightforward candidate for the first orientation can be defined by the means of the two groups. Since this does not yield a complete transformation matrix, it is complemented by orientations computed using each of the aforementioned techniques.

2.1   Notations

For a general matrix $M \in \mathbb{R}^{d \times p_M}$

- d : the original dimension of the data (number of attributes)
- $Mean(M) \in \mathbb{R}^{d \times 1}$: the mean of the instances of M
- $Cov(M) \in \mathbb{R}^{d \times d}$: the covariance matrix of M
- $Mom(M) \in \mathbb{R}^{d \times d}$: the matrix of second moments (around the origin) of M

- $Eig(M) \in \mathbb{R}^{d \times d}$: the matrix of eigenvectors of M

Note: $Cov(M) = Mom(M) - Mean(M).Mean(M)^t$

2.2 Data

- A : the matrix of p_A columns representing the instances of the first set
- B : the matrix of p_B columns representing the instances of the second set
- $T = [A, B]$: the matrix of $p_T = p_A + p_B$ columns representing the instances of both sets

2.3 Reduction Operation

- R : the transformation matrix
- $n < d$: the dimension after reduction

R is assumed to be ordered row-wise. Usually the rows of R are the eigenvectors of some matrix, ordered by decreasing eigenvalues.

The dimension reduction consists of calculating RT and dropping all rows except the first n. The result is a new feature space.

2.4 Principal Components

We define the transformation matrix based on principal components as

$$R = Eig(Cov(T))$$

2.5 Linear Discriminants

Let

$$S_W = \frac{p_A Cov(A) + p_B Cov(B)}{p_T}$$

$$S_B = Cov(T) - S_W$$

Then we define the transformation matrix based on linear discriminants as

$$R = Eig(S_W^{-1} S_B)$$

2.6 Principal Separation Components

Define the $d \times (p_A p_B)$ matrix $A \ominus B$, as consisting of all d-vectors $a - b$ for any pair of d-vectors $a \in A$ and $b \in B$.

We want to keep the 'spread'

$$\sum_{a-b \in A \ominus B} \|a - b\|^2$$

as high as possible after reduction. In a way similar to principal components analysis, this is obtained using transformation matrix

$$R = Eig(Mom(A \ominus B))$$

Since the complexity of calculating $Mom(M)$ is in general $O(p_M d^2)$ the calculation of $Mom(A \ominus B)$ seems at first glance to be an ominous $O(p_A p_B d^2)$. This complexity is however strongly reduced to $O((p_A + p_B)d^2) = O(p_T d^2)$ thanks to the following result.

Theorem 1. $Mom(A \ominus B) = Mom(A) + Mom(B) - Mean(A)Mean(B)^t - Mean(B)Mean(A)^t$

Proof
For any $1 \leq i, j \leq d$ we have:

$$Mom(A \ominus B)_{ij} = \frac{1}{p_A p_B} \sum_{a \in A} \sum_{b \in B} (a_i - b_i)(a_j - b_j)$$

$$= \frac{1}{p_A p_B} \sum_{a \in A} \sum_{b \in B} (a_i a_j - b_i a_j - a_i b_j + b_i b_j)$$

$$= \frac{1}{p_A} \sum_{a \in A} a_i a_j + \frac{1}{p_B} \sum_{b \in B} b_i b_j - \frac{1}{p_A p_B} \sum_{a \in A} \sum_{b \in B} a_i b_j - \frac{1}{p_A p_B} \sum_{a \in A} \sum_{b \in B} b_i a_j$$

$$= \frac{1}{p_A} \sum_{a \in A} a_i a_j + \frac{1}{p_B} \sum_{b \in B} b_i b_j - (\frac{1}{p_A} \sum_{a \in A} a_i)(\frac{1}{p_B} \sum_{b \in B} b_j) - (\frac{1}{p_B} \sum_{b \in B} b_i)(\frac{1}{p_A} \sum_{a \in A} a_j)$$

$$= Mom(A)_{ij} + Mom(B)_{ij} - Mean(A)_i Mean(B)_j^t - Mean(B)_i Mean(A)_j^t$$

$\square$

2.7 Mean Component Methods

Let

$$p = Mean(A) - Mean(B)$$

We define the first row of the transformation matrix based on means as

$$R_1 = \frac{p}{||p||}$$

We define the remaining rows $R_{2..n}$ as the $n - 1$ first rows of the aforementioned techniques after projection of the instances on the hyperplane perpendicular on R_1. This yields the following three variants:

- principal mean components
- linear mean discriminants
- principal mean separation components

3 Classification Algorithms

3.1 Optimal Distance Separating Hyperplane

Here we use a linear classifier, chosen so as to minimize sum of the euclidean distances of misclassified instances to the separating hyperplane as proposed in [5]. By reducing the dimension, we hope not only to solve the problem of the high complexity the algorithms have concerning the dimensionality of the feature space [4,7], but also hope to reduce overfitting. The classifier is obtained by way of the Grid-Cell VNS algorithm as was proposed in [7].

3.2 Eigenvalue-Based Classification Tree

Since the ranking of RT indicates the importance of the features of the new feature space, it is straightforward to make a selection for a split in a hierarchical structure. We therefore we propose a new kind of classification tree in which the split in the top node is done based on the first feature, in the nodes on the second level the splits are done based on the second feature etc. The split value is calculated by taking that midpoint between two consecutive instances that minimizes the number of misclassifieds. The expansion of the tree ends either when only instances of one class remain for the given node or when the level of the node equals the reduced dimension n. Note that no feature is used more than once in each branch.

4 Computational Results

Table 1 shows the best average results of ten 10-fold cross validations on six data sets from the UCI [8] database when applying all six reduction techniques and varying dimensionality. As a reference, the results of some industry standards such as support vector machines with linear kernels (SVM) and C4.5 classification trees (C4.5), as well as a 1-dimensional principal component (PCA) or a linear discriminant analysis (LDA) are also presented. We can see that, combined with a good dimensionality reduction, our new algorithms (Best ODSH, Best EVCT) can compete with these standards.

Table 2 shows the optimal dimensionalities and reduction techniques for each pair of algorithm and data set. No dimensionality reduction technique seems

Table 1. Cross Validations

Data set	d	p_T	Best ODSH	Best EVCT	SVM	C4.5	PCA	LDA
Cancer	9	683	96.8%	97.5%	97.0%	95.4%	97.5%	97.1%
Diabetes	8	768	76.1%	75.6%	76.8%	74.4%	68.1%	75.6%
Echocardiogram	7	74	76.5%	73.4%	70.9%	70.9%	65.2%	67.5%
Glass windows	9	214	93.7%	96.1%	92.2%	93.3%	92.2%	93.2%
Hepatitis	16	150	83.6%	84.5%	84.6%	77.6%	80.9%	84.5%
Housing	13	506	86.8%	81.7%	86.4%	81.9%	77.1%	79.9%

Table 2. Optimal Dimension Reduction

Data Set	d	p_T	ODSH		EVCT	
			Best Tech	Best Dim	Best Tech	Best Dim
Cancer	9	683	LD	1	PC/PSC	1
Diabetes	8	768	PMC	6	LD	1
Echocardiogram	7	74	PSC	2	PMSC	2
Glass windows	9	214	PMC	2	PMC	2
Hepatitis	16	150	PC	1	LD	1
Housing	13	506	PMSC	10	PSC	6

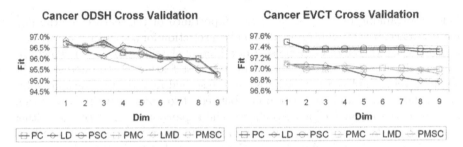

Fig. 1. Cancer set cross validations

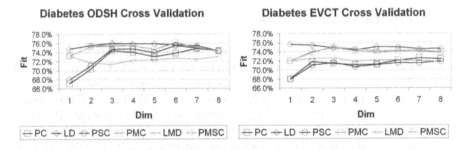

Fig. 2. Diabetes set cross validations

superior or inferior to the others, which makes a selection difficult. Although severe dimensionality reductions often yield good results, finding a pattern for an effective selection is difficult. It should also be noted that no clear correlation was found between the results and the eigenvalues yielded by the dimensionality reduction techniques.

Full results can be found in the figures below. Although an optimal selection is difficult without full results, the impact of good pre-processing can be clearly seen here. A reduction to one dimension can give good results, but in many cases a reduction of this magnitude seems too drastic and moving up to two or three dimensions can result in a very significant improvement. On the other hand, the results can decrease rapidly when choosing a higher dimensionality, although

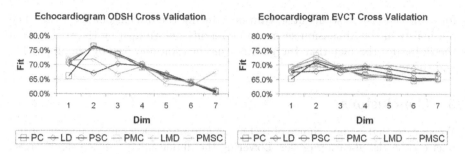

Fig. 3. Echocardiogram set cross validations

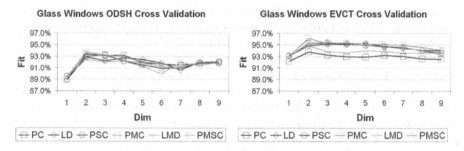

Fig. 4. Glass windows set cross validations

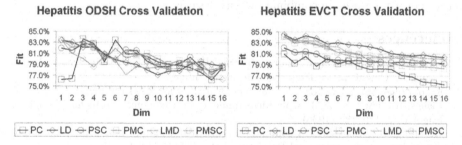

Fig. 5. Hepatitis set cross validations

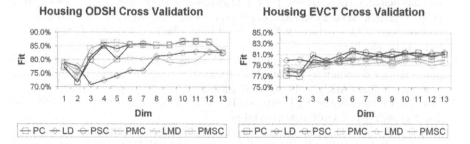

Fig. 6. Housing set cross validations

for some sets, there seems little gain in reducing the dimensionality at all. The optimality of the dimension seems to be mainly determined by the structure of the data and the fact that the goal is classification and less by the algorithm and the reduction technique.

5   Conclusions

We showed that a good choice of technique and dimension can have a major impact on the classification power. Lowering the dimensionality often significantly reduces the overfitting by an algorithm. On the other hand, one should be careful not to lower the dimensionality too much as the information loss can then rapidly overtake the reduction in overfitting. However, we observe that neither a single superior dimensionality reduction technique nor a straightforward way to select the optimal dimension can be identified.

We conclude that dimensionality reduction should not only be used for visualisation or as pre-processing on very high dimensional data, but also as a general pre-processing technique on numerical data to raise the classification power. The difficult choice of both the dimensionality reduction technique and the reduced dimension however, should be directly based on the effects on the classification power. We are currently researching methods to incorporate the choice of the dimensionality reduction into the algorithm itself [1].

Many of these findings can also be extended to problems with more than two classes or can be used in combination with kernels.

References

1. De Bruyne, S., Plastria, F.: 2-class Internal Cross-validation Pruned Eigen Transformation Classification Trees. Optimization Online,
   http://www.optimization-online.org/DB_HTML/2008/05/1971.html
2. Fisher, R.: The Use of Multiple Measurements in Taxonomic Problems. Annals of Eugenics 7, 179–188 (1936)
3. Hotelling, H.: Analysis of a complex of statistical variables into principal components. Journal of Educational Psychology 24, 417–441 (1933)
4. Karam, A., Caporossi, G., Hansen, P.: Arbitrary-norm hyperplane separation by variable neighbourhood search. IMA J. Management Math. 2007 18, 173–189 (2007),
   http://imaman.oxfordjournals.org/cgi/content/abstract/18/2/173?etoc
5. Mangasarian, O.L.: Arbitrary-Norm Separating Plane. Operations Research Letters 24, 15–23 (1999)
6. Peres-Neto, P., Jackson, D., Somers, K.: How many principal components? stopping rules for determining the number of non-trivial axes revisited. Computational Statistics & Data Analysis 49, 974–997 (2005)
7. Plastria, F., De Bruyne, S., Carrizosa, E.: Alternating local search based VNS for linear classification. Optimization Online,
   http://www.optimization-online.org/DB_HTML/2008/02/1910.html
8. Newman, D.J., Hettich, S., Blake, C.L., Merz, C.J.: UCI Repository of machine learning databases. University of California, Department of Information and Computer Science, Irvine (1998),
   http://www.ics.uci.edu/~mlearn/MLRepository.html

Trajectories Mining for Traffic Condition Renewing

Danhuai Guo

Institute of Remote Sensing Applications, Chinese Academy of Sciences, Beijing 100101,
China
guodanhuai@gmail.com

Abstract. Advances in wireless transmission and increasing quantity of GPS in
vehicles flood us with massive amount of trajectory data. The large amounts of
trajectories imply considerable quantity of interesting road condition that current traffic database lacks. Mining live traffic condition from trajectories is a
challenge due to complexity of road network model, uncertainty of driving behavior as well as imprecision of trajectories. In this paper, road linear reference
system, road segmentation and road condition models are employed in preprocessing trajectory data to lower dimension of trajectory mining problems and reduce uncertainties and imprecision of raw trajectories. The trajectory mining
problem includes the one near road intersection and the one in general road
segment. The former focuses on finding turn information of road intersection,
while the latter focuses on extracting road live condition. The experimental results show that the mining algorithm is effective and efficient in traffic condition mining.

1 Introduction

Live traffic condition reporting, as one important part of LBS (Location Based Service), has achieved widening application. But the information it provides hardly meets
the demand of intelligent traffic applications limited by data obtaining method and
data update mechanism. The flaw of current live traffic condition reporting systems
includes low precision in spatial and temporal scale, lack of road spatio-temporal
information, and lack of traffic information in lane granularity level. GPS and other
positioning devices carried by vehicles can track a vehicle as it moves. These consequently recorded location and velocity data of specific vehicle in specific time interval form trajectory[1]. The trajectories hide a large amount of interesting and valuable
knowledge of trajectories' surroundings. In recent years, mining moving objects has
emerged as a hot topic both academically and practically. [2] employed differential
GPS receivers and spatial clustering algorithm to extract road centerline, lane position, and intersection structure and road segments. But the application of this method
was limited as most of GPS receivers embedded in vehicles are not differential GPS
receivers in decimeter accuracy level but navigational ones in a few ten's meters accuracy level. [3] and [4] provided REMO to detect four spatio-temporal patterns
namely flock, leadership, convergence, and encounter. [5] provided FlowScan that
was density-based algorithms to mine hot routes in road network. The database

C. Tang et al. (Eds.): ADMA 2008, LNAI 5139, pp. 419–426, 2008.
© Springer-Verlag Berlin Heidelberg 2008

projection based association rule mining method described in [6] was efficient to extract long, sharable frequent routes. The spatio-temporal similarity calculation of trajectories provided in [7] are effective and adopted in our experiment. [8] proposed a new data mining algorithm to extract identity temporal patterns from series of locations of moving objects in LBS, and used spatial operation to generalize a location of moving object, applying time constraints between locations of moving objects to make valid moving sequences. [9] proposed a model of trajectories patterns and a novel measure to represent the expected occurrences of pattern in a set of imprecise trajectories, and mined sequential patterns from imprecise trajectories of moving objects. [10] proposed an approach to predict future location of moving objects from their long-term moving behavior history. [11] provided ST-DBSCAN to calculate spatio-temporal clustering of trajectories.

The rest of the paper is organized as follows. Section 2 gives the notations and definitions of trajectory mining. Section 3 describes the data preprocessing, mining algorithms and mining implementation. The conclusion and future work is discussed in section 4.

2   Problem Statement and Definition

Most of drivers tend to choose the optimal (shortest in most cases) route to his/her destination if there is no obstacle, traffic light or traffic regulations constraints. The trajectories are mixed result of drivers' subjective will and circumstance constraints. In this paper, it is supposed that there is a GPS receiver in moving vehicles, the collected trajectories will be transferred to and stored in trajectories database timely. Before mining, it is necessary to confirm some related notation and definition.

Definition 1. To road linear reference system and road segment all road segments in road network are numbered by spatial index, $R=\{R_1, R_2,...R_n\}$. All lanes are numbered by offset distance from centerline, the lanes in the road direction are set positive value, and the others are assigned to negative number. $l=\{ l_{-i}, l_{1-i} ...l_{-1}, l_1 ...l_{j-1}, l_j\}$. The n-lane of m-road can be notated as $R_m\text{-} l_n$.

Definition 2. If $R_m\text{-} l_n$ and $R_i\text{-} l_j$ have the spatio-temporal connection relationship, i.e. a vehicle can get $R_i\text{-} l_j$ directly from $R_m\text{-}l_n$ not through any other road, it is notated as Connect($R_m\text{-}l_n$, $R_i\text{-}l_j$). Its support is notated as Support(Connect($R_m\text{-} l_n$, $R_i\text{-}l_j$)). If Support(Connect($R_m\text{-}l_n$, $R_i\text{-} l_j$)) > threshold, it can be described that n-lane of m-road is connected with j-lane of i-road. Or roughly speaking, i-road is connected with m-road.

Definition 3. If Support(Connect $(R_m\text{-}l_n$, $R_k\text{-} l_l))$ > threshold in the road intersection and one of following conditions is satisfied, the lane can be described in natural language as:

$$\theta\left(\vec{R}_m, \vec{R}_k\right) \approx 0 \Rightarrow \text{ the lane is ``Straight through lane''} \tag{1}$$

$$\theta\left(\vec{R}_m, \vec{R}_k\right) \approx \frac{\pi}{2} \Rightarrow \text{ the lane is ``Left-turn lane''} \tag{2}$$

$$\theta\left(\vec{R}_m,\vec{R}_k\right) \approx \pi \Rightarrow \text{the lane is "U-turn lane"} \tag{3}$$

$$\theta\left(\vec{R}_m,\vec{R}_k\right) \approx \frac{3\pi}{2} \Rightarrow \text{ the lane is "Right-turn lane"} \tag{4}$$

Where θ is the angle of vector $\vec{R}_m$ to vector $\vec{R}_k$. And in formula (3), in fact m-Road and k-Road is the same road. The lane which has max support value is the turn lane. If there is any $l_i \in \{ l_1 , l_2 ,\dots l_j \}$ of R_m, its Support(Connect(R_m- l_i, R_k- l_j)) > threshold and one of above angle conditions is satisfied, the road intersection can be described as "No Straight through", "No Left-turn", "No U-turn" and "No Right-turn" respectively.

Definition 4. If the sum of vehicles in one road in one direction in the time interval$[t_1, t_2]$is much greater than the one in opposite direction:

$$\sum_{k=1}^{i} Sum\_Vehicle(l_k) >> \sum_{l=-j}^{-1} Sum\_Vehicle(l_l), (l_k, l_l \in R_m) \tag{5}$$

the road can be described in natural language as "One way road".

Definition 5. If the sum of vehicles of one road in both directions in the time interval $[t_1, t_2]$ < threshold

$$\sum_{k=1}^{i} Sum\_Vehicle(l_k) + \sum_{l=-j}^{-1} Sum\_Vehicle(l_l) < threshold, (l_k, l_l \in R_m) \tag{6}$$

the road is a "Closure road". The closure road includes abandon road and closing road.

Definition 6. If the amount of vehicle running in a road > threshold and the vehicles' average velocity < threshold in $[t_1, t_2]$, the road is a "Hot road".

The thresholds mentioned above have various values in various cases for various mining objective expected.

3 Moving Objects Trajectory Data Mining

In this paper, the term "moving object" is restricted to denote an object to which we can associate a trajectory, and in the following experiment it is restricted as moving vehicle carrying GPS receiver and data transferring device. Location trajectory and velocity trajectory are the two types of trajectory shape. Location trajectory includes the moving object location's spatial dimension (x_i, y_i) maybe including h_i, and temporal dimension (t_i). The velocity trajectory records the velocity (V_i), direction (d_i), and temporal value (t_i). Location trajectory is usually sampled by linear interpolation and has the advantage of fast and easy constructing and precise trajectory location, as well as the disadvantage of abruption discontinuing of speed and direction. Velocity trajectory is usually sampled by Bezier curves interpolation and has the advantage of smooth and nice trajectory graph, and accurate and continuous speed and direction, as well as disadvantage of high computing complexity. Being limited by GPS receiver's precision and variety of GPS receivers install position, it is difficult to extract all lanes position precisely from trajectories. What people concern in general road segment and near road intersection is different. The former focuses on finding whether the intersection is specific turn-allowed, and if it is, which lane is turn lane. The latter focuses on finding the live road information i.e. hot road, one-way road, and closure road etc.

3.1 Data Preprocessing

The road spatial data in traffic map are usually organized in Arc-Node model, which is not sufficient in road and lane representation[12]. The trajectories collected by GPS receivers and other positioning devices store the location 2- or 3-D geo-coordinate that requires a spatial reference system. In road network applications, it was verified that the road linear referencing system and road segment are more efficient in road indexing and location querying than spatial reference system [12]. The raw trajectories should be transformed to linear referencing systems and road segment. $(x_i, y_i, t_i) \Rightarrow (R_m, l_n, D_i, t_i)$. In this transformation, R_m and l_n represent the road and lane which the moving objects is located in time instant t_i respectively; D_i is the segment length along the road between the perpendicular point of trajectory sample point to road centerline and the road start point.

The GPS recorded coordinate sometimes "drifts" caused by GPS satellites signal sheltering, multi-way effect or other reasons. When GPS "drifts", it is actually difficult to determine the road and lane number. There are two methods to process these imprecise trajectories data: the first one is to get rid of those trajectories segment, the other one is to transform imprecise trajectories sample points to their corresponding most-probable positions. The former can raise mining efficiency but lost some useful data. The latter tries to transform the imprecise data to its most-probable position according to moving object moving inertia and moving trend predicting models. [9] provided an improved probable position algorithm based on equation *predict_loc=last_loc +v*t*. We adopt that algorithm and extend it as: 1)If the moving object is in i-road in time t_1 and the time interval Δt is small enough, in the moment of $t_2=t_1+\Delta t$, the moving object will keep in the same road i.e. i-road; 2) There are trajectory sample points sorted by offset distances from the centerline in different lanes of same road in the same direction and in the same moment, if any sample point is beyond the range of reasonable lane position, the lane number of the innermost trajectory is set to the innermost lane number and the other trajectories are assigned according to variant offset distance, and vice versa.

3.2 Traffic Condition Extraction Near Road Intersection

There are many interesting road and lane information can be extracted from moving objects trajectories. But the expected mining objective is different in different cases. When driving to a road intersection, what the drivers concerned is whether the coming intersection is straight through, left-turn, right-turn or u-turn, and if it is turn-allowed, which lane is turn lane? In way-finding and other transporting planning applications, the road intersection turn information in various time intervals is a crucial factor. In data mining from trajectories near road intersection, the key is to find the correlations of different road and lane and calculate their supports.

The first procedure is to select all trajectories and trajectory segments which are near the road intersection Road_Int$_i$ in specific time interval $[t_1, t_2]$.

```
Select trajectory from trajectories where
trajectory.interpoint is near Road_Int_i and t_1 <=
trajectory.time and trajectory.time <= t_2
```

Where the operator "near" is a buffering spatial calculation centered in the intersection of Road_Int$_i$ with user specific buffer distance. In the trajectory mining near road intersection, what we concerned is which roads and lanes the trajectory connects, so the middle part of trajectory can be ignored. The selected trajectories can be simplified as:

$$Trajectory(Point_1, Point_2,...)$$
$$\Rightarrow Trajectory(Point_i, Point_{i+1},...Point_j)$$
$$\Rightarrow Point_i, Point_j \tag{7}$$
$$\Rightarrow (R_{mi}, l_{ni}, D_{ki}, t_{li}), (R_{mj}, l_{nj}, D_{kj}, t_{lj})$$

Point$_i$ and *Point$_j$* are the start point and end point of trajectory segment respectively. Formula (7) can be simplified further: D_{ki} and D_{kj}, can be ignored as they are not the interesting point in the mining application. It usually takes very short time for drivers to pass the road intersection, so $t_{li} \approx t_{lj}$. Table 1 lists one part of simplified result of trajectories near a road intersection.

Table 2. An example of simplified trajectories

Trajectory ID	Start_road	Start_lane	End_road	End_lane	Time
D00034	23	1	103	-1	20060506123118
D00311	23	2	24	1	20060506123120
D00228	23	1	23	-2	20060506123124
D00115	23	2	104	2	20060506123128
D00341	23	2	24	1	20060506123130
...					

The connection support of road or lane is defined as the ratio of the turning vehicle amount compared with the sum of vehicle passing the road intersection from this road. In support calculation, we are interesting in the trajectory total amount which is composed of one or more destination lanes. So the destination lane information can be ignored too.

$$Support(R_m, R_i) = \frac{Connect\_Sum(R_m - l_n, R_i)}{Sum(R_m)} \tag{8}$$

Since the mining problem in spatio-temporal database is transformed to the one in relational database, the mining algorithm can be achieved in standard query language (SQL) statement:

```
Connect_Sum (Rm-ln, Ri): select count(Traj_ID) FROM
Traj_Table where Start_road=m and Start_lane=n and
End_road=  i and Time >= t1 and Time <= t2
```

```
Sum(Rm-ln):   select count(Traj_ID) FROM Traj_Table
where Start_road=m and Time >= t1 and Time <= t2
```

If the support > threshold, and one of premises of 0 is satisfied, the road can be described in natural language as: the road with "Straight through Lane", "Left-turn Lane", "U-turn Lane" and "Right-turn Lane" respectively. The lane which has the max support value is the turn lane.

We choose Kunming, the capital of Yunnan province, southwest of China as the experimental region. Nearly 100 cars were employed in the 30-day experiment. 20 road intersections mining results were selected randomly as comparison with field survey figures. Fig. 2 shows the mining result compared with field survey figures.

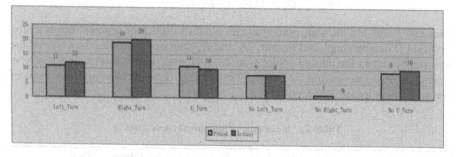

Fig. 2. Mining result of trajectory near road intersection (the blue column is figure of mining result, the violet one is figure of filed survey)

3.3 Traffic Condition Extraction in General Road Segment

In the general road segments away from road intersection, what drivers concerned is whether the road is clear, whether the road is closed, and whether there is traffic jam in the road. So we focus on not only the location trajectory but the velocity trajectory. And the lane information can be ignored. The location and velocity trajectories need to be transformed as:

$$Trajectory((Point_1,V_1,t_1),(Point_2,V_2,t_2),...(Point_j,V_j,t_j))$$

$$\Rightarrow Trajectory((R_{m1},l_{n1},D_{k1},V_1,t_1),(R_{m2},l_{n2},D_{k2},V_2,t_2),...(R_{mj},l_{nj},D_{kj},V_j,t_j)) \qquad (9)$$

$$\Rightarrow Trajectory((R_{m1},S_1,t_1),(R_{m2},S_2,t_2),...(R_{mj},S_j,t_j)$$

Where S is represented as trajectory speed, which absolute value is equal to velocity and is signed by the trajectory direction. If the trajectory is in the same direction with

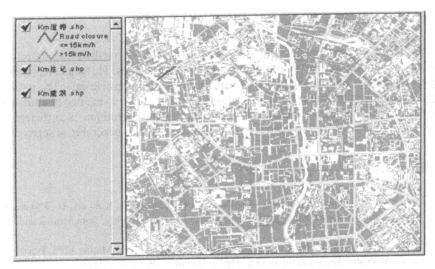

Fig. 3. Live road condition mining result in the rush hour. (The green lines are clear roads with driving speed > 15km/h; the yellow ones are hot road with driving speed ≤ 15km/h; and the red one is closure road.)

the road vector, S is positive. On the contrary, it is negative. The SQL statement of counting the amount of vehicles in a "road closure" is:

```
SELECT DISTINCT count(Trajectory_ID)FROM Traj_Table
where Start_road=m and Time >= t₁ and Time <= t₂;
```

If the count<threshold, the m-Road is "road closure" in time interval $[t_1, t_2]$. The SQL statement of counting the amount of vehicles in a "hot road" is:

```
SELECT DISTINCT count(Trajectory_ID)FROM Traj_Table
where Start_road=m and abs(Speed) < threshold and Time
>= t₁ and Time <= t₂;
```

If the count > threshold, the m-Road is "hot road" in time interval $[t_1,t_2]$. The SQL statement of counting the number of vehicle in a "one-way road" of positive direction count(PC) and negative direction count (NC) list follow:

```
SELECT DISTINCT count(Trajectory_ID) FROM Traj_Table
where Start_road=m and Speed > 0 and Time >= t1 and
Time <= t2;
```

```
SELECT DISTINCT count(Trajectory_ID) FROM Traj_Table
where Start_road=m and Speed < 0 and Time >= t₁ and Time
<= t₂
```

If PC >> NC, the road is a "one-way road", and the passable way is in same direction with the road direction, and vice versa. Fig. 3 is a snapshot of mining result of traffic condition of Kunming in the rush hour on April 6, 2006.

4 Conclusion and Future Work

In this paper, we propose the trajectory data preprocessing method and trajectory mining algorithms in different traffic condition extraction cases. This data preprocessing lowers trajectories mining dimension and revise some imprecise data. The mining algorithms convert the mining task of spatio-temporal database to the one of relational database. The experimental results show that the mining algorithm is sufficient to extract live road information near road intersections as well as general road segments.

References

1. Macedo, J., Vangenot, C., Othman, W., Pelekis, N., Frentzos, E., Kuijpers, B., Ntoutsi, I., Spaccapietra, S., Theodoridis, Y.: Trajectory Data Models. Mobility, Data Mining and Privacy, 123–150 (2008)
2. Schroedl, S., Wagstaff, K., Rogers, S., Langley, P., Wilson, C.: Mining GPS Traces for Map Refinement. Data mining and knowledge Discovery 9, 59–87 (2004)
3. Gudmundsson, J., Kreveld, M.v., Speckmann, B.: Effient Detection of Patterns in 2D Trajectories of Moving Points. Geoinformatica 11, 195–215 (2007)
4. Laube, P., van Kreveld, M., Imfeld, S.: Finding REMO - Detecting relative motion patterns in geospatial lifelines. In: Fisher, P. (ed.) Developments in Spatial Data Handling, pp. 201–215 (2005)
5. Li, X., Han, J., Lee, J.-G., Gonzalez, H.: Traffic Density-Based Discovery of Hot Routes in Road Networks. Advances in Spatial and Temporal Databases, 441–459 (2007)
6. Gidófalvi, G., Pedersen, T.: Mining Long, Sharable Patterns in Trajectories of Moving Objects. GeoInformatica (2007)
7. Hwang, J.-R., Kang, H.-Y., Li, K.-J.: Spatio-temporal similarity analysis between trajectories on road networks. In: Akoka, J., Liddle, S.W., Song, I.-Y., Bertolotto, M., Comyn-Wattiau, I., van den Heuvel, W.-J., Kolp, M., Trujillo, J., Kop, C., Mayr, H.C. (eds.) ER Workshops 2005. LNCS, vol. 3770, pp. 280–289. Springer, Heidelberg (2005)
8. Lee, J.W., Paek, O.H., Ryu, K.H.: Temporal moving pattern mining for location-based service. Journal of Systems and Software 73, 481–490 (2004)
9. Yang, J., Hu, M.: TrajPattern: Mining sequential patterns from imprecise trajectories of mobile objects. In: Ioannidis, Y., Scholl, M.H., Schmidt, J.W., Matthes, F., Hatzopoulos, M., Böhm, K., Kemper, A., Grust, T., Böhm, C. (eds.) EDBT 2006. LNCS, vol. 3896, pp. 664–681. Springer, Heidelberg (2006)
10. Jin, M.-H., Horng, J.-T., Tsai, M.-F., Wu, E.H.-K.: Location query based on moving behaviors. Information Systems 32, 385–401 (2007)
11. Birant, D., Kut, A.: ST-DBSCAN: An algorithm for clustering spatial-temporal data. Data and Knowledge Engineering 60, 208–221 (2007)
12. Scarponcini, P.: Generalized Model for Linear Referencing in Transportation. GeoInformatica 6, 35–55 (2002)

Mining Bug Classifier and Debug Strategy Association Rules for Web-Based Applications

Lian Yu, Changzhu Kong, Lei Xu, Jingtao Zhao, and HuiHui Zhang

The School of Software and Microelectronics, Peking University
Daxing District, Beijing, 102600, P.R. China
lianyu@ss.pku.edu.cn, {xzlkcz,xulei8310}@gmail.com

Abstract. The paper uses data mining approaches to classify bug types and excavate debug strategy association rules for Web-based applications. Chi-square
algorithm is used to extract bug features, and SVM to model bug classifier
achieving more than 70% predication accuracy on average. Debug strategy association rules accumulate bug fixing knowledge and experiences regarding to
typical bug types, and can be applied repeatedly, thus improving the bug fixing
efficiency. With 575 training data, three debug strategy association rules are
unearthed.

Keywords: bug mining, bug classification, debug strategy, association rule,
Chi-square algorithm, SVM.

1 Introduction

Web-based applications have become so popular that they have been fundamentally
changing human's life styles. The trend will keep continuing and become ever more spec-
tacular. However, developing Web-based applications is still facing a lot of challenges,
indicated by hundreds and thousands of bug reports deluging the bug tracking systems.

When a new bug is reported to a bug tracking system, it will trigger a series of
tasks: 1) figure out what bug types the report belongs to; 2) choose who is going to
fix; and 3) decide how to fix the bugs.

The first task faces a lot of challenges. The ways to define bug types vary from
people to people. There are some research works that try to handle the second task,
such as Anvik et al. [1], Cubranic and Murphy [2]. There are great difficulties with
the third task. It is essentially a hard job to derivate the crux of the problem from
symptoms of an error, and debuggers must be well-equipped with a wide range of
Web development knowledge and experience.

This paper proposes to use data mining approach to obtain a bug classifier to automatically predicate bug types of Web-based applications; and to acquire debug strategy association rules which directly indicate the relations between bug types and bug
fixing solutions. Debug strategy can provide clues to locate the erroneous part of the
source code. Once the mistake is found, correcting it is usually easy.

We are aware that there are few researches on the relationship between the description of fixing bugs and category of bugs. Haran et al. [3] analyze data from deployed

C. Tang et al. (Eds.): ADMA 2008, LNAI 5139, pp. 427–434, 2008.
© Springer-Verlag Berlin Heidelberg 2008

software to classify executions as success or failure. They use tree-based classifiers and association rules to model "failure signals". Zimmermann et al. mined source version histories to determine association rules which can then be used to predict files (or smaller program elements, such as functions and variables) that usually change together [4]. In addition, Kim focused on predicting faults from cached history [5]. Arumuga used compound Boolean predicates to implement statistical debugging [6]. The statistical debugging uses dynamic instrumentation and machine learning to identify predicates on program state that are strongly predictive of program failure.

The paper is organized as follows. Section 2 describes the process of mining bug classifier and debug strategy association rules. Section 3 presents the pre-process on bug reports from Mozilla open bug repository. Section 4 depicts the bug feature extraction using Chi-square algorithm. Section 5 trains bug classifier using Support Vector Machine (SVM) algorithm, and predicts bug types with testing data. Section 6 mines debug strategy association rules to obtain the relationship between bug types and bug fixing solutions. Section 7 demonstrates several experimental results on bug classifier and debugs strategy association rules. Finally, Section 8 concludes the paper and scratches the future work.

2   Process of Bug Classification and Debug Strategy Association

Figure 1 shows the data mining based process of bug classification and debug strategy association rules.

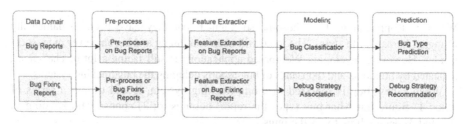

Fig. 1. Data Mining Process of Bug Classification and Debug Strategy Association Rules

1) Getting data set from problem domain: We choose Mozilla bug repository as data resources. JavaScript technique is used to automatically obtain bug information, including "Category", "Summary" and "Comments", which will be used for bug feature extraction.

2) Data pre-processing: The pre-process on bug reports is to manually refine categories of bug reports and sort out the useless information from "Summary". We use Regular Expression rules to filter the punctuations and use stop-words dictionary to filter useless words.

3) Feature extraction: Feature extraction is to take out words which can best represent the characteristics of the bugs, and are used as "features" in the feature extraction algorithm. We choose Chi-square algorithm to calculate these values of bug features.

4) Modeling of bug classification and debug strategy association: We model bug classification using Support Vector Machine (SVM) with training data set (a set of bug category and bug features) obtained in the previous step; and model debug strategy association rules using Apriori algorithm with training data set (a set of bug fixing solutions and bug features) obtained in the previous step as well.

5) Prediction of bug category and Recommendation of debug strategy: We use testing data to evaluate the prediction accuracy of the bug classification model. The bug classification model can be used to predict the type of a new bug report. When a new bug report comes, the bug features are extracted firstly. With the bug features and association rules as inputs, a rule engine can produce a debug strategy recommendation as guidance for a bug fixing engineer. We do not report the experiment results on predictions and recommendations in this paper, but as our ongoing research.

3 Pre-process on Bug Report Data

In data pre-process stage, there are three tasks: raw data preparation, data cleaning, and manually categorizing bug. The goal is to get clean, meaningful, and reasonable data for the extraction of bug features and bug fixing solutions.

3.1 Raw Data Preparation

In the Mozilla open bug repository, a bug report consists of many fields, including product, classification, component, hardware platform, operating system, summary, and comments. Among them, we combine "search options" of four classifications (Client Software, Components, Server Software, Client Support), three products (add-ons, bugzilla, calendar), and three components (API, add-ons, accessibility), and get about 6,700 bug reports. A program we developed using JavaScript takes out "Classification", "Summary" and "Comments" from each original bug report.

3.2 Data Cleaning

In this paper, data cleaning is to eliminate the punctuations and the stop-words. The former can be filtered by regular expression" [^a-zA-Z0-9-] +". The later are stored in a dictionary to tell programs which words should be deleted in the bug summaries and bug fixing comments.

3.3 Manually Labeling Bug Types

This paper divides bug types of Web-based applications into seven categories, and each type is further decomposed into sub-types as needed, shown in Table 1.

The way to define bug types serves the purpose for establishing debug strategy. The clearer the bug type is, the more specific the debug strategy is.

Manually labeling bug types for each bug report in the selected bug data set serves two purposes: 1) prepare training data set for feature extraction, bug classification and

Table 1. Bug Types and Sub-types of Web-based Applications

Bug Type	Sub-type	Bug Type	Sub-type
Content	Static Content	Navigation	Redirect
	Data Transmission		Bookmark
	Data Management		Frames and Framesets
	Data Access		Site Maps
User Interface	Layout		Internal Search Engines
	Links	Component	Style
	Readability		Storage
	Accessibility		Validation
	Compatibility		Exception
	Cookie	Security	Security
	Streaming Content	Configuration	Configuration
	Client-side Scripting	Performance	Performance

debug strategy association rules; 2) prepare testing data set for evaluating the accuracy of data mining models.

4 Bug Feature Extraction

Bug feature extraction aims at identifying the terms/features that best describe bug characteristics from pre-processed data and associating with bug types using Chi-square algorithm.

Chi-square measures the relationship between feature and category, and calculates the maximum chi-value and the average chi-value. The maximum chi-value is used to determine which category a feature belongs to; and the average chi-value can distinguish whether the word is an invalid bug feature. Table 2 shows the chi-values of features "character" and "compatible", and a feature belongs to a bug type where the feature has the highest chi-value.

From pre-processed bug reports, 1,605 individual features are taken out. By carefully observing, we discover that the features whose chi-values are lower than 0.5 contain lots of invalid information. For example, as shown in Table 3, the three features "com", "Thunderbird" and "Dev" have low average chi-values. With the literal meanings of the features, they are unhelpful for the bug classification and even decline the prediction accuracy; therefore we define them as invalid features for bug classification, and scrub out such words.

Table 2. The Relation between Features Chi-Values and Categories

Bug Type / Feature	Content	User Interface	Navigation	Security
character	11.8	5.19	0.33	0.02
compatible	1.47	5.89	0.39	0.02

Table 3. Invalid Features Scrubbed out

Feature	Category	Average chi-value
com	Component	0.017577484306667425
Thunderbird	Content	0.06389555770005631
Dev	Performance	0.13736511334578255

Consequently we set the threshold of average chi-value as 0.5. Retain the features with chi-values above the threshold, and obtain number of 1,384 features with 13.8% of features removed.

5 Bug Classification

The paper selects SVM classification algorithm for the two reasons: 1) SVM supports text classification and multi-label classification; 2) SVM can solve high-dimensional and non-linear problems. The quality of bug classification is measured by prediction accuracy, which is the ratio of the number of bug reports with correct types classified to the total number of bug reports to be classified. We improve the prediction accuracy of bug classification from the following four aspects.

1) Handling stop-words and punctuations: In the early experiment, we find there are still some stop-words and punctuations in the bug summaries, which worsen the prediction accuracy. Accordingly, we append more stop-words to the dictionary and more punctuations to the regular expressions.

2) Managing data unbalance and incorrect labeling by human being: In order to balance training data, we increase the amount of the types of bug data which account for small proportions. In addition, we define a weight for each bug type during the feature extraction. As for labeling, inspection meeting, which is arranged among the members to reconcile each other's opinion, is critical to improve accuracy.

3) Decontaminating bug reports: Some bug summaries are useless and have negative impact on the prediction accuracy, which have been excluded manually.

4) Tuning parameters of SVM tool: During modeling bug classification, we can obtain different prediction accuracy with the same data by varying the threshold of the feature value, or adjusting the parameters which is obtained by cross validation, or changing the proportion between training data and testing data.

6 Mining Debug Strategy Association Rules

The goal of association rule mining is to find debug strategy for Web-based applications. Generally, association rules identify collections of data attributes that are statistically related in the underlying data. Here are two terms that describe the significance of the association rule: 1) the confidence of the rule, a percentage of data sets that contain the antecedent; and 2) the support of the rule, a percentage of the data sets with the antecedent that also contain the consequent. Here probability is taken to be the observed frequency in the data set.

Finding frequent item sets is one of the most investigated fields of association mining. The Apriori algorithm is the most established algorithm for frequent item sets mining (FIM), which is used in this paper. We preprocess bug reports to improve the quality of mining association rules and use confidence to evaluate the results.

When it comes to our research domain, antecedent is the bug feature set and consequent is the bug fixing solutions. Debug strategy association rules can tell us the relationship between bug features and bug fixing solutions. Bug fixing solutions can be seen as accumulation of debug knowledge and experience. In the experiment, debug knowledge and experience come from two sources: extracting comments of bug reports and manually adding bug fixing recommendations.

Different from Apriori algorithm, frequent pattern growth, or simply FP-growth, generates frequent itemsets without candidate generation, which adopts a divide-and-conquer strategy. Our future work will explore the application of FP-growth in our problem domain.

7   Experiments

In order to analyze the behavior and quality of bug classifier (SVM) and debug strategy association rules, we perform several experiments by varying different aspects of models.

7.1   Experiments with Bug Classifier

Using bug classifier based on SVM, experiments are carried out from the following three aspects, where cost (c) is the penalty/parameter of the error term and gamma (g) is a kernel parameter, which controls the sensitivity of kernel function.

1) Adjusting feature threshold: The threshold can be used to cut off invalid features. With the other parameters remaining the same, accuracy will change corresponding to the threshold, as shown in Table 4. Then we choose the threshold value with the highest accuracy.

2) Tuning parameter g: SVM produces parameters c and g through cross validation (32.0 and 8.0 in Table 5). Manually tuning parameter g influences the prediction accuracy, i.e., parameters obtained by SVM are not optimal.

Table 4. Adjusting Feature threshold

Training data	Testing data	Feature #	Threshold	Cost	gamma	Accuracy
474	100	22 per line	0	8.0	8.0	67%
474	100	20 per line	0.266	32.0	8.0	74%
474	100	20 per line	0.3	32.0	8.0	70%
474	100	19 per line	0.5	32.0	8.0	77%

Table 5. Varying Parameter *g*

Training data	Testing data	Feature #	Threshold	Cost	gamma	Accuracy
474	100	19	0.5	32.0	9.0	75%
474	100	19	0.5	32.0	8.0	77%
474	100	19	0.5	32.0	7.0	78%
474	100	19	0.5	32.0	6.0	76%

3) Adjusting ratio of training data to testing data: When keeping parameters *c* and *g* the same, increasing the proportion of training data against testing data boosts the prediction accuracy, as shown in Table 6. This conforms to intuition, and indicates that we should enlarge the size of overall raw data that will be our future work.

Table 6. Varying Ratio of Training Data to Testing Data

Proportion	Training data	Testing data	Feature #	Threshold	Accuracy
3:1	431	143	19	0.5	67%
4:1	459	115	19	0.5	73%
6:1	492	82	19	0.5	78%
10:1	522	52	19	0.5	85%

7.2 Experiments with Debug Strategy Association Rules

There are two experiments with debug strategy association rules. In the first experiment, input data includes 454 bugs with 1,277 features obtained from pre-process. With the support (occurrence frequency of an association rule) being 1%, three association rules are excavated out as shown in Table 7:

Table 7. Three Association Rules Mined From 454 Training Data

Association Rule		Confidence
Features	Bug Fixing Solution	
ranges, compatibility, multiple	Check CSS documents and know the difference between Firefox and IE.	100%
install, rdf, extension	(S1) Check JavaScript statements, such as string concatenation operation. (S2) Give meaningful warnings before installing add-ons.	100%
update, mozilla, org	In model layer, data is accessed or updated correctly.	57.14%

The second experiment increases data amount to include 575 bugs with 1,629 features. With the support 1%, three association rules are quarried out. The result shows that the first association rule is replaced by a new one, because the support of the old rule doesn't increase with the bug total number whereas that of the new rule increases up to and over the support threshold, as a result, substituting the old one. Our future work will continue increasing the size of training data with high quality.

8 Conclusion and Future Work

This paper uses data mining approaches to classify bug types and excavate debug strategy association rules for Web-based applications. Chi-square algorithm is used to extract features that properly characterize bugs of Web-based application; and SVM is used to model classifier, which achieves more than 70% of prediction accuracy on average in our experiments. Bug classification is useful for our future research on analysis of the relation between bug types and developer skills as well as bug fixing solutions. We use Apriori algorithm to excavate debug strategy association rules, which describe that with what kinds of bug features, what kinds of actions should be taken to handle the bugs. With 575 training data, three debug strategy association rules are unearthed. Our future work will collect more bug reports and bug fixing solutions to dig out more association rules.

Acknowledgement. The work presented in this article is partly sponsored by the National High-Tech Research and Development Plan of China (No. 2006AA01Z175) and by IBM Joint Research Program (No. JS200705002).

References

[1]   Anvik, J., Hiew, L., Murphy, G.C.: Who should fix this bug? In: Proceeding of the 28th international conference on Software engineering, pp. 361–370 (2006)

[2]   Cubranic, D., Murphy, G.C.: Automatic bug triage using text categorization. In: The 16th International Conference on Software Engineering & Knowledge Engineering (SEKE 2004), pp. 92–97 (2004)

[3]   Haran, M., Karr, A., Last, M., Orso, A., Porter, A.A., Sanil, A., Fouché, S.: Techniques for classifying executions of deployed software to support software engineering tasks. IEEE Transactions on Software Engineering 33(5), 287–304 (2007)

[4]   Zimmermann, T., Weissgerber, P., Diel, S., Zeller, A.: Mining version histories to guide software changes. In: Proc. of ICSE 2004. IEEE Press, Los Alamitos (2004)

[5]   Kim, S., Zimmermann, T., James Whitehead Jr., E., Zeller, A.: Predicting Faults from Cached History. In: Proceedings of the 29th International Conference on Software Engineering, pp.489–498 (2007)

[6]   Arumuga, P., Nainar,, Chen, T., Rosin, J., Liblit, B.: Statistical Debugging Using Compound Boolean Predicates. In: Proceedings of the 2007 international symposium on Software testing and analysis, pp. 5–15 (2007)

Test the Overall Significance of p-values by Using Joint Tail Probability of Ordered p-values as Test Statistic

Yongxiang Fang* and Ernst Wit

Department of Mathematics and statistics
Lancaster University
Lancaster, LA1 4YF, UK
y.fang@lancaster.ac.uk

Abstract. Fisher's combined probability test is the most commonly used method to test the overall significance of a set independent p-values. However, it is very obviously that Fisher's statistic is more sensitive to smaller p-values than to larger p-value and a small p-value may overrule the other p-values and decide the test result. This is, in some cases, viewed as a flaw. In order to overcome this flaw and improve the power of the test, the joint tail probability of a set p-values is proposed as a new statistic to combine and make an overall test of the p-values. Through the development of a method and a practical application, this study reveals that the new method has plausible properties and more power.

Keywords: p-values, joint tail probability, combined probability test.

1 Introduction

The p-value is the probability of obtaining a value of the test statistic at least as extreme as the one that was actually observed, given that the null hypothesis is true. In many cases of statistical analysis, taking the p-values from a set of independent hypothesis tests as statistics and combining their significance is required. There are several methods for combining p-values available, for example Fisher's combined probability test [1], minimum p-value test [2], sum p-value method [3], [4], Wilkinson method [5], and inverse normal method [6]. There are also some review and comparative studies of methods for combining p-values. For example, Birnbaum [7], Littell and Folks [8], [9] and Berk and Cohen [10]. These studies essentially agree that Fisher's method is generally best and efficient among the methods mentioned above, however, none of the methods are uniformly more powerful then the others and different methods are usually sensitive in different pattern of outliers.

---

* Please note that the LNCS Editorial assumes that all authors have used the western naming convention, with given names preceding surnames. This determines the structure of the names in the running heads and the author index.

C. Tang et al. (Eds.): ADMA 2008, LNAI 5139, pp. 435–443, 2008.
© Springer-Verlag Berlin Heidelberg 2008

Fisher's statistic is $T_{fk} = -2ln(\Pi_{i=1}^{k}p_i)$, while k is the number of p-values. Since the statistic is a logarithm transformed product of p-values, it is more sensitive to small p-value than large p-value. This property is viewed as a flaw especially in certain applications [11]. Furthermore, Fisher's statistic is actually also a transformed joint tail probability of the p-values, because the p-values are supposed from independent hypothesis tests. Therefore, we introduce and discuss a slightly different statistic from Fisher's for combining p-values, The new statistic is defined as the joint tail probability of **ordered p-values**. The value of Fisher's statistic depends only on the product or geometric mean of a set of p-values, no matter how alike or different between the individual elements. Our statistic is different from this. To say there are two different sets of p-values with the same product, in the first set of p-values all the elements have the same value, in the second set of p-values the elements have different values, then the the first set of p-values will be valued smaller than the second set of p-values under our statistic. Therefore, we expect that testing on our statistic shows some plausible properties and higher power.

2   Methods

Let's start from the computation of our statistic for given p-values. Denote by $p_1, p_2, ..., p_k$ k p-values from independent hypothesis tests. Let $p_{[1]} \leq p_{[2]} \leq \cdots \leq p_{[k]}$ be the ordered k p-values and V_k the joint tail probability of the ordered k p-values, V_k can be expressed by:

$$V_k = k! \int_0^{p_{[1]}} \int_{x_1}^{p_{[2]}} \cdots \int_{x_{k-1}}^{p_{[k]}} dx_k dx_{k-1}...dx_1 \tag{1}$$

Let $V_0 = 1$ and V_j (j=1, 2,...,k) be the joint tail probability of $p_{[k-j+1]}, p_{[k-j+2]}, ..., p_{[k]}$, obviously $V_1 = p_{[k]}$. We can have:

$$V_j = \sum_{i=1}^{j} (-1)^{i-1} \binom{j}{i} p_{[k-j+1]}^i V_{j-i} \tag{2}$$

Proof. When $j = 1$ equation (2) is correct, because it simply becomes $V_1 = p_{[k]}$. Suppose when $j = n < k$ equation (2) stands. For $j = n + 1$, we have

$$V_{n+1} = (n+1)! \int_0^{p_{[k-n]}} \int_{x_{k-n}}^{p_{[k-n+1]}} \cdots \int_{x_{k-1}}^{p_{[k]}} dx_k dx_{k-1}...dx_{k-n}$$

and it can be written as:

$$V_{n+1} = (n+1) \int_0^{p_{[k-n]}} (n! \int_0^{p_{[k-n+1]}} \cdots \int_{x_{k-1}}^{p_{[k]}} dx_k dx_{k-1}...d_{k-n+1}) dx_{k-n}$$

$$-(n+1) \int_0^{p_{[k-n]}} (n! \int_0^{x_{k-n}} \cdots \int_{x_{k-1}}^{p_{[k]}} dx_k dx_{k-1}...d_{k-n+1}) dx_{k-n}$$

Making use of the definition of V_j and equation (2), we can have:

$$V_{n+1} = (n+1)p_{[k-n]}V_n - (n+1)\int_0^{p_{[k-n]}} (\sum_{i=1}^n (-1)^{i-1} \binom{n}{i} x_{k-n}^i V_{n-i}) dx_{k-n}$$

On integration and simplification we have

$$V_{n+1} = \sum_{i=1}^{n+1} (-1)^{i-1} \binom{n+1}{i} p_{[k-(n+1)+1]}^i V_{(n+1)-i}$$

Equation (2) is proved.

Hence for a given set of p-values, the value of our statistic can be computed recursively by using equation (2). The computation starts with $n=1$ and increases n by 1 for a new iteration until $n=k$. V_k as a statistic has its own probability density function (p.d.f) and cumulative probability function (c.d.f). There are two useful properties about V_k and its c.d.f $F(x) = Pr(V_k \leq x \mid null)$. First one is obvious $0 \leq V_k \leq 1$, because V_k is defined as joint tail probability of ordered k p-values. The second is $F(x) \geq x$, because the equation below:

$$k! \int_0^{1-\sqrt[k]{1-x}} \int_{x_1}^1 ... \int_{x_k}^1 dx_k dx_{k-1}...dx_1 = x \tag{3}$$

In fact, let $\mho$ be the collection of all the ordered p-value sets which satisfy $V_k \leq x$, then integration limits of the definite integral in the left hand side of equation (3) pick out a subset $\mathcal{C}$ from the collection $\mho$. That is under null hypotheses, the chance for a set of ordered p-values P_o being a member of $\mathcal{C}$ is $Pr(V_k \leq x \mid P_o \in \mathcal{C}) = x$. Therefore, $F(x) \geq x$ stands.

Now we discuss the distribution function for our statistic. The simplest case is when there are two p-values. Based on equation (2) and by some simplification, the statistic can be formulated as:

$$V_2 = 2p_{[1]}p_{[2]} - p_{[1]}^2 \tag{4}$$

Based on equation (4), we can transfer $V_2 \leq x$ for ($0 \leq x \leq 1$) into constraints to $p_{[1]}$ and $p_{[2]}$. The constraint of $p_{[1]}$ is obviously that:

$$0 \leq p_{[1]} \leq \sqrt{x} \tag{5}$$

There are two different constants on $p_{[2]}$ when equation (5) is satisfied.

$$p_{[1]} < p_{[2]} \leq 1 \ when \ 0 < p_{[1]} \leq 1 - \sqrt{1-x} \tag{6}$$

$$p_{[1]} < p_{[2]} \leq \frac{x + p_{[1]}^2}{2p_{[1]}} \ when \ 1 - \sqrt{1-x} < p_{[1]} \leq \sqrt{x} \tag{7}$$

Hence the cumulative distribution function of our statistic for $k=2$ can be worked out through integrals below:

$$Pr(V_2 \le x) = 2 \int_0^{1-\sqrt{1-x}} \int_{x_1}^1 dx_2 dx_1 + 2 \int_{1-\sqrt{1-x}}^{\sqrt{x}} \int_{x_1}^{\frac{x+x_1^2}{2x_1}} dx_2 dx_1 \qquad (8)$$

From equation (8) we have the c.d.f of our statistic for $k=2$.

$$F(x) = 1 - \sqrt{1-x} + x ln \frac{\sqrt{x}}{1 - \sqrt{1-x}} \qquad (9)$$

Hence we have its corresponding p.d.f:

$$f(x) = ln \frac{\sqrt{x}}{1 - \sqrt{1-x}} \qquad (10)$$

Due to V_2 is the tail probability of given two ordered p-values and equation (9) is its distribution function, replacing x in equation (9) with V_2 produces actually the extremity of a set of two ordered p-values. That is to put the value of V_2 into equation (9), we directly get the p-value of testing on V_2.

For $k = 3$, we have

$$V_3 = 6p_{[1]}p_{[2]}p_{[3]} - 3p_{[1]}p_{[2]}^2 - 3p_{[1]}^2 p_{[3]} + p_{[1]}^3 \qquad (11)$$

Similarly, from equation (11) we can transfer $V_3 \le x$ into constraints to $p_{[1]}$, $p_{[2]}$ and $p_{[3]}$ and formulate the probability distribution V_3 as the sum of four integrals:

$$F(x) = Pr(V_3 < x) = I_1 + I_2 + I_3 + I_4 \qquad (12)$$

while $I_1 = 6 \int_0^{b_{11}} \int_{x_1}^1 \int_{x_2}^1 dx_3 dx_2 dx_1$, $I_2 = 6 \int_{b_{11}}^{b_{12}} \int_{x_1}^{b_{21}} \int_{x_2}^1 dx_3 dx_2 dx_1$, $I_3 = 6 \int_{b_{11}}^{b_{12}} \int_{b_{21}}^{b_{22}} \int_{x_2}^{b_{31}} dx_3 dx_2 dx_1$, $I_4 = 6 \int_{b_{12}}^{b_{13}} \int_{x_1}^{b_{22}} \int_{x_2}^{b_{31}} dx_3 dx_2 dx_1$.

while $b_{11} = 1 - \sqrt[3]{1-x}$, b_{12} **is solution of** $b_{12}^3 - \frac{3}{2}b_{12}^2 + \frac{x}{2} = 0$ **in [0,1]**,

$b_{13} = \sqrt[3]{x}$, $b_{21} = 1 - \sqrt{1 + \frac{x_1^3 - 3x_1^2 - x}{3x_1}}$, $b_{22} = \frac{1}{2}(1 + \sqrt{\frac{4x - x_1^3}{3x_1}})$, $b_{31} = \frac{x + 3x_1 x_2^3 - x_1^3}{6x_1 x_2 - 3x_1^2}$.

Due to there is no analytical solution for the integral I_3, the computation of $F(V_3)$ (the c.d.f of V_3) cannot be done without numeric integration. This makes the test on V_3 complicate. Obviously, when the number of p-values $k > 3$, the test on our statistic becomes more difficult. Therefore, how to test on our statistic in a simple way is the problem should be first solved in the practical application of our statistic.

A solution can be developed based on two properties of V_k which are $0 \le V_k \le 1$ and $Pr(V_k \le x \mid null) \ge x$. Denote by α the significance level and $V_{k,\alpha}$ the critical value, then a power scale $\gamma_{k,\alpha}$ for V_k exists so that:

$$Pr(V_k \le V_{k,\alpha} \mid null) = Pr(V_k^{\gamma_{k,\alpha}} \le \alpha \mid null) = \alpha \qquad (13)$$

Table 1. $\gamma_{k,\alpha}$ values

k	$\gamma_{k,0.01}$	$\gamma_{k,0.05}$	k	$\gamma_{k,0.01}$	$\gamma_{k,0.05}$
1	1	1	16	0.4069	0.3452
2	0.762	0.7159	17	0.4016	0.3400
3	0.6602	0.5995	18	0.3970	0.3350
4	0.5982	0.5368	19	0.3929	0.3306
5	0.5560	0.4935	20	0.3890	0.3264
6	0.5244	0.4635	21	0.3852	0.3224
7	0.5023	0.4395	22	0.3816	0.3187
8	0.4848	0.4204	23	0.3783	0.3152
9	0.4697	0.4062	24	0.3749	0.3121
10	0.4569	0.3937	25	0.3715	0.3092
11	0.4460	0.3830	26	0.3682	0.3064
12	0.4365	0.3735	27	0.3647	0.3038
13	0.4276	0.3653	28	0.3615	0.3014
14	0.4201	0.358	29	0.3587	0.2992
15	0.4131	0.3514	30	0.3561	0.2971

Table 2. Simulated rejecting rate to null cases

k	$P^*_{0.01}$	CI of $P^*_{0.01}$	$P^*_{0.05}$	CI of $P^*_{0.05}$
1	0.0117	(0.0095799, 0.013820)	0.0504	(0.048280, 0.052520)
2	0.0112	(0.0091257, 0.013274)	0.0517	(0.049626, 0.053774)
3	0.0086	(0.0067824, 0.010418)	0.0490	(0.047182, 0.050818)
4	0.0100	(0.0080400, 0.011960)	0.0516	(0.049640, 0.053560)
5	0.0110	(0.0089443, 0.013056)	0.0490	(0.046944, 0.051056)
6	0.0098	(0.0078597, 0.011740)	0.0449	(0.042960, 0.046840)
7	0.0097	(0.0077696, 0.011630)	0.0499	(0.047970, 0.051830)
8	0.0106	(0.0085821, 0.012618)	0.0508	(0.048782, 0.052818)
9	0.0094	(0.0074997, 0.011300)	0.0493	(0.047400, 0.051200)
10	0.0101	(0.0081302, 0.012070)	0.0513	(0.046861, 0.055739)

From equation (14) we have:

$$\gamma_{k,\alpha} = \frac{\ln(\alpha)}{\ln(V_{k,\alpha})} \tag{14}$$

Based on equation (13) and (14), we can simplify the test as a simple comparing the power scaled our statistic with the significance level, if the critical value $V_{k,\alpha}$ is available. Due to the c.d.f of V_k (when $k \geq 3$) is not analytical, we proposed to work out $V_{k,\alpha}$ using simulation technique and then get $\gamma_{k\alpha}$ from equation (14). The simulation is simply drawing a large number N sets of p-values from $U(0,1)^k$ and computing V_k's value from each set of them. Order these values and take the one being ordered as $N \times \alpha$ to be a realization of $V_{k,\alpha}$. The process is repeated M times then $\hat{V}_{k,\alpha}$ is valued by the mean of M realizations.

Our simulation takes N=10000 and M=100, for k=3 to k=30, $\alpha = 0.05$ and $\alpha = 0.01$, the results are shown in table 1. Where for $k=1$ and $k=2$ the power

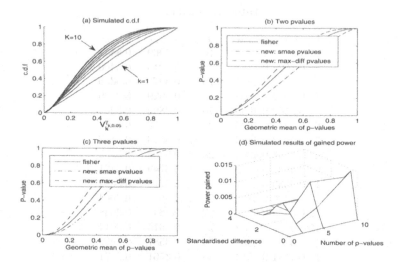

Fig. 1. Results from methods comparisons

scale is computed from the corresponding distribution function, therefore no confidence interval is required.

A simulation of the application of the proposed technique is conducted for $k = 1, 2, ..., 10$ and $\alpha = 0.05$. For each value of k, 10000 sets of p-values are drawn from $U(0,1)^k$, then V_k is computed and it is power scaled by corresponding $\gamma_{k,0.01}$ (and $\gamma_{k,0.05}$) so that to get $V_k^{\gamma_k,\alpha}$. The $V_k^{\gamma_k,\alpha}$ with values smaller than α are the null hypotheses should be rejected. For the cases in this simulation, the expected rejecting rate is α. The simulated rates of rejection are shown in Table 2, which are very encouraging on comparing them with the corresponding α. We plot the simulated c.d.f of the power scaled our statistic in Figure 1 subplot(a) for $\alpha = 0.05$. It shows that for all $k = 1, 2, ..., 10$, when $x < 0.05$, $Pr(V_k^{\gamma_k,\alpha} \leq x) < x$ and $Pr(V_k^{\gamma_k,\alpha} \leq x) \simeq x$. when $x > 0.05$, $Pr(V_k^{\gamma_k,\alpha} \leq x) > x$.

3   Discussion

We expected our method has some plausible behaviors which pictures the difference from Fisher's combined probability test, hence a comparison is made in this section. Let $\wp$ contain all different sets of p-values whose products equal a given value $c \in (0,1)$. Let $V_k(\wp)$ be collection of their corresponding values under our statistic. Hance, a set of p-values whose all elements have the same value $\sqrt[k]{c}$ will be in $\wp$ and its corresponding value under our statistic will be the smallest one in $V_k(\wp)$. On the other hand, if a set of p-values has the biggest variation among their elements and belongs $\wp$, combining this set of p-values under our approach, will produce the biggest value in $V_k(\wp)$.

When $k=2$, the two sets of p-values being the smallest and largest under our statistic are correspondingly $(\sqrt{c}, \sqrt{c})$ and $(1 - \sqrt{(1-c)}, 1)$. We test them by

Fisher's method and ours. By changing c's value we get three sets results, one is from Fisher's, the other two are from our method. They are illustrated in Figure 1 subplot (b). Similar work is done for number of p-values $k=3$, and the results is shown in Figure 1 subplot (c). From the two subplots we can see that if two sets of p-values are with the same value of product they are tested no difference under Fisher's test. However, the one which has smaller variation among their elements will be tested with smaller p-values under our test. In another words, our method is more sensitive to p-value sets which their elements are uniformly small. This means our test are more plausible for testing where the null hypotheses are commonly true in the k independent tests.

A simulation based comparison between Fisher's with ours confirms the above analysis. In the simulation, we suppose the variation is normally distributed, the null hypothesis is that the original individual test statistic is with zero mean, the alternative hypothesis is that the mean of the original test statistics moves away from zero and the distance of the move is scaled by standard deviation. We select the distance as $0.5 \times d$ where $d = 1, 2, ..., 8$. The number of p-values are 2, 5 and 10 respectively and the significance level α are 0.01 and 0.05 respectively. The results shows our method is more powerful than Fisher's. We present the power gained by our method, compared to Fisher's, in Figure 1 subplot(d).

Finally, we make two comparisons by using practical examples. The first is a simple one which has been used by William Rice [11]. A biological study were conducted twice in two different years respectively, and two p-values are 1/120 and 1 respectively. The product of he two p-values is 1/120 and using Fisher's method produces a p-values 0.049 which is significant at 0.05 level. Due to the two element are extremely different, under our method the test results shows it is not significant at 0.05. level, because the p-value from our test is 0.0538.

The second example is an microarray study on the effects of treating roach with chemicals of three different concentrations 0.1 ng EE2/L, 1 ng EE2/L and 10 ng EE2/L. In the study, besides the three treatment groups, a control group is also employed, and we use L0, L1, L2 and L3 to represent the groups from control to highest level of treatment respectively. In addition, except L3 group animals whose gender is not clear, the other three groups have both male and female samples. A major outcome of the study is that the objects under highest level treatment tend to be female like. Therefore, an interesting question is that which genes expressed differently in common between the L3 subjects and other samples. Let L3/L0, L3/L1 and L3/L2 denote the expression ratio on log2 scale, then we want to know which genes are with significantly non zero values cross the three parameters. Due to p-values (from two-side test) for three parameters of each gene are available, both Fisher's method and our method are used to find such genes. Without loss generality, we simply take significance level $\alpha = 0.01$. The outcomes are that our method identified 2049 genes and Fisher's method identified 1831 genes. In the union of the two lists of genes, most of them are identified by both method, however, still a considerable number of them are identified by only Fisher's method or our method. The results also shows that almost all the genes identified only by our test are genes whose three parameters are not close to zero. In contrast, if a gene is only identified by Fisher's methods, at least one of its three parameters has a value closing to zero. This is evident that our method performs better than Fisher's.

4   Conclusion

The comparative study of our method with Fisher's combined probability test confirm our method has a plausible property and stronger power. The point is shows by not only theoretical analysis, but also simulation results and application to practical cases.

The computation required by the proposed method becomes more and more intensive as the the increase of the number of p-values k. For very large k the application of our method is not as easy as Fisher's. Another problem is the availability of probability distribution function when $k > 3$, we hope there is a better way to get it in the future.

Funding

Y.F. was supported by NERC grants (NE/D000602/1) and NE/F001355/1.

Acknowledgement

We thank C. Tyler and L. Anke and A. Cossins, for providing and allowing to use their roach microarray data.

References

1. Fisher, R.A.: Statistical Methods for Research Workers, 4th edn. Oliver and Boyd (1932)
2. Tippett, L.H.C.: The method of Statistics. Williams and Norgate (1931)
3. Edgington, E.S.: An additive method for combining probability values from independent experiments. Journal of Psychology 80, 351–363 (1972)
4. Edgington, E.S.: A normal curve method for combining probability values from independent experiments. Journal of Psychology 82, 85–89 (1972)
5. Wilkinson, B.: A statistical consideration in psychological research. Psychological Bulletin 48, 156–157 (1951)
6. Stouffer, S.A., Suchman, E.A., DeVinney, L.C., Star, S.A., Williams Jr., R.M.: The American Soldier. In: Adjustment during Army Life, vol. I. Princeton University Press, Princeton (1949)
7. Birnbaum, A.: Combining independent tests of significance. Journal of the American Statistical Association 49, 559–574 (1954)
8. Littell, R.C., Folks, J.L.: Asymptotic optimality of Fisher's method of combining independent tests. Journal of the American Statistical Association 66(336), 802–806 (1971)

9. Littell, R.C., Folks, J.L.: Combining Independent Tests of Significance. Journal of the American Statistical Association 68(341), 193–194 (1973)
10. Berk, R.H., Cohen, R.: Asymptotically optimal methods of combining tests. Journal of the American Statistical Association 74, 812–814 (1979)
11. William, R.: A Consensus Combined P-Value Test and the Family-Wide Significance of Component Tests. Biometrics 46(2), 303–308 (1990)

Mining Interesting Infrequent and Frequent Itemsets Based on MLMS Model

Xiangjun Dong[1,2], Zhendong Niu[3], Donghua Zhu[1],
Zhiyun Zheng[4], and Qiuting Jia[2]

[1] School of Management and Economics, Beijing Institute of Technology,
Beijing 100081, China
dxj@sdili.edu.cn, zhudh111@bit.edu.cn
[2] School of Information Science and Technology, Shandong Institute of Light Industry,
Jinan 250353, China
[3] School of Computer Science and Technology, Beijing Institute of Technology,
Beijing 100081, China
zniu@bit.edu.cn
[4] School of Information & Engineering, Zhengzhou University,
Zhengzhou 450052, China
iezyzheng@zzu.edu.cn

Abstract. MLMS (Multiple Level Minimum Supports) model which uses multiple level minimum supports to discover infrequent itemsets and frequent itemsets simultaneously is proposed in our previous work. The reason to discover infrequent itemsets is that there are many valued negative association rules in them. However, some of the itemsets discovered by the MLMS model are not interesting and ought to be pruned. In one of Xindong Wu's papers [1], a pruning strategy (we call it Wu's pruning strategy here) is used to prune uninteresting itemsets. But the pruning strategy is only applied to single minimum support. In this paper, we modify the Wu's pruning strategy to adapt to the MLMS model to prune uninteresting itemsets and we call the MLMS model with the modified Wu's pruning strategy IMLMS (Interesting MLMS) model. Based on the IMLMS model, we design an algorithm to discover simultaneously both interesting frequent itemsets and interesting infrequent itemsets. The experimental results show the validity of the model.

1 Introduction

Mining association rules in database has received much attention recently. Many efforts have been devoted to design algorithms for efficiently discovering association rules of the form $A \Rightarrow B$, whose support (s) and confidence (c) meet a minimum support (ms) threshold and a minimum confidence (mc) respectively. This is the famous support-confidence framework [2]. The rules of the form $A \Rightarrow B$ have been studied widely since then, while the rules of the form $A \Rightarrow \neg B$ have only been attracted a little attention until recently some papers proposed that the rules of the form $A \Rightarrow \neg B$ could play the same important roles as the rules of the form $A \Rightarrow B$. The rules of the form $A \Rightarrow \neg B$, which suggests that a customer may not buy item B after the customer buys

C. Tang et al. (Eds.): ADMA 2008, LNAI 5139, pp. 444–451, 2008.

item *A,* together with the rules of the forms $\neg A \Rightarrow B$ and $\neg A \Rightarrow \neg B$, are called **negative association rules** (**NARs**) and the rules of the form $A \Rightarrow B$ **positive association rules** (**PARs**) [1].

Discovering infrequent itemsets is one of the new problems that would occur when we study NARs. The reason to discover infrequent itemsets is that there are many valued negative association rules in them. How to discover infrequent itemsets, how-ever, is still an open problem. Theoretically, infrequent itemsets are the complement of frequent itemsets and the number of infrequent itemsets is too large to be mined completely. So in real application, some constraints must be given so as to control the number of infrequent itemsets in a moderate degree. The constraints to infrequent itemsets in different applications are different. MLMS (Multiple Level Minimum Supports) model [3], which is proposed in our previous work, can be used to discover infrequent itemsets and frequent itemsets simultaneously. The details about the MLMS model are mentioned in section 3.1.

Another new problem is how to prune uninteresting itemsets because some item-sets are not interesting. In one of Xindong Wu's papers [1], a pruning strategy (we call it Wu's pruning strategy here) which concerns the support, the confidence, and interestingness of a rule $A \Rightarrow B$ is used to prune uninteresting itemsets. But the Wu's pruning strategy is only applied to single minimum support. In this paper, we modify the Wu's pruning strategy to adapt to the MLMS model to prune uninteresting item-sets and we call the MLMS model with the modified Wu's pruning strategy IMLMS (Interesting MLMS) model.

The main contributions of this paper are as follows:

1. We modify the Wu's pruning strategy to adapt to the MLMS model.
2. We design an algorithm *Apriori_IMLMS* to discover simultaneously both interest-ing infrequent itemsets and interesting frequent itemsets based on the IMLMS model.

The rest of the paper is organized as follows: Section 2 discusses the related works. Section 3 discusses the modified Wu's pruning strategy and the algorithm *Apriori_IMLMS*. Experiments are discussed in section 4. Section 5 is conclusions and future work.

2 Related Work

Negative relationships between two itemsets were first mentioned in [4]. [5] proposed a new approach for discovering strong NARs. [6] proposed another approach based on taxonomy for discovering PARs and NARs. In our previous work [7], we proposed an approach that can discover PARs and NARs by chi-squared test and multiple mini-mum confidences. [8] proposed an approach to discover confined PARs and NARs. In [9], a MMS (multiple minimum supports) model was proposed to discover frequent itemsets using multiple minimum supports to solve the problems caused by a single minimum support, [10] proposed an approach of mining multiple-level association rules based on taxonomy information.

These works, however, do not concentrate on discovering infrequent itemsets. There are many mature techniques to discover frequent itemsets, while few papers study the approach of how to discover infrequent itemsets. In our previous work [11], a 2LS (2-Level Supports) model was proposed to discover infrequent itemsets and frequent itemsets, however, the 2LS model only used the same two constraints to divide the infrequent itemsets and frequent itemsets and did not prune uninteresting itemsets. In [1], the Wu's pruning strategy was used to prune uninteresting itemsets, however, the constrains to infrequent itemsets and frequent itemsets are still a single minimum support.

3 Mining Interesting Infrequent and Frequent Itemsets

3.1 Review of the MLMS Model

Let $I=\{i_1, i_2,..., i_n\}$ be a set of n distinct literals called items, and TD a transaction database of variable-length transactions over I, and the number of transactions in TD is denoted as $|TD|$. Each transaction contains a set of item $i_1, i_2,...,i_m \in I$ and each transaction is associated with a unique identifier TID. A set of distinct items from I is called an itemset. The number of items in an itemset A is the length of the itemset, denoted by $length(A)$. An itemset of length k are referred to as k-itemset. Each itemset has an associated statistical measure called support, denoted by s. For an itemset $A \subseteq I$, $s(A)=A.count / |TD|$, where $A.count$ is the number of transactions containing itemsets A in TD. The support of a rule $A \Rightarrow B$ is denoted as $s(A \cup B)$ or $s(A \Rightarrow B)$, where $A, B \subseteq I$,and $A \cap B = \Phi$. The confidence of the rule $A \Rightarrow B$ is defined as the ratio of $s(A \cup B)$ over $s(A)$, i.e., $c(A \Rightarrow B) = s(A \cup B) / s(A)$.

In the MLMS model, different minimum supports are assigned to itemsets with different lengths. Let $ms(k)$ be the minimum support of k-itemsets ($k=1,2,...,n$), $ms(0)$ be a threshold for infrequent itemsets, $ms(1) \geq ms(2) \geq ..., \geq ms(n) \geq ms(0) > 0$, for any itemset A,

if $s(A) \geq ms(length(A))$, then A is a frequent itemset; and
if $s(A) < ms(length(A))$ and $s(A) \geq ms(0)$, then A is an infrequent itemset.

The MLMS model allows users to control the number of frequent and infrequent itemsets easily. The value of $ms(k)$ can be given by users or experts.

3.2 The Modified Wu's Pruning Strategy

The Wu's pruning strategy uses different methods to prune uninteresting itemsets from frequent and infrequent itemsets. The following equations are used to prune uninteresting frequent itemsets.

M is a *frequent itemset of potential interest* if

$$fipi(M) = s(M) \geq ms \wedge (\exists A, B: A \cup B = M) \wedge fipis(A, B), \tag{1}$$

$$\text{where} \quad fipis(A, B) =(A \cap B)=\Phi \ \wedge \ f(A,B, ms, mc, mi) = 1, \tag{2}$$

$$f(A, B, ms, mc, mi) \tag{3}$$

$$= \frac{s(A \cup B) + c(A \Rightarrow B) + interest(A,B) - (ms + mc + mi) + 1}{|s(A \cup B) - ms| + |c(A \Rightarrow B) - mc| + |interest(A,B) - mi| + 1},$$

where *interest(A,B)* is a interestingness measure and *interest(A,B)*=|*s(A∪B)* - *s(A)s(B)*|, *mi* is a minimum interestingness threshold given by users or experts, and *f* () is a constraint function concerning the support, confidence, and interestingness of *A⇒B* .

Since *c(A⇒B)* is used to mine association rules after discovering frequent itemsets and infrequent itemsets, here we replace *f* (*A,B, ms, mc, mi*) with *f* (*A,B, ms, mi*) as [1] did.

From the equations 1-3 we can see that the Wu's pruning strategy is only applied to single minimum support *ms*. Considering that there are different minimum support s *ms(k)* for *k*-itemsets in the MLMS model, we must modify the Wu's pruning strategy by replacing corresponding variables as follows.

M is a *frequent itemset of potential interest* in the MLMS model if

$$fipi(M) = s(M) \geq ms(length(M)) \wedge (\exists A, B: A \cup B = M) \wedge fipis(A, B), \tag{4}$$

where $fipis(A, B) = A \cap B = \Phi \wedge f(A,B, ms(length(A \cup B)), mi) = 1,$ (5)

$$f(A, B, ms(length(A \cup B)), mi)$$

$$= \frac{s(A \cup B) + interest(A,B) - (ms(length(A \cup B)) + mi) + 1}{|s(A \cup B) - ms(length(A \cup B))| + |interest(A,B) - mi| + 1}. \tag{6}$$

Equations 4-6 can be used to prune uninteresting frequent itemsets in the MLMS model. As for pruning uninteresting infrequent itemsets in the MLMS model, we can not use the methods of pruning uninteresting infrequent itemsets in the Wu's pruning strategy because the constraints to infrequent itemsets in the MLMS model and in [1] are different. Fortunately, according to the above discussion, we can get the following equations by modifying the equations 4-6.

N is an *infrequent itemset of potential interest* if

$$iipi(N) = s(N) < ms(length(N)) \wedge s(N) \geq ms(0) \wedge$$

$$(\exists A, B: A \cup B = N) \wedge iipis(A, B), \tag{7}$$

where $iipis(A, B) = A \cap B = \Phi \wedge f(A,B, ms(0), mi) = 1,$ (8)

$$f(A, B, ms(0), mi) = \frac{s(A \cup B) + interest(A,B) - (ms(0) + mi) + 1}{|s(A \cup B) - ms(0)| + |interest(A,B) - mi| + 1}. \tag{9}$$

The IMLMS model is to use equation 4 -9 to prune the uninteresting frequent itemsets and the uninteresting infrequent itemsets discovered by the MLMS model.

3.3 Algorithm Design

```
Algorithm Apriori_IMLMS
Input:   TD:   Transaction   Database;   ms(k)(k=0,1,…,n):
         minimum support threshold;
Output:  FIS: set of interesting frequent itemsets;inFIS:
         set of interesting infrequent itemsets;
(1) FIS=Φ; inFIS=Φ;
(2) temp₁ = {A|A∈1-itemsets,s(A)≥ms(0)};
    FIS₁ = {A|A∈temp₁ ∧ s(A)≥ms(1)};
    inFIS₁ = temp₁-FIS₁;
(3) for (k=2;temp_{k-1}≠Φ;k++) do
  begin
    (3.1) C_k = apriori_gen(temp_{k-1}, ms(0));
    (3.2) for each transaction t∈TD do
        begin
           /*scan transaction database TD*/
           C_t=subset(C_k, t);
           for each candidate c ∈ C_t
               c.count++;
        end
    (3.3) temp_k = {c|c∈C_k (c.count/|TD|)≥ms(0)};
          FIS_k = {A|A∈temp_k ∧ A.count/|TD|≥ms(k)};
          inFIS_k = temp_k - FIS_k;
    (3.4) /*prune all uninteresting k-itemsets in FIS_k */
          for each itemset  M in FIS_k do
              if NOT (fipi(M)) then
              FIS_k =FIS_k - { M }
    (3.5)/*prune all uninteresting k-itemsets in inFIS_k */
          for each itemset N in inFIS_k do
                if NOT (iipi(N)) then
                inFIS_k =inFIS_k - { N }
  end
(4) FIS = ∪FIS_k; inFIS = ∪inFIS_k;
(5) return FIS and inFIS;
```

The algorithm $Apriori\_IMLMS$ is used to generate all interesting frequent and interesting infrequent itemsets in a given database TD, where FIS is the set of all interesting frequent itemsets, and $inFIS$ is the set of all interesting infrequent itemsets. There are four kinds of sets: FIS_k, $inFIS_k$, $temp_k$ and C_k. $Temp_k$ contains the itemsets whose support meets the constraint $ms(0)$. C_k contains the itemsets generated by the procedure $apriori\_gen$. The procedure $apriori\_gen$ is the same as the procedure in traditional $Apriori$ [2] and is omitted here. The main steps of the algorithm $Apriori\_IMLMS$ are the same as the $Apriori\_MLMS$ except steps (3.4) and (3.5).

In step (3.4), if an itemset M in FIS_k does not meet $fipi(M)$, then M is an uninteresting frequent itemset, and is removed from FIS_k. In step (3.5), if an itemset N in $inFIS_k$

does not meet *iipi(N)*, then *N* is an uninteresting infrequent itemset, and is removed from *inFIS*$_k$.

3.4 An Example

The sample data is shown in Table 1. Let $ms(1)=0.5$, $ms(2)=0.4$, $ms(3)=0.3$, $ms(4)=0.2$ and $ms=0.15$. FIS_1, FIS_2, $inFIS_1$, and $inFIS_2$ generated by the MLMS model are shown in Table 2, where the itemsets with gray background are infrequent itemsets with non background are frequent itemsets and the itemsets.

Table 1. Sample Data

TID	itemsets
T_1	A, B, D
T_2	A, B, C, D
T_3	B, D
T_4	B, C, D, E
T_5	A, C, E
T_6	B, D, F
T_7	A, E, F
T_8	C, F
T_9	B, C, F
T_{10}	A, B, C, D, F

Table 2. FIS_1, FIS_2, $inFIS_1$, and $inFIS_2$ generated by the MLMS model from the data in table 1

1-itemsets	$s(*)$	2- itemsets	$s(*)$		$s(*)$
A	0.5	BD	0.6	CD	0.3
B	0.7	BC	0.4	CF	0.3
C	0.6	AB	0.3	AE	0.2
D	0.6	AC	0.3	AF	0.2
E	0.3	AD	0.3	CE	0.2
F	0.5	BF	0.3	DF	0.2

Take FIS_2 ={ BD, BC }and $inFIS_2$={$AB,AC,AD,BF,CD,CF,AE,AF,CE,DF$} for example. Suppose $mi=0.05$. The results are shown in Fig. 1.

$f(B, D, ms(length(B \cup D)), mi)$ $= \dfrac{0.6+0.18-(0.4+0.05)+1}{\|0.6-0.4\|+\|(0.18-0.05\|+1} =1$	$f(B, C, ms(length(B \cup C)), mi)$ $= \dfrac{0.4+0.02-(0.4+0.05)+1}{\|0.4-0.4\|+\|0.02-0.05\|+1} <1$
$f(A, B, ms(0), mi)= \dfrac{0.3+0.05-(0.2+0.05)+1}{\|0.3-0.2\|+\|0.05-0.05\|+1} =1$	$f(C, F, ms(0), mi)= \dfrac{0.3+0-(0.2+0.05)+1}{\|0.3-0.2\|+\|0-0.05\|+1} <1$
$f(A, C, ms(0), mi)= \dfrac{0.3+0-(0.2+0.05)+1}{\|0.3-0.2\|+\|0-0.05\|+1} <1$	$f(A, E, ms(0), mi) = \dfrac{0.2+0.05-(0.2+0.05)+1}{\|0.2-0.2\|+\|0.05-0.05\|+1} =1$
$f(A, D, ms(0), mi)= \dfrac{0.3+0-(0.2+0.05)+1}{\|0.3-0.2\|+\|0-0.05\|+1} <1$	$f(A, F, ms(0), mi) = \dfrac{0.2+0.05-(0.2+0.05)+1}{\|0.2-0.2\|+\|0.05-0.05\|+1} =1$
$f(B, F, ms(0), mi)= \dfrac{0.3+0.05-(0.2+0.05)+1}{\|0.3-0.2\|+\|0.05-0.05\|+1} =1$	$f(C, E, ms(0), mi) = \dfrac{0.2+0.02-(0.2+0.05)+1}{\|0.2-0.2\|+\|0.02-0.05\|+1} <1$
$f(C, D, ms(0), mi)= \dfrac{0.3+0.06-(0.2+0.05)+1}{\|0.3-0.2\|+\|0.06-0.05\|+1} =1$	$f(D, F, ms(0), mi) = \dfrac{0.2+0.1-(0.2+0.05)+1}{\|0.2-0.2\|+\|0.1-0.05\|+1} =1$

Fig. 1. The results of calculation for the itemsets in FIS2 and inFIS2

BC is not interesting, and therefore is removed from FIS_2. *AC, AD, CF, CE* are not interesting, and therefore are removed from $inFIS_2$. Other itemsets can be analyzed in the same way.

4 Experiments

The real dataset records areas of www.microsoft.com that each user visited in a one-week timeframe in February 1998. Summary statistical information of the dataset is: 32711 training instances, 5000 testing instances, 294 attributes and the mean area visits per case is 3.0 (http://www.cse.ohio-state.edu/~yanghu /CIS788_dm_proj.htm# datasets).

Table 3. The number of the interesting inFISand the interesting FIS with different mi.(ms(1) =0.025, ms(2)=0.02, ms(3)=0.017, ms(4)=0.013, ms(0)=0.01)

mi		$k=1$	$k=2$	$k=3$	$k=4$	Total	
0	FIS	-	37	24	3	64	150
	inFIS	-	43	40	3	86	
0.005	FIS	-	30	24	3	57	119
	inFIS	-	21	38	3	62	
0.01	FIS	-	23	21	3	47	63
	inFIS	-	7	8	1	16	
0.015	FIS	-	20	13	1	34	34
	inFIS	-	0	0	0	0	

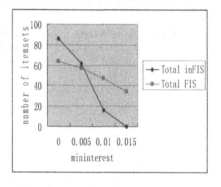

Fig. 2. The changes of total *inFIS* and total *FIS* with different *mi*

Table 3 shows the number of the interesting infrequent itemsets and the interesting frequent itemsets with different *mi* when *ms*(1)=0.025, *ms*(2)=0.02, *ms*(3)=0.017, *ms*(4)=0.013, and *ms*(0)=0.01. From table 3 we can see that the total number of *FIS* is 64,57,47,34, and total number of *inFIS* is 86,62,16,0 when *mi*=0, 0.005, 0.01, 0.015 respectively. With *mi* increasing, the total number decreases obviously. Figure 2 illustrates these changes. Table 3 also gives the number of *FIS* and *inFIS* in different *k*. These data show that *fipi(M)* and *iipi(N)* can efficiently prune the uninteresting itemsets in the IMLMS model, i.e., the modified Wu's pruning strategy can efficiently work on the MLMS model.

5 Conclusions and Future Work

When we study negative association rules, infrequent itemsets become very important because there are many valued negative association rules in them. In our previous work, a MLMS model is proposed to discover both infrequent itemsets and frequent itemsets. Some of the itemsets, however, are not interesting and ought to be pruned. In this paper, a new model IMLMS is proposed by modifying the Wu's pruning strategy to adapt to the MLMS model to prune the uninteresting itemsets. An algorithm Apriori_IMLMS is also proposed to discover simultaneously both interesting frequent itemsets and interesting infrequent itemsets based on the IMLMS model. The experimental results show the validity of the model.

For future work, we will work on finding interesting infrequent itemsets with some new measures and use some better algorithms than *Apriori*, FP-growth, for example, to discover infrequent itemsets and frequent itemsets.

Acknowledgements

This work was supported by Program for New Century Excellent Talents in University, China; Huo Ying-dong Education Foundation, China (91101); Excellent Young Scientist Foundation of Shandong Province, China (2006BS01017); and Natural Science Foundation of Shandong Province, China (Y2007G25).

References

1. Wu, X., Zhang, C., Zhang, S.: Efficient Mining of both Positive and Negative Association Rules. ACM Transactions on Information Systems 22, 381–405 (2004)
2. Agrawal, R., Imielinski, T., Swami, A.: Mining Association Rules between Sets of Items in Large Database. In: Proceedings of the 1993 ACM SIGMOD International Conference on Management of Data, pp. 207–216. ACM Press, New York (1993)
3. Dong, X., Zheng, Z., Niu, Z., Jia, Q.: Mining Infrequent Itemsets based on Multiple Level Minimum Supports. In: Proceedings of the Second International Conference on Innovative Computing, Information and Control (ICICIC 2007), Kumamoto, Japan (September 2007)
4. Brin, S., Motwani, R., Silverstein, C.: Beyond Market: Generalizing Association Rules to Correlations. In: Processing of the ACM SIGMOD Conference, pp. 265–276 (1997)
5. Savasere, A., Omiecinski, E., Navathe, S.: Mining for Strong Negative Associations in a Large Database of Customer Transaction. In: Proceedings of the 1998 International Conference on Data Engineering, pp. 494–502 (1998)
6. Yuan, X., Buckles, B.P., Yuan, Z., Zhang, J.: Mining Negative Association Rules. In: Proceedings of The Seventh IEEE Symposium on Computers and Communications, pp. 623–629 (2002)
7. Dong, X., Sun, F., Han, X., Hou, R.: Study of Positive and Negative Association Rules Based on Multi-confidence and Chi-Squared Test. In: Li, X., Zaïane, O.R., Li, Z. (eds.) ADMA 2006. LNCS (LNAI), vol. 4093, pp. 100–109. Springer, Heidelberg (2006)
8. Antonie, M.-L., Zaiane, O.: Mining Positive and Negative Association Rules: An Approach for Confined Rules. In: Boulicaut, J.-F., Esposito, F., Giannotti, F., Pedreschi, D. (eds.) PKDD 2004. LNCS (LNAI), vol. 3202, pp. 27–38. Springer, Heidelberg (2004)
9. Liu, B., Hsu, W., Ma, Y.: Mining Association Rules with Multiple Minimum Supports. In: Proceedings of the ACM SIGKDD International Conference on Knowledge Discovery & Data Mining (KDD 1999), San Diego, CA, USA, August 15-18, 1999, pp. 337–341 (1999)
10. Han, J., Fu, Y.: Mining Multiple-Level Association Rules in Large Databases. IEEE Transactions on Knowledge and Engineering 11(5), 798–805 (1999)
11. Dong, X., Wang, S., Song, H.: 2-level Support based Approach for Mining Positive & Negative Association Rules. Computer Engineering 31(10), 16–18 (2005)

Text Learning and Hierarchical Feature Selection in Webpage Classification

Xiaogang Peng, Zhong Ming, and Haitao Wang

College of Information Engineering(Software College),
Shenzhen University, 518060 P.R. China
patrickpeng@126.com

Abstract. One of the solutions of retrieving information from the Internet is by classifying web pages automatically. In almost all classification methods that have been published, feature selection is a very important issue. Although there are many feature selection methods has been proposed. Most of them focus on the features within a category and ignore that the hierarchy of categories also plays an important role in achieving accurate classification results. This paper proposes a new feature selection method that incorporates hierarchical information, which prevents the classifying process from going through every node in the hierarchy. Our test results show that our classification algorithm using hierarchical information reduces the search complexity from n to log(n) and increases the accuracy by 6.2% comparing to a related algorithm.

Keywords: text learning, web page classification, category hierarchy, feature selection.

1 Introduction

The World Wide Web is growing at a great speed but the documents in the Web do not form a logical organization and inevitably making the manipulation and retrieval difficult. The need for mechanisms to assist in locating relevant information becomes more and more urgent. One of the solutions to assist in retrieving documents on the Web is provided by classified directories [1]. However, current systems, such as Yahoo [2] still require human labor in doing the classification. Whether manual classification is able to keep up with the growth of the Web remains a question. First, manual classification is slow and costly since it relies on skilled manpower. Second, the consistency of categorization is hard to maintain since different human experiences are involved. Finally, the task of defining the categories is difficult and subjective since new categories emerge continuously from many domains. Considering all these problems, the need of automatic classification becomes more and more important.

Although there are many automatic classification algorithms and systems[1,3,4] that have been proposed, most of them focus on the classifier itself and ignore the hierarchy of categories also plays an important role in achieving accurate classification results. The algorithm, unlike others, considers the hierarchical structure information for improving the classification accuracy. The core of the algorithm is a hierarchical classification technique that assigns a web page to a category. One of the most important

C. Tang et al. (Eds.): ADMA 2008, LNAI 5139, pp. 452–459, 2008.
© Springer-Verlag Berlin Heidelberg 2008

issues in text classification is deciding document representation. In order to be classified, each document should be turned into a certain machine comprehendible format. In order to achieve the hierarchical classification goal, this paper proposed a new feature selection method to incorporate the feature as well as the structure of the hierarchy into the document representation.

2 Related Research

Text learning is a machine-learning method on text data that also combines information retrieval techniques and is often used as a tool to extract the true content of text data. The product of any text learning process is a machine-readable form of a given document, which is called its document representation. A common and widely used document representation in the information retrieval and text learning area is the bag-of-words text document representation, the idea of which is found in Koller and Sahami [5] and Lang [6]. One of the drawbacks of this document representation is that word order and text structure are ignored. Many experiments have been done to improve the performance of the text document representation. For example, Mladenic [7] extended the bag-of-words representation to a bag-of-features representation. She defined the features of a text document as a word or a word sequence. Chan [8] also suggested that using word sequences other than single words is a better choice. The goal of using word sequences as features is to preserve the information left out of the bag-of-words. This representation, which is also called "feature vector representation" in Chan [8], uses a feature vector to capture the characteristics of the document by an "n-gram" feature selection, which extracts word sequences with i consecutive words from the entire document during the i-th run, and the range of i is from 1 to n.

Automatic text document classification is the task of assigning a text document to the most relevant category or several relevant categories by using computers. In information retrieval, TFIDF (Term Frequency–Inverse Document Frequency) classification algorithm is well studied [9]. Based on the document vector model, the distance between vectors is calculated by the cosine of the angle between them for the purpose of classification. Joachims [10] analyzed the TFIDF classifier in a probabilistic way based on the assumption that the TFIDF classifier is as explicit as the Naïve Bayes classifier. Other more sophisticated classification algorithms and models were proposed including: multivariate regression models [11], nearest neighbor classifiers [12], Bayesian classifiers [13], decision tree [13], Support Vector Machines [4]. Tree structures appear with all of these systems. Some proposed systems focus on classification algorithms to improve the accuracy of assigning testing documents to related catalogs [10], while others go even further by taking the classifier structure into account [5].

3 Classification by Using Hierarchical Feature Selection

In this section, we started with a well-grained text-learning method modified from normal N-gram selection which is used to extract more appropriate useful features from documents. Then a new classification algorithm using hierarchical feature selection is discussed.

3.1 Well-Grained Text-Learning Method

To extract appropriate features from documents, we incorporate two additional steps that are ignored by most known feature extraction methods. The first step is segmenting the whole document into smaller text units. A text unit can be a sentence or part of a sentence. The second step is to assign different weights to the text unit. We realize that not all the text units are equally important. The content, HTML tags, and URL of a text document might help in deciding a correct importance rate on different text units and enabling the acquisition of a better document representation.

In order to segment a document to smaller units, we analyze the entire document and find all the delimiters such as ',' '.' '!' '?' '"' ':' ';' and other delimiting symbols except spaces. Then, the text between two delimiters is considered as a text unit. In this way, a document is turned into a number of smaller text units. Segmenting the document will reduce the number of word sequences when applying the n-gram selection because the words separated by a delimiter will not be combined to form a word sequence. The second advantage is that segmenting the document will reduce unrelated words. For example, a sentence fragment like "...spiders are known world wide. The web of different kinds of spiders..." might contribute a word sequence "World Wide Web" after removing stop word "the" and applying 3-gram feature selection technique on the entire sentence. The problem is obvious that the topic of the document is about insects and has nothing to do with the World Wide Web.

Table 1. Different Weights of Text Units

Text unit type	Weight	Text unit type	Weight
Normal body text	1	<title>	4
First and last paragraph of a document	2	<H1>	2
Beginning sentence of a paragraph	2	URL	4
Sentences with bonus words and indicator phrases as pointed out in Paice [13]	3	<EM>	2
<Meta >	3	<Strong>	3

After the document is segmented to smaller text units, we need to recognize different levels of importance between text units. A text unit is considered to be more important in a text document, meaning that it can describe the main topic of the document better. For example, the text units within the title line are usually considered more important than those text units in the normal body text. The common way to specify different importance of text units is by assigning higher weights to text units that are more important. Several different sources of information within the text document itself will help with assigning weights to different text units in a text document. To be more specific, the information from document context, HTML tags, and URLs are three major information sources that can be used to determine the weights for text units. We analyze the text document and assign different weights listed in Table1. according to different types of text units.

3.2 Extracting Category Information

The first step of a classification system is to define the categories. If categories are regarded as separated nodes, a document representation for each category should be decided. The characteristics of each category are represented as a "bag of words" or a feature list based on the text-learning method described above. If categories are arranged in a hierarchical tree structure, say each tree node represents one category and a child note of any given node represents a subcategory under the given node, the hierarchical information should be also taken into consideration using the step that follows.

3.3 Capturing Hierarchical Information

Tree structures are used extensively nowadays to depict all kinds of taxonomic information. In this kind of application on a tree structure, the child node is a subdivision of the parent node, which usually represents information that is more general. Then, the information in the child node should also be considered as part of the information of the parent node because of the parent-child relationship. For example, if the parent node is "fruit," then one of the children nodes can be "apple" because "apple" is a subdivision of "fruit." Then the information "green apple" existing in the "apple" node should also be considered as information of the "fruit" node since "green apple" is a "fruit."

If the presence of the information in a child node can be represented by an *original weight*, then one way to present the existence of this information in the parent node is to assign a scale factor to the original weight and propagate it to the parent node. The scale factor reflects the parent-child relationship. If an original weight is in each tree node of a tree structure, then the propagated weight in the tree structure, which contains the hierarchical information, can be estimated by propagating all the original weights following the parent-child relationships from the leaf nodes to the root. The value is called the *propagated weight* of the tree and is assigned to the root of the tree structure.

Many existing category structures are unbalanced hierarchical structures. In order to ensure the actual containment relation, the feature information of a category is propagated upward from leaf nodes to the root node of our classification tree. For example, Mladenic [14] studied Yahoo unbalanced structure and proposed an algorithm for featuring propagation. The algorithm takes care of the structure of the tree hierarchy. As proposed in [14], with a tree T rooted at node N having k sub-trees (SubTi $_{(i=1...k)}$), we can calculate the probability for a feature w belonging to a category after propagation as follow:

$$P(w \mid T) =$$

$$\sum_{i=1}^{k} P(w \mid SubTi) * P(SubTi \mid T) + P(w \mid N) * P(N \mid T)$$

Where $P(w|T)$ is the propagated feature probability given tree T and $P(w|N)$ is the probability of the feature w in the node N before the propagation, which can be calculated by dividing the particular term frequency by the total term frequency. $P(SubT_i|T)$ and $P(N|T)$ are the weight factor of the sub-tree $SubTi$ given tree T and the probability of current node given tree T.

In the generated classification tree (from stage 1), each node represents a category by a feature list. The propagated feature list is generated by adding the original feature list of the current node and all the propagated feature lists of the sub-categories and by assigning different weights. By propagating in this way, the feature list captures the characteristics of a sub-tree rooted in the current node rather than in an isolated category set.

3.4 Selecting Good Features for Category

What really contributed in distinguish between categories are those features in a category that are much less likely exist in other categories. We call these features as "good features". Because of the feature propagation, these good features will be weighted and propagated upwards and become the features of the parent category. In this case, by tracing these features it is easy to locate the correct category. Due to this reason, following a path with higher weited sum of good features, we can find the destination. This phenomenon provides a foundation for our single path classification algorithm.

The goal of our feature selection is to compare the features in a node to its sibling nodes and try to distinguish the good features. In order to do this, we take advantage of the feature propagation and use the features of the parent node as negative examples to determine a ranking. After propagation, each propagated feature probability is actually the weighted sum of the same feature probability from the sub-trees and the current node itself. We proposed the following formula for determining the "uniqueness ranking" $R_c(w)$ of a feature w of a category c.

$$R_c(w) = P(SubTc|T)*P(w|c)/P(w|parent)$$

Where c is the current node and parent is the parent node of c. P(SubTc|T) is the weight factor that assigned to node c when it is propagated to the parent. If a feature is unique in one node, it is the only source that can propagate to the parent feature list. In this case, we get the maximum value of the formula, which is 1. The unique features will be considered as key features that differentiate the node from its siblings and forms the basis for our single path traversal algorithm.

3.5 Classifying in a Single Path

Text classification requires the use of a classifier to assign a similarity values to a document for each category. A global maximum value is considered the correct place to hold the document. Most automatic classification researches concentrated on the global search algorithm. They treat all categories in a flat structure when trying to find the maximum. It follows that in order to find the category with the greatest value, it is necessary to compare all the categories.

In the tree structure that we have configured, we claim that traveling one path is sufficient to achieve this goal. If there are N categories in the tree, the complexity of searching all categories is $\theta(N)$, but by our single path algorithm it is merely $\theta(\log (N))$.

The first step of the single path traversal is to discriminate sibling nodes in each level and find a correct path for the incoming web page. In order to determine the discriminating probability for each node, we only consider the nodes at each level and apply the PrTFIDF formula described in section 2 on the features with a ranking of 1 of the category information using the formula mentioned in section 3.4, which indicate a unique feature. At each level, we chose the node with the maximum discriminating probability as the starting point for the next iteration. Recursively applying this rule creates a path from the root of the tree to one of the leaf nodes.

Then following this path we apply the PrTFIDF classifier again using all the features of the nodes belonging to the path, to get the actual probability for the page with categories within this path. By picking the node along the classification path with maximum actual probability value, we determine the candidate category for the page.

4 Experiments and Results

To test the performances of the single path traversal, we design a experiment as follow. The root of our category hierarchy is set to Yahoo /Science/Engineering/, one of the sub-categories of Yahoo's classification tree[2]. We also chose the categories that are strictly following the levels of this root category; that is, we eliminated those categories that either go to another root category or do not follow the level structure. As we have noticed, many of the outgoing URLs in Yahoo are not accessible. Our expectation is that it will somewhat reduce the number of outdated outgoing URLs and provide enough testing examples for our system. We also ignored the categories with less than 20 unique features after feature selection as stated in section 3.4.

Considering processing time for testing purposes, we direct our program in getting the category information of three levels in the Yahoo "Science/Engineering" sub-tree. Labrou and Finin [15] compared several different ways in describing the category information and the web page information. By their experiments, they pointed out that, the best way of describing category was entry summaries and entry titles; correspondingly the best choice of web page description (called entry in their paper) was the entry summaries. Because of this, when generating the category information, we use summaries that are generated by man power and already there in Yahoo website, instead of using the actually website contents to generate the category information tree.

The testing examples of our system are actual website contents whose URLs are taken from three levels of the Yahoo sub-tree rooted in "Science/ Engineering." Some non-text format paged associated with the URLs cannot yet be classified, for example, jpeg, swf, and gif files. We only use the URLs whose pages having more than 70 unique features after our well grain 3-gram feature extraction and these URLs are called "good" URLs.

In order to test the accuracy of single path algorithm, we compare the actual classification results of the single path algorithm to the one that searches all categories (thorough search) using the same classifier. We randomly selected 464 of all the web pages with good URLs in Yahoo "Science/Engineering" tree as testing web pages, we compare the two algorithms by the accuracy and the effectiveness, and the result is shown in Table 2.

By the results, we can see that the two algorithms have the same result is more than 73% of all testing cases, of which 333 are correctly predicted and only 6 are wrong. In different classification results, 58 are correctly predicted by sigle path comparing to 30 by thorough search. By calculating the correct rate, even most of the branches of the tree are ignored, the single path classification still has an accuracy of 84.52%, which outperforms by more than 6.2% the accuracy that was achieved by the thorough search algorithm. From these results, we can see the advantage of classifying in a single path.

Table 2. Results of comparing two algorithms

Same classification results by two algorithms		
Correct results	Wrong results	
333	6	
Different classification results		
Correct results by Single path algorithm	Correct results by thorough search algorithm	Wrong results either by single or thorough search
58	30	37

5 Conclusion

In this paper, we describe an approach to select features utilizing the class hierarchies as well as a classification system for improving text classification. The single path classification algorithm, in the hierarchical classification module, reduces the computational expense compared to the thorough search algorithm that is used by most of the existing classification algorithms. By distinguishing the siblings, the algorithm recognizes a correct path containing the destination category. The algorithm is successful not only in saving computational resources but even improving the correct hits to a higher percentage. Our experiment also shows that because of the diversity of contents of the pages, the thorough search algorithm sometimes cannot tell the key information from the common information since it treats all the information equally. The single path algorithm avoids this problem by only considering unique features in discriminating siblings. Our experiments support that the single path algorithm is more competent both in time and in accuracy.

Acknowledgement. This paper is funded by NSFC#60673122.

References

1. Rousu, J., Saunders, C., Szedmak, S., Shawe-Taylor, J.: Learning Hierarchical Multi-Category Text Classification Models. In: Proceedings of 22nd International Conference on Machine Learning (ICML 2005), Bonn, Germany (2005)
2. Yahoo.: http://www.Yahoo.com
3. Kan, M.-Y., Thi, H.O.N.: Fast webpage classification using URL features. In: Proc. of Conf. on Info. and Knowledge Management (CIKM 2005), Germany (2005)

4. Dumais, S., Chen, H.: Hierarchical Classification of Web Content. In: Proceedings of SIGIR 2000, 23rd ACM International Conference on Research and Development in Information Retrieval (2000)
5. Koller, D., Sahami, M.: Hierarchically classifying documents using very few words. In: Proceedings of the 14th international Conference on Machine Learning ECML 1998 (1998)
6. Lang, K.: Newsweeder: Learning to filter news. In: Proceedings of the 12th International Conference on Machine Learning, pp. 331–339 (1995)
7. Mladenic, D., Grobelnik, M.: Word sequences as features in text-learning. In: Proceedings of ERK 1998, the Seventh Electro-technical and Computer Science Conference, pp. 145–148 (1998)
8. Chan, P.K.: A non-invasive learning approach to building web user profiles. In: KDD 1999 Workshop on Web Usage Analysis and User Profiling (1999)
9. Salton, G., Buckley, C.: Term Weighting Approaches in Automatic Text Retrieval. Technical Report, COR-87-881, Department of Computer Science, Cornell University (1987)
10. Joachims, T.: A probabilistic analysis of the Rocchio algorithm with TFIDF for text categorization. In: International Conference on Machine Learning (ICML) (1997)
11. Dominggos, P., Pazzani, M.: On the optimality of the simple Baysian classifier under zero-one loss. Machine learning 29, 103–130 (1997)
12. Yang, Y., Pedersen, O.J.: A comparative Study o Feature Selection in Text Categorization. In: Proc. of the fifth International Conference on Machine Learning ICML 1997, pp. 412–420 (1997)
13. Paice, C.D.: Constructing Literature Abstracts by Computer: Techniques and Prospects. Information Processing and Management 26(1), 171–186 (1990)
14. Mladenic, D.: Machine Learning on non-homogeneous, distributed text data. Ph.D thesis. University of Ljubljana, Slovenia (1998)
15. Labrou, Y., Finin, T.: Yahoo! as an ontology – using Yahoo! Categories to Describe Document. In: CIKM 1999. Proceedings of the Eighth International Conference on Knowledge and Information Management, pp. 180–187. ACM, New York (1999)

The RSO Algorithm for Reducing Number of Set Operations in Association Rule Mining

Muhammad Sarwar and Onaiza Maqbool

Department of Computer Science Quaid-i-Azam University Islamabad, Pakistan
sarwar@cs.qau.edu.pk, onaiza@qau.edu.pk

Abstract. Association rule mining is a data mining technique used to find interesting associations between items in a transaction database. Well known algorithms for association rule mining include Apriori and FP-tree. Apriori is a level wise algorithm and works by scanning the database multiple times. In an attempt to optimize the performance of Apriori, many variations of basic Apriori algorithm have been proposed. These variations exploit different approaches including reducing the number of database scans performed, using special data structures, using bitmaps and granular computing. Majority of these approaches are improvements in implementation of the same basic algorithm. In this paper we propose the RSO (Reduced Set Operations) algorithm, based on reducing the number of set operations performed. RSO is an algorithmic improvement to the basic Apriori algorithm; it is not an implementation improvement. Our analysis shows that RSO is asymptotically faster than Apriori. Experimental results also validate the efficiency of our algorithm.

1   Introduction

Data Mining has been defined as "The process of employing one or more computer learning techniques to automatilly analyze and extract knowledge from data" [1]. Data mining methods include clustering, prediction, estimation, outlier analysis and association rule mining. Association rule mining (ARM) may be used to identify sets of items that often occur together. An example of such an association rule might be that 90% of customers who purchased computer also purchased printer.

Some well known algorithms for ARM include AIS [2], SETM [3], Apriori [4], Apriori TID [4], Apriori Hybrid [4], and FP-tree [5]. Researchers have used various techniques to improve the speed of ARM task [6]-[13]. These approaches have been categorized by [14] as: (a) Reducing number of passes over database. (b) Sampling the database. (c) Adding extra constraints on the structure of patterns. (d) Through parallelization.

Our approach is different from the above methods. We have proposed an algorithm called RSO (Reduced Set Operations) based on the idea of reducing number of set operations needed during mining process. Our approach is general and can be combined with most of the existing enhancements to Apriori. The asymptotic analysis given in Section 3 and experimental results given in Section 4 show that RSO is faster than Apriori.

C. Tang et al. (Eds.): ADMA 2008, LNAI 5139, pp. 460–468, 2008.

Rest of the paper is organized as follows. Background of ARM and Apriori are discussed in Section 2. Section 3 contains RSO and its running time analysis. Experimental results are presented in section 4. Finally we present conclusions in Section 5.

2 Background

We describe ARM and Apriori briefly in this section. For details the reader may refer to [14] and [15].

Let $I=\{i_1, i_2, i_3, \dots, i_n\}$ be a set of items. A transaction T is a subset of I and a transaction database DB is a set of transactions. If $X \subseteq I$ and $|X|=k$ then X is called a *k-itemset*. If X is an itemset then the number of transactions containing X is called *support* of X. If X is an itemset and support of X is greater than a predefined minimum support threshold (*minsup*) then X is called a *frequent itemset*. If $X \subseteq I$, $Y \subseteq I$ and $X \cap Y = \phi$ then an implication of the form $X \Rightarrow Y$ is an *association rule*.

$$Support(X \Rightarrow Y) = Support\ of\ (X \cup Y) \quad Confidence(X \Rightarrow Y) = \frac{Support\ of\ (X \cup Y)}{Support\ of\ X}$$

An association rule is said to be *interesting* if its support and confidence are above some user defined thresholds. Since confidence and support of an association rule can be calculated from support of itemsets included in the rule, therefore main task of ARM is to calculate support of itemsets.

Number of all possible itemsets is exponentially large, so counting support for all of them is intractable. We need some algorithm that only considers a reasonable number of itemsets and still possesses completeness.

Apriori [2] is an algorithm that does not need to consider every possible itemset to find all frequent itemsets. To reduce the potential number of itemsets to consider, it uses the *apriori* property. According to apriori property *an itemset cannot be frequent if any of its subsets is not frequent*. Once we know that a certain itemset is not frequent we can ignore all its supersets. Apriori is a level wise algorithm. It first finds frequent 1-itemsets by scanning the database, then frequent 2-itemsets by again scanning the database and continues until no further frequent itemsets are found.

Let the set of frequent itemsets of size $k-1$ be denoted by F_{k-1}. Apriori first finds candidate (potentially frequent) itemsets of size k, denoted by C_k, from F_{k-1}. Generation of C_k using F_{k-1} consists of two steps namely *join* and *eliminate*. Two sets are joined if they have same elements except the last. Thus joining any two sets of size $k-1$ produces a set of size k. The generated set is included in C_k only if all of its subsets are frequent.

Figure 1 presents the pseudo code for the Apriori algorithm, as given in [2]. Since our work involves improvements to the AprioriGenerate function; we will analyze the complexity of this function only. For simplicity we will consider a single set operation like testing two sets for equality, joining two sets or generating a subset of a given set as the basic cost unit. Suppose $|F_{k-1}|=n$

HasInfrequentSubsets: - Line 1: k times because C will have k subsets of size $k-1$. Line 2: n times since it is searching for s in F_{k-1} and $|F_{k-1}|=n$. Total cost=$n \times k$.

1.	$C_1 \leftarrow$ {candidate 1-itemsets} //all 1-itemsets are considered as candidates
2.	$F_1 \leftarrow$ {$c \in C_1$	c.count$\geq$minsupp}//remove infrequent candidates
3.	for ($k \leftarrow 2$; $F_{k-1} \neq \phi$; k++)/repeat until no more frequent itemsets are found
4.	$C_k \leftarrow$ AprioirGenerate(F_{k-1})
5.	for each transaction $t \in D$
6.	$C_t \leftarrow$ Subsets (C_k, t)//get subsets that are candidates
7.	for all candidates $c \in C_t$
8.	c.count++
9.	end
10.	$F_k \leftarrow$ {$c \in C_k$	c.count$\geq$minsupp}//remove infrequent candidates
11.	end
12.	return $F \leftarrow U_k F_k$

AprioriGenerate(F_{k-1})	HasInFrequentSubsets(C)
1. for $i \leftarrow 1$ to $\| F_{k-1} \|$	1. for each k−1 subsets s of C
2. for $j \leftarrow 1$ to $\| F_{k-1} \|$	2. if $s \notin F_{k-1}$
3. if JoinAble(F_{k-1}[i], F_{k-1}[j])	3. return true
4. $C \leftarrow F_{k-1}$[i] $U F_{k-1}$[j]	4. return false
5. if HasInfrequentSubsets(C)	
6. delete (C)	
7. else C_k.add(C)	
8. return C_k	

Fig. 1. Pseudo code for Apriori

Joinable: - It is a single set operation so its cost is constant.

AprioriGenerate. Line 1, 2: n times. Line 3, 4: constant time. Line 5: $n \times k$ times. Line 6, 7: constant time (One of them will execute). Line 8: constant time.

$$\text{Total cost of Apriori Generate} = \sum_{i=1}^{n} \sum_{j=1}^{n} (1+1+nk+1)+1 = O(n^3 k)$$

3 RSO Algorithm

Majority of improvements in Apriori made by other researches are implementation improvements; the basic algorithm remains the same. We have changed the basic algorithm itself. The idea behind RSO is general and can be combined with most of the other approaches to improve the performance of Apriori. The RSO algorithm that we propose works by reducing the number of set operations required.

In the discussion that follows we assume that all itemsets and sets of itemsets are sorted lexicographically. If 1-itemsets are kept sorted then AprioriGenerate function will generate the candidates in such a way that subsequent itemsets and sets of itemsets will be automatically sorted and no overhead is involved.

Notations: - The operator "<" will be used to denote that a certain itemset occurs before the other in lexicographic order. Two itemsets S_i & S_j of size k.are said to be *joinable* if (a) $S_i[1]=S_j[1]$, $S_i[2]=S_j[2]$,..., $S_i[k-1]=S_j[k-1]$ (b) $S_i[k]<S_j[k]$. Note that if condition (a) holds and $S_i<S_j$, then condition (b) will hold automatically. *Similarity* between any two itemsets of same size is the count of initial elements that are same in both itemsets. Two itemsets of size k will be joinable if similarity between them is equal to $k-1$. Similarity between two itemsets depends on their proximity in lexicographic order.

Theorem 1:- Let S_i & S_j be elements of F_{k-1}, where $S_i<S_j$. Let S_i be joinable with S_j & let $X=S_i$ join S_j. Let R be any subset of X of size $k-1$other than S_i & S_j. If $R \in F_{k-1}$ then $R=S_m$ for some $m>j$

Proof: - If we generate subsets of X of size $k-1$ in lexicographic order, then first subset will be S_i and second will be S_j. All other subsets will be greater than S_j. Therefore if $R \subseteq X$ other than S_i & S_j and if $R \in F_{k-1}$ then $R = S_m$ for some $m>j$.

Theorem 2:- Let S_i & S_j be elements of F_{k-1}, where $S_i < S_j$ and let $X= S_i$ join S_j. If X is frequent then $i \leq n-k+1$

Proof: - For X to be frequent it must have apriori property. Since $|X|=k$ therefore for apriori property, X must have k subsets of size $k-1$in F_{k-1}. S_i is automatically a subset X, so there remain $k-1$ subsets to be searched for. As proved in theorem 1 the remaining $k-1$ subsets must exist after index i therefore there must be $k-1$ elements after index i. The remaining elements after index i are $n-i$. Therefore

$n-i \geq k-1 \Rightarrow i \leq n-k+1$. So if $i > n-k+1$then X cannot be frequent.

Theorem 3:- Let S_i & S_j be elements of F_{k-1}. If S_i is not joinable with S_j then S_i cannot be joined with any $S_m \in F_{k-1}$ where $m>j$

Proof: - Since S_i & S_j are elements of F_{k-1}, therefore for $|S_i|=|S_j|=k-1$. For S_j to be joinable with S_j, the similarity between them must be equal to $k-2$. Now if S_i is not joinable with S_j then similarity between S_i & S_j will be less than $k-2$.

Sim $(S_i, S_j) <k-2$-------- (1)

Since S_m comes after S_j in lexicographic order therefore similarity between S_i and S_m will be less than or equal to similarity between S_i and S_j

Sim $(S_i, S_m) \leq$ Sim (S_i, S_j)

$\Rightarrow$ Sim$(S_i, S_m)<k-2$ Using (1)

Hence S_i is not joinable with S_m.

The modified AprioriGenerate function is given in Figure 2. Using theorem 2, line number 1 needs only to be executed $n-k+1$ times. Using theorem 3, line number 3 stops checking for joinability as soon as first non joinable set is found. And by using theorem 1 searching of subsets starts from index $j+1$. Let us calculate the running time of AprioiGenerate2

Join: - Running time is constant.

AprioriGenerate2: - It contains three nested loops. Suppose loop on line 1 executes p times, loop on line 3 executes q times and loop on line 5 executes r times then.

$$Cost = p \times q \times r, \text{ Since } p < n, q < n \text{ \& } r < n \Rightarrow Cost < n^3 = O(n^3)$$

AprioriGenerate2(F_{k-1})
```
1.   for i ←1 to n–k+1 //Theorem 2
2.      j ←i+1
3.      while ( j ≤ n–k+2 & ( C←Join ( F_{k-1}[i], F_{k-1}[j] ) ≠ null ))// Theorem 3
4.         l ←2 //counter for counting number of subsets
5.         for (m ← j+1 ; l ≠ k & m≤ n ; m++) // Theorem 1
6.            if (F_{k-1}[m] ⊂ C )
7.               l ← l+1
8.         if ( l=k)
9.            C_k.add(C)
10.        j ← j+1
11.  return C_k
Join( A, B)
1.   for i ← 1 to k–1
2.      if A[i]≠B[i]
3.         return null
4.   reutn A∪B
```

Fig. 2. The proposed version of AprioriGenerate function used by RSO

Hence RSO algorithm is asymptotically faster than Apriori.

We now compare RSO and Apriori with the help of an example. Let I={A, B, C, D, E, F}. Let us suppose that all 1, 2, 3 & 4 itemsets are frequent. We will generate candidate 5-itemsets from frequent 4-itemsets. Frequent 4-itemsets are given in Table 1, and generated candidate 5-itemsets are given in Table 2.

Table 1. Frequent 4-itemsets

Index	Itemset	Index	Itemset	Index	Itemset
1	ABCD	6	ABEF	11	BCDE
2	ABCE	7	ACDE	12	BCDF
3	ABCF	8	ACDF	13	BCEF
4	ABDE	9	ACEF	14	BDEF
5	ABDF	10	ADEF	15	CDEF

Table 2. Candidate 5-itemsets

Index	Itemset
1	ABCDE
2	ABCDF
3	ABCEF
4	ABDEF
5	ACDEF
6	BCDEF

USING APRIORI: - Each member of F_4 will be tested for join ability with every member of F_4. So 15 operations will be performed for each set and there are 15 total sets. Therefore total number of joinable operations performed will be 15x15=225. As a result of these 225 joinable tests 6 candidates will be generated. Next we need to see whether all subsets of these candidates are also frequent or not. For this purpose subsets of each member of C_5 will be generated and searched in F_4.

Since each member of C_5 has 5 elements, 5 subsets will be generated for each, requiring 5 set operations. So a total of 30 operations are required to produce subsets. Let us see how many operations are performed during searching the subsets in F_4. Table 3 gives the number of comparisons needed for subsets.

Table 3. Number of comparisions needed for subsets of each candidate set

Candidate Itemset	Number of comparisons needed fo each subset					Total
ABCDE	ABCD	ABCE	ABDE	ACDE	BCDE	25
	1	2	4	7	11	
ABCDF	ABCD	ABCF	ABDF	ACDF	BCDF	29
	1	3	5	8	12	
ABCEF	ABCE	ABCF	ABEF	ACEF	BCEF	33
	2	3	6	9	13	
ABDEF	ABDE	ABDF	ABEF	ADEF	BDEF	39
	4	5	6	10	14	
ACDEF	ACDE	ACDF	ACEF	ADEF	CDEF	39
	7	8	9	10	15	
BCDEF	BCDE	BCDF	BCEF	BDEF	CDEF	65
	11	12	13	14	15	

Joinable operations=225. Subset generation operations=30
Comparisons=25+29+33+39+39+65=230. Total =225+30+230=485

USING RSO: - First element in F_4 is ABCD. ABCD is joinable with ABCE producing ABCDE. ABCD is also joinable with ABCF, producing ABCDF. ABCD is not joinable with ABDE. No further test will need to be performed for ABCD. Therefore a total of 3 joinable operations will be required for ABCD. Number of joinable operations performed for each member of F_4 including the last unsuccessful operation are listed in Table 4. Note that no comparison will be made for BCDF, BCEF, BDEF & CDEF because they occur after index $(n-k+1)$.

Table 4. Number of joinable operations required for each set

Itemset	Number of operations	Itemset	Number of operations
ABCD	3	ACEF	1
ABCE	2	ADEF	1
ABCF	1	BCDE	1(j becomes > n-k+2)
ABDE	2	BCDF	0
ABDF	1	BCEF	0
ABEF	1	BDEF	0
ACDE	2	CDEF	0
ACDF	1		

Table 5. Elements of C_5 and cost of testing apriori property

Set	# of Comparisons	Set	# of comparisons
ABCDE	9	ABDEF	8
ABCDF	9	ACDEF	7
ABCEF	10	BCDEF	3

ABCD was joined with ABCE producing ABCDE. ABCD & ABCE are automatically subsets of ABCDE, we only need to search for 3 more subsets. Start comparing ABCDE with elements of F_4 from index 3. First subset ABDE is found at index 4, second ACDE is found at index 7 and third subset BCDE is found at index 11. Since the required 3 subsets are found, we do not need to search any more and so we need 9 set operations. Set operations required for each generated set are listed in Table 5.

Joinable operations=16. Comparisons=9+9+10+8+7+3=46. Total =16+46=62.

For the above example Apriori performed 485 set operations where as RSO has performed only 62 set operations.

4 Experimental Results

Since our work only involves improvement to AprioriGenerate function, we will compare AprioriGenerate functions of Apriori and RSO. Two types of comparisons are being presented; execution time and number of set operations performed. Data sets were obtained from [16]; details are given in Table 6. Results are shown in Figure 3 and Figure 4 for different support thresholds. Reducing the support increases the required number of set operations. Therefore, for lower support the difference in efficiency between the two algorithms is more in comparison to higher support.

Table 6. Details of data sets

Data Set	Name	Size in KB	No. of transactions	No of items
1	Chess	335	3196	75
2	Mushroom	558	8124	119

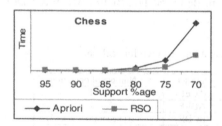 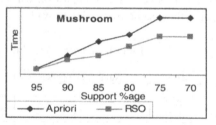

Fig. 3. Comparison of candidate generation time for Chess & Mushroom datasets

	95	90	85	80	75	70
Apriori	2325	99618	2E+06	1E+07	8E+07	4E+08
RSO	896	61644	9E+05	7E+06	4E+07	2E+08

	95	90	85	80	75	70
Apriori	37	69	125	263	401	401
RSO	5	10	24	63	98	98

Fig. 4. Comparison of set operations performed for Chess & for Mushroom datasets

5 Conclusion

In this paper we present RSO algorithm for improving the running time of Apriori algorithm. A number of improvements have been proposed by different researchers, our method adopts a different approach. We have changed the basic Apriori algorithm itself. We provide three theorems about the properties of frequent itemsets.

By using these theorems, number of set operations required during the mining process is considerably reduced. Our method can be combined with most of the other methods that use different techniques to improve the performance of Apriori algorithm. According to the running time analysis and experimental results, RSO outperforms the classical Apriori algorithm. The set operation reduction approach used by RSO can be used to improve other steps within Apriori. We are currently working on these improvements.

References

1. Roiger, R.J., Geatz, M.: Data Mining: A Tutorial Based Primer. Addsion Wesley (2002)
2. Agrawal, R., Imielinski, T., Swami, A.: Mining association rules between sets of items in very large databases. In: Proceedings of the ACM SIGMOD Conference on Management of Data, pp. 207–216 (1993)
3. Houtsma, M., Swami, A.: Set-oriented mining of association rules. Research Report RJ 9567, IBM Almaden Research Center, San Jose, California (1993)
4. Agrawal, R., Srikant, R.: Fast Algorithms for Mining Association Rules. In: Proceedings of 20th Conference on Very Large Databases, pp. 487–499 (1994)
5. Han, J., Pei, J., Yin, Y.: Mining Frequent Patterns without Candidate Generation. In: SIGMOD Conference, pp. 1–12 (2000)
6. Zaki, M., Parthasarathy, S., Li, W.: A Localized Algorithm for Parallel Association Mining. In: 9th Annual ACM Symposium on Parallel Algorithms and Architectures, pp. 321–330 (1997)
7. Jamali, M., Taghi, F., Rahgozar, M.: Fast Algorithm for Generating Association Rules with Encoding Databases Layout. PWASET 4, 167–170 (2005)
8. Das, A., Keong, W., Kwong, Y.: Rapid Association Rule Mining. In: Proceedings of 10th International Conference on Information and Knowledge Management, pp. 474–478 (2001)
9. Park, J.S., Chen, M.S., Yu, P.S.: An Effective Hash-Based Algorithm for Mining Association Rules. In: Proceedings of ACM SIGMOD International Conference on Management of Data, pp. 175–186 (1995)
10. Wang, Y.Y., Hu, X.G.: A fast algorithm for mining association rules based on concept lattice. In: Proceedings of Third International Conference on Machine Learning and Cybernetics, pp. 1687–1692 (2004)
11. Bodon, F.: A fast APRIORI implementation. In: Proceedings of IEEE ICDM Workshop on Frequent Itemset Mining Implementations, vol. 90 (2003)
12. Lin, T.Y., Hu, X., Louie, E.: A Fast Association Rule Algorithm Based On Bitmap and Granular Computing. In: Proceedings of the IEEE International Conference on Fuzzy Systems, pp. 678–683 (2003)

13. Liu, X.W., He, P.L.: The research of improved association rules mining Apriori Algorithm. In: Proceedings of the Third International Conference on Machine Learning and Cybernetics, pp. 1577–1579 (2004)

14. Kotsiantis, S., Kanellopoulos, D.: Association Rules Mining:A Recent Overview. GESTS International Transactions on Computer Science and Engineering 32(1), 71–82 (2006)

15. Han, J., Kamber, M.: Data Mining Concepts and Techniques, 2nd edn. Morgan Kaufman Publishers, San Francisco (2006)

16. http://mlearn.ics.uci.edu/MLRepository.html

Predictive Performance of Clustered Feature-Weighting Case-Based Reasoning

Sung Ho Ha*, Jong Sik Jin, and Jeong Won Yang

School of Business Administration, Kyungpook National University,
1370 Sangyeok-dong, Buk-gu, Daegu, Korea, 702-701
{hsh,jjs,jeongwonyang}@knu.ac.kr

Abstract. Because many factors are complexly involved in the production of semiconductors, semiconductor manufacturers can hardly manage yield precisely. We present a hybrid machine learning system, i.e., a clustered feature-weighting case-based reasoning, to detect high-yield or low-yield lots in semiconductor manufacturing. The system uses self-organizing map neural networks to identify similar patterns in the process parameters. The trained back-propagation neural networks determine feature weights of case-based reasoning. Based on the clustered feature-weighting case-based reasoning, the hybrid system predicts the yield level of a new manufacturing lot. To validate the effectiveness of our approach, we apply the hybrid system to real data of a semiconductor company.

1 Introduction

Yield management in the semiconductor industry is understood as a very important management practice that has to be monitored and controlled completely. Yield is defined as the ratio of normal products to finished products.

Semiconductor companies can achieve a certain degree of yield by applying statistical process control and six-sigma to a semiconductor. Yield enhancement employing statistical measurements, however, has difficulty in detecting low-yield lots effectively. This is because manufacturing process variables have a non-linear complex relationship with the yield.

Thus manufacturers need an intelligent approach to pinpoint the relationship between process parameters in time and to detect the main process variables which seriously affect changes in the yield. We have developed a clustered feature-weighting case-based reasoning as a complement to the existing statistical approach. This system is based on a hybrid application of machine learning techniques to effectively depict multiple process variables concerned with predicting the production yield in semiconductor manufacturing.

The hybrid system adopts a case-based reasoning (CBR) which can be directly applied to prediction purposes. However, CBR suffers from feature weighting; when it measures the distance between cases, some features should be weighted differently [1]. In order to weigh features and guide CBR, the hybrid system adopts four feature-weighting methods: Sensitivity, Activity, Saliency, and Relevance. In addition, this

---

* Corresponding author.

C. Tang et al. (Eds.): ADMA 2008, LNAI 5139, pp. 469–476, 2008.
© Springer-Verlag Berlin Heidelberg 2008

system also adopts a self-organizing map (SOM) to cluster cases in order to improve the predictive performance. In order to validate this hybrid approach, it is applied to a semi-conductor company and is compared with other methods that have been used.

2   Literature Review

Sobrino and Bravo [11] embodied an inductive algorithm to learn the tentative causes of low quality wafers from manufacturing data. Last and Kandel [6] presented the Automated Perceptions Network for accurate planning of yield through automated construction of models from noisy data sets. Kang et al. [5] integrated inductive decision-trees and neural networks with back-propagation and SOM algorithms to manage yields over major semiconductor manufacturing processes. Shin and Park [10] integrated neural networks and memory based reasoning to develop a wafer yield prediction system for semiconductor manufacturing. Yang, Rajasekharan, and Peters [13] mixed tabu search and simulated annealing to integrate layout configuration and automated material handling system in a wafer fabrication. Chien, Wang, and Cheng [3] included k-means clustering and a decision tree to infer possible causes of faults and manufacturing process variations from the semiconductor manufacturing data. Hsu and Chien [4] integrated spatial statistics and adaptive resonance theory neural networks to extract patterns from wafer bin maps and to associate with manufacturing defects. Li and Huang [8] integrated the SOM and support vector machine (SVM): the SOM clusters the wafer bin maps; the SVM classifies the wafer bin maps to identify the manufacturing defects. Wang [12] presented a spatial defect diagnosis system for semiconductor manufacturing, which combines square-error based fuzzy clustering and kernel-based spectral clustering, and a decision tree.

3   Methodology

In order to improve the ability of predicting yield accurately, a methodology, called a clustered feature-weighting case-based reasoning, is developed. It is a hybrid method combining several machine learning techniques, such as SOM, back-propagation network (BPN), CBR, and k-NN (k-Nearest Neighbor) (see Fig. 1). The hybrid system consists of five phases: clustering yield cases, neural learning about clustered cases, feature weighting, extracting k similar cases, and weighted averaging of extracted yields.

The first phase uses a SOM to cluster the cases in the Yield case base into several homogeneous groups. When a Yield case base contains historical yield-related information, a case in the case base is defined as $(\mathbf{x}, y)$, if $\mathbf{x} = (x_1, x_2, \ldots, x_N)$ and x_i represents case variables and y indicates the production yield rate. A SOM performs competitive learning. It uncovers patterns in the input fields set (i.e., $\mathbf{x}$ of case variables) and clusters the case set into distinct groups without a target field. The connection weights of the SOM, $\mathbf{v}$, represent the input patterns. Cases within a cluster tend to be similar to each other, and cases in different groups are dissimilar.

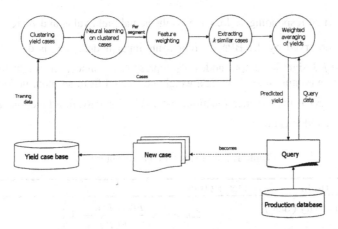

Fig. 1. The architecture of a clustered feature-weighting case-based reasoning

The second phase finds the relative importance of independent variables (i.e., manufacturing variables) within each case cluster. The importance is derived from the relationship between independent variables and a dependent variable (i.e., yield). When the training of a BPN is finished in the unbiased samples from the Yield case base, the connection weights of a trained neural network reveal the importance of the relationship between the process variables and yield.

To obtain a set of feature weights from the trained network, four feature-weighting methods are utilized: Sensitivity, Activity, Saliency, and Relevance [9]. Each of these methods calculates the degree of each feature's importance by using the connection weights and activation patterns of the nodes in the trained neural network. The feature-weighting algorithms are briefly described as follows:

- Sensitivity method: An input node i's sensitivity is calculated by removing the input node from the trained neural network. The sensitivity of an input node is the difference in error between the removal of the feature and when it is left in place.
- Activity method: Node activity is measured by the variance of the level of activation for the training data. When the activity value of a node varies significantly according to its input value, the activity of the node is high.
- Saliency method: Saliency is measured by estimating the second derivative of the error with respect to weight. Saliency is used to prune neural networks iteratively: that is, to train to reasonable error levels, compute saliencies, delete low saliency weights, and resume training.
- Relevance method: The variance of weight in a node is a good predictor of the node's Relevance. This relevance is a good predictor of the expected increase in error when the node's largest weight is deleted.

Table 1 summarizes the four feature-weighting algorithms. Notice that $E(0)$ indicates the amount of error after removing an input node i and $E(w^{j})$ means the error value when the node is left untouched. CB is a case base which contains case variables (features) and corresponding yield. y means the actual yield value and o_y represents the yield value observed by the BPN. x_i represents input nodes, Act_j^h is the activity of a hidden node j, k signifies output nodes, w_{kj} represents a connection weight from a hidden node j to an output node k, w_{ji} is a weight connected from an input node i to a hidden node j, var() is the variance function, and $\sigma()$ is the activation function. Rel_j^h is the relevance of a hidden node j.

Table 1. Four feature-weighting algorithms

Algorithm	Description	
Sensitivity (Sen_i)	$Sen_i = \max\left(\dfrac{E(0) - E(w^j)}{E(w^j)},\ 0 \right)$	(1)
	$E = \sum_{CB} \lvert y - o_y \rvert$	
Activity (Act_i)	$Act_i = \sum_{j=1}^{H} w_{ji}^2 Act_j^h$	
	$Act_j^h = \sum_{k=1}^{o} w_{kj}^2 \cdot \mathrm{var}\left(\sigma\left(\sum_{i=1}^{N} w_{ji} x_i \right) \right)$	(2)
Saliency (Sal_i)	$Sal_i = \sum_{j=1}^{H} \sum_{k=1}^{o} w_{kj}^2 w_{ji}^2$	(3)
Relevance (Rel_i)	$Rel_i = w_{ji} \cdot Rel_j^h$	
	$Rel_j^h = \sum_{k=1}^{o} w_{kj}^2 \cdot \mathrm{var}\left(w_{ji} \right)$	(4)

After weighting features based on the trained neural network and four weighting methods, a k-NN algorithm finds the most similar k cases from the case base. When a new query comes in from a manufacturing database, the normalized Euclidean distance between the query and the case, $\Delta(\mathbf{q}, \mathbf{x})$, is calculated as follows:

$$\Delta(\mathbf{q}, \mathbf{x}) = \sqrt{\sum_{i=1}^{N} w_i \delta(q_i, x_i)^2} \qquad (5)$$

where $\mathbf{q}$ is the query and $\mathbf{x}$ is a case which is stored in the case base, q_i and x_i are the ith input feature values of $\mathbf{q}$ and $\mathbf{x}$. In this case, w_i is one of the Sensitivity, Activity, Saliency, and Relevance weights, which is assigned to the ith feature. $\delta(q_i, x_i)$ is the difference between the two values q_i and x_i. It is $\lvert q_i - x_i \rvert$ if attribute i is numeric, zero if attribute i is symbolic and $q_i = x_i$, and otherwise, one.

Finally, in order to calculate the predicted value of yield, the hybrid system calculates the weighted average of yields from those k similar cases. At this time, the normalized distances to the query are used as the weights. The predicted value of yield is calculated as follows:

$$\text{Predicted yield} = \frac{\sum_{l=1}^{k} \Delta(\mathbf{q}, \mathbf{x})_l^{-1} y_l}{k} \tag{6}$$

where y_l is the lth production yield which is discovered from the feature-weighted case retrieval.

4 Application

In order to verify the effectiveness of the hybrid method, it was applied to the production data collected from the manufacturing lots of a semiconductor company. We could gather 622 lot data from the company. They consisted of 311 high-yield lots, 311 low-yield lots, and 21 process variables. By definition, a high-yield lot delivers more than 90% yield from a lot and a low-yield lot conveys less than 35% yield from a lot. Among the real lot data sampled, 400 lots (64%) were utilized as training data and 186 lots (30%) were utilized as testing data, and 36 lots (6%) were utilized as evaluation data.

4.1 Cases Clustering

In order to cluster 400 training data in accordance with the 21 process variables, a SOM with 21 input nodes and nine output nodes was prepared. Several techniques speed up the self-organizing process and make it more reliable. One method to improve the performance of the SOM during training is to vary the size of the neighborhoods: from large (one, in our case) to small enough to include only the winning neuron. The learning rate also varies over time. An initial rate of 0.9 allows neurons to learn input vectors quickly. It then shrinks asymptotically toward zero. In training a SOM, 10,000 epochs continue through the training data.

After being trained with the 400 lot data, the three-by-three SOM revealed patterns of the process variables and divided the cases into nine distinct segments (see Table 2).

Table 2. Training results of SOM

Case segment	Number of cases	No. of member cases
CS1	38	2, 3, ..., 309, 376
CS2	22	21, 42, ..., 321, 389
CS3	46	12, 43, ..., 229, 302
CS4	47	51, 63, ..., 367, 371
CS5	65	27, 31, ..., 359, 396
CS6	74	22, 30, ..., 311, 316
CS7	36	1, 4, ..., 300, 363
CS8	34	5, 9, ..., 399, 400
CS9	38	6, 7, ..., 299, 305

Nine BPNs were constructed for nine segments and were trained to learn the relationship between the process variables and yield of member cases in each segment. Akaike Information Criterion (AIC) determined the optimal number of hidden nodes of the BPN through heuristic search [2]. When the number of input nodes is set to 21, the number of hidden layers is one, and the number of output nodes is two, AIC suggested 21 hidden nodes as an optimal topology of the BPNs. Therefore nine BPNs with 21 input nodes, 21 hidden nodes, and two output nodes, were utilized.

4.2 Feature-Weighting CBR

For each segment, to weigh features of CBR with the Sensitivity weighting scheme (cwCBR_Sen), member cases from each segment flowed through the BPN. Nine training data sets were arranged for nine case segments, one data set per segment. When a series of training were done, the Sensitivity weights of the 21 input nodes (i.e., manufacturing process variables) were frozen for each segment. Using these weights, a k-NN algorithm acquired the k-nearest cases from the Yield case base. The weighted average of yields was calculated from these k similar cases.

Following the weighting procedure done for the cwCBR_Sen, the CBR with the Activity weighting scheme (cwCBR_Act), the CBR with the Relevance weighting scheme (cwCBR_Rel), and the CBR with the Saliency weighting scheme (cwCBR_Sal) were constructed, trained, and evaluated against the testing data. The k-nearest cases were obtained by using these weights and the weighted averages of yields were calculated for the cwCBR_Act, cwCBR_Rel, and cwCBR_sal.

4.3 Evaluation

The evaluation procedure for the clustered feature-weighting CBRs is as follows:

1. Choose an evaluation data and identify to which case segment it belongs. A similarity score is used to determine a belonging segment. It is obtained by calculating an inner product of input nodes of an evaluation data (**x**) and the connection weights (**v**) of the SOM [7]. An evaluation data is regarded as to belong to the case segment which has the highest similarity score.
2. Utilize the feature weights (Sensitivity, Activity, Relevance, and Saliency) trained for that segment.
3. Calculate the predicted yield values for each weighting scheme.
4. Reiterate the same procedure while varying k and calculate the average predictive performance of the cwCBR_Sen, cwCBR_Act, cwCBR_Rel, and cwCBR_sal.

These cwCBR methods were compared with non-clustered feature-weighting CBR (i.e., wCBR) methods in order to show performance comparison. Fig. 2 depicts the average prediction accuracy of all feature-weighting methods, according to varying k.

As k increases, the prediction errors decreased in all of hybrid CBR methods. The clustered feature-weighting methods excelled the non-clustered feature-weighting methods in every experiment. The mean errors of cwCBR methods were lower than those of the wCBR methods. Furthermore, the cwCBR_Act showed the highest prediction accuracy, followed by cwCBR_Sal, cwCBR_Rel, and cwCBR_Sen. Adopting the cwCBR_Act weighting method is an acceptable solution to predict the yield rate

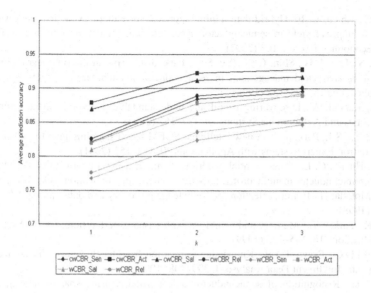

Fig. 2. Average prediction accuracy of each weighting scheme

in semiconductor manufacturing. There are, however, small differences in the prediction accuracy among these four clustered feature-weighting methods.

5 Conclusion

We applied a hybrid method, combining SOM and feature-weighting CBR, to predicting yield of the target semiconductor manufacturing company. In the system, the SOM clustered the Yield cases into several homogeneous segments and the BPN assigned relative weights to manufacturing process features of each instance in the Yield case base. There was no previous similar research of predicting the yield rate of the semiconductor company, with utilizing the clustered and neural feature-weighting CBR. The hybrid system showed that the clustered CBR with the Activity weighting method had a better prediction rate, outperforming the entire hybrid CBRs and the existing statistical approach having been utilized at the target company (Prediction accuracy of the statistical approach reached around 80%).

References

1. Ahn, H., Kim, K., Han, I.: Global optimization of feature weights and the number of neighbors that combine in a case-based reasoning system. Expert Systems 23, 290–301 (2006)
2. Burnham, K.P., Anderson, D.R.: Model selection and multimodel inference: A practical-theoretic approach, 2nd edn. Springer, Heidelberg (2002)
3. Chien, C.-F., Wang, W.-C., Cheng, J.-C.: Data mining for yield enhancement in semiconductor manufacturing and an empirical study. Expert Systems with Applications 33, 192–198 (2007)

4. Hsu, S.-C., Chien, C.-F.: Hybrid data mining approach for pattern extraction from wafer bin map to improve yield in semiconductor manufacturing. International Journal of Production Economics 107, 88–103 (2007)
5. Kang, B.-S., Lee, J.-H., Shin, C.-K., Yu, S.-J., Park, S.-C.: Hybrid machine learning system for integrated yield management in semiconductor manufacturing. Expert Systems with Applications 15, 123–132 (1998)
6. Last, M., Kandel, A.: Discovering useful and understandable patterns in manufacturing data. Robotics and Autonomous Systems 49, 137–152 (2004)
7. Lee, J.H., Yu, S.J., Park, S.C.: A new intelligent SOFM-based sampling plan for advanced process control. Expert Systems with Applications 20, 133–151 (2001)
8. Li, T.-S., Huang, C.-L.: Defect spatial pattern recognition using a hybrid SOM–SVM approach in semiconductor manufacturing. Expert Systems with Applications (October 2007)
9. Liu, H., Motoda, H.: Feature selection for Knowledge discovery and data mining. Kluwer, Norwell (1998)
10. Shin, C.K., Park, S.C.: Memory and neural network based expert system. Expert Systems with Applications 16, 145–155 (1999)
11. Sobrino, M.D.C., Bravo, L.J.B.: Knowledge acquisition from batch semiconductor manufacturing data. Intelligent Data Analysis 3, 399–408 (1999)
12. Wang, C.-H.: Recognition of semiconductor defect patterns using spatial filtering and spectral clustering. Expert Systems with Applications 34, 1914–1923 (2008)
13. Yang, T., Rajasekharan, M., Peters, B.A.: Semiconductor fabrication facility design using a hybrid search methodology. Computers & Industrial Engineering 36, 565–583 (1999)

Selecting the Right Features for Bipartite-Based Text Clustering

Chao Qu[1], Yong Li[1], Jie Zhang[1], Tianming Hu[1,2,*], and Qian Chen[1]

[1] Dongguan University of Technology, China
[2] East China Normal University, China
tmhu@ieee.org

Abstract. Document datasets can be described with a bipartite graph where terms and documents are modeled as vertices on two sides respectively. Partitioning such a graph yields a co-clustering of words and documents, in the hope that the cluster topic can be captured by the top terms and documents in the same cluster. However, single terms alone are often not enough to capture the semantics of documents. To that end, in this paper, we propose to employ hyperclique patterns of terms as additional features for document representation. Then we use F-score to select the top discriminative features to construct the bipartite. Finally, the extensive experiments indicated that compared to the standard bipartite formulation, our approach is able to achieve better clustering performance at a smaller graph size.

1 Introduction

The high dimension in text clustering is a major difficulty for most probabilistic methods such as Naive Bayes. To circumvent this problem, graph-theoretic techniques have been considered for clustering. They model the document similarity by a graph whose vertices correspond to documents and weighted edges give the similarity between vertices. Graphs can also model terms as vertices and similarity between terms is based on documents in which they co-occur. Partitioning the graph yields a clustering of terms, which is assumed to be associated with similar concepts [1]. The duality between document and term clustering can also be naturally modeled using a bipartite, where documents and terms are modeled as vertices on two sides respectively and only edges linking different types of vertices are allowed in the graph [2]. Finding an optimal partitioning in such a bipartite gives a co-clustering of documents and terms. It is expected that top documents and terms in the same cluster can represent its topic, where top vertices usually mean the ones with highest degrees within the cluster.

However, such claims may fail if the cluster is not pure enough or it includes terms/documents with very general topics. To perform natural clustering and to precisely capture the cluster topic, we need to identify those micro-sets of terms, which, as semantic units, are able to embody their respective topics clearly. Besides, we need to ensure that they would not be separated into different clusters

---

* Corresponding author.

C. Tang et al. (Eds.): ADMA 2008, LNAI 5139, pp. 477–484, 2008.

during the clustering process. In this paper, we propose to augment the original single terms with term hypercliques as additional features for document representation. Then we perform feature selection over this mixed feature set to enhance the subsequent bipartite-based text clustering. As a special kind of frequent itemsets with confidence constrains, hyperclique patterns truly possess such desirable property: the objects in a hyperclique pattern have a guaranteed level of global pairwise similarity to one another as measured by the cosine or Jaccard similarity measures [3,4]. Compared to the standard bipartite formulation, the extensive experiments show that our approach, HABIP(Hyperclique-Augmented BIpartite Partitioning), is able to yield better clustering results at smaller graph sizes, which were validated with various clustering criteria.

Overview. Section 2 describes the necessary background. Section 3 presents the details of our algorithm. Section 4 reports extensive experimental results. Finally, we draw conclusions in Section 5.

2   Related Work

In this section, we first review text clustering. Then we introduce hyperclique patterns, which serve as additional features for document representation.

2.1   Document Clustering

In general, clustering algorithms can be divided into two categories: hierarchical and partitional [5]. Hierarchical clustering approaches falls into two classes: divisive and agglomerative. A recent study [6] found Group Average (UPGMA) to be the best in this class for clustering text. As for the partitional category, probably K-means is the most widely used method. As a modification, bisecting K-means has been proposed in hierarchical clustering of documents and produces competitive results [7]. For more robust clustering, another direction is to combine multiple candidate clustering into a consolidated one, which is often referred to as consensus clustering or clustering ensembles [8]. Graph-theoretic techniques have also been considered for clustering [9]. They model the word-document datasets by a graph whose vertices correspond to documents or words. The duality between document and word clustering can be naturally modeled using a bipartite, where documents and words are modeled as vertices on two sides respectively [10].

2.2   Term Hypercliques

In this paper, term hypercliques are employed as additional features for capture of semantics. They are based on the concepts on frequent itemsets. Let $I = \{i_1, i_2, ..., i_m\}$ be a set of distinct items. Each transaction T in database D is a subset of I. We call $X \subseteq I$ an itemset. The support of X, denoted by $supp(X)$, is the fraction of transactions containing X. If $supp(X)$ is no less than a user-specified threshold, X is called a frequent itemset. The confidence of association rule $X_1 \rightarrow X_2$ is defined as $conf(X_1 \rightarrow X_2) = supp(X_1 \cup X_2)/supp(X_1)$. To measure the overall affinity among items within an itemset, the h-confidence was proposed in [3]. Formally, the h-confidence of an itemset $P = \{i_1, i_2, ..., i_m\}$ is defined as $hconf(P) = min_k\{conf(i_k \rightarrow P - i_k)\}$. Given a minimum threshold h_c, an itemset $P \subseteq I$ is a hyperclique pattern if and only if $hconf(P) \geq h_c$. A hyperclique pattern P can be interpreted as that the presence of any item $i \in P$ in a transaction implies the presence of all other items $P - \{i\}$ in the same transaction with probability at least h_c. A hyperclique pattern is a maximal hyperclique pattern if no superset of this pattern is a hyperclique pattern.

Table 1 shows examples of term hypercliques from one of datasets used in our experiments, k1a, whose documents are from categories like people, television, etc. Apparently, the first two rows are from class technology and sports, respectively. Martina Hingis is a star player of woman tennis. WaveTop is a data broadcast software by WavePhor Inc. that allows users with TV tuner-enabled PCs to watch cable TV. Although their h-confidence is high, their support is low, which means there are few edges between them and the documents. Thus it is very possible for graph partitioning algorithms to assign terms of a hyperclique into different clusters. Taking them as initial clusters, however, prevents them from being separated.

Table 1. Examples of term hypercliques

pattern	support	h-confidence
solaris, unix, sparc	0.19%	100%
wnba, lineman	0.19%	75%
martina, hingis	0.51%	80%
wavetop, wavephore, tuner	0.51%	75%

3   The HABIP Algorithm

As shown in Fig. 1, our approach HABIP is divided into three step. We first mine term hypercliques and then perform feature selection over the mixed set of features. Finally we generate the bipartite graph and partition it to yield the clustering. Detailed description is given later in this section.

3.1   Feature Generation

To apply clustering algorithms, a document data set is usually represented by a matrix by extracting words from documents. The matrix A's non-zero entry A_{ij} indicates the presence of term w_j in document d_i, while a zero entry indicates an absence. Given A, if we treat documents as transactions and terms as items, we can find maximal hyperclique patterns of terms. For mining maximal hyperclique patterns, we employ a hybrid approach proposed in [11], which exploited key advantages of both the depth first search strategy and the breadth first search strategy for efficient computation.

Input:
D: a data set represented by a document-term matrix.
K: the desired number of clusters.

Output: C: the clustering result.

Variables:
TH: the set of maximal term hypercliques.
ST: the selected set of terms and term-hypercliques for graph construction.
BG: a bipartite graph.

Steps
  1. TH = MaximalHypercliquePattern(D)
  2. ST = SelectFeature(MT, D)
  3. BG = GenerateBipartite(ST, D)
  4. C = GraphPartition(BG, K)

Fig. 1. Overview of the HABIP Algorithm

Term weighting schemes determine the value of non-zero entry A_{ij} in the document-term matrix when term w_j appears in document d_i. In this paper, we use the classic $tf \times idf$ [12] for single terms. As for term hypercliques, we compute the $\bar{tf} \times idf$, where $\bar{tf}$ is the average of tf for those terms in the hyperclique.

Now we have a mixed feature set of terms and term hypercliques. Although the introduction of term hypercliques brings more semantics, they increase the feature size. Besides, there are some noisy words in the original set of single features. For more efficient and effective bipartite partitioning subsequently, we employ the F-score to select the optimal subset of features. It is a direct technique which measures the discrimination of two sets of real numbers. In detail, suppose feature(terms or term hypercliques) i appears in m instances(documents), n_+ from class + and n_- from class -. Let x_k denote its value at k-th instance, $\bar{x}_+/\bar{x}_-$ the average value over class +/-, $\bar{x}$ the total average value. Then, the F-score of feature i is defined as

$$F(i) = \frac{\left(\bar{x}_+ - \bar{x}\right)^2 + \left(\bar{x}_- - \bar{x}\right)^2}{\frac{1}{n_+-1} \sum_{k=1}^{n_+} \left(x_{+_k} - \bar{x}_+\right)^2 + \frac{1}{n_--1} \sum_{k=1}^{n_-} \left(x_{-_k} - \bar{x}_-\right)^2}$$

A large value of F-score means feature i is more discriminative. Because our datasets are from $K > 2$ classes, we treat them as K two-class problems and compute the average of K scores as the final score. After that, we select the top n fraction of features for subsequent clustering.

3.2   Bipartite-Based Text Clustering

A graph $G = (V, E)$ is composed of a vertex set $V = \{1, 2, ..., |V|\}$ and an edge set $\{(i, j)\}$ each with edge weight E_{ij}. The graph can be stored in an adjacency matrix M, with entry $M_{ij} = E_{ij}$ if there is an edge (i, j), $M_{ij} = 0$ otherwise. Given the $n \times m$ document-(term/term hyperclique) matrix A, the bipartite graph $G = (V, E)$ is constructed as follows. First we order the vertices such that the first m vertices index the terms while the last n index the documents, so $V = V_W \cup V_D$, where V_W contains m vertices each for a term/term hyperclique, and V_D contains n vertices each for a document. Edge set E only contains edges linking different kinds of vertices, so the adjacency matrix M may be written as $\begin{pmatrix} 0, A \\ A^T, 0 \end{pmatrix}$.

Given a weighted graph $G = \{V, E\}$ with adjacency matrix M, clustering the graph into K parts means partitioning V into K disjoint clusters of vertices $V_1, V_2, ..., V_K$, by cutting the edges linking vertices in different parts. The general goal is to minimize the sum of the weights of those cut edges. Formally, the cut between two vertex groups V_1 and V_2 is defined as $cut(V_1, V_2) = \sum_{i \in V_1, j \in V_2} M_{ij}$. Thus the goal can be expressed as $min_{\{V_1, V_2, ..., V_K\}} \sum_{k=1}^{K} cut(V_k, V - V_k)$. To avoid trivial partitions, often the constraint is imposed that each part should be roughly balanced in terms of part weight $wgt(V_k)$, which is often defined as sum of its vertex weight. That is, $wgt(V_k) = \sum_{i \in V_k} wgt(i)$. The objective function to minimize becomes $\sum_{k=1}^{K} \frac{cut(V_k, V - V_k)}{wgt(V_k)}$. Given two different partitionings with the same cut value, the above objective function value is smaller for the more balanced partitioning. Here, we select the normalized cut criterion [13] that defines $wgt(i) = \sum_j M_{ij}$. It favors clusters with equal sums of vertex degrees, where vertex degree refers to the sum of weights of edges incident on it. For graph partitioning, we employ Graclus [14], a fast kernel based multilevel algorithm.

4   Experimental Evaluation

In this section, we present an extensive evaluation of HABIP. First we introduce the experimental datasets and cluster validation criteria, then we report comparative results.

4.1   Experimental Setup

For evaluation, we selected seven real datasets from different domains used in [6]. The RE0 and RE1 datasets are from the Reuters-21578 text categorization test collection Distribution 1.0. The datasets K1a and K1b are from the WebACE project; each document corresponds to a web page listed in the subject hierarchy of Yahoo. The LA1, LA2 and LA12 datasets were obtained from articles of the Los Angeles Times that was used in TREC. For all data sets, we used a stoplist to remove common words, stemmed the remaining words using Porter's suffix-stripping algorithm, and discard those with very low document frequencies. Some characteristics of them are shown in Table 2.

Because the true class labels of documents are known, we can measure the quality of the clustering solutions using external criteria that measure the discrepancy between the structure defined by a clustering and what is defined by

Table 2. Characteristics of data sets

data	re0	re1	k1a	k1b	la1	la2	la12
#doc	1504	1657	2340	2340	3204	3075	6279
#word	2886	3758	21839	21839	31472	31472	31472
#class	13	25	20	6	6	6	6
source	Reuters-21578		WebACE		TREC		

Table 3. Comparison of clustering results

data	method	NMI	CE	ERR	F	sup/hconf
k1a	STD	0.51	1.72	0.52	0.44	NA
	HABIP	0.59	1.39	0.50	0.50	0.005/0.1
k1b	STD	0.58	0.54	0.37	0.64	NA
	HABIP	0.66	0.57	0.23	0.84	0.0015/0.1
la1	STD	0.25	0.87	0.52	0.42	NA
	HABIP	0.47	1.28	0.31	0.65	0.002/0.2
la2	STD	0.32	0.84	0.57	0.47	NA
	HABIP	0.42	1.42	0.38	0.58	0.0015/0.2
la12	STD	0.27	1.15	0.56	0.46	NA
	HABIP	0.37	1.42	0.55	0.45	0.005/0.2
re0	STD	0.32	2.53	0.40	0.36	NA
	HABIP	0.33	1.79	0.43	0.36	0.0015/0.1
re1	STD	0.37	2.98	0.49	0.32	NA
	HABIP	0.40	2.13	0.45	0.32	0.02/0.2

the true class labels. We use the following four measures: normalized mutual information(NMI), conditional entropy(CE), error rate(ERR) and F-measure [15]. NMI and CE are entropy based measures. Error rate $ERR(T|C)$ computes the fraction of misclassified data when all data in each cluster is classified as the majority class in that cluster. F-measure combines the precision and recall concepts from information retrieval.

4.2 Clustering Results

First we compare the clustering results between the standard bipartite formulation(STD) and HABIP without feature selection. Detailed results are shown in Table 3, where NMI and F are preferred large while ERR and CE are preferred small. The two parameters of HABIP in the last column, support threshold and h-confidence threshold, were tuned separately for each dataset, but not for each criterion. One can see that HABIP is able to achieve improvement on nearly all datasets in terms of most measures.

Next, we evaluate HABIP by varying top n fraction of features. Although a smaller subset of features would lead to a smaller bipartite graph and an easier partitioning subsequently, too much deletion of features would harm the clustering results. Therefore we need a tradeoff here. Due to lack of space, we only

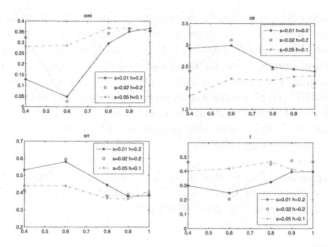

Fig. 2. re0: clustering results with top n fraction of features

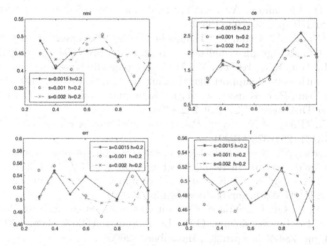

Fig. 3. k1a: clustering results with top n fraction of features

report results on re0 and k1a. Fig. 2 and 3 illustrate the results with different support threshold and h-confidence threshold around optimal values for full feature set (reported in Table 3). One can see that it is not the case the clustering performance would improve with increase of n. For re0, there is little change in the performance once n exceeds around 90%. For k1a, the results oscillates considerably. In general, the optimal value of n appears in the range of $[0.7, 0.9]$, where it yields the best clustering results at a relatively smaller graph size.

5   Concluding Remarks

The performance of text clustering depends on both the document representation and the clustering model. In this paper, we studied feature selection for bipartite-based text clustering. Because single terms are not enough to capture the semantics, we propose to augment the feature set with hyperclique patterns of terms. After feature selection with F-score, these micro-set of semantics serve as starting points in the bipartite and would not be separated during the graph partitioning process. Our experiments on real datasets showed that our approach, HABIP (Hyperclique-Augmented BIpartite Partitioning), not only is able to achieve better clustering performance than the standard bipartite formulation, but also leads to a smaller graph size. These gains were validated by various external clustering criteria.

Acknowledgments. This work was partially supported by SRF for ROCS, Sci. Tech. Plan Foundation of Guangdong(No. 20070328005), and Sci. Tech. Plan Foundation of Dongguan(No. 2007108101022).

References

1. Baker, L.D., McCallum, A.: Distributional clustering of words for text classification. In: SIGIR, pp. 96–103 (1998)
2. Usui, S., Naud, A., Ueda, N., Taniguchi, T.: 3d-SE viewer: A text mining tool based on bipartite graph visualization. In: IJCNN, pp. 1103–1108 (2007)
3. Xiong, H., Tan, P.N., Kumar, V.: Mining strong affinity association patterns in data sets with skewed support distribution. In: ICDM, pp. 387–394 (2003)
4. Xiong, H., Tan, P.N., Kumar, V.: Hyperclique pattern discovery. Data Mining and Knowledge Discovery 13(2), 219–242 (2006)
5. Jain, A.K., Murty, M.N., Flynn, P.J.: Data clustering: A review. ACM Computing Surveys 31(3), 264–323 (1999)
6. Zhao, Y., Karypis, G.: Empirical and theoretical comparisons of selected criterion functions for document clustering. Machine Learning 55(3), 311–331 (2004)
7. Steinbach, M., Karypis, G., Kumar, V.: A comparison of document clustering techniques. In: KDD Workshop on Text Mining (2000)
8. Hu, T., Liu, L., Qu, C., Sung, S.Y.: Joint cluster based co-clustering for clustering ensembles. In: Li, X., Zaïane, O.R., Li, Z. (eds.) ADMA 2006. LNCS (LNAI), vol. 4093, pp. 284–295. Springer, Heidelberg (2006)
9. Strehl, A., Ghosh, J., Mooney, R.: Impact of similarity measures on web-page clustering. In: Proc. AAAI: Workshop of Artificial Intelligence for Web Search, pp. 58–64 (2000)
10. Dhillon, I.S.: Co-clustering documents and words using bipartite spectral graph partitioning. In: SIGKDD, pp. 269–274 (2001)
11. Huang, Y., Xiong, H., Wu, W., Zhang, Z.: A hybrid approach for mining maximal hyperclique patterns. In: ICTAI, pp. 354–361 (2004)
12. Baeza-Yates, R., Ribeiro-Neto, B.: Modern Information Retrieval. Addison-Wesley, Reading (1999)
13. Shi, J., Malik, J.: Normalized cuts and image segmentation. IEEE Trans. Pattern Analysis and Machine Intelligence 22, 888–905 (2000)
14. Dhillon, I.S., Guan, Y., Kulis, B.: A fast kernel-based multilevel algorithm for graph clustering. In: SIGKDD, pp. 629–634 (2005)
15. Larsen, B., Aone, C.: Fast and effective text mining using linear-time document clustering. In: SIGKDD, pp. 16–22 (1999)

Image Emotional Classification Based on Color Semantic Description

Kaiping Wei, Bin He, Tao Zhang, and Wenya He

Department of Computer Science, Huazhong Normal University
430079 Wuhan, China
binh2008@sina.com

Abstract. Describing images in semantic terms is an important and challenging problem in content-based image retrieval. According to the strong relationship between colors and human emotions, an emotional image classification model based on color semantic terms is proposed in this paper. First, combined with PSO, fuzzy c-means clustering is implemented for color segmentation, and eight color clusters can be obtained to describe the main color of an image. Secondly, based on Wundt's theory, a 3D emotional model is constructed and a novel approach for describing image color semantic is proposed. Finally, we present a trial classification system which allows users to query images using emotional semantic words. Experimental results demonstrate that this model is effective for sentimental image classification.

1 Introduction

Content-based image retrieval (CBIR) system supports image searches based on perceptual features, such as color, texture, and shape [1], [2]. However, this sort of query is unnatural. In recent years, great progress has been made in this filed [3], [4], Due to the difficulties in recognizing and classifying images on general level, there are few existing methods that have been achieved in identifying high-level semantic descriptors for image retrieval or classification.

In this paper, an improved method for image emotional classification based on color features representation and similarity measuring is proposed. The rest paper is organized as follows. The color image clustering algorithm is described in detail in Section 2. Section 3 describes the method of image semantic description. The experimental results are presented in Section 4 followed by the conclusion and future work in Section 5.

2 Color Segmentation

Color image segmentation is very important in image processing. From the segmentation results, it is possible to identify regions of interest and objects in the scene. In this paper, we propose an effective image segmentation method, which involves three stages: 1) Image preprocessing. Edges are removed and the images are smoothed by

C. Tang et al. (Eds.): ADMA 2008, LNAI 5139, pp. 485–491, 2008.
© Springer-Verlag Berlin Heidelberg 2008

Gauss kernel. 2) Color space conversion. The color space is converted from RGB space into L*a*b* space. 3) Color clustering using fuzzy c-means clustering based on PSO algorithm (PSFCM) in L*a*b* space.

2.1 Image Preprocessing

Based on the observations [5], we eliminate the edges whose color content is perceptually unimportant and we do not process or care about. After that, we perform Gaussian low-pass filtering on the pixels to detect the object edges which can be removed from the original images. In our algorithm, these removed edge pixels are filled with (0, 0, 0) in RGB space which means emotionless in affective computing.

2.2 Color Space Conversion

Segmentation validity is obtained through an appropriate selection of the color space so that small feature distances correspond to similar colors in the perceptual domain [6]. This condition, which is not exhibited by the standard RGB space, has been accomplished with the adoption of the L*a*b* space. The L*a*b* color space is colorimetric and perceptually uniform. The color space is therefore converted from RGB space into L*a*b* space.

2.3 Color Clustering

1)   Alogorithm 1: fuzzy c-means clustering algorithm (FCM)

The Fuzzy C-means (FCM) algorithm [7] is an iterative clustering method that produces an optimal c partition, which minimizes the weighted within group sum of squared error objective function $J_q(U,V) = \sum_{g=1}^{n}\sum_{i=1}^{c}(u_{ig})^q d^2(x_g,v_i)$.

Where $X = \{x_1, x_2, \cdots, x_n\} \subseteq R^p$, n is the number of data items, c is the number of clusters with $2 \le c < n$, u_{ig} is the degree of membership of x_g in the ith cluster, q is a weighting exponent on each fuzzy membership, v_i is the prototype of the centre of cluster i , $d^2(x_g, v_i)$ is a distance measure between object x_g and cluster centre v_i .

Since FCM algorithm is an iterative operation, it is very time consuming in image segmentation. To cope with this problem, the color level histogram of image is applied to the algorithm.

Define color descriptor E in L*a*b* space as follows:

$$E = \left[(L*)^2 + (a*)^2 + (b*)^2 \right]^{1/2} \qquad (1)$$

The non-negative integrate set $E = \{E_{min}, E_{min+1}, \cdots, E_{max}\}$ is color level, where E_{min} is the minimum color level, E_{max} is the maximum color level, so the color scale is

$E_{max} - E_{min}$. For image size $M \times N$, at point (m,n), $f(m,n)$ is the color value with $0 \le m \le M-1, 0 \le n \le N-1$. Let $His(e)$ denotes the number of pixels having color level e ($e \in E$). The statistical histogram function is as follows:

$$His(e) = \sum_{m=0}^{M-1} \sum_{n=0}^{N-1} \delta(f(m,n) - e) \qquad (2)$$

Where $e \in E$, $\delta(0) = 1$ and $\delta(\sigma \neq 0) = 0$.

2) FCM based on PSO Algorithm-PSFCM

In PSO [8], a fitness function f is evaluated, using the particle's positional coordinates as input values. The velocity and position update equations for the pth dimension of ith particle in the swarm may be given as follows:

$$v_{ip}(t+1) = w \cdot v_{ip}(t) + C_1 \cdot \varphi_1 \cdot (p_{ibest} - Z_{ip}(t)) + C_2 \cdot \varphi_2 \cdot (p_{gbest} - Z_{ip}(t)) \qquad (3)$$

$$Z_{ip}(t+1) = Z_{ip}(t) + v_{ip}(t+1) \qquad (4)$$

The variables φ_1 and φ_2 are random positive numbers with an upper limit φ_{max}, C_1 and C_2 are acceleration constants, and ω is the inertia weight. P_{ibest} is the best solution found so far by an individual particle, while P_{gbest} represents the fittest particle found so far in the entire community.

Define partition entropy V_{pe} and the fitness f as follows,

$$V_{pe} = \frac{\sum_{i=1}^{c} [v_i \log v_i]}{E_{max}}, \quad f = \max_{E_{min} \le e \le E_{max}} \{ \frac{1}{V_{pe} + eps} \} \qquad (5)$$

The idea of the validity function is that the partition with less fuzziness means better performance. Consequently, the best clustering is achieved when the value V_{pe} is minimal.

For a user-specified maximum number of clusters C_{max}, a particle is a vector of real numbers of dimension $2 * C_{max}$. The first C_{max} entries are positive floating-point numbers in $(0, 1)$, each of which controls whether the corresponding cluster is to be activated (i.e. to be really used for classifying the data) or not. The remaining entries are reserved for C_{max} cluster centers, each p-dimensional. A single particle is illustrated as [10]:

$$\vec{Z}_i(t) = (T_{i,1}, T_{i,2}, \cdots, T_{i,C_{max}}; V_{i,1}, V_{i,2}, \cdots, V_{i,C_{max}})$$

Step 1) Initialization

(a) Set constants $K_{max}, C_1, C_2, \omega$ and particle size *SwarmSize*.

(b) For particle i, position $T_{i,j} (1 \le j \le C_{max})$ can be initialized by

$$T_{i,j} = rand() * (E_{max} - E_{min}) + E_{min}.$$

Where, E_{min}, E_{max} , resulted from Eq.(1), represents the minimum and maximum color level respectively.

(c) For particle i , velocity $V_{i,j} (1 \le j \le C_{max})$ can be initialized by

$$V_{i,j} = rand() * (E_{max} - E_{min}) .$$

(d) Set $k = 1$.

Step 2) Optimization

(a) For each particle, evaluate the fitness value f_k defined in Eq. (5).

(b) If $f_{best}^i \le f_k^i$ then $f_{best}^i = f_k^i, \overrightarrow{P_{ibest}} = \overrightarrow{T_i}$, where f_{best}^i is the best fitness value found so far by an individual particle.

(c) If $f_{best}^g \le f_k^i$ then $f_{best}^g = f_k^i, \overrightarrow{P_{gbest}} = \overrightarrow{T_i}$, where f_{best}^g is the fittest value found so far in the entire community.

(d) If $k > K_{max}$, go to Step 3).

(e) Update particle velocity and position using Eq. (3) and Eq. (4).

(f) Increment i . If $i > I$ then increment k ,and set $i = 1$.

(g) Go to Step 2 (a).

Step 3) Report results

Cluster centre $\overrightarrow{V} = Uniform(\overrightarrow{p_{gbest}})$.

The parameters in this algorithm are as follows:

$$SwarmSize = 20, K_{max} = 8, C_{max} = 2, C_1 = C_2 = 2.05 , \omega = 0.729 .$$

In our algorithm, 8 basic colors, called color terms, have been chosen to establish emotional space. Following table shows the clustering results for picture 'rose'□

Table 1. Clustering centers described as color center E

Terms	I1	I2	I3	I4	I5	I6	I7	I8
rose	0	89.7902	51.2280	106.4020	70.8947	1.0000	18.8547	6.8156

In our system, eight color terms have been selected to describe emotions of images. For picture 'rose', the terms are: *Black, Dark Blue, Dark Green, Red, Purple, White, Pink and Linen* as shown in Table 1.

3   Emotion Semantic Descriptions of Colors

In this section, we propose a color description model which can automatically generate the semantic terms of image segmentations and the whole image through a fuzzy clustering algorithm.

3.1 Emotional Model

In our work, eight emotional states are described by eight emotion semantic terms: anger, despair, interest, pleasure, sadness, irritation, joy and pride.

3.2 Emotion Mapping

Based on the results of section 2, image can be divided into eight color regions. Get areas of each region and implement the following classification algorithm.

At the beginning of comparison, emotion distance $DE(i, j)$ is proposed and is defined as follows:

$$DE(i, j) = |Region(I_{i,j}) - I_{i,j}| < \sigma_{i,j}, (i, j = 1, 2, \cdots, 8) \tag{6}$$

Where, $Region(I_{i,j})$ is the current region size of each cluster and $I_{i,j}$ is the region size of each cluster defined in Table 3. $\sigma_{i,j}$ is a constant integer.

The key to classification algorithm is the definition of emotional-color mapping, which is how to accurately define the color distribution of emotion among eight clusters. Through numerous experiments, we have got a set of mapping data for reference. In practical application, users can also update the dataset by interactive training. The results of same data are presented in Table 2, in which, for example, "Interest" is described as follows: $I(3, j) = \{0.2280, 16.7902, 0, 24.4020, 3.8947, 0, 44.2789, 10.4054\}$.
$$1 \leq j \leq 8$$

Table 2. Emotion-Color mapping Table

	E1	E2	E3	E4	E5	E6	E7	E8
1 Anger	0	1.1532	0	10.3721	27.3437	2.1130	58.9283	0.0898
2 Despair	0	0	0	0	50.3139	48.5754	0.2760	0.8348
3 Interest	0.2280	16.7902	0	24.4020	3.8947	0	44.2789	10.4054
4Irritation	8.1442	30.1156	0.2535	31.8286	10.1973	1.2368	18.1621	0.0618
5 Joy	0	2.0594	0	0.6251	57.3984	3.7956	35.9370	0.1846
6 Pleasure	0.0187	7.3263	0	5.1290	17.4198	24.8880	32.9111	12.3072

4 Experiments and Analysis

4.1 Training

To meet the user's emotional bias, the following method can be used for training Clustering

Step 1: Choose emotion terms of a new image I_new by user's interaction;

Step 2: On I_new, implement *algorithm 1* and get new clusters $E\_new(i)$;

Step 3: Update $E(i)$ using $E(i) = (E(i) + E\_new(i))/2$;

Where, $E\_new(i) = \{I1, I2, \cdots, I8\}$ is the same as $E(i)$ described in Table 1.

4.2 Experimental Result and Analysis

In order to evaluate our method, we have implemented a trial classification system on windows XP platform, 200 images are collected as image database. These images are collected from Internet which contain more colors and express more complex feelings with wide range of lightness and color distributions.

Fig.1 shows the results of query "Pleasure" images, based on the experience of color and emotion, while the bright image and the warm colors will induce the happiness feelings, so the images which are bright and contain more warm colors will induce the pleasure feelings.

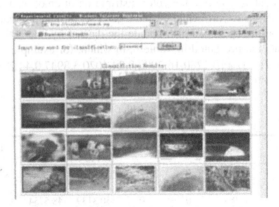

Fig. 1. Classification results of "Pleasure" images

Table 3. Confusion matrix of the classification system based on Color Semantic Description.

	Anger	Despair	Interest	Irritation	Joy	Pleasure	Pride	Sadness
	a	b	c	d	e	f	g	h
a	**48.75**	6.25	4.25	15.25	6.75	6.75	12.75	6.25
b	12	**38**	12.25	8.75	0	13.25	3.25	10
c	5.75	5.25	**45**	3.75	6.75	10	16.75	0
d	10	6.75	10	**46.25**	3.25	6.75	6.25	6.75
e	5.25	0	12.25	16.75	**50.25**	10	8.25	3.25
f	7.75	10.25	6.75	3.25	12.75	**33.25**	13.25	0
g	10.25	5.25	14.75	6.75	10.25	13.25	**33.75**	0
h	6.75	8.75	3.25	3.75	0	6.75	5.75	**43.75**

Table 3 shows the confusion matrix of the emotion recognition system based on Color Semantic Description. The overall performance of this classifier was 42.3 %. The most recognized emotions were joy (50.25 %), anger (48.75%), and irritation (46.25 %). Pride is misclassified with interest (16.75%), while irritation is misclassified with joy (16.75 %).

5 Conclusions and Future Work

In this paper, we propose an emotional semantic classification model. Compared with the existing image classification methods, we present an image classification scheme and define a natural classification language, which bridge the high level semantic templates and the low level semantic indicators. Thus the classification keywords can be constructed to describe high level semantics according to the accumulated knowledge and experience. The system is general and is able to satisfy classifies simple color images.

The approach presented in this paper is only the first step, more work should be performed in the future. First, more features and semantic indictors can be fulfilled into this scheme. Second, how to describe the complex emotion using color clustering and make the scheme more useful for end users is a challenging and hard work.

References

1. Smeulders, A.W.M., Worring, M., Santini, S., Gupta, A., Jain, R.: Content-based image retrieval: the end of the early years. IEEE Trans, Pattern Analysis and Machine Intelligence 22, 349–1380 (2001)
2. Li, Y., Shapiro, L.: Consistent Line Clusters for Building Recognition in CBIR. In: Proc. Int'l Conf. Pattern Recognition, vol. 3, pp. 952–956 (2002)
3. Carneiro, G., Vasconcelos, N.: Formulating Semantic Image Annotation as a Supervised Learning Problem. In: IEEE Conference on Computer Vision and Pattern Recognition (CVPR), pp. 1–6 (2005)
4. Carneiro, G., Chan, A.B., Moreno, P.J., Vasconcelos, N.: Supervised learning of semantic classes for image annotation and retrieval. IEEE Trans. on PAMI 29, 394–410 (2007)
5. Kandel, E.R., Schwartz, J.H., Jessel, T.M.: Principles of Neural Science. Appleton and Lange, New York (1991)
6. Wang, W.-N., Yu, Y.-L.: Image Emotional Semantic Query Based on Color Semantic Description. In: International Conference on Machine Learning and Cybernetics, vol. 7, pp. 4571–4576 (2005)
7. Wang, X., Wang, Y., Wang, L.: Improving fuzzy c-means clustering based on feature-weight learning. Pattern Recognit. Lett., 1123–1132 (2004)
8. Eberhart, R.C., Shi, Y.: Particle swarm optimization: Developments, applications and resources [J]. In: International Conference on Evolutionary Computation, vol. 1, pp. 81–86 (2001)

A Semi-supervised Clustering Algorithm Based on Must-Link Set

Haichao Huang, Yong Cheng*, and Ruilian Zhao

Computer Department, College of Information Science and Technology,
Beijing University of Chemical Technology, 100029, Beijing, China
chengsiyong@gmail.com
http://www.buct.edu.cn

Abstract. Clustering analysis is traditionally considered as an unsupervised learning process. In most cases, people usually have some prior or background knowledge before they perform the clustering. How to use the prior or background knowledge to imporve the cluster quality and promote the efficiency of clustering data has become a hot research topic in recent years. The Must-Link and Cannot-Link constraints between instances are common prior knowledge in many real applications. This paper presents the concept of Must-Link Set and designs a new semi-supervised clustering algorithm MLC-KMeans using Musk-Link Set as assistant centroid. The preliminary experiment on several UCI datasets confirms the effectiveness and efficiency of the algorithm.

Keywords: Semi-supervised Learning, Data Clustering, Constraint, MLC-KMeans Algorithm.

1 Introduction

Data mining is the analysis of (often large) observational data sets to find unsuspected relationships and to summarize the data in novel ways that are both understandable and useful to the data owner[1]. One of the basic tasks in data mining is clustering data which can be formulated to identify the distribution of patterns and intrinsic correlations in large datasets by partitioning the data instances into similar clusters. Traditionally, clustering analysis is usually considered as an unsupervised learning problem. However, in the real application domains, it is often the case that people have some prior or background knowledge about the domains and the dataset which can be useful for clustering. Traditional clustering algorithms have no ways to use the information or knowledge. Therefore, how to use these background information to improve the clustering analysis is the focus of recent studies[3,8,4,9].

Wagstaff[3] introduces two types of background information that can be expressed as set of instance-level constraints, the Must-Link and Cannot-Link. The former constraint specifies that two data instances have to be in the same cluster,

---

* Communication author.

C. Tang et al. (Eds.): ADMA 2008, LNAI 5139, pp. 492–499, 2008.
© Springer-Verlag Berlin Heidelberg 2008

the later constraint specifies that two data instances must not be placed in the same cluster. Wagstaff also modified the K-Means algorithm and proposed a constrained clustering algorithm COP-KMeans[3]. The experiment result confirms that COP-KMeans can improve clustering quality. In [4], Sugato Basu presents a pairwise constrained clustering method PCKMeans for actively selecting informative pairwise constraints to improve clustering performance. The basic idea of PCKMeans algorithm is configuring the energy of Hidden Markov Random Field (HMRF) using a well-designed cost function. The clustering process is equal to find the minimal energy configuration of HMRF. In order to maximize the utility of the limited supervised data available in a semi-supervised setting, PCKMeans algorithm can actively select the supervised training examples. Other advantages of the learning are the PCKMeans algorithm is not only easily scalable to large datasets but also can handle very high dimensional data. The experiment shows that the active selection strategy can significantly improve the accuracy of clustering. In most cases, finding a clustering solution that satisfies all constraints is often a NP complete problem[5].

This paper is organized as follows. In section 2, we introduce basic concepts and the ideas of COP-KMenas algorithm. In the following, we analyze the disadvantages of COP-KMeans, and introduce Must-Link Set and Cannot-Link Set concepts. Based upon Must-Link Set, the MLC-KMeans algorithm is proposed and described in detail. In section 4, we present experimental results and show MLC-KMeans algothm is effective and efficient compared with COP-KMeans. Finally, section 5 summarizes our contributions.

2   Background

Assume $X = \{x_1, x_2, \cdots, x_n\} \subset \Re^d$ is a vector space of d dimensions. The element x_i in X is a d dimension data instance that can be described by a vector $[x_{i1}, x_{i2}, \cdots, x_{id}]^T$, the size of the dataset is n. The partitioned result of clustering is a set $\prod = C_1, C_2, \cdots, C_k$ that satisfies $X = C_1 \cup C_2 \cup \cdots \cup C_k$ and $C_1 \cap C_2 \cap \cdots \cap C_k = \varnothing$.

Definition 1 (Must-Link). *For two data instances x_i and x_j in the dataset, $x_i, x_j \in X (1 \leq i, j \leq n)$, if x_i and x_j satisfy the Must-Link constraint, then after finishing the clustering, x_i and x_j satisfy $x_i \in C_m \wedge x_j \in C_m, C_m \in \prod, 1 \leq m \leq k$, or else the clustering fails. The constraint can be described as $x_i \mathsf{ML} x_j$.*

Definition 2 (Cannot-Link). *For two data instances x_i and x_j in the dataset, $x_i, x_j \in X (1 \leq i, j \leq n)$, if x_i and x_j satisfy the Cannot-Link constraint, then after finishing the clustering, x_i and x_j satisfy $x_i \in C_m \wedge x_j \in C_n, C_m, C_n \in \prod, 1 \leq m, n \leq k, m \neq n$, or else the clustering fails. The constraint can be described as $x_i \mathsf{CL} x_j$.*

Definition 3 ($Con_=$). *$Con_=$ is a set that includes all Must-Link constraints in the clustering.*

$$Con_= = \{x_i \mathsf{ML} x_j | x_i, x_j \in X, 1 \leq i, j \leq n\}$$

Definition 4 ($Con_{\neq}$). $Con_{\neq}$ *is a set that includes all Cannot-Link constraints in the clustering.*

$$Con_{\neq} = \{x_i CL x_j | x_i, x_j \in X, 1 \leq i, j \leq n\}$$

According to the definitions above, the clustering problem with Must-Link and Cannot-Link constraints can be formulated as follows. Given the data space $X = \{x_1, x_2, \cdots, x_n\} \subset \mathfrak{R}^d$, $x_i \in X (1 \leq i \leq n)$ is an instance in the data space X. $Con_{=}$ and $Con_{\neq}$ are the Must-Link constraint and Cannot-Link constraint set respectively. The semi-supervised clustering is trying to partition the data space into cluster set $\prod = \{C_1, C_2, \cdots, C_k\}$ and to minimize the object function, $E = \sum_{i=1}^{k} \sum_{j=1}^{n_i} ||x_{ij} - m_i||^2$ under the $Con_{=}$ and $Con_{\neq}$ constraints. Here k is the cluster number, $x_{ij} \in C_i$, m_i is the centroid of cluster i.

3   MLC-KMeans Clustering Algorithm

3.1   The Disadvantage of COP-KMeans Algorithm

The COP-KMeans algorithm may fail when it assigns the instance to cluster. Here, we suppose the cluster num $k = 2$. As shown in Fig 1, the cluster and instance are represented by ellipse and circle respectively. The solid line between the instances is Must-Link constraint, while the broken line is Cannot-Link constraint. The figure illustrates three situations in which the algorithm may fail and derive incorrect result. Especially, when the number of Must-Link and Cannot-Link constraint is large and the cluster num k is small, the COP-KMeans algorithm will frequently fail.

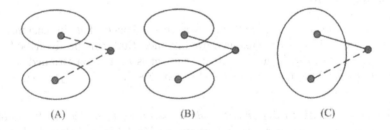

(A)   (B)   (C)

Fig. 1. Failures in COP-KMeans Algorithm

3.2   Basic Idea of Algorithm

To overcome the disadvantage of COP-KMeans and enhance the quality and efficiency of clustering, we propose a semi-supervised clustering algorithm MLC-KMeans based on the Must-Link Set. To illustrate clearly, we firstly define the Must-Link Set and the Cannot-Link Set concepts in the following.

Definition 5 (Must-Link Set). *Must-Link Set (MLSet) is defined as a set that includes all instances that satisfy the Must-Link constraint.*

$$MLSet = \{x_i, x_j, x_r | \forall x_i, x_j, x_r \in X \wedge x_i ML x_j \wedge x_j ML x_r, 1 \leq i, j, r \leq n\}$$

Definition 6 (Cannot-Link Set). *Cannot-Link Set (CLSet) is defined as a set that includes all instances that satisfy the Cannot-Link constraint.*

$$CLSet = \{x_i, x_j, x_r | \forall x_i, x_j, x_r \in X \wedge x_i CL x_j \wedge x_j CL x_r, 1 \leq i, j, r \leq n\}$$

Theorem 1. *The Must-Link relation on Must-Link Set is transitive.*

Proof. For instances $x_p, x_q, x_r \in X$, $(1 \leq p, q, r \leq n)$. If $x_p ML x_q \in Con_=$ and $x_q ML x_r \in Con_=$, According to the definition of Must-Link Set, $x_p, x_r \in MLSet$, we can conclude the Must-Link relation on Must-Link Set is transitive.

To make full use of the knowledge contained in the constraints, we use the centroid of MLSet allocated to the cluster as an assistant centroid to calculate the similarity of instance and cluster. Assume the data space is an euclidean space. C_i and $C_j, (1 \leq i, j \leq k)$ are two clusters whose centroids are m_i and m_j respectively. $MLSC_i$ and $MLSC_j$ are Must-Link Set assigned to C_i and C_j. Now suppose O is an instance to assign, if $dist(O, C_i) > \beta * dist(O, MLSC_j)$ and $dist(O, MLSC_i) > dist(O, MLSC_j)$, or $dist(O, C_i) > dist(O, C_j)$ and $\beta * dist(O, MLSC_i) > dist(O, C_j)$, then allocates O to C_j, or else to C_i. β is regulative coefficient, usually a constant $(\beta > 0)$. β can be adjusted to regulate the importance of assistant centroid, when $\beta > 1$, the centroid has dominant effect, otherwise the assistant centroid has dominant effect in clustering. In our experiments, the β is set to 2. The MLC-KMeans algorithm is described in detail as follows.

Input: Must-Link Constraint Set: $Con_= \subseteq X \times X$, Cannot Link
       Constraint Set: $Con_{\neq} \subseteq X \times X$
Output: $NewCon_=$, $NewCon_{\neq}$
1   initialize $NewCon_= = \varnothing, NewCon_{\neq} = \varnothing$;
2   **for** $X_i, X_j \in Con_=$ **do**
3   **if** $\exists S \in NewCon_= \wedge x_i \in S$ **then**
4 | $S = S \cup X_j$;
5   **else if** $\exists S \in NewCon_= \wedge x_j \in S$ **then**
6 | $S = S \cup X_i$;
7   **else if** $\exists S1 \in NewCon_= \wedge x_i \in S1 \wedge \exists S2 \in NewCon_= \wedge x_j \in S2$ **then**
8 | $S1 = S1 \cup S2$;
9   **else**
10 | $NewCon_= = NewCon_= \cup \{x_i, x_j\}$;
11   **end**
12 **end**
13 **for** $(x_p, x_q) \in NewCon_{\neq}$ **do**
14   **if** $\exists S1, S1 \in NewCon_= \wedge \exists S2, S2 \in NewCon_= \wedge x_p \in S1 \wedge x_q \in S2$
       then
15 | remove (x_p, x_q) from $Con_{\neq}$;
16 | $NewCon_{\neq} = NewCon_{\neq} \cup \{S1CLS2\}$;
17   **end**
18 **end**

Algorithm 1. ConstraintConverter Algorithm

The constraint converter algorithm converts the Must-Link and Cannot-Link to Must-Link and Cannot-Link Set.

Input: MLS, C_m, $NewCon_=$, $NewCon_{\neq}$
Output: $Boolean$
1 **for** $S \in NewCon_=$ **do**
2   **if** $MLS \subseteq C_m \wedge MLSCLS \in NewCon_{\neq}$ **then**
3   **return** true;
4   **end**
5 **end**
6 **return** false;

Algorithm 2. ViolateNewConstraints Algorithm

The constraint violation algorithm judges whether the allocation of Must-Link Set violates the constraints in $NewCon_=$ and $NewCon_{\neq}$.

Input: Dataset: X, Must-Link Constraint Set: $Con_= \subseteq X \times X$, Cannot Link Constraint Set: $Con_{\neq} \subseteq X \times X$, Cluster number: k
Output: $C_1, C_2, \cdots, C_k$
1 $\{NewCon_=, NewCon_{\neq}\} = ConstraintConverter(Con_=, Con_{\neq})$;
2 **if** $k < |NewCon_{\neq}|$ **then**
3   **return** ERROR;
4 **end**
5 initialize C_i with S, $S \in NewCon_{\neq}, (1 \leq i \leq k)$;
6 **repeat**
7   **for** $S \in NewCon_=$ **do**
8   find the closest cluster C_m,
        $dist(S, C_m)$=min$dist(S, C_j), (1 \leq m, j \leq k)$;
9   **if** $!ViolateNewConstraints(S, C_m, NewCon_=, NewCon_{\neq})$ **then**
10              $C_m = C_m \cup S$;
11   update the assistant centroid of $C_i(1 \leq i \leq k)$;
12   **else**
13   **return** ERROR;
14   **end**
15   **end**
16   **for** $x_i \in \{X - \bigcup S | S \in NewCon_=\}$ **do**
17   find the closest cluster C_n,
        $dist(S, C_n)$=min$dist(x_i, C_j), (1 \leq n, j \leq k)$;
18   **if** $!ViolateConstraints(x_i, C_n, Con_{\neq})$ **then**
19              $C_n = C_n \cup \{x_i\}$;
20   **else**
21   **return** ERROR;
22   **end**
23   **end**
24   update the centroid of $C_i(1 \leq i \leq k)$;
25 **until** $convergence$;
26 **return** $C_1, C_2, \cdots, C_k$;

Algorithm 3. MLC-KMeans Algorithm

4   Experiment Result

4.1   Datasets and Evaluation Method

We use four datasets in UCI machine learning repository [6] to test MLC-KMeans algorithm and compare the performance of COP-KMeans with our algorithm. The datasets are described in the table 1.

Table 1. The experimental dataset

Name	Attribute Type	Attribute Num	Instance Num	Class Num	Source
iris	numeric	4	150	3	UCI
xor	nominal	2	40	2	UCI
wine	numeric	13	178	3	UCI
balance-scale	numeric	4	625(200)	3	UCI

In the experiment, the Must-Link and Cannot-Link constraints are generated randomly. We generate a pair of random numbers that associate two instances each time. If the classes of the instances are same, a Must-Link constraint is labeled and added to $Con_=$, or else a Cannot-Link constraint is labeled and added to $Con_{\neq}$. The process continues until the size of constraint set is satisfied. For a given number of constraints, the algorithm is executed for 20 times. Each uses 10-folds cross validation that the constraints are generated in 90 percentage of the dataset, clustering result is evaluated on the whole dataset. We also choose Rand Index [3] which calculates the percent of correctly assigned instances with the whole dataset to evaluate the clustering quality. Generally, the larger the Rand Index is, the better the clustering result is. The max iteration number is set to 1000 in each experiment.

4.2   Experimental Result

Four datasets are selected to compare the quality of clustering obtained from COP-KMeans with MLC-KMeans algorithm. As Figure 2 illustrated, the abscissa axis represents the number of constraints, the ordinate axis represents the Rand Index. The regulative coefficient of MLC-KMeans β is set to 2.

Table 2 compares the times of failure when COP-KMeans and new MLC-Kmeans algorithms cluster on different datasets.

4.3   Analysis of Experiment Result

From Fig 2, we can conclude that the new algorithm achieves good performance compared with COP-KMeans. The trend of RI curve is monotonously increasing for the new algorithm. The more constraints given the better the performance tends to be. For $\beta = 2$, the performance of MLC-KMeans is much better than that of COP-KMeans, especially when the number of constraints is large on the datasets. For xor dataset, the value of RI for the two algorithm is alternately larger than the other with the increasing number of constraints.

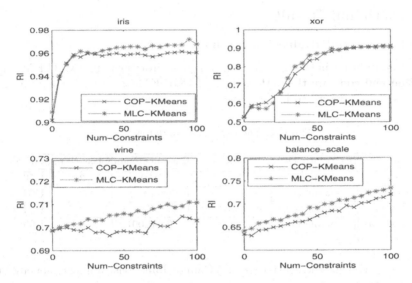

Fig. 2. Rand index analysis of clustering

Table 2. Times of Failure

Dataset	Const.Num	10	20	30	40	50	60	70	80	90	100
iris	COP	.04	.28	.93	1.40	3.02	5.52	13.4	29.8	112.0	221.2
	MLC	.0	.01	.02	.07	.09	.15	.25	.41	.59	.95
xor	COP	1.44	23.7	342.5	1093.3	1743.7	1143.5	504.3	300.4	193.7	104.3
	MLC	.14	0.90	1.29	0.72	0.35	0.12	0.08	0.02	0.02	0.01
wine	COP	.08	.41	1.02	2.65	6.41	13.58	34.15	102.1	224.7	773.8
	MLC	.0	.02	.02	.06	.21	.3	.54	.83	1.30	1.77
balance-scale	COP	.07	.62	1.99	4.88	13.6	47.2	129.1	595.6	2639.8	35782.4
	MLC	.01	.01	.02	.04	.05	.06	0.14	0.3	0.40	0.57

Table 2 shows the average number of failure for the two algorithm under certain number of constraints. Because the MLC-KMeans algorithm is also a partition-based algorithm, the less the algorithm fails, the better it gets the good clusters. So the failure times are a good measurement of algorithm's efficiency. From the tables we can see with the increasing number of constraints the failure of COP-KMeans is always hundreds of times to that of MLC-KMeans which means that if we have certain number of constraints, it can be more easily to get an clustering result that satisfies all constraints using the new algorithm. It is crucial for algorithm's practicability.

5   Conclusion

Traditional clustering analysis views the clustering as an unsupervised learning process and finds no ways to use background knowledge people have before clustering. We study the clustering problem with prior knowledge in the form of

Must-Link and Cannot-Link constraint between instances. Based upon the new concept Must-Link Set and Cannot-Link Set coined, a new semi-supervised clustering algorithm MLC-KMeans is proposed that uses Must-Link Set as assistant centroid.

The algorithm improves the COP-KMeans by transforming the original constraints to Must-Link Set and allocating it as a whole. The algorithm also makes good use of the knowledge between instances contained in the dataset. The effect of constraints is extended by using Must-Link Set as assistant centroid to lead instances assign to clusters. Experimental results confirm that the new algorithm is effective and valid in clustering data with instance-level constraints.

There still have several issues should be addressed further. For example, How to improve and optimize the algorithm so that it can more effective in clustering larger and high dimension dataset; How to use the knowledge using other semi-supervised learning methods to imporve the clustering quality.

Acknowledgments

The work is is supported by Beijing Natural Science Foundation under Grant 4072021. We also thank Qingyong Li for his insightful advice and suggestions on the work as it progressed.

References

1. Hand, D., Mannila, H., Smyth, P.: Principles of Data Mining. The MIT Press, Massachusetts (2001)
2. Tan, P.-N., Steinbach, M., Kumar, V.: Introduction to Data Mining. Addison Wesley, Reading (2005)
3. Wagstaff, K., Cardie, C., Rogers, S., Schroedl, S.: Constrained k-means clustering with background knowledge. In: Brodley, C., Danyluk, A. P. (eds.) Proc. of the 18th Int'l Conf. on Machine Learning (ICML 2001), pp. 577–584. Morgan Kaufmann Publishers, San Francisco (2001)
4. Basu, S., Banerjee, A., Mooney, R.J.: Active semi-supervision for pairwise constrained clustering. In: Proceedings of the SIAM International Conference on Data Mining, pp. 333–344 (2004)
5. Davidson, I., Ravi, S.S.: Clustering with constraints: feasibility issues and the k-Means algorithm. In: 5th SIAM Data Mining Conference, pp. 138–149 (2005)
6. Blake, C., Keogh, E., Merz, C.J.: UCI repository of machine learning databases. University of California, Irvine (1998), http://www.ics.uci.edu/~mlearn/MLRepository.html
7. Shin, K., Abraham, A.: Two phase semi-supervised clustering using background knowledge. In: Corchado, E., et al. (eds.) IDEAL 2006. LNCS, vol. 4224, pp. 707–712. Springer, Heidelberg (2006)
8. Basu, S., Banerjee, A., Mooney, R.: Semi-Supervised clustering by seeding. In: Sammut, C., Hoffmann, A. (eds.) Proc. of the 19th Int'l Conf. on Machine Learning (ICML 2002), pp. 19–26. Morgan Kaufmann Publishers, San Francisco (2002)
9. Basu, S.: Semi-supervised clustering: probabilistic models, algorithms and experiments. Ph.D. Thesis, Department of Computer Sciences, University of Texas at Austin (2005)

T-rotation: Multiple Publications of Privacy Preserving Data Sequence

Youdong Tao, Yunhai Tong, Shaohua Tan, Shiwei Tang, and Dongqing Yang

Key Laboratory of Machine Perception (Peking University), Ministry of Education,
100871 Beijing, China
{taoyd,yhtong,shtan,tsw,dqyang}@pku.edu.cn

Abstract. In privacy preserving data publishing, most current methods are limited only to the static data which are released once and fixed. However, in real dynamic environments, the current methods may become vulnerable to inference. In this paper, we propose the t-rotation method to process this continuously growing dataset in an effective manner. T-rotation mixes t continuous periods to form the dataset and then anonymizes. It avoids the inference by the temporal background knowledge and considerably improves the anonymity quality.

1 Introduction

Privacy preservation in data publishing tries to preserve the individual privacy against re-identifying by joining external dataset. Avoiding re-identifying, k-anonymity model was proposed [6,7]. That requires each tuple be indistinguishable from at least (k-1) other tuples. Other models, such as *l*-diversity[4], have been proposed. But all these models don't consider the situation of multiple publications of data sequence. They always assume that data are published once and fixed. However in real world, this condition can't be met. Many departments need to publish incremental dataset periodically.

In fact, multiple publications naturally form a time sequence of datasets. If the adversary knows the individual's QI attributes and published time, he may draw an inference and narrow down the extent of possible QI attribute values, even to discover the individual's sensitive value.

For instance, a medical management board needs to publish the patient table every month. To preserve the privacy, the table has to be anonymized for publishing. Suppose Table 1 contained the patient tuples in the first month and Table 3 contained the patient tuples in the second month. Suppose that the number of tuples in each period varies little.

The two basic ideas are independent anonymity and accumulative anonymity. Independent anonymity method is just to anonymize and publish the tuples in the current period. Each publication has to meet the k-anonymity requirement. Table 2 is the 2-anonymity table in the first period and Table 4 is the 2-anonymity table in the second period. It's a natural and naive method. But if the adversary knows someone appears in the two continuous publications, he may compare the corresponding QI groups and narrow down the extent of possible tuples, even to discover the individual's sensitive value.

C. Tang et al. (Eds.): ADMA 2008, LNAI 5139, pp. 500–507, 2008.

Table 1. The first period table

Name	Zipcode	Sex	Age	Disease
Ally	10375	F	24	Insomnia
Billy	10379	M	35	Heart
Bob	10375	M	46	Cancer
Carl	10379	M	40	HIV

Table 2. 2-anonymity of Table 1

Seq	Zipcode	Sex	Age	Disease
1-1	1037*	*	[24-35]	Insomnia
1-2	1037*	*	[24-35]	Heart
1-3	1037*	M	[40-46]	Cancer
1-4	1037*	M	[40-46]	HIV

Table 3. The second period table

Name	Zipcode	Sex	Age	Disease
Jerry	10379	M	55	Bird-flu
Frank	10375	M	42	Tracheitis
Peter	10377	M	38	Coprostasis
Tracy	10373	F	21	Gastritis

Table 4. 2-anonymity of Table 3

Seq	Zipcode	Sex	Age	Disease
2-1	1037*	*	[21-38]	Gastritis
2-2	1037*	*	[21-38]	Coprostasis
2-3	1037*	M	[42-55]	Tracheitis
2-4	1037*	M	[42-55]	Bird-flu

Table 5. 2-rotation mixed table

Name	Zipcode	Sex	Age	Disease
Bob	10375	M	46	Cancer
Frank	10375	M	42	Tracheitis
Carl	10379	M	40	HIV
Peter	10377	M	38	Coprostasis

Table 6. 2-anonymity table of Table 5

Seq	Zipcode	Sex	Age	Disease
1	10375	M	[42-46]	Cancer
2	10375	M	[42-46]	Tracheitis
3	1037*	M	[38-40]	HIV
4	1037*	M	[38-40]	Coprostasis

Accumulative anonymity method is to anonymize and publish all tuples till the current period. Each publication has to meet the k-anonymity requirement. These are two channels to inferences. If an adversary knows that someone doesn't exist in the former publication but exists in the later one, he compare two corresponding QI groups according to someone's QI attribute values in the two publications. If the tuples which exist in the later QI group but don't exist in the former are less than k, they become vulnerable to inference. The other channel is that an adversary knows that someone exists both in the former and later publications. If the tuples which exist in the corresponding QI groups of two publications are less than k, they also become vulnerable to inference.

In the analysis of two methods, we notice that temporal background knowledge helps inferences. We should eliminate this background knowledge to avoid inferences. In this paper, we propose a method, called t-rotation, to form and anonymize the multiple publications of datasets.

T-rotation means that each publication contains tuples from t continuous periods datasets and then is anonymized to meet anonymity requirement. Thus published tuples avoid being recognized by temporal background knowledge.

We have a great number of combinations to form a publication from t continuous periods, so we may choose an adapted combination to reduce information loss. For example, in Table 5, we choose Frank and Peter from the second period with the left tuples of the first period to form the table for anonymity. Compared to independent anonymity method, our method helps to improve the anonymity quality.

The remainder of the paper is organized as followings. In section 2, we review the related work. In section 3, we describe our method in detail. The algorithm is described in section 4. We present an empirical study in section 5. Then we conclude in section 6.

2   Related Work

In privacy preserving data publishing, Samarati and Sweeney proposed a principle called k-anonymity [6,7]. Beyond the k-anonymity, Machanavajjhala et al. proposed l-diversity principle [4]. That requires each quasi-identifier group should have at least l "well-represented" sensitive values. All these methods release dataset once and fixed. There are two main approaches in anonymity. One is generalization[1,3,6], and the other is lossy join[11].

Dynamic publication has attracted research recently. Wang and Fung proposed a method to process the "horizontal" increment of data set by lossy join [9]. The lossy join method is now adopted to achieve anonymity and improve the utility [11]. Pei et al. proposed a refineness method to process incremental update [5]. Refineness is to insert the new tuples into the old QI groups and then split the groups which contain too much tuples. But this method doesn't take temporal background knowledge attack into account. Xiao and Tao proposed an m-invariance model to process incremental update [12]. This model maintains the sensitive values consistence of QI groups between two publications. But it introduces the pseudo tuples to meet the sensitive values consistence. Byun et al. researched the inference channels by comparing publications and proposed secure method for incremental datasets avoiding these channels [2].

To evaluate the result of anonymity, several metrics are proposed to measure the information loss. Distortion ratio [10] evaluates the generalization height ratio between the result table and the full generalization table. The normalized certainty penalty (NCP) evaluates the extent of generalized value in a QI group [13]. That is, if a tuple $t=(x_1,\ldots,x_n)$ on QI attributes $(A_1,\ldots,A_n)$ is generalized to $([y_1, z_1],\ldots,[y_n, z_n])$, NCP value of t is $NCP_t = \sum_{i=1}^{n} w_i \cdot |z_i - y_i|/|A_i|$, w_i is the weight of attribute A_i and $|A_i|$ is the extent of values on A_i.

3   T-rotation

We consider that a table sequence, called as $T_1, T_2, \ldots, T_i, \ldots$, needs to publish periodically. Table T_i contains the tuples happened in period i. We assume that all these T_is share the same schema T and have approximate number of tuples. We consider that a publication sequence, called $P_t, P_{t+1}, \ldots, P_i, \ldots$, is the released result periodically.

We consider that a function F transforms the original dataset to the released dataset. According to the independent anonymity method, $P_i = F(T_i)$. But in t-rotation method, $P_i = F(T_i, T_{i-1}, \ldots, T_{i-t+1})$, t is a positive integer. For each table T_j, T_j contributes its $|T_j|/t$ tuples into the P_i. For table T_{i-t+1}, it only left $|T_{i-t+1}|/t$ tuples without release since other tuples have been anonymized and published in the $P_{i-t+1}, P_{i-t+2}, \ldots, P_{i-1}$. For table T_i, it has $|T_i|$ tuples without release.

We have a great number of combinations to choose adapted tuples into P_i. For each $T_j (i-t+1 \leq j \leq i)$, T_j contains $|T_j| \cdot (j-i+t)/t$ tuples without release. So there are $C_j = \dbinom{|T_j| \cdot (j-i+t)/t}{|T_j|/t}$ combinations to choose tuples from T_j into P_i. So the total number of combinations for P_i is $Q_i = \prod_{j=i-t+1}^{i} C_j$. We evaluate Q_i approximately. Since each table is acquired within the same time interval, we suppose that each of them contains the same number of tuples, here represented by m. To simplify the inference, we suppose $m = t \cdot n$. So

$$C_j = \binom{|T_j| \cdot (j-i+t)/t}{|T_j|/t} = \binom{(j-i+t)n}{n}$$

$$Q_i = \prod_{j=i-t+1}^{i} C_j = \prod_{j=i-t+1}^{i} \binom{(j-i+t)n}{n} = \binom{n}{n} \cdot \binom{2n}{n} \cdot \ldots \cdot \binom{tn}{n} = \frac{(tn)!}{(n!)^t}$$

According to the Stirling Formula, $lnN! = NlnN - N + 0.5ln(2N\pi)$, Q_i is approximately evaluated as

$$Q_i = t^m \cdot \sqrt{\frac{2m\pi}{(\frac{2m\pi}{t})^t}}$$

So we have a great number of combinations to form the release dataset. Among them, we choose an adapted combination to reduce the information loss. But it's hard to search all possible combinations to achieve the optimal result, so we present a greedy algorithm in the section 4.

T-rotation method avoids temporal background knowledge attack by the mixture of t continuous periods datasets. Each publication contains tuples from t periods and a tuple in period T_i may be anonymized in any of t publications. If an individual appears in the several continuous periods with the same sensitive value, we just remove the redundant tuples in the release dataset.

For instance, if an adversary knows an individual's QI value and his period T_i, there are t publications $P_i, P_{i+1}, \ldots, P_{i+t-1}$ that may contain the individual. Each publication has at most one QI group that contains the individual. So there are at most t QI groups that may contain the individual.

At the worst case, only one QI group in these t publications contains the individual. The possibility is at most 1/k to find the corresponding tuple according to k-anonymity. We don't take the distribution of sensitive attribute value into account here. If we consider the distribution of sensitive attribute value, we may adopt l-diversity to anonymity the publication instead of k-anonymity.

On average, a half of publications have the QI groups which may contain the individual and each QI group meets the k-anonymity. The possibility is $2/(k \cdot t)$, much less than the common k-anonymity.

T-rotation method can't process and release data at the first (t-1) periods since it needs t periods to mix up. The first publication releases at the tth period and contains $|T_j| \cdot (t-j+1)/t$ tuples of T_j, where j=1,2,...,t. The first publication contains $m \cdot \sum_{j=1}^{t}(t-j+1)/t = m \cdot (t+1)/2$ tuples. Later publication $P_i(i > t)$ contains $|T_j|/t$ tuples of T_j, as we have described before. According to that assumption, the size of later publications is m, less than the first publication.

4   Algorithm

It's hard to search all combination space and we propose a greedy algorithm for local optimization. Publication P_i comes from t continuous datasets, T_{i-t+1}, ..., T_i. For table T_{i-t+1}, it only left $|T_{i-t+1}|/t$ tuples without release. So P_i must contain these unreleased tuples. Then for table T_{i-t+2}, we choose half of the unreleased tuples. We greedily require the tuples selected should be close to prior tuples every time. Until to T_i, we finish the process and get all tuples to anonymize. Since these tuples are close to each other, anonymity result will have a narrow extent in QI attributes and improve the information quality of publication.

To measure whether the two tuples are close, we define the distance between two tuples. We only take the QI attribute into account.

First, we consider the case of numeric attributes. Let attribute A be numeric. Suppose two values a_1,a_2 on A. Let the distance of two values on A be

$$d_A = \frac{|a_1 - a_2|}{|A|}, \ where \ |A| = max_{t \in T}\{T.A\} - min_{t \in T}\{T.A\}$$

is the range of all tuples on attribute A. For example, attribute Age is numeric. a_1 is 32 and a_2 is 45. Max and min values are 90 and 17, respectively. So the distance between a_1 and a_2 is d=(45-32)/(90-17)=0.18.

Second, we consider the case of category attributes. Since generalization hierarchy exists in a category attribute, we make use of hierarchy to define the

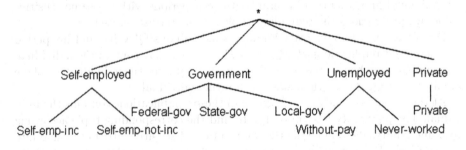

Fig. 1. The hierarchy tree of attribute Employment

distance of category attribute. Let B be a category attribute and $b_1,\ldots,b_w$ be the set of leaf nodes in hierarchy tree of attribute B. For two values on B, b_1 and b_2, let u be the node in the hierarchy tree of the attribute B such that u is an ancestor of b_1 and b_2 and u contains no descendant node that is the ancestor of b_1 and b_2. Node u is called the minimal ancestor of b_1 and b_2, and size(u) means the number of distinct leaf nodes covered by u. Define the distance of b_1 and b_2 as

$$d_B = \frac{size(ancestor(b_1, b_2)) - 1}{|B| - 1},$$

where $|B|$ is the number of distinct values on attribute B. For example, the hierarchy tree of attribute Employment is listed in the figure 1. The number of all values is 8. Distance between "Federal-gov" and "Local-gov" is 2/7 because the "Government" is their minimal ancestor and the value "government" contains 3 nodes.

For two tuples, t_1 and t_2, let tuple distance be $d = \sum_{i=1}^{n} w_i \cdot d_i$, $(w_1 + \ldots + w_n = 1)$ where n is the number of QI attributes, w_i is the weight on the ith attribute of QI and d_i is the distance on the ith attribute of QI. Clearly, when all weights are set equally, the distance is $d = \sum_{i=1}^{n} d_i/n$.

Based on tuple distance, we define the distance between a tuple t and a dataset T as the shortest distance between t and any tuple in T. That is, $d_{t,T} = \min\{d_{t,s}|s \in T\}$.

For tuple choice, we first define the tuples without release in T_{i-t+1} as fixedset since these tuples must be contained in the P_i. Then we evaluate other tuples in the $T_j(i - t + 1 < j \leq i)$ on the distance to the fixedset. We choose the tuples which correspond to the shortest $|T_j|/t$ distances. So each T_j contributes $|T_j|/t$ tuples to P_i. All these chosen tuples and fixedset form the P_i. The time complexity of tuple choice is $O(m^2)$ which is acceptable.

At last, we anonymize all tuples in P_i. Anonymity model can be k-anonymity or l-diversity, according to application requirement.

5   Experiments

In this section, we report an empirical study on the effectiveness of our proposed method on multiple publications of data sequence. We compare our method to the independent anonymity and accumulative anonymity. Experimental data come from the Adult database of UCI Machine Learning Repository[8]. The Adult database contains 45,222 tuples from US census data. We remove tuples with missing values.

We choose 7 attributes as QI, including Age, Sex, Race, Marital, Education, Country and Employment. We choose Occupation as sensitive attribute.

To examine the effectiveness on multiple publications, we partitioned all tuples into 20 disjoined parts for 20 periods. Each part contains the same number of tuples. We marked these parts with sequence number from 1 to 20. Thus we had total 20 tables for 20 periods.

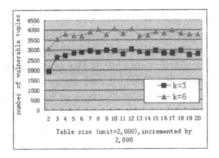

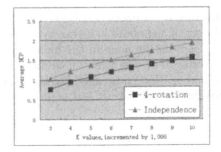

Fig. 2. Vulnerable tuples   **Fig. 3.** Anonymity quality

We first investigated the vulnerable tuples number in the accumulative method. For simplicity, we only compared two continuous publications to find the vulnerable tuples. If we found an inference channel, we counted the number of tuples which were vulnerable by it. Our rotation method are free of these inference channels.

Figure 2 shows the number of vulnerable tuples when k=3 and 6 among datasets incremented by 2,000. As expected, more tuples become vulnerable as the k parameter of anonymity get larger.

Then we adopted the NCP metric (described in Section 2) to evaluate the quality of anonymity. When the NCP value is lower, the anonymity quality is higher. We compared anonymity quality resulted by independent anonymity method and our t-rotation method.

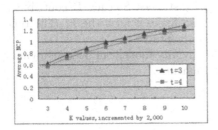

Fig. 4. Anonymity quality on t   **Fig. 5.** Anonymity quality on size

We compared the average NCP value of 20 periods incremented by 1,000 when parameter k gets different values. Figure 3 shows that result. We notices that t-rotation (t=4) method gets much lower average NCP value than the independent method. Because t-rotation method chooses close tuples together from t periods, our method achieves much higher anonymity quality. Then we compared the effect of different t values. Figure 4 shows that larger t gets lower NCP but its influence is not much. That is because larger t means more combinations for a better choice. Last we compared the effect of the incremental size. Figure 5 shows that larger increment size gets lower NCP because larger size means much more combinations for a better choice.

6   Conclusions

In this paper, we presented an approach to securely anonymize a continuous growing dataset while assuring higher anonymity quality. We propose t-rotation method to process the multiple publications of privacy preserving data sequence. T-rotation is to mix and regroup t continuous datasets periodically and then anonymizes the data. This method avoids the inferences by temporal background knowledge. Choosing an adapted combination from continuous periods also considerably improves the anonymity quality of publication.

Acknowledgements

This work was supported by the National Science Foundation of China under Grant No.60403041 and 863 Projects under No.2006AA01Z230 & 2007AA01Z191.

References

1. Aggarwal, G., Feder, T., Kenthapadi, K., Motwani, R., Panigrahy, R., Thomas, D., Zhu, A.: Anonymizing Tables. In: The 10th International Conference on Database Theory, pp. 246–258 (2005)
2. Byun, J.W., Sohn, Y., Bertino, E., Li, N.: Secure Anonymization for Incremental Datasets. In: Secure Data Management, 3rd VLDB Workshop, pp. 48–63 (2006)
3. LeFevre, K., DeWitt, D.J., Ramakrishnan, R.: Incognito: Efficient Full-domain K-anonymity. In: ACM International Conference on Management of Data, pp. 49–60 (2005)
4. Machanavajjhala, A., Gehrke, J., Kifer, D.: l-diversity: Privacy beyond K-anonymity. In: The 22nd International Conference on Data Engineering, pp. 24–35 (2006)
5. Pei, J., Xu, J., Wang, Z., Wang, W., Wang, K.: Maintaining K-anonymity against Incremental Updates. In: 19th International Conference on Scientific and Statistical Database Management, pp. 5–14 (2007)
6. Samarati, P.: Protecting Respondents' Identities in Microdata Release. IEEE Transactions on Knowledge and Data Engineering 13, 1010–1027 (2001)
7. Sweeney, L.: Achieving K-anonymity Privacy Protection Using Generalization and Suppression. International Journal on Uncertainty, Fuzziness and Knowledge Based Systems 10, 571–588 (2002)
8. UCI Machine Learning Repository,
   http://www.ics.uci.edu/~mlearn/MLRepository.html
9. Wang, K., Fung, B.C.M.: Anonymizing Sequential Releases. In: 12th ACM SIGKDD, pp. 414–423 (2006)
10. Wong, R.C., Li, J., Fu, A.W., Wang, K. (α, k)-anonymity: an Enhanced K-anonymity Model for Privacy-preserving Data Publishing. In: 12th ACM SIGKDD, pp. 754–759 (2006)
11. Xiao, X., Tao, Y.: Anatomy: Simple and Effective Privacy Preservation. In: The 32nd international conference on Very large data bases, pp. 139–150 (2006)
12. Xiao, X., Tao, Y.: M-Invariance: Towards Privacy Preserving Re-publication of Dynamic Datasets. In: ACM International Conference on Management of Data, pp. 689–700 (2007)
13. Xu, J., Wang, W., Pei, J., Wang, X., Shi, B., Fu, A.W.: Utility-based Anonymization Using Local Recoding. In: 12th ACM SIGKDD, pp. 785–790 (2006)

The Integrated Methodology of KPCA and Wavelet Support Vector Machine for Predicting Financial Distress

Jian-guo Zhou, Tao Bai, and Ji-ming Tian

School of Business Administration, North China Electric Power University,
Baoding, 071003, China
dldxzjg@126.com, ncepubaitao@126.com

Abstract. In this paper, a hybrid intelligent system, combining kernel principal component analysis (KPCA) and wavelet support vector machine (WSVM), is applied to the study of predicting financial distress. KPCA method is used as a preprocessor of classifier to extract the nonlinear features of input variables. Then a method that generates wavelet kernel function of the SVM is proposed based on the theory of wavelet frame and the condition of the SVM kernel function. The Mexican Hat wavelet is selected to construct the SVM kernel function and form the wavelet support vector machine (WSVM). The effectiveness of the proposed model is verified by experiments through the contrast of the results of SVMs with different kernel functions and other models.

Keywords: Financial Distress; Kernel Principal Component Analysis; Wavelet Support Vector Machine.

1 Introduction

In recent three decades, predicting financial distress has been an important topic in accounting and finance [1]. Creditors, stockholders and senior management are all interested in predicting financial distress because it affects all of them alike. As a forecasting tool, an accurate financial distress prediction model can provide them with timely warnings. From a managerial perspective, financial distress forecasting tools allow to take timely strategic actions so that financial distress can be avoided. For stakeholders, efficient and automated credit rating tools allow to detect client that are to default their obligations at an early stage.

Originally, Statistical methods had been used to developing more accurate financial distress prediction models. In order to develop a more accurate and general applicable prediction approach, data mining and machine learning techniques are employed [2]. Recently, new algorithms in machine learning, support vector machines (SVMs) [3], developed by Boster, Guyon, and Vapnik (1992) provide better solutions to design boundary than that of neural network. Since the new model was proposed, SVM has been successfully applied to numerous fields, including digital image identification, time series forecasting and bankruptcy prediction.

But there exists a problem in the practical application of SVM. In the real financial prediction, there are usually many irrelevant variables in the sample data spoiling the

C. Tang et al. (Eds.): ADMA 2008, LNAI 5139, pp. 508–515, 2008.

classification of the SVM classifier, increasing many unwanted calculations and decreasing the real-time capacity of the financial prediction. A feasible option to solve this problem is to use some dimensionality-reducing methods such as the kernel principle component analysis (KPCA) [4] to extract the nonlinear features of the sample data. Consequently, the efficiency of the financial distress prediction model can be improved further.

On the other hand, kernel function selection is another problem to form an efficient SVM classifier. If the kernel function is not selected correctly, the performance of the classifier will be influenced. In this paper, a method that generates wavelet kernel function [5] with the SVM is propose, based on the theory of wavelet frame and the SVM kernel function. Then, the Mexican Hat wavelet is selected to construct the SVM kernel function and form the wavelet support vector machine (WSVM).

2 Basic Concept of Models

2.1 Kernel Principal Component Analysis

The basic ideal of KPCA is using $x_t \to \varnothing(x_t)$ to map the original input data $X \in R^{m \times l}\ (m < l)$ into a n-dimensional feature space $H(n \gg l > m)$, and $\varnothing(x_t)$ has been standardized by column in H, and so the Covariance matrix of $\varnothing(x_t)$ is:

$$\tilde{C} = \frac{1}{l}\sum\nolimits_{t=1}^{l}\varnothing(x_t)\varnothing(x_t)^{T} \tag{1}$$

Decomposing the $\tilde{C}$ eigenvalue, (1) can be transformed to the eigenvalue problem (2):

$$\lambda_i u_i = \tilde{C}u_i, i = 1,\dots,l, \tag{2}$$

λ_i denotes one of the non-zero eigenvalue of $\tilde{C}$, u_i denotes the corresponding eigenvector of λ_i, equation (2) can be transformed to the eigenvalue problem (3):

$$\tilde{\lambda}_i \alpha_i = K\alpha_i, i = 1,\dots,l, \tag{3}$$

K denotes the $l \times l$ kernel matrix. $\tilde{\lambda}_i$ denotes the eigenvalue of K, satisfying $\tilde{\lambda}_i = l\lambda_i$, α_i denotes the corresponding eigenvector of K, satisfying:

$$u_i = \sum_{j=1}^{l}\alpha_i(j)\varnothing(x_j)\quad \alpha_i(j), j = 1,\dots,l \tag{4}$$

$\alpha_i(j), j$ are the components of α_i. The value of each element of K is equal to the inner product of two high dimensional feature vectors $\varnothing(x_i)$ and $\varnothing(x_j)$. That is:

$$K(x_i, x_j) = \varnothing(x_i)\cdot\varnothing(x_j) \tag{5}$$

For assuring the previous hypothesis $\varnothing(x_t)$ is of unit length, namely $u_i \cdot u_j = 1$, α_i must be normalized using the corresponding eigenvalue by:

$$\tilde{\alpha}_i = \frac{\alpha_i}{\sqrt{\tilde{\lambda}_i}}, i = 1, \ldots, l \tag{6}$$

At last, based on the estimated $\tilde{\alpha}_i$, the principal component for x_t is calculated by:

$$s_t(i) = u_i^T \varnothing(x_t) = \sum_{j=1}^{l} \tilde{\alpha}_i(j) K(x_j, x_t), i = 1, \ldots, l \tag{7}$$

In addition, for making the input samples $\sum_{t=1}^{l} \varnothing(x_t) = 0$, centralizing, in (4), the kernel matrix on the training set K and on the testing set K_t are respectively modified by:

$$\tilde{K} = \left(I - \frac{1}{l} 1_l 1_l^T\right) K \left(I - \frac{1}{l} 1_l 1_l^T\right) \tag{8}$$

$$\tilde{K}_t = \left(K_t - \frac{1}{l} 1_{l_t} 1_l^T K\right)\left(I - \frac{1}{l} 1_l 1_l^T\right) \tag{9}$$

where I denotes l-dimensional matrix, l_t denotes the number of testing data points, 1_l and 1_{l_t} represent the vectors whose elements are all ones, with length l and l_t respectively, K_t represents the $l_t \times l$ kernel matrix for the testing data points.

It has been found that, inputting data set to $X \in R^{m \times l}$, the maximal number of principal components is extracted better by KPCA. If several eigenvectors be used to determine the eigenvalues, KPCA can decrease the dimensions.

2.2 Non-linear Support Vector Machine

The basic idea of designing a non-linear SVM model is to map the input vector $X \in R^n$ into vectors z of a higher-dimensional feature space F ($Z = \varphi(X)$, where φ denotes the mapping $R^n \rightarrow R^f$), and to solve a nonlinear classification problem in this feature space:

$$X \in Rn \rightarrow Z(X) = [a_1 \varphi_1(X), a_2 \varphi_2(X), \ldots, a_n \varphi_n(X)]^T \in R^f \tag{10}$$

The mapping function $\varphi(X)$ (also called kernel function) selected by the user in advance. By replacing the inner product for non-linear pattern problem, the kernel function can perform a non-linear mapping to a high-dimensional feature space.

The learning algorithm for a non-linear classifier SVM follows the design of an optimal separating hyper plane in a feature space. Accordingly, the dual Lagrangian in z-space is:

$$L_d(\alpha) = \sum_{i=1}^{l} \alpha_i - \frac{1}{2} \sum_{i,j=1}^{l} y_i y_j \alpha_i \alpha_j z_i z_j \tag{11}$$

And using the chosen kernel, the Lagrangian is maximized as follows:

Maximize: $L_d(\alpha) = \sum_{i=1}^{l} \alpha_i - \frac{1}{2} \sum_{i,j=1}^{l} y_i y_j \alpha_i \alpha_j K(x_i, x_j)$

Subject to: $C \geq \alpha_i \geq 0, i = 1, \cdots, l$

$$\sum_{i=1}^{l} \alpha_i y_i = 0 \tag{12}$$

In this way, the influence of the training data point will be limited and remained on the wrong side of a separating non-linear hyper plane. The decision hyper plane $d(x)$ and the indicator are as follows:

$$d(x) = \sum_{i=1}^{l} y_i \alpha_i K(x_i, x) i_F = sign(d(x)) = sign(\sum_{i=1}^{l} y_i \alpha_i K(x_i, x) + b) \tag{13}$$

Depending upon the chosen kernel, the bias term b may implicitly be a part of the kernel function. For example, the bias term b is not required when Gaussian RBFs are used as kernels.

2.3 Wavelet Kernel Function

In Hilbert space H, there is a function family $\{\psi_k\}_{k \in K}$. If there exists $0 < A < B < \infty$ for all $f \in H$, then

$$A\|f\|^2 \leq \sum_k |< f, \psi_k >|^2 \leq B\|f\|^2 \tag{14}$$

$\{\psi_k\}_{k \in K}$ is named as a frame in H. While A and B are called the lower and the upper boundary of the frame, respectively. Especially, it is called tight frame if $A = B$, and orthogonal frame if $A = B = 1$. When $\|\psi_k\| = 1$, $\{\psi_k\}_{k \in K}$ is the standard orthogonal basis. For each f, which belongs to H, can be decomposed to the following form:

$$f = \sum_k < f, \overline{\psi}_k > \psi_k = \sum_k < f, \psi_k > \overline{\psi}_k \tag{15}$$

Wherein, $\overline{\psi}_k$ is dual frame of ψ_k.

In square integrable space $L^2(\Omega)$, $F = \{\psi_i\}$ is a frame, which has a increasing positive sequence $\{\lambda_i\}$. And the function of $K(x, y)$ can be expressed in the following form:

$$K(x, y) = \sum_i \lambda_i \psi_i(x) \psi_i(y) \tag{16}$$

In the above formula, definite function is semi-positive.

Mercer Theorem: The necessary and sufficient condition that symmetric function $K(x, x')$ under L_2 being inner producer of the characteristic space is:

To all $g \neq 0$ and $\int_{R^d} g^2(\xi) d\xi < \infty$, condition $\iint_{R^d \oplus R^d} K(x, x') f(x) f(x') dx dx' \geq 0$ is holding.

This theorem provided the straightforward procedure to judge and construct the kernel function. The formula (16) is to be allowed to be used as kernel function in SVM so long as it satisfies the Mercer condition.

3   The KPCA-WSVM Model

Prior knowledge is not necessary when applying kernel principal component analysis approach. It can deal with imperfect information only based on the information of the data itself. Through mapping the original data into higher-dimensional features space, the nonlinear features of input variables could be attained, then the noisy data can be removed and the performance of classifier be optimized. In this paper, kernel principal component analysis approach is used as a preprocessor to attain principal components of input variables.

Previously, we have already made out the general kernel function of SVM based on the wavelet. After determining wavelet kernel function, the model can be determined. In this paper, we choose the commonly Mexican Hat wavelet function $\psi(x) = (1 - x^2)\exp(-\frac{x^2}{2})$ to construct the translation Invariant wavelet kernel function.

As mentioned above, the translation Invariant kernel function produced by the Mexican Hat wavelet is:

$$K(x, x') = K(x - x') = \prod_{i=1}^{d} \psi\left[\frac{x_i - x_i'}{a_i}\right] = \prod_{i=1}^{d}\left[1 - \frac{\|x_i - x_i'\|^2}{a_i^2}\right]\exp\left[-\frac{\|x_i - x_i'\|^2}{2a_i^2}\right] \quad (17)$$

$$x_i, x_i', a_i \in R; a_i \neq 0; x, x' \in R^d$$

It is one kind of permission SVM kernel function.

This structure between WSVM and standard SVM are consistent, but the nonlinear mapping and the kernel function are different. Suppose that training sample is $G = \{(x_i, y_i)\}_{i=1}^{n}$, $x_i \in R^d$ is input vectors, $y_i \in R$ is the expected value, n is the number of points. And the number of suppose vectors is N, they are $SV_1, SV_2, \ldots, SV_n$. Then the corresponding wavelet frame that satisfies the Mercer condition is attained by wavelet transformation. And the kernel function is attained by formula (16). The non-linear SVM classifier is as follows:

$$i_F = sign(d(x)) = sign\left(\sum_{i=1}^{l} y_k \alpha_k \prod_{i=1}^{d}\left[1 - \frac{\|x_k^i - x^i\|^2}{(a_k^i)^2}\right]\exp\left[-\frac{\|x_k^i - x^i\|^2}{2(a_k^i)^2}\right]\right) \quad (18)$$

In this formula, x_k^i denotes the *ith* component in the *kth* training data. Thus, based on the wavelet kernel function and SVM we form a new classifier. But SVM cannot optimize the kernel function parameter. In this paper, a_k^i is fixed as a, therefore, the number of kernel function parameter turns to be 1. The wavelet kernel ultra-parameter a can be selected by using the Cross-Validation method.

4   Experiment and Analysis

Experiments were performed to examine three kinds of validation: (1) interval validation (matched samples), (2) external validation (holdout sample prediction) and (3) external validation (simulated sample prediction). The experiments were made using different model: Fisher, Probit, BPN, SVM with RBF kernel function (RBF-SVM), SVM with Polynomial kernel function (PSVM), SVM with Sigmoid kernel function (SVM) and Wavelet SVM (WSVM). Besides the accuracy of the prediction of financial distress, Type I and Type II error were analyzed among these experiments.

4.1 Research Data

In this study, 50 financial ratios and 460 listed companies are selected to be our analysis samples. These companies are divided into distressed and non-distressed sets. In this paper, the distressed companies are defined as ST companies. In order to increase the rationality, we selected the ST and non-distress companies in pairs.

In cases of SVM, Fisher and Probit, each data set is split into two subsets: a training set of 80% (368) and a holdout set of 20% (92) of the total data (460), respectively. The holdout data is used to test the results.

In case of BPN, each data set is split into three subsets: a training set of 60% (276), a validation set of 20% (92), and a holdout set of 20% (92) of the total data (460) respectively, where the validation data is used to check the results.

4.2 Application of Kernel Principal Component Analysis

There are many redundant information and noises in the data for the firms' difference in trade or asset scale. In order to intensify the anti-interference ability of classifier, in this paper, we selected KPCA strategy to attain the principal components of original 9 financial ratios. It projects the data to a higher-dimensional feature space, and then removes the noisy data. At last, we get 7 principle components in which 94.18% information is included. The principal components are shown in Table 1.

Table 1. List of tested principal components

Principal component	Elucidative financial ratio	Contribution rate
Z_1	Cash ratio	0.711
	Return rate on main business	0.817
	Earnings Before Interest	0.767
Z_2	assets and liabilities ratio	0.644
Z_3	inventory turnover ratio	0.596
Z_4	inventory turnover ratio	0.443
	account receivable velocity	0.422
	Growth rate of net cash flow on business	0.410
	Cash rate on main business	0.516
Z_5	account receivable velocity	0.724
Z_6	Growth rate on main business	0.706
Z_7	Growth rate of net cash flow on business	0.489

4.3 Prediction Accuracies of Matched Samples

The average   prediction   accuracy of the failing company model is 97.17% in the first year before failure, 96.31% in the second year, and 94.14% in the third year as presented in Table 2. Artificial intelligence models (BPN, RBF-SVM, PSVM, SSVM and WSVM) are able to perfectly predict financial failure (100% accuracy), in the

Table 2. Prediction accuracies of models in matched sample

Models	Year-1			Year-2			Year-3		
	Accuracy	Type I error	Type II error	Accuracy	Type I error	Type II error	Accuracy	Type I error	Type II error
Fisher	0.8696	0.1087	0.1522	0.8397	0.1304	0.1902	0.7907	0.2609	0.1576
Probit	0.9321	0.125	0.0109	0.9022	0.1522	0.0435	0.7989	0.2391	0.1631
BPN	1.0000	0.0000	0.0000	1.0000	0.0000	0.0000	1.0000	0.0000	0.0000
RBF-SVM	1.0000	0.0000	0.0000	1.0000	0.0000	0.0000	1.0000	0.0000	0.0000
PSVM	1.0000	0.0000	0.0000	1.0000	0.0000	0.0000	1.0000	0.0000	0.0000
SSVM	1.0000	0.0000	0.0000	1.0000	0.0000	0.0000	1.0000	0.0000	0.0000
WSVM	1.0000	0.0000	0.0000	1.0000	0.0000	0.0000	1.0000	0.0000	0.0000
Average	0.9717	0.0334	0.0233	0.9631	0.0404	0.0334	0.9414	0.0714	0.0458

first year, second and third years before failure. Fisher exhibited the lowest predictive accuracies of all the models. Fisher and Probit models yielded the highest Type I and Type II errors, respectively, in all years before failure.

4.4 Prediction Accuracies of Holdout Samples

The holdout method, sometimes called test sample estimation. In this paper, two thirds of the data are commonly used as the training set and the remaining one third are then used as the test set. The models used to predict financial distress were trained using the preceding years' data. As it is shown in Table 3, the average predictive accuracy was 87.53% in the first year before financial distress, and 83.54%, 80.28% in the second and third year. The proposed model, WSVM, outperformed other models in the three situations. The WSVM had the highest predictive accuracy, the lowest Type I error and Type II error.

Table 3. Prediction accuracies of models in holdout sample

Models	Year-1			Year-2			Year-3		
	Accuracy	Type I error	Type II error	Accuracy	Type I error	Type II error	Accuracy	Type I error	Type II error
Fisher	0.7826	0.174	0.2609	0.7609	0.1739	0.2609	0.7283	0.2391	0.3043
Probit	0.8152	0.1522	0.2174	0.7717	0.1522	0.3043	0.7500	0.1739	0.3261
BPN	0.8261	0.1087	0.2391	0.8043	0.1087	0.2826	0.7717	0.1522	0.3043
RBF-SVM	0.9239	0.0652	0.0870	0.8696	0.1087	0.1522	0.8261	0.0652	0.2826
PSVM	0.9022	0.0870	0.1087	0.8587	0.1522	0.1304	0.8043	0.1739	0.2174
SSVM	0.9130	0.6522	0.1087	0.8587	0.1739	0.1087	0.8369	0.1304	0.4957
WSVM	0.9639	0.0217	0.0435	0.9239	0.0652	0.0869	0.9021	0.0435	0.1522
Average	0.8753	0.1801	0.1522	0.8354	0.1335	0.1894	0.8028	0.1397	0.2975

4.5 Prediction Accuracies of Stimulated Samples

In this section, the simulated samples are constructed by bootstrap technique elucidated by Efron (1993). The original sample of 84 enterprises is divided into a training sample 56 enterprises and a validation sample 28 enterprises. The financial distress

Table 4. Prediction accuracies of models in stimulated sample

Bootstrap times	Prediction accuracies of financial models						
	Fisher	Probit	BPN	RBF-SVM	PSVM	SSVM	WSVM
100	0.68	0.68	0.71	0.72	0.75	0.79	0.8
200	0.72	0.68	0.71	0.73	0.76	0.77	0.75
300	0.71	0.71	0.7	0.73	0.77	0.76	0.81
400	0.7	0.72	0.72	0.75	0.76	0.79	0.78
500	0.73	0.71	0.74	0.74	0.77	0.78	0.82

models are predicting for varying samples, by bootstrapping from 100 to 500 times, to evaluate the reliability of validation. As the Table 4 shows, WSVM performed well when applied to the simulated sample when bootstrapping was performed various numbers of times. The result implied that the predictive accuracy of the SVM was dramatically increased by using the wavelets kernel function.

5   Conclusion and Future Work

This study pioneered on applying kernel principal component analysis to attain financial features and wavelets frame as kernel function of support vector machine for financial distress prediction. Therefore, the primary target of this study is to apply this new model to increase the predictive accuracy of financial failure. Experiment results reveal that the proposed WSVM model is a very promising hybrid SVM model for predicting financial distress in terms of both predictive accuracy and generalization ability. The contribution of this study demonstrate that the proposed model performed well when applied in the holdout sample, revealing the generalization of this model to forecast financial distress firms in various industries.

References

1. Tay, F.E.H., Shen, L.: Economic and financial prediction using rough set model. European Journal of Operational Research 141, 641–659 (2002)
2. Wilson, R.L., Sharda, R.: Bankruptcy prediction using neural networks. Decision Support Systems 11, 545–557 (1994)
3. Cristiamini, N., Shawe-Taylor, J.: An Introduction to Support Vector Machines. Cambridge university press, Cambridge (2000)
4. Scholkopf, B., Smola, A., Muller, K.R.: Nonlinear Component Analysis as a Kemel Eigenvalue Problem. Neural Computation 10, 1299–1319 (1998)
5. Strauss, D.J., Steidl, G.: Wavelet-support vector classification of waveforms. Journal of Computational and Applied Mathematics 56(12), 375–400 (2002)

Outlier Detection Based on Voronoi Diagram[*]

Jilin Qu

School of Computer and Information Engineering
Shandong University of Finance, Jinan, China
qujilin@126.com

Abstract. Outlier mining is an important branch of data mining and has attracted much attention recently. The density-based method LOF is widely used in application. However, selecting *MinPts* is non-trivial, and LOF is very sensitive to its parameters *MinPts*. In this paper, we propose a new outlier detection method based on Voronoi diagram, which we called Voronoi based Outlier Detection (VOD). The proposed method measures the outlier factor automatically by Voronoi neighborhoods without parameter, which provides highly-accurate outlier detection and reduces the time complexity from $O(n^2)$ to $O(n\log n)$.

1 Introduction

Outlier detection has many important applications in financial surveillance, marketing, fraud detection and intrusion discovery. Mining outliers in database is to find exceptional objects that deviate from the rest of the data set [1].

Methods for outlier detection in large data sets are drawing increasing attention. Various data mining algorithms for outlier detection have been proposed. The approaches can be classified into distribution-based[2], depth-based[3], clustering[4], distance-based[5], and density-based[6].

The density-based outlier mining algorithm was proposed by Breunig et al [6]. It relies on the Local Outlier Factor (LOF) to measure the degree of outlying for an object with respect to its surrounding neighbors. The LOF value depends on how the data points are closely packed in its local reachable neighborhood. The neighborhood is defined by the distance to the *MinPts-th* nearest neighbor, where *MinPts* is the minimum number of points of the nearest neighbors. The LOF algorithm is able to detect all forms of outliers including those that could not be detected by the distance-based algorithms.

The density-based methods are the current state of the art in outlier detection and widely used in many domains. But they have some common problems.

(1) The biggest hurdle of effectively applying the density-based outlier mining algorithms is the determination of their input parameter *MinPts*. The parameter should be either known a priori or estimated and optimized by trial-and-error with the help of expert opinions.

---

[*] Supported by the Science and Technology Key Projects of Shandong Province under Grant No.2007GG3WZ10010; Doctoral Scientific Research Foundation of Shandong University of Finance under Grant No.06BSJJ09.

C. Tang et al. (Eds.): ADMA 2008, LNAI 5139, pp. 516–523, 2008.

(2) LOF is very sensitive to its parameter *MinPts*. Because LOF ranks points only considering the neighborhood density of the points, thus it may miss the potential outliers whose densities are close to those of their neighbors [7, 10].

(3) LOF must calculate *k*-distance neighborhoods of all objects. Computing *k*-distance of *p* involves computing distances of all objects within *p*'s neighborhood, which is very expensive when *MinPts* is large. The time complexity of LOF is $O(n^2)$ for all the *n* objects in the database.

In this paper, we propose a new VOD method to overcome the problems of density-based outlier detection method. The main contributions of this paper are as follows:

- We introduce the Voronoi neighbor outlier factor (VNOF), and use the Voronoi nearest neighbor instead of a fixed number nearest neighbor to calculate the outlier factor of a data point. With respect to the existing density-based outlier detection method, the VNOF performs better in identifying local outliers that deviate from the main patterns.
- We propose a nonparametric outlier detection method. The candidate outliers are ranked based on the outlier score assigned to each data point.
- We propose a new outlier detection algorithm base on Voronoi diagram, which is more efficient and effective than density-based method. The running time of our algorithm is $O(n\log n)$, where *n* is the size of dataset.

The rest of this paper is organized as follows. In section 2, we discuss related work on outlier detection and their drawbacks. Section 3 introduces the basic properties of Voronoi diagram and describes our VOD method. Section 4 presents an experimental evaluation, and we conclude in Section 5.

2 Related Work

Researchers have developed various algorithms to improve the density-based method.

Papadimitirou et al. proposed a LOCI outlier detection method [7]. This method selects a point as an outlier if its multi-granularity deviation factor (MDEF) deviates three times from the standard deviation of MDEF in a neighborhood. However, the cost of computing the standard deviation is high.

LSC-Mine proposed in [8] improves upon the response time of LOF by avoiding the computation of reachability distances and local reachability densities. In addition, data objects that are not likely outlier candidates are pruned as soon as they are identified. But it is need to determine the parameter *k*.

A connectivity-based outlier factor (COF) scheme was introduced in [9], which improves the effectiveness of an existing local outlier factor (LOF) scheme when a pattern itself has similar neighborhood density as an outlier. However, it is also need to determine the prior parameter *k*.

A spatial local outlier measure (SLOM) was proposed to discern local spatial outliers that are usually missed by global techniques [11]. The final cost of the SLOM is $O(nk \log n + kdn)$, where *k* is a prior parameter.

In [12], a reference based outlier detection method was proposed, which uses the relative degree of density with respect to a fixed set of reference points to calculate the neighborhood density of a data point. The running time of the algorithm based on this approximation is $O(Rn\log n)$ where *n* is the size of dataset, and *R* is the number of reference points to be determined prior.

A histogram method was proposed in [13] to efficiently approximate densities rather than explicit computation using nearest neighbors. By discarding points within these regions from consideration, the histograms method significantly reduce the number of nearest neighbor calculations for local outliers. But it also need a prior parameter k.

The above algorithms reduce the computation of LOF to some extent. However, they need the determination of the prior parameters.

Some nonparametric outlier mining algorithm was proposed recently. Fan et al proposed a nonparametric outlier mining algorithm which can efficiently identify top listed outliers from a wide variety of datasets [14], and generates reasonable outlier results by taking both local and global features of a dataset into consideration. A mutual-reinforcement-based local outlier detection approach was proposed in [15], which attempts to find local outliers in the center rather than around the boarder. For categorical/ordinal data, it does not need to use a *MinPts* parameter. Another nonparametric outlier detection approach was proposed, which based on a local density estimation using kernel functions [16].

These nonparametric outlier mining methods have overcome the prior parameters problem, but the running time of the algorithms has not been improved.

3   Proposed Method

In this section we first introduce the basic properties of Voronoi diagram, and then describe our VOD method.

3.1 Preliminaries

Definition 1 (Voronoi diagram). *Given a set S of n points p_1, p_2. . . p_n in the plane, the Voronoi diagram, denoted as Vor(S), is a subdivision of the plane into Voronoi cells. The Voronoi cell, denoted as $V(p_i)$ for p_i, to be the set of points q that are closer or as close to p_i than to any other point in S . That is*

$$V(p_i)=\{ \; q\mid dist(\; p_i, \; q \;) \le dist(\; p_j, \; q \;) , \; \forall \; j{\neq}i \; \}$$

where dist is the Euclidian distance function.

See Figure 1 for an example.

The Voronoi diagram decomposes the plane into n convex polygonal regions, one for each p_i. The vertices of the diagram are the *Voronoi vertices*, and the boundaries between two Voronoi cells are referred to as the *Voronoi edges*. The boundaries of a Voronoi cell $V(p_i)$ is a Voronoi polygon having no more than n-1 edges.

Voronoi diagram contains all of the proximity information defined by the given set [17]. It is one of the most important structures in computational geometry, and has been widely used in clustering, learning, graphics, and other applications. We focus on the properties of the Voronoi diagram related to the nearest neighbor problem in outlier detection.

Theorem 1. *Every nearest neighbor of p_i defines an edge of the Voronoi polygon $V(p_i)$[17].*

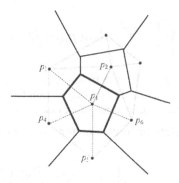

Fig. 1. Voronoi diagram

Theorem 2. *Every edge of the Voronoi polygon $V(p_i)$ defines a nearest neighbor of p_i* [17].

Theorem 3. *For $n \geq 3$, A Voronoi diagram on n points has at most 2n-5 vertices and 3n-6 edges* [17].

Theorem 4. *The Voronoi diagram of a set of n points can be constructed in O(nlogn) time and this is optimal* [17].

There are four fairly well-known algorithms for constructing Voronoi diagrams, including divide-and-conquer, randomized incremental, plane sweep, and reduction to convex hulls.

Theorem 5. *With the Voronoi diagram, nearest neighbor search can be performed in O(logn) time, which is optimal* [17].

3.2 The VOD Method

The Voronoi diagram captures the proximity uniquely. We address the outlier detection by refining the concept of a neighborhood with the Voronoi diagram.

Given a data set S, the neighborhood relationship is the inherent properties of the data set. For a point $p_i \in S$, each edge of the Voronoi polygon $V(p_i)$ defines a nearest neighbor of p_i. The numbers of nearest neighbor vary for different points; it can't be of a fixed number k. Once the polygons are formed, it creates a periphery of the immediate neighborhood in the form of neighborhood. Therefore, the k nearest neighbor definition in the existing density-based method is not reasonable, and results in a quadratic number of pair wise distance evaluations.

To solve the problems, we propose a Voronoi based Outlier Detection (VOD) method based on the Voronoi diagrams to define the neighborhood relationship.

Definition 2 (Voronoi nearest neighbor). *For a point p_i of set S, the nearest neighbors of p_i defined by the Voronoi polygon $V(p_i)$ are the Voronoi nearest neighbor of p_i, denoted as $V_{NN}(p_i)$.*

In Figure 1, the Voronoi nearest neighbors of point p_1 are p_2, p_3, p_4, p_5 and p_6.

Definition 3 (Voronoi reachability density). *The Voronoi reachability density of point p_i defined as*

$$V_{RD}(p_i) = 1 \Bigg/ \left(\sum_{o \in V_{NN}(p_i)} dist(p_i, o) \Big/ \left|V_{NN}(p_i)\right| \right) \tag{1}$$

where $| V_{NN}(p_i)|$ *is the number of points in* $V_{NN}(p_i)$.

Intuitively, the Voronoi reachability density of point p_i is the inverse of the average distance based on the Voronoi nearest neighbors of p_i.

Definition 4 (Voronoi neighbor outlier factor). *The Voronoi neighbor outlier factor of* p_i *is defined as*

$$V_{NOF}(p_i) = \frac{1}{\left|V_{NN}(p_i)\right|} \sum_{o \in V_{NN}(p_i)} \frac{V_{RD}(o)}{V_{RD}(p_i)} \tag{2}$$

The Voronoi neighbor outlier factor of p_i is the average of the ratio of the local Voronoi density of p_i and those of p_i's Voronoi nearest neighbors.

The VOD outlier detection algorithm based on the discussion is illustrated below.

Algorithm1. VOD outlier detection
Input. Data set S
Output. Outlier factor of the points in S, in descending order
1. Constructing Voronoi diagrams Vor(S) of data set S.
2. For each $p_i \in S$, compute Voronoi reachability density $V_{RD}(p_i)$ by Eq. (1)
3. For each $p_i \in S$, compute Voronoi neighbor outlier factor $V_{NOF}(p_i)$ by Eq. (2)
4. Sort the data by $V_{NOF}(p_i)$ in descending order

3.3 Complexity Analysis

Given a data set of S points $p_1, p_2 \ldots p_n$, computing the outlier factor of the data set in descending order involves the following steps:

The first step is to construct the Voronoi diagrams Vor(S) of data set S. By theorem 4, the computational cost is $O(n\log n)$.

The second step is to compute the Voronoi reachability density $V_{RD}(p_i)$ for p_i, we need to find the Voronoi nearest neighbors of p_i and calculate the distance between them. By theorem 5, with the Voronoi diagram, a single nearest neighbor query can be performed in $O(\log n)$, the cost of all nearest neighbor query is $O(n\log n)$. By theorem 2, each edge of the Voronoi polygon $V(p_i)$ defines a nearest neighbor of p_i. Each edge shared between two polygons is an explicit representation of a neighborhood relation between two points. By theorem 3, a Voronoi diagram on n points has at most $3n$-6 edges. The times to calculate the distance between the points is at most $2(3n$-6); the cost of computing the distance is $O(n)$. Thus, the cost of the second step is $O(n\log n)$, so is the third step.

Finally, we sort the data by $V_{NOF}(p_i)$ in descending order, for which the cost is $O(n\log n)$.

Thus, the final cost of the algorithm is $O(n\log n)$. Compared with the LOF method, the time complexity is reduced from $O(n^2)$ to $O(n\log n)$.

4   Experimental Evaluation

In this section, we will perform an experimental evaluation to show that the proposed VOD outlier detection method can efficiently identify local outliers, and compare the performance of the proposed method with the existing density-based methods.

The experiments are executed on P4 2.0GHz CPU with 768Mb RAM running WIN XP. The algorithm is implemented by MATLAB 7.1. Our experiment considered the outlier detection in IBM stock daily closing prices time series, which can downloaded from http://www-personal.buseco.monash.edu.au/~hyndman/TSDL/ korsan/dailyibm. dat. The time series contains 3333 data points from 1/1/1980 to 10/8/1992. By piece-wise-linear representation [18], the time series is transformed into 826 linear segments, which represented by points (length, slope), where slope is the volatility of the closing prices.

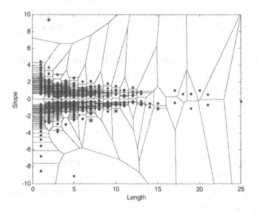

Fig. 2. Outlier detection result from LOF, $k=3$ and *MinPts* = 3. There are 7 outliers in the high density region, which is obviously wrong.

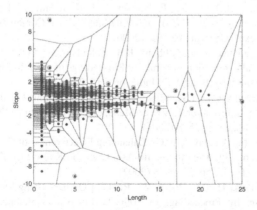

Fig. 3. Outlier detection result from VOD. All the 10 outliers are detected correctly by VOD.

Figure 2 shows the outlier detection result from LOF, where we set $k=3$ and *MinPts* = 3. The 10 outliers are denoted by red small circle. There are 7 outliers in the high density region, which is obviously wrong. When we set k and *MinPts* varying from 4 to 10, the outlier detection results from LOF are not improved obviously. The result of VOD method showed in figure 3 captures all the 10 outliers correctly.

With the 826 data points, the running time of VOD is 2.6 seconds while that of LOF is 416.8 seconds, which shows VOD is more efficient than LOF.

5 Conclusions

In this paper, we have proposed an efficient VOD outlier detection method that uses the Voronoi nearest neighbor instead of a k nearest neighbor to calculate the outlier factor of a data point. With respect to the popular LOF outlier detection, the proposed method performs better in identifying local outliers that deviate from the main patterns in a given dataset, and need no parameter. The running time of our algorithm is $O(n\log n)$ where n is the size of dataset, which shows VOD method is more efficient than LOF.

In performing the VOD algorithms for high-dimensional dada set, we can construct an approximate Voronoi diagram of near linear size [19], which ensures the VOD method perfectly in the same way.

References

1. Hawkins, D.: Identification of Outliers. Chapman and Hall, London (1980)
2. Barnett, V., Lewis, T.: Outliers in Statistical Data. John Wiley, England (1994)
3. Johnson, T., Kwok, I., Ng, R.: Fast Computation of 2-Dimensional Depth Contours. In: Proceedings of the KDD, pp. 224–228 (1998)
4. Jain, A.K., Murty, M.N., Flynn, P.J.: Data Clustering: A Review. ACM Comp. Surveys 31(3), 264–323 (1999)
5. Knorr, E.M., Ng, R.T.: Algorithms for Mining Distance-Based Outliers in Large Datasets. In: Proceedings of the VLDB, pp. 392–403 (1998)
6. Breunig, M.M., Kriegel, H.-P., Ng, R., Sander, J.: LOF: Identifying Density-Based Local Outliers. In: Proceedings of the ACM SIGMOD International Conference on Management of Data, Dallas, Texas, USA, pp. 93–104 (2000)
7. Papadimitirou, S., Kitagawa, H., Gibbons, P.B., Faloutsos, C.: LOCI: Fast Outlier Detection Using the Local Correlation Integral. In: Proceedings of the 19th International Conference On Data Engineering, Bangalore, India, pp. 315–326 (2003)
8. Agyemang, M., Ezeife, C.I.: LSC-Mine: Algorithm for Mining Local Outliers. In: Proceedings of the 15th Information Resource Management Association (IRMA) International Conference, New Orleans, pp. 5–8 (2004)
9. Tang, J., Chen, Z., Fu, A., David, W.C.: Enhancing Effectiveness of Outlier Detections for Low Density Patterns. In: The 6th Pacific-Asia Conf. on Knowledge Discovery and Data Mining (PAKDD), Taipei, pp. 535–548 (2002)
10. Jin, W., Tung, A.K.H., Han, J., Wang, W.: Ranking Outliers Using Symmetric Neighborhood Relationship. In: Proceedings of 10th Pacific-Asia Conference on Advances in Knowledge Discovery and Data Mining, Singapore, pp. 577–593 (2006)

11. Sanjay, C., Pei, S.: SLOM: A New Measure for Local Spatial Outliers. Knowledge and Information Systems 9(4), 412–429 (2006)

12. Yaling, P., Osmar, R.Z., Yong, G.: An Efficient Reference-Based Approach to Outlier Detection in Large Datasets. In: Proceedings of the Sixth International Conference on Data Mining (ICDM), Washington, DC, USA, pp. 478–487 (2006)

13. Matthew, G., Raymond, K.W.: An Efficient Histogram Method for Outlier Detection. Advances in Databases: Concepts, Systems and Applications, 176–187 (2007)

14. Fan, H., Zaïane, O.R., Foss, A., Wu, J.: A Nonparametric Outlier Detection for Effectively Discovering Top-n Outliers from Engineering Data. In: Proceedings of the 10th Pacific-Asia Conference on Knowledge Discovery and Data Mining(PAKDD), Singapore, pp. 557–566 (2006)

15. Yu, J.X., Qian, W., Lu, H., Zhou, A.: Finding Centric Local Outliers in Categorical/Numerical Spaces. Knowledge and Information Systems 9(3), 309–338 (2006)

16. Latecki, L.J., Lazarevic, A., Pokrajac, D.: Outlier Detection with Kernel Density Functions. In: Perner, P. (ed.) MLDM 2007. LNCS (LNAI), vol. 4571, pp. 61–75. Springer, Heidelberg (2007)

17. Preparata, F.P., Shamos, M.I.: Computational Geometry-An Introduction. Springer, Heidelberg (1985)

18. Fink, E., Pratt, K.B.: Indexing of Time Series by Major Minima and Maxima. In: Proceedings of the IEEE International Conference on Systems, Man, and Cybernetics, pp. 2332–2335 (2003)

19. Sariel, H.-P.: A Replacement for Voronoi Diagrams of Near Linear Size. In: Proceedings of the 42nd IEEE Symposium on Foundations of Computer Science, Las Vegas, Nevada, USA, pp. 94–103 (2001)

Jilin Qu, born in 1963, Ph.D., Professor. His research interests include data mining and computational geometry.

AWSum – Data Mining for Insight

Anthony Quinn[1], Andrew Stranieri[1], John Yearwood[1], and Gaudenz Hafen[2]

[1] University of Ballarat, Australia
[2] Department of Pediatrics, University Hospital CHUV, Lausanne, Switzerland
9952146@students.ballarat.edu.au, a.stranieri@.ballarat.edu.au,
j.yearwood@.ballarat.edu.au, gaudenz.hafen@gmx.ch

Abstract. Many classifiers achieve high levels of accuracy but have limited use in real world problems because they provide little insight into data sets, are difficult to interpret and require expertise to use. In areas such as health informatics not only do analysts require accurate classifications but they also want some insight into the influences on the classification. This can then be used to direct research and formulate interventions. This research investigates the practical applications of **A**utomated **W**eighted **Sum**, (AWSum), a classifier that gives accuracy comparable to other techniques whist providing insight into the data. AWSum achieves this by calculating a weight for each feature value that represents its influence on the class value. The merits of AWSum in classification and insight are tested on a Cystic Fibrosis dataset with positive results.

1 Introduction

In an ideal situation a classifier would be able to not only classify accurately but convey to the user, who may not be an expert in data mining, the contribution that the various feature values make to the classification. If this were able to be achieved it would allow a greater understanding of the problem area and help point to areas for possible investigation and intervention. This is particularly pertinent in health informatics and medical research. Medical researchers want to be able to accurately classify a disease and also gain insight that leads to further research or possible interventions. In order to achieve this a classifier would need to be transparent in its process and provide insights that accurately conveyed meaning to the analyst. In striving for accuracy, many classifiers have become complex and difficult to interpret. Bayesian approaches [2] require the analyst to compare probabilities for each class in order to see any influences on the classification. Connectionist approaches [6] provide little meaningful visualisation of influences. Geometric approaches, such as Support Vector Machines [8], are difficult to interpret as the problem space has been transformed. Trees and rules [4] provide a visual representation of the influences on classification that don't necessarily contain all feature values or quantify the influence. They are also not always easy to interpret. While regression can indicate the importance of features it doesn't easily provide insight into its processes.

C. Tang et al. (Eds.): ADMA 2008, LNAI 5139, pp. 524–531, 2008.

This research investigates the, **A**utomated **W**eighted **Sum** (AWSum) classification technique [5]. AWSum provides insight into the data that is simple and visual to interpret whist maintaining accuracy comparable with other classifiers. It does this by formulating a weight for each feature value that indicates its relative influence on the classification. The application of AWSum to parts of The Australian Cystic Fibrosis Data Registry (ACFDR) database [11] is investigated demonstrating potentially valuable insights that can be obtained by applying this approach.

When we discuss insight we mean that the technique provides an analyst with an appreciation of the influence that a feature value has on the class value. For example it is intuitive to ask the question: what influence does high blood pressure have on the prospects of having heart disease? A classifier that provides answers to these sorts of questions in a simple and easily interpreted fashion could be expected to provide a degree of insight. The influences identified by AWSum are not intended to imply any causality. They are simply indicators of the strength of association between feature values and class values. The investigation of causality is left to the domain expert.

The intuition behind AWSum's approach is that each feature value has an influence on the classification that can be represented as a weight and that combining these influence weights gives an influence score for an example. This score can then be compared to a threshold in order to classify the example. The algorithm for calculating and combining weights, and determining thresholds is briefly described in section 2.

2   The Algorithm

The following section briefly describes the algorithm. It consists of 2 steps; the first involves the calculation of influence weights for each feature value and the second involves the classification of new examples.

2.1   Influence Weights

The first phase of the AWSum approach lays the foundations for classification by calculating influence weights for each feature value. Calculating the conditional probability of the outcome given the feature value gives the level of association between the feature value and the outcome. To calculate an influence weight the level of association for each class value, for a given feature value, is combined into a single figure. This is illustrated with a binary classifier.

A feature value's influence weight, W represents its influence on each class value and so it needs to simultaneously represent the feature value's association with both class values. To achieve this, one association is considered positive and the other negative. This leads to a range for the influence weight of -1 to 1, where a certainty of one class value produces a weight of -1 and a certainty of the other class value a weight of 1. By summing the two associations we arrive at a single influence weight that represents the feature value's influence on one

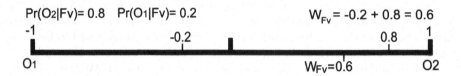

Fig. 1. Binary class example

class value relative to the other. Equation 1 demonstrates this calculation and figure 1 shows an example where $Pr\,(O_1|Fv) = 0.2$, or -0.2 when mapped and $Pr\,(O_2|Fv) = 0.8$.

$$W = Pr\,(O_1|Fv) + Pr\,(O_2|Fv) \qquad (1)$$

This process has some similarities with logistic regression. where the natural log of the odds of a class are adjusted by parameters in order to find a model to describe the outcome. It differs because we are calculating a simple scaled weight that indicates a feature value's influence on the class value rather than trying to fit the data to a mathematical model. This allows the process to be described in simple intuitive terms.

2.2   Classification

Classification of an example is achieved by combining the influences weights for each of the example's feature values into a single score. By summing and averaging influence weights we are able to arrive at a scaled score that represents a combination of the evidence that the example belongs to one class and not to another. Equation 2 depicts this. Performing the combination by summing and averaging assumes each feature value's influence is equally comparable. Although this is a relatively naive approach, it is quite robust as described later in this section. It also leaves open the possibility of using other functions for the combining of influence weights, much the same as different kernel functions can be used in support vector machines.

$$e_1 = \frac{1}{n} \sum_{m=1}^{n} W_m \qquad (2)$$

e_1 = the influence weight of the ith example
n = the number of features

The influence score for an example is compared to threshold values that divide the influence range into as many segments as there are class values. For instance, a single threshold value is required for a binary classification problem so that examples with an influence score above the threshold are classified as one class value, and those with a score below the threshold are classified as the other class value. Each threshold value is calculated from the training set by ordering the

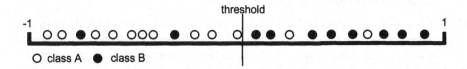

Fig. 2. Threshold optimisation

examples by their influence weight and deploying a search algorithm based on minimising the number of incorrect classifications. For instance, the examples with total influence scores that fall to the left of the threshold in Figure 2 are classified as class outcome A. This however includes two examples that belong to class B in the training set and so these two examples are misclassified but the number of misclassifications has been minimised. Two examples to the right of the threshold are misclassified as class B when they are A's. In cases where there are equal numbers of correctly and incorrectly classified examples the threshold is placed at the mid-point under the assumption that misclassification of class A and B is of equal cost. New examples can be classified by comparing the example's influence score to the thresholds. The example belongs to the class in which its influence score falls.

AWSum is suited to nominal feature values and class outcomes although it is not necessary that they are ordinal. Continuous numeric features require discretisation before use in AWSum. While there is a potential for developing a distinct method of discretisation in AWSum the research to date has used Fayyad and Irani's MDL method [12].

2.3 Combinations of Feature Values

The combining of influence weights for single feature values into a total influence score for an example and using this to classify is intuitively based however, it is plausible that feature values may not individually be strong influences on a class outcome but when they occur together the combination is a strong influence. For example both *drug A* and *drug B* may individually be influential toward low blood pressure but taken together lead to an adverse reaction that results in exceedingly high blood pressure.

The influence weights for each feature value combination can be calculated in the same way as they were for the single feature values. These combinations of feature values can contribute to an increase in accuracy and provide insight. Analysts can use them to identify feature values that have interesting interactions. This is achieved by comparing the influence weights of the individual component feature values of the combination to the influence weight of the combination. If they are markedly different this indicates a level of interaction between the feature values. This is useful, for example, in identifying things such as adverse drug reactions.

2.4 Model Selection

Model selection has also been kept very simple. Combinations of feature values are ordered according to the magnitude of the difference between their influence weight as a combination and the average of their influence weights as individual feature values. The first N combinations, where N ranges from 1 to the number of possible combinations, are added and N incremented until classification is maximised.

3 Experiments

Four datasets were sourced from the UCI Repository [1] for the comparative evaluation of the AWSum approach. In addition, the Cystic Fibrosis dataset [11], with 17 categorical features, 6 continuous features, 3 classes, 212 instances, and many missing values, was used. Ten fold stratified cross validation was used in all experiments. Table 1 shows the classification accuracy by other techniques using the Weka [9] suite alongside results from AWSum. AWSum Single refers to the results using single feature feature values independently, without considering any interaction between feature values. AWSum Triples shows the classification accuracies achieved by including the influence weights for combinations of feature values up to a combination of three feature values. Table1 illustrates that AWSum performs comparably on all datasets.

Table 1. Classifier comparison using single feature value influence weights only

Data	AWSum Single	AWSum Triple	NBC	TAN	C4.5	SVM	Logistic
Heart	83.14	**89.90**	84.48	81.51	78.87	84.16	84.48
Iris	94.00	**96.76**	94.00	94.00	96.00	96.67	93.33
Mush	95.77	99.37	95.83	99.82	**100**	**100**	**100**
Vote	86.00	**97.48**	90.11	94.25	96.32	96.09	94.94
CF	48.40	**64.24**	60.38	59.91	60.85	55.66	60.84
Avg	81.46	**93.93**	89.53	84.96	85.90	86.41	86.52

To represent three or more class values on a linear scale assumptions need to be made. The class values need to be treated as ordinal, and the conditional probabilities scaled by a simple mapping value as per 3. This approach can be demonstrated to classify well on the Iris dataset and CF, which indicates a potential for the approach to work on both ordinal and non ordinal data although further work needs to be done on more complex datasets to confirm this potential.

$$M_i = \left(\frac{2}{c-1} \times (i-1) \right) - 1 \tag{3}$$

where: c = the number of class values and i is the mapping value for the ith class value.

4   Insight in the Cystic Fibrosis Data

AWSum's ability to convey meaningful insights to the user has been tested using Cystic Fibrosis data supplied by the ACFDR [11].

In order to be useful in real world situations the insights presented need to convey meaning to the user and be easy to interpret. This was tested by giving a domain expert the output from AWSum for the CF data and analyzing their interpretation of the information. The second criteria measured was the accuracy of the insight. AWSum's measure of influence for single feature values and combinations of feature values was presented to a CF expert for comments on the appropriateness of the influence measure. Preliminary results are encouraging.

4.1   Ease of Interpretation

The expert was presented with diagrams in the form seen in figure 3. There were: 21 single feature values, 25 combinations of 2 feature values and 16 combinations of 3 feature values presented. For the single feature values the expert interpreted the figure as telling him that if a patient had the feature value concerned this would lead to a level of severity of CF as indicated by the influence weight. For the combinations of feature values the expert interpreted the combination influence weight as being the level of severity that could be expected when these factors occurred together in a patient. The expert was able to determine that this was potentially different to the way that the constituent feature values may act when occurring independently.

These interpretations indicate that the information presented is being interpreted correctly by our expert. It needs to be noted that the expert was always keen to interpret causality. For instance, he noted influence weights such as *presence of yeast infection candida albicans* (CA) and *breath volume* (FVCP<95.85) where he considered that the association was not causal. This is to be expected in a field where interventions and diagnosis are the focus.

4.2   Accuracy of Insights

When an insight is being assessed it falls into one of several categories: *Correct and expected, Correct and unexpected* or *incorrect*. Insights that are correct and expected, help verify the insight process and confirm domain knowledge. Those that are unexpected need further explanation. It could be that they are incorrect, although as the weights are heavily based on conditional probabilities this would need further investigation and may imply that the data is unrepresentative of the population. The unexpected influence weights may also reflect new domain knowledge and uncover associations that may or may not be causal.

It is difficult in a field such as this to quantify exactly the level of agreement between the influence weight and the experts domain knowledge. For this experiment the expert was simply asked to comment on the appropriateness of the influence weights presented. Of the 62 influence weights the expert deemed 60 or 96.8 percent to be appropriate. It can be said that these influence weights were

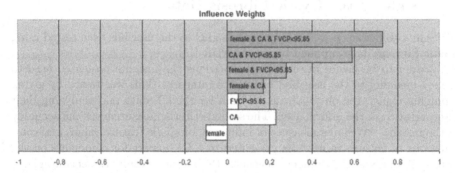

Fig. 3. Influence weights for feature values and combinations of feature values

both correct and expected, although they do give the additional advantage of scaling and quantifying the influences, which the expert found informative and helpful.

The two influence weights that were unexpected to the expert involve the presence of Candida Albicans (CA). They were, *CA and FVCP<95.85* and *Female, CA and FVCP<95.85*. Individually CA and FVCP<95.85 are not strong indicators of severe CF having influence weights of 0.23 and 0.05 respectively. The expert concurred with these weights. When they occur together the influence weight jumps to 0.59. This increases again to 0.73 for females with CA and FVCP<95.85. This can be seen graphically in figure 3. In was not in the experts experience that CA had a clinical link with the severity of CF. His suggestion was that perhaps severe CF caused CA, although this explanation doesn't fully cover what is seen in the data, as CA seems to compound the CF severity when association with and FVCP<95.85. The explanation for the increase for females may be that females more often have CA. This data has proven interesting enough to the expert that further enquiries are being made of experts in the CA area to try and determine an explanation for the observation. There has also been microbiological research identified [10,13] that suggests a possible causal link between CA and the severity of CF. While no link has causal link has been established at this stage and may well not be the insight provided by AWSum has proved interesting to our expert and prompted him to expand his domain knowledge by consulting other related experts. This indicates that AWSum can reveal insights that are complex and of interest in real world research.

5   Conclusion

AWSum demonstrates that classification accuracy can be maintained whist providing insight into the problem domain. The insights into the CF data have been shown to confirm domain knowledge. It has also been shown that AWSum can elicit non trivial insights that can be of interest to domain experts. Given the ease of use and interpretation of AWSum's insights it would seem that it would be of use in real world data mining situations. Future work involves redesigning the algorithm for the streaming of data.

References

1. Blake, C.L., Newman, D.J., Hettich, S., Merz, C.J.: UCI repository of machine learning databases (1988)
2. Duda, R., Hart, P.: Pattern Classification and scene analysis. John Wiley, Chichester (1973)
3. Friedmann, N., Goldszmidt: Building classifiers using bayesian intelligence. In: Proceedings of the National Conference on Artificial Intelligence, pp. 207–216. AAAI Press, Portland (1993)
4. Quinlan, J.: Programs for Machine Learning. Morgan Kaufmann, San Francisco (1993)
5. Quinn, A., Stranieri, A., Yearwood, J.: Classification for accuracy and insight. A weighted sum approach. In: Proceedings of 6th Austalasian data mining conference, Gold Coast, Australia, vol. 70 (2007)
6. Setiono, R., Liu, H.: Symbolic Representation of Neural Networks, Computer, vol. 29, pp. 71–77. IEEE Computer Society Press, Los Alamitos (1973)
7. Shafer, G.: A Mathematical theory of evidence. Princeton University Press, Princeton (1993)
8. Vapnik, V.: The nature of statistical learning theory. Springer, Heidelberg (1999)
9. Witten, I.H., Frank, E.: Data Mining: Practicle machine learning tools and techniques with java implementations. Morgan Kaufmann, San Francisco (2000)
10. Klotz, S., Nand, K., Richard De Armond, R., Donald Sheppard, D., Khardori, N., Edwards Jr., J.E., Lipkee, P.N., El-Azizi, M.: Candida albicans Als proteins mediate aggregation with bacteria and yeasts Medical Mycology, vol. 45, pp. 363–370 (2007)
11. Australian Cystic Fibrosis Data Registry: Cystic Fibrosis database (1999–2003)
12. Fayyad, U.M., Irani, K.B.: Multi-interval discretization of continuousvalued attributes for classification learning. In: Thirteenth International Joint Conference on Articial Intelligence, pp. 1022–1027 (1993)
13. Maiz, M., Cuevas, M., Lamas, A., Sousa, A., Santiago, Q., Saurez, S.: Aspergillus fumigatus and Candia Albicans in Cystic Fibrosis: Clinical Significance and Specific Immune Response Involving Serum Immunoglobulins G, A and M. Arch Bronconeumol, vol. 44(3), pp. 146–151 (2008)

Integrative Neural Network Approach for Protein Interaction Prediction from Heterogeneous Data

Xue-wen Chen[1,*], Mei Liu[1], and Yong Hu[2]

[1] Bioinformatics and Computational Life-Sciences Laboratory, ITTC, Department of Electrical Engineering and Computer Science, The University of Kansas, 1520 West 15th Street, Lawrence, KS 66045, USA
{xwchen,meiliu}@ku.edu

[2] Department of Management Science, School of Business Management, Sun Yat-sen University, Guangdong University of Foreign Studies, Guangzhou, Guangdong 510275, China
henryhu200211@163.com

Abstract. Protein interactions are essential in discovery of protein functions and fundamental biological processes. In this paper, we aim to create a reliable computational model for protein interaction prediction by integrating information from complementary data sources. An integrative Artificial Neural Network (ANN) framework is developed to predict protein-protein interactions (PPIs) from heterogeneous data in Human. Performance of our proposed framework is empirically investigated by combining protein domain data, molecular function and biological process annotations in Gene Ontology. Experimental results demonstrate that our approach can predict PPIs with high sensitivity of 82.43% and specificity of 78.67%. The results suggest that combining multiple data sources can result in a 7% increase in sensitivity compared to using only domain information. We are able to construct a protein interaction network with proteins around mitotic spindle checkpoint of the human interactome map. Novel predictions are made and some are supported by evidences in literature.

Keywords: Protein-Protein Interaction, Interaction Network Prediction, Heterogeneous Data Integration, Integrative Neural Network.

1 Introduction

Proteins are major components of living organisms that exhibit variety of roles in cellular processes and biochemical events which are mainly attributed to their interactions with other proteins. Over the years, high throughput technologies have deposited tremendous amount of protein interaction data into databases [1-5]. Unfortunately, these experiments are labor-intensive and often associated with high error rates. In addition, the number of possible protein interaction pairs within one cell is enormous, which makes experimental verification impractical. Hence, it is vital to seek reliable

---

* Corresponding author.

C. Tang et al. (Eds.): ADMA 2008, LNAI 5139, pp. 532–539, 2008.

complementary *in silico* methods. Various computational methods for protein interaction discovery have been developed, and among them, domain-based models have attracted growing interests. Protein domains are the structural and/or functional units of proteins that are conserved through evolution to represent protein functions or structures. It is widely believed that proteins interact with each other through their domains. One of the pioneering works is the association method [6], and numerous other methods soon followed [7-9]. Nevertheless, most of those methods do not consider the fact that multiple domains in a protein can form a unit to participate in interactions as a whole, and they assume independence between domain pairs. In an effort to address such concerns, we considered contributions of all domain combinations in protein interactions, yielding promising results [10, 11].

In this paper, by extending our previous work in domain-based models, we argue that integration of domain information with other complementary data sources will further improve prediction accuracy. Here, we propose an integrative Artificial Neural Network (ANN) framework to combine multiple data sources for protein-protein interaction (PPI) prediction. The proposed integrative framework includes learning models for each complementary data source and a model for integrating prediction results from these heterogeneous sources that contain intrinsic errors and noises. Experimental results demonstrate that comparing to a model using only domain information; the integrative ANN framework can lead to a 7% increase in accuracy. Furthermore, we are able to construct an interaction network with proteins around the mitotic spindle checkpoint, and results indicate that our predicted network has a large overlap with the existing network. Novel predictions are also made, and supporting evidences for some can be found in literatures.

2 Method

2.1 Feature Representation

Protein Domain Feature. Essentially, protein pairs can be characterized by the domains that exist in each protein. Let $D=[X_1, X_2, \cdots, X_n]$ represent n training samples and $X_i = [x_1^{(i)}, x_2^{(i)}, \cdots, x_k^{(i)}, y_i]$ represent the ith sample with k features (attributes) x_i belonging to the class y_i. Among all proteins in our dataset, there are 8,642 protein domains. In our problem formulation, $y_i = 1$ refers to the "interaction" class and 0 to the "non-interaction" class. Each feature x_i has a discrete value of 0, 0.5, or 1. If a protein pair does not contain a particular domain, then the associated feature value is 0. If one of the proteins contains the evidence, then the value is 0.5. Finally, if both proteins have them, then it is 1. The ternary-valued system was introduced in our previous research [11]. It distinguishes between protein pairs with interaction evidences existing in one protein and those existing in both proteins. Some domains often interact with themselves. With a binary-valued system, it will classify all protein pairs containing this self-interacting domain as interacting even though only one protein contains it. Furthermore, it is protein order independent.

Features Derived from Molecular Function and Biological Process. A protein may execute variety of functions in different biological processes. Two proteins often come together through interaction to achieve a common goal, which implies that interacting proteins are more likely to exhibit similar functions and perform their functions in similar biological processes than non-interacting proteins. There are 3,672 and 3,892 GO [12] 'molecular function' and 'biological process' terms among our datasets, respectively. A discrete value is assigned to each feature x_i in which if both proteins contain a particular function or process term, then the associated feature value is 1. If one of the proteins contains the evidence, then the value is 0.5 and otherwise 0. This feature representation enables our model to capture similarities between two proteins' GO annotations through learning. Existing methods require two proteins to have at least one annotation term in common to draw any conclusion. Our model tackles the problem through pattern matching rather than term matching.

2.2 Integrative ANN

Different genomic features can be viewed as puzzle pieces in which each piece holds some information to the whole picture of protein interaction network. Here, we propose an integrative ANN model to glue the pieces together. Unlike existing methods where different features are mixed together and classifiers are then applied, our integrative framework starts classification on a low-level with each specific data feature independently. Classifications of the individual pieces of data are then combined systematically and a final output is produced on a higher level.

For the lower level classification task, we propose to employ a multilayer feed-forward neural network and use the error back-propagation learning algorithm that contains two passes: a forward pass and a backward pass. In the forward pass, effects of input instances propagate throughout the network layer-by-layer producing a set of network outputs. In the backward pass, the network synaptic weights are calibrated according to the Delta learning rule. The neural network has three layers: input, hidden, and output. In our application, each processing elements in the input layer represents a feature or attribute of a particular data type. The non-linearity of ANN arises from the hidden layer through its hidden units. Sigmoid transfer function was used in input-to-hidden and hidden-to-output layers. Finally, the output units assign values to each input instance. The nodes between layers are fully connected. There are no connections between nodes in the same layer. All connections point to the same direction from the input toward the output layer. The weights associated with each connection are real numbers in the range of [0, 1]. The connection weights are initialized to random small real numbers, and are adjusted during network training. This structure can capture various combinations between attributes such as domains, instead of only one feature pair at a time. Each feature will contribute to the network output, depending on the weights associated with the nodes. In this application, we only have one output unit, where it assigns real numbers between 0 and 1 to each input sample.

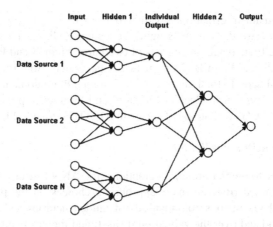

Fig. 1. General view of our integrative neural network structure. It can be applied to N different data sources, where one ANN is trained for each data source independently and outputs from those individual networks are treated as inputs to the second neural network for data integration.

In the higher level, to incorporate multiple data sources into the prediction process, we propose to use another ANN to systematically combine the classifications of each piece of data rather than heuristic rules. A general structure of our integrative ANN is shown in Fig. 1. The most important benefit of using ANN is its natural ability in estimating reliability of each data source by adjusting its connection weights between the input layer (Individual Output) and the hidden layer (Hidden 2) (Fig. 1). Also since each data source is learned independently, it can handle uneven distribution problem for the numerous data sources.

3   Experimental Results

3.1   Data Sources

The proposed framework is evaluated empirically over the Human proteome. Protein interaction data was collected from the Human Protein Reference Database (HPRD) [13], which is manually curated by trained biologists who read and interpret each and every scientific paper related to the molecule of interest. The final interaction dataset contain 12,645 protein interaction pairs. The negative samples are randomly generated. A protein pair is considered to be a negative sample if the pair does not exist in the interaction set. The interaction and non-interaction data are then split into training, validation, and testing datasets. The final training dataset contains 16,890 samples with 8,445 positives and 8,445 negatives. Each of the validation and testing datasets contains 4,200 samples (2,100 positives and 2,100 negatives). In order to avoid data separation bias, data samples are randomly selected. A sample belongs to one and only one dataset (training, validation, or testing). Training data are used to learn the ANN models and validation data are used for parameter selection.

The protein domain information is gathered from Pfam [14], which is a protein domain family database that contains multiple sequence alignments of common domain families. The Pfam database consists of two parts: Pfam-A and Pfam-B. Pfam-A is manually curated, and Pfam-B is automatically generated. Both Pfam-A and Pfam-B families are used here. In total, there are 8,642 unique Pfam domains defined by our set of proteins. The protein 'molecular function' and 'biological process' annotations are retrieved from the Gene Ontology Consortium (GO) February, 2006 release [12].

3.2 Protein Interaction Prediction

Training. In order to predict protein interactions, the ANN learning models for each data source are trained first. To make appropriate choices on the parameters, each network is trained via various combinations of hidden neurons and training cycles. Each model is validated over the validation dataset, and the errors are plotted against different number of training cycles for different number of hidden neurons. For illustration, Fig. 2 shows validation errors for the classifiers trained with domain information. ANNs with different number of hidden neurons all converge after certain number of training epochs. In fact, all of them converge after 5000 training cycles. At last, parameter pairs that result in the lowest validation errors are chosen. After parameter selection, we combined the training and validation datasets and used them to train each network again with the fixed parameters. Finally, training outputs from the individual networks are fed into the final integrative neural network as training inputs for information fusion.

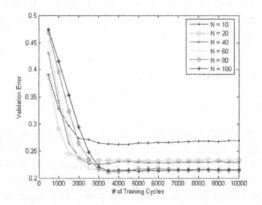

Fig. 2. Parameter selection process for the ANN with protein domain information. Validation errors are plotted against different parameter pairs (i.e. number of neurons and number of training cycles). N is the number of neurons. The parameters chosen for this protein domain ANN are N = 60 and # of training cycles = 6500 (validation error = 21.3%).

Test Results. To classify a new protein pair as either interacting or non-interacting, the pair is first converted to three feature vectors according to the information sources as described in Section 2.1. These feature vectors are then used as inputs to the individual networks and outputs are subsequently used as input to the final ANN. A protein pair is classified as interacting if the output value is larger than or equal to certain threshold. We use both specificity and sensitivity to evaluate the performance of our method in predicting protein interactions. Specificity is defined as the percentage of matched non-interactions between the predicted set and the observed set over the total number of non-interactions. Sensitivity is defined as the percentage of matched interactions (true positives) over the total number of known interactions. Fig. 3 illustrates ROC curves of the ANN trained with domain data only and the integrative ANN. It is clear that the integrative ANN performs better than the single domain ANN, especially when the specificity is high between 72% and 95%. When we fix their specificities at approximately the same level (~78%), our integrative framework achieves 82.43% in sensitivity, which yields an increase of roughly 7% from the classifier trained with only domain information (75.48%).

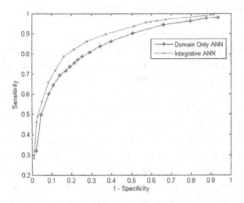

Fig. 3. ROC comparisons between integrative ANN and ANN trained with the protein domain data source. Y-axis is sensitivity and X-axis is 1-specificity. Therefore, we want the curve to be as close to the upper left corner as possible.

3.3 Human Interaction Network Analysis

With the trained prediction system, we are able to construct a small protein interaction network from proteins around one specific area of the human interactome map, namely the mitotic spindle checkpoint. The mitotic spindle checkpoint pathway is important in aneuploidy and cancer [15, 16]. Beginning with some well characterized members of the mitotic spindle checkpoint (e.g. CDC20, BUB1, and BUB3), Rhodes et al. [17] predicted and analyzed a focused view of the human interactome. With the proteins, we applied our model to predict interactions between them and created an interaction network of our own (Fig. 4). In the network, each node corresponds to a protein, and edges specify the interactions between two proteins. All edges in the network reflect interaction predictions that our model has made. None of the interactions belong to the datasets we used for training, validating, or testing. As shown in Fig. 4, our predicted network has a large overlap with the known interactions and

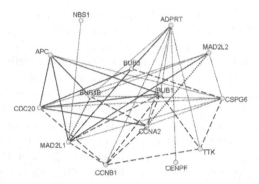

Fig. 4. Small human protein interaction network constructed by our model using proteins in the mitotic spindle checkpoint and surrounding proteins [17]. Known interactions are shown in solid edges. The long dashed edges characterize predicted interactions in [17]. Lastly the remaining square dot dashed edges are our novel predictions.

predicted interactions in [17]. In addition, we were able to make novel predictions and find supports for those discoveries in literatures. For instance, an interaction is predicted between MAD2L2 (mitotic spindle assembly checkpoint protein MAD2B) and CDC20 (cell division cycle protein 20 homolog). In [18], it was shown that MAD2B inhibits both CDH1-APC and CDC20-APC. The inhibition is targeted to CDH1 and CDC20, but not directly to APC. Moreover, our model identified APC (adenomatous polyposis coli protein) and CSPG6 (Structural maintenance of chromosomes protein 3 – SMC3) to be interacting. Ghiselli et al. found SMC3 expression to be elevated in a large fraction of human colon carcinomas [19]. Additional findings suggest that the protein is significantly increased in the intestinal polyps of ApcMin/+ mice, which led them to believe that SMC3 expression is linked to activation of the APC/beta-catenin/TCF4 pathway.

4 Conclusion

Evidences of protein interactions may be found in diverse data sources. These evidences may cover different parts of an interactome, and each may be a weak predictor of protein interactions. However, combining these complementary data sources may increase prediction accuracy. In this paper, we introduced an ANN-based integrative system to predict protein interactions from heterogeneous data. The experimental results indicate that adding GO molecular function and biological process information can increase prediction accuracy of the domain-based model by 7%. We further validated our model by creating an interaction network from a list of proteins that are related to mitotic spindle checkpoint. More data sources such as protein sequence and gene expression profiling can be readily incorporated into the integrative system for better predictions.

Acknowledgments. This work was supported by NSF award IIS-0644366.

References

1. Uetz, P., Giot, L., Cagney, G., Mansfield, T.A., Judson, R.S., et al.: A comprehensive analysis of protein-protein interactions in Saccharomyces cerevisiae. Nature 403, 623–627 (2000)
2. Ito, T., Tashiro, K., Muta, S., Ozawa, R., Chiba, T., et al.: Toward a protein-protein interaction map of the budding yeast: A comprehensive system to examine two-hybrid interactions in all possible combinations between the yeast proteins. Proc. Natl. Acad. Sci. USA 97, 1143–1147 (2000)
3. Bader, G.D., Hogue, C.W.: Analyzing yeast protein-protein interaction data obtained from different sources. Nat. Biotechnol. 20, 991–997 (2000)
4. Ho, Y., Gruhler, A., Heilbut, A., Bader, G.D., Moore, L., et al.: Systematic identification of protein complexes in Saccharomyces cerevisiae by mass spectrometry. Nature 415, 180–183 (2002)
5. Gavin, A.C., Bosche, M., Krause, R., Grandi, P., Marzioch, M., et al.: Functional organization of the yeast proteome by systematic analysis of protein complexes. Nature 415, 141–147 (2002)
6. Sprinzak, E., Margalit, H.: Correlated sequence-signatures as markers of protein-protein interaction. J. Mol. Biol. 311, 681–692 (2001)
7. Kim, W.K., Park, J., Suh, J.K.: Large scale statistical prediction of protein-protein interaction by potentially interacting domain (PID) pair. Genome Inform. 13, 42–50 (2002)
8. Han, D., Kim, H.S., Seo, J., Jang, W.: A domain combination based probabilistic framework for protein-protein interaction prediction. Genome Inform. 14, 250–259 (2003)
9. Deng, M., Mehta, S., Sun, F., Chen, T.: Inferring domain-domain interactions from protein-protein interactions. Genome Res. 12, 1540–1548 (2002)
10. Chen, X.W., Liu, M.: Prediction of protein-protein interactions using random decision forest framework. Bioinformatics 21, 4394–4400 (2005)
11. Chen, X.W., Liu, M.: Domain Based Predictive Models for Protein-Protein Interaction Prediction. In: EURASIP (2006)
12. Ashburner, M., Ball, C.A., Blake, J.A., Botstein, D., Butler, H., et al.: Gene ontology: tool for the unification of biology. The Gene Ontology Consortium. Nat. Genet. 25, 25–29 (2000)
13. Peri, S., Navarro, J.D., Amanchy, R., Kristiansen, T.Z., Jonnalagadda, C.K., et al.: Development of human protein reference database as an initial platform for approaching systems biology in humans. Genome Res. 13, 2363–2371 (2003)
14. Bateman, A., Coin, L., Durbin, R., Finn, R.D., Hollich, V., et al.: The Pfam protein families database. Nucleic Acids Res. 32, D138-141 (2004)
15. Cahill, D.P., Lengauer, C., Yu, J., Riggins, G.J., Willson, J.K., et al.: Mutations of mitotic checkpoint genes in human cancers. Nature 392, 300–303 (1998)
16. Bharadwaj, R., Yu, H.: The spindle checkpoint, aneuploidy, and cancer. Oncogene 23, 2016–2027 (2004)
17. Rhodes, D.R., Tomlins, S.A., Varambally, S., Mahavisno, V., Barrette, T., et al.: Probabilistic model of the human protein-protein interaction network. Nat. Biotechnol. 23, 951–959 (2005)
18. Chen, J., Fang, G.: MAD2B is an inhibitor of the anaphase-promoting complex. Genes Dev. 15, 1765–1770 (2001)
19. Ghiselli, G., Coffee, N., Munnery, C.E., Koratkar, R., Siracusa, L.D.: The cohesin SMC3 is a target the for beta-catenin/TCF4 transactivation pathway. J. Biol. Chem. 278, 20259–20267 (2003)

Rules Extraction Based on Data Summarisation Approach Using DARA

Rayner Alfred

School of Engineering and Information Technology,
Universiti Malaysia Sabah,
Locked Bag 2073, 88999, Kota Kinabalu, Sabah, Malaysia
ralfred@ums.edu.my

Abstract. This paper helps the understanding and development of a data summarisation approach that summarises structured data stored in a non-target table that has *many-to-one* relations with the target table. In this paper, the feasibility of data summarisation techniques, borrowed from the Information Retrieval Theory, to summarise patterns obtained from data stored across multiple tables with one-to-many relations is demonstrated. The paper describes the Dynamic Aggregation of Relational Attributes (DARA) framework, which summarises data stored in non-target tables in order to facilitate data modelling efforts in a multi-relational setting. The application of the DARA algorithm involving structured data is presented in order to show the adaptability of this algorithm to real world problems.

1 Introduction

Algorithms that summarise structured data stored in relational databases have become essential tools in knowledge discovery processes. An important practical problem in contemporary data mining is that users often want to discover models and patterns over data that resides in multiple tables. Most of the structured data in the world is stored across multiple tables, in a relational database [3,2]. In this multi-relational setting, a user often needs to find records or tuples related to certain target records. It is often infeasible to analyse all possible relationships among entities in a database manually. Therefore it is highly desirable to summarise records that are related to a specific target record automatically.

Data summarisation methods, such as aggregation operators, are popular in relational data mining because they can be used to capture information about the value distributions in a multi-relational setting with one-to-many relations between tables. This is a very useful operation in order to reduce a set of tuples that corresponds to a unique record to a single tuple. The traditional way to summarise one-to-many relationships between tables in statistics and on-line analytical processing (OLAP) [7] is through aggregates that are based on histograms, such as *count, mode, sum, min, max* and *avg*. However, these basic

C. Tang et al. (Eds.): ADMA 2008, LNAI 5139, pp. 540–547, 2008.

aggregation operators provide simple summaries of the distributions of features of related entities [5,4] and aggregation has received little direct attention [6].

The overall motivation of this paper is to explore the feasibility of summarising structured data stored in relational databases with one-to-many relations between entities. In this paper, we propose a data summarisation approach called Dynamic Aggregation of Relational Attributes (DARA) that can be applied to summarise data stored in non-target tables. Section 2 will introduce the framework of $DARA$ [1]. The $DARA$ algorithm employs the TF-IDF weighted frequency matrix (vector space model [13])to represent the relational data model, where the representation of data stored in multiple tables will be analysed and it will be transformed into data representation in a vector space model. Section 3 describes the experimental design and presents an application area of the $DARA$ algorithm in medical domain. The results are discussed in the context of applying data summarisation to summarise structured data and finally, this paper is concluded in section 4.

2 Dynamic Aggregation of Relational Attributes ($DARA$)

In order to classify records stored in the target table that have one-to-many relations with records stored in non-target tables, the $DARA$ algorithm transforms the representation of data stored in the non-target tables into an $(n \times p)$ matrix in order to cluster these records (see Fig. 1), where n is the number of records to be clustered and p is the number of patterns considered for clustering. As a result, the records stored in the non-target tables are summarised by clustering them into groups that share similar charateristics.

In Fig. 1, the target relation has a one-to-many relationship with the non-target relation. The non-target table is then converted into bags of patterns associated with records stored in the target table. After the records stored in the non-target relation are clustered, a new column, F_{new}, is added to the set of original features in the target table. This new column contains the cluster identification number for all records stored in the non-target table. In this way, we aim to map data stored in the non-target table to the records stored in the target table. There are three main stages in the $DARA$ algorithm (see Fig. 1): *data preparation (A)*, *data transformation (B)* and *data summarisation(C)*.

2.1 Data Preparation Stage

The $DARA$ algorithm performs two types of data preparation; features discretisation and features construction. Feature discretisation is a process of transforming continuous-valued features to nominal. Alfred and Kazakov [16] discussed the discretisation methods for continuous attributes in a multi-relational setting in greater detail. Feature construction involves constructing new attributes, based on some functional expressions that use the values of original features, that describe

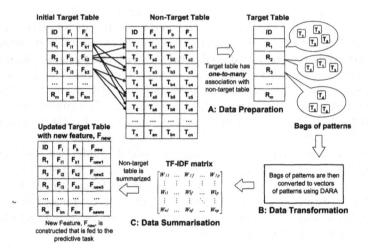

Fig. 1. Data transformation for data stored in a Non-Target table for prediction task (*A*: Data Preparation, *B*: Data Transformation, *C*: Data Summarisation)

the hypothesis at lease as well as the original set. Alfred [17,18] discussed how feature construction affects the performance of the proposed *DARA* method in summarising data stored in a multi-relational setting with one-to-many relations.

2.2   Data Transformation

At this stage, the representation of data stored in a relational database is changed to a vector space data representation. We will describe the data transformation process and explain the data representation of relational data with high cardinality attributes in a vector space representation.

Data Transformation Process. In a relational database, a single record, R_i, stored in the target table can be associated with other records stored in the non-target table. Let R denote a set of m records stored in the target table and let S denote a set of n records $(T_1, T_2, T_3, ..., T_n)$, stored in the non-target table. Let S_i be a subset of S, $S_i \subseteq S$, associated through a foreign key with a single record R_a stored in the target table, where $R_a \in R$. Thus, the association of these records can be described as $R_a \longleftarrow S_i$. In this case, we have a single record stored in the target table that is associated with multiple records stored in the non-target table. The records stored in the non-target table that correspond to a particular record stored in the target table can be represented as vectors of patterns. As a result, based on the vector space model [15], a unique record stored in non-target table can be represented as a vector of patterns. In other words, a particular record stored in the target table that is related to several records stored in the non-target table can be represented as a *bag of patterns*, i.e., by the patterns it contains and their frequency, regardless of their order.

Data Representation in a Vector Space Model. In this subsection, we describe the representation of data for objects stored in multiple tables with one-to-many relations. Let DB be a database consisting of n objects. Let $R := R_1,...,R_m$ be the set of different representations existing for object O_i in DB and let each object O_i have zero or more representations of each R_i, such that $|R_i| \geq 0$, where $i = 1,...,m$. Each object $O_i \in DB$, where $i = 1,...,n$ can be described by maximally m different representations where each representation having its frequency,

$$O_i := R_1(O_i) : |R_1(O_i)| : |O_b(R_1)|, ..., R_m(O_i) : |R_m(O_i)| : |O_b(R_m)| \quad (1)$$

where $R_j(O_i)$ represents the jth representation of the ith object and $|R_j(O_i)|$ represents the frequency of the jth representation of the ith object, and finally $|O_b(R_j)|$ represents the number of objects exist in the data that have the jth representation. If all different representations exist for O_i, then the total different representations for O_i is $|O_i| = m$ else $|O_i| < m$. In the $DARA$ approach, the vector-space model [15] is applied to represent each object. In this model, each object O_i is considered as a vector in the representation-space. In particular, the TF-IDF weighted frequency matrix borrowed from [15] is employed, in which each object O_i, $i = 1,...,n$ can be represented as

$$\left(rf_1 \cdot log\left(\frac{n}{of_1}\right), rf_2 \cdot log\left(\frac{n}{of_2}\right), ..., rf_m \cdot log\left(\frac{n}{of_m}\right) \right) \quad (2)$$

where rf_j is the frequency of the jth representation in the object, of_j is the number of objects that contain the jth representation and n is the number of objects.

2.3 Data Summarisation Using Clustering

After transforming the dataset, the newly transformed data (in the form of vector space model) is taken as an input to a clustering algorithm. The idea of this approach is to transform the data representation for all objects in a multi-relational environment into a vector space model and find the similarity distance measures for all objects in order to cluster them. These objects are then grouped based on the similarity of their characteristics, taking into account all possible representations and the frequency of each representation for all objects.

The next section presents an application area of the $DARA$ algorithm to evaluate the adaptability of the proposed data summarisation method to real world problem. The results are discussed in the context of applying data summarisation to summarise structured data.

3   STULONG Dataset and Experimental Design

3.1   STULONG Dataset

STULONG is a data set concerning the twenty year long longitudinal study of the factors of *atherosclerosis* in the population of 1419 middle aged men. The dataset STULONG was prepared for the Discovery Challenge PKDD/ECML 2002 conference. In this dataset, two data matrices are included: the *ENTRY* and *CONTROL* data matrices.

The *ENTRY* data matrix stores the values of 219 attributes that have been surveyed in 1,419 men during the entry examination. The *CONTROL* data matrix contains results of observation of 28 attributes, selected from the 66 attributes, at 10,610 examinations made in the years 1976 − 1999. In this work, the attributes considered for the *ENTRY* and *CONTROL* data matrices can be divided into groups. The entity-relationship diagram of the *CONTROL* data matrix are shown in Fig. 2.

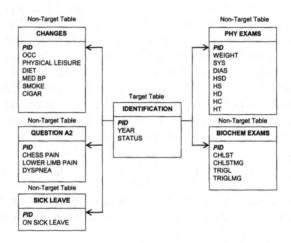

Fig. 2. CONTROL dataset: Table IDENTIFICATION has *one-to-many* relationships with tables CHANGES, SICK LEAVE, QUESTION A2, PHY EXAMS, BIOCHEM EXAMS

The goal of the discovery challenge is to extract knowledge or patterns from the STULONG data stored in the *CONTROL* matrix. Not many studies have focused on mining the *CONTROL* data and most data mining on the STU-LONG dataset has been based on the *ENTRY* table [8,9]. These patterns can help physicians to know if a patient is at risk of having cardiovascular disease. This work focused on the *CONTROL* table that stores records that have a *many-to-one* relationship with the record stored in *ENTRY* table.

3.2   Experimental Design and Results

In this work, records stored in the *CONTROL* table are summarised by using the *DARA* algorithm based on the distribution of patterns for each set of attributes (see Fig. 3). All data stored in the non-target tables that have many-to-one relationships with the data stored in the target table are summarised in order to form an attribute-value table format. The Weka [10] tool is applied to extract patterns (e.g. association and classification rules) from the summarised data, by

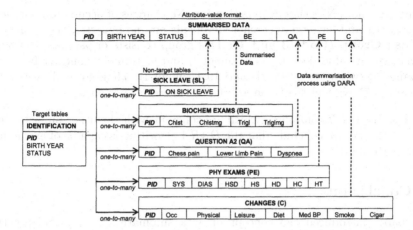

Fig. 3. Data Summarisation performed by *DARA* algorithm to convert data stored in multiple tables into an attribute-value (*AV*) format

using the *J*48 classifier and *PredictiveApriori* respectively and these patterns are compared with other published results. Below are some of the association and classification and rules obtained from the *J*48 and *PredictiveApriori* classifiers, which are consistent with other results [11,12].

Association Rules

- No changes in cigarette consumption $\rightleftharpoons$ No sickness since the last visit and No physical activities after the job (consistent with [12]).
- High cholesterol and low triglycerides $\rightleftharpoons$ No diet changes and No medication to control the blood pressure.
- High cholesterol and low triglycerides $\rightleftharpoons$ Hypercholesterolemia, Hypertriglyceridemie, Systolic-diastolic Hypertension, Systolic Hypertension and Diastolic Hypertension.
- Weighing 73.8 − 83.4 Kg $\rightleftharpoons$ No diet changes and No medication to control their blood pressure.
- Risk Group $\rightleftharpoons$ High cholesterol, low triglycerides, has chest and lower limb pains, has Dyspnea.
- Risk Group $\rightleftharpoons$ No diet changes and No medication to control blood presure (BP) and No sickness since the last visit.

Classification Rules. Below are the classification rules extracted from the summarised *CONTROL* data matrix.

- **Normal Group (Code 1 and 2):** This group consists of patients who do not have any chest and lower limb pains, no dyspnea, and do not have any changes in cigarette, have cholesterol values that are less than 5.9 (mmol/l), triglycerides values that are less than 9.8 (mmol/l), and No changes in Job, physical activities, and No systolic-diastolic hypertension, No Systolic

hypertension, No diastolic hypertension, No changes of occupation, physical activities and have no hypercholesterolemia and no hypertriglyceridemie.
- **Risk Group (Code 3 and 4):** This group consists of patients who have cholesterol values between 5.9 (mmol/l) and 9.3(mmol/l) and triglycerides values between 9.8 (mmol/l) and 19.4 (mmol/l). They normally weigh on average 77 Kg and smoke on average 15 cigarettes per day.

Based on the results obtained, which are coherent with the other published results [11,12], we can conclude that the $DARA$ algorithm is capable of extracting useful patterns.

4   Conclusion

This paper introduced the concept of data summarisation that adopts the $TF\text{-}IDF$ weighted frequency matrix concept borrowed from the information retrieval theory [15] to summarise data stored in relational databases with a high number of one-to-many relationships among entities, through the use of a clustering technique. Clustering algorithms can be used to generate summaries based on the information contained in the datasets that are stored in a multi-relational environment. This paper described the proposed data summarisation approach called *Dynamic Aggregation of Relational Attributes* ($DARA$) that transforms the representation of data stored in relational databases into a vector space format data representation that is suitable in clustering operations. By clustering these multi-association occurrences of an individual record in the multi-relational database, the characteristics of records stored in non-target tables are summarised by putting them into groups that share similar characteristics.

It is shown in the experimental results that the $DARA$ algorithm can be applied to summarise data stored in the $CONTROL$ table that has a many-to-one relationship with the $ENTRY$ table in order to facilitate the task of predictive and descriptive modelling. The $CONTROL$ table is transformed into an attribute-value (AV) table, by summarising the data using the $DARA$ algorithm. As a result, one can apply any AV data mining tools to extract both the association and classification rules from the summarised data. The classification and association rules were used to analyse the differences of the correlations concerning the characteristics of the patients from each group. The results shown in this experiment are quite promising and consistent with other researchers' results on the STULONG dataset.

References

1. Alfred, R., Kazakov, D.: Data Summarisation Approach to Relational Domain Learning Based on Frequent Pattern to Support the Development of Decision Making. In: Li, X., Zaïane, O.R., Li, Z. (eds.) ADMA 2006. LNCS (LNAI), vol. 4093, pp. 889–898. Springer, Heidelberg (2006)
2. Kuentzer, J., Backes, C., Blum, T., Gerasch, A., Kaufmann, M., Kohlbacher, O., Lenhof, H.P.: BNDB - The Biochemical Network Database. BMC Bioinformatics 8(1) (2007)

3. Soon, M.C., Pyeong, S.M., Junguk, L.K.: Integration of a Relational Database with Multimedia Data. Compsac., vol. 00. IEEE Computer Society, Los Alamitos (1996)
4. Claudia, P., Foster, P.: Distribution-based Aggregation for Relational Learning with Identifier Attributes. Machine Learning 62(1-2), 65–105 (2006)
5. Claudia, P., Foster, P.: Aggregation-Based Feature Invention and Relational Concept Classes. In: KDD, pp. 167–176 (2003)
6. Knobbe, A.J., de Haas, M., Siebes, A.: Propositionalisation and Aggregates. In: Siebes, A., De Raedt, L. (eds.) PKDD 2001. LNCS (LNAI), vol. 2168, pp. 277–288. Springer, Heidelberg (2001)
7. Tremblay, M.C., Fuller, R., Berndt, D., Studnicki, J.: Doing More with More Information: Changing Healthcare Planning with OLAP tools. Decision Support System 43(4), 1305–1320 (2007)
8. Couturier, O., Delalin, H., Fu, H., Edouard, G.: A Three Step Approach for STULONG Database Analysis: Characterisation of Patients's Groups. In: Proceeding of the ECML/PKDD 2004 Challenge (2004)
9. Correa, E., Plastino, A.: Mining Strong Associations and Exceptions in the STULONG Data Set. In: Proceeding of the ECML/PKDD 2004 Challenge (2004)
10. Witten, I.H., Frank, E.: Data Mining: Practical Machine Learning Tools and Techniques with Java Implementations. Morgan Kaufmann, San Francisco (1999)
11. Blatak, J.: Mining First-Order Frequent Patterns in the STULONG Database. In: Proceeding of the ECML/PKDD 2004 Challenge (2004)
12. Van Assche, A., Verbaeten, S., Krzywania, D., Struyf, J., Blockeel, H.: Attribute-Value and First Order Data Mining within the STULONG Project. In: Proceedings of the ECML/PKDD 2003 Workshop on Discovery Challenge, pp. 108–119 (2003)
13. Salton, G., Wong, A., Yang, C.S.: A Vector Space Model for Automatic Indexing. Commun. ACM 18(11), 613–620 (1975)
14. Witten, I.H., Frank, E.: Data Mining: Practical Machine Learning Tools and Techniques with Java Implementations. Morgan Kaufmann, San Francisco (1999)
15. Salton, G., McGill, M.: Introduction to Modern Information Retrieval. McGraw-Hill Book Company, New York (1984)
16. Alfred, R., Kazakov, D.: Discretisation Numbers for Multiple-Instances Problem in Relational Database. In: Eleventh East-European Conference on Advances in Databases and Information Systems, pp. 55–65 (2007)
17. Alfred, R., Kazakov, D.: Clustering Approach to Generalised Pattern Identification Based on Multi-Instanced Objects with DARA. In: Eleventh East-European Conference on Advances in Databases and Information Systems (2007)
18. Alfred, R.: DARA: Data Summarisation with Feature Construction. In: Second Asia International Conference on Modelling and Simulation AMS 2008, Kuala Lumpur, Malaysia (2008)

A Rough-Apriori Technique in Mining Linguistic Association Rules

Yun-Huoy Choo, Azuraliza Abu Bakar, and Abdul Razak Hamdan

Department of Science and System Management, Faculty of Information Science and Technology, National University of Malaysia, 43600 Bangi, Selangor, Malaysia
huoy@utem.edu.my, {aab,arh}@ftsm.ukm.my

Abstract. This paper has proposed a rough-Apriori based mining technique in mining linguistic association rules focusing on the problem of capturing the numerical interval with linguistic terms in quantitative association rules mining. It uses the rough membership function to capture the linguistic interval before implementing the Apriori algorithm to mine interesting association rules. The performance of conventional quantitative association rules mining algorithm with Boolean reasoning as the discretization method was compared to the proposed technique and the fuzzy-based technique. Five UCI datasets were tested in the 10-fold cross validation experiment settings. The frequent itemsets discovery in the Apriori algorithm was constrained to five iterations comparing to maximum iterations. Results show that the proposed technique has performed comparatively well by generating more specific rules as compared to the other techniques.

1 Introduction

Srikant and Agrawal's algorithm [1] discretizes the quantitative attributes sufficiently from large databases, laying out the appropriate interval range for rules mining process. Knowledge is more suitable to be presented in natural language. Quantitative rules that are conveyed in numbers are sometimes less practical. Research in linguistic association rules mining branched into different research focus, i.e. mining the linguistic summaries, hedges, quantitative intervals, linguistic support and confidence, etc. This paper only looks into the linguistic association rules via quantitative intervals. Recently, researchers have suggested a number of techniques and algorithms in mining linguistic based association rules, mostly involving fuzzy theory because of its ability in capturing fuzzy boundaries in linguistic association rules [2], [3]. Besides fuzzy theory, rough sets suggested by Zdzislaw Pawlak is another technique dealing with ambiguous boundary data sets [4]. Rough sets theory uses the upper and lower approximation as well as the rough membership function to determine the items in a set which can be obtained through self discovery in learning data. Thereby, it has gained the interest of researchers in the development of rough sets techniques as a complement of fuzzy techniques. This paper attempts to investigate the opportunity and strength of rough sets theory in linguistic association rules mining from the perspective of rough membership function.

C. Tang et al. (Eds.): ADMA 2008, LNAI 5139, pp. 548–555, 2008.
© Springer-Verlag Berlin Heidelberg 2008

Linguistic association rules convey the messages in linguistic terms instead of numerical values in quantitative attributes. Linguistic association rules mining task is generally being divided into two phases, which are firstly to create the intervals from the continuous data and represent those intervals with a suitable linguistic term [5], while the second phase is the rules mining process. However, partitioning continuous attributes are needed in most of the mining models. These attributes are discretized into intervals and presented by linguistic terms before the mining process. Partitioning the numeric values into interval sets causes crisp boundary problems. In contrast, linguistic association rules need a soft boundary instead of crisp boundary. Thus, fuzzy sets are used to soften the boundary of interval sets in association rules mining.

Data discretization has arisen since the earlier work on quantitative association rule mining, while the linguistic terms representation is always being related to Fuzzy sets theory. Although typical analysis such as binning, statistical and evolutionary techniques have contributed to a certain extent in dealing with quantitative attribute partitioning, the advancement in fuzzy algorithm has made it the most prominent technique in dealing with linguistic representation on soft boundary interval. Rough sets theory introduced by Pawlak on the other hand also deals with vagueness and uncertainty. With embedded foundation of classical theory, rough sets theory has its own perspective towards vagueness which is similar to fuzzy set theory [6]. Hence, it is gradually gaining attention in association rules mining research involving vagueness.

2   The Proposed Rough Membership Reference Association Rules Mining (RMRARM) Technique

A fusion of rough sets theory and the Apriori algorithm, RMRARM technique combines the rough membership reference (RMR) generation and the linguistic association rules mining task into one complete process flow. Figure 1 shows the step-by-step procedures of the RMRARM technique. The principal concepts applied in the RMRARM technique are described in the following sections.

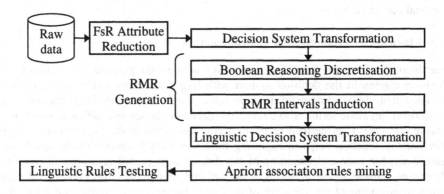

Fig. 1. The RMRARM technique

2.1 Boolean Reasoning (BR) Discretization

The BR discretization method is implemented as a necessary step in RMR generation. The ultimate goal of RMR generation is to obtain the rough membership values corresponding to each discretised interval. The basic concepts of the discretization based on the rough sets Boolean reasoning was summarized by Zhong & Skowron [7]. In certain cases, a single pass of BR discretization process may not fully discretize all the attributes in the dataset. This is due to the characteristic of BR discretization technique of which will only identify the prime attributes needed in the discernibility function. In the proposed RMRARM technique, BR discretization technique is implemented twice, i.e. in the FsR [8] and in RMR generation. In RMR generation, all attributes need to be discretized in order to avoid unique rule in rules generation later [9]. Hence, multiple passes of BR discretization has to be applied till all the attributes in the dataset are fully discretized.

2.2 Rough Membership Function

For every important attribute, the discretised intervals were named the rough membership reference (RMR) intervals. Rough membership value (RMV) from rough sets theory indicates the probability of an object being classified in a set [10], [11], [12]. In our research, RMV was regarded as the probability of a particular RMR interval that was categorised into the set of an output class in this research in line to its original proposal in rough sets theory. RMV derived from accuracy of the rules will be used as the membership reference in transforming numerical values into linguistic variable [13], [14]. The generated RMR and intervals and RMV were applied in transforming the attribute values into rough region in linguistic rules mining. The RMV for each RMR interval is shown in equation 1 as follows:

$$RMV_i = \frac{Card(O_j)}{Card(i)} ; \; repeat \; for \; every \; 0 < i = x \; and \; 0 < j = y \qquad (1)$$

Let x denote the number of RMR interval and i is the i-th RMR interval. Card (i) is the total instance in the i-th RMR interval. *Card (O_j)* is the total instance from i-th RMR interval that concludes to output class O_j while j is the j-th output class and y is the total output class.

2.3 Linguistic Decision System Transformation

The linguistic decision transformation serves a two fold purpose, i.e. replaces the decision classes in the decision system with linguistic terms and to transform the decision table into a linguistic decision table. Replacing the decision classes with predefined linguistic terms is to change the decision classes into different rough linguistic sets [15]. User-defined linguistic terms were used in the experiments. Rough membership function helps in capturing the uncertainty boundary of the rough linguistic set, but user understanding of the dataset used is still necessary in order to determine suitable linguistic terms to be replaced. Imprecise terms chosen will only result in deviation of the meaning of the rules. However, this would not affect the process of generation and performance testing of the rules. Choosing suitable linguistic terms with expert knowledge was not the focus of this research. Thus, the precision of linguistic terms chosen in the experiments were not evaluated in the performance evaluation. The second part of the linguistic decision system transformation is to convert the original decision system into a linguistic decision system. The attributes in the linguistic decision system are the linguistic terms chosen previously while the attributes values are the RMV attained from the RMR intervals induction. All the instances that fall in the same RMR interval will be assigned the same RMV.

2.4 Association Rules Mining and Linguistic Rules Testing

The Apriori algorithm was used in RMRARM technique. The difference in linguistic association rules mining and conventional Boolean association rules mining lies in the support value of each item. The support in Boolean association rules is the number of occurrence supporting a particular item in the dataset. The support in linguistic association rules adapted in this research is interpreted as the probability ratio of occurrence described as graded membership values of the respective item in the dataset, reflecting the degree of support to the particular item [14], [16], [17]. The main intention of the linguistic rules testing is to obtain the accuracy of the generated linguistic association rules set, here; we called it the predictive strength. The performance measurements were the predictive ratio (PR), the dimension of rules (DR), rules confidence (Conf.) and number of rules generated (NR). All the measurements are as suggested in conventional quantitative association rules [1] except the PR. The PR is defined as in equation 2 below:

$$PR = \frac{matching\ c\ ase\ by\ rul\ es\ set}{Total\ case}\%$$

(2)

3 Experimental Study

In this research, FGMA technique [16] with MMFF [18] method and the BRQARM technique had been chosen as the comparison techniques to RMRARM. The minimum support threshold was set to 10% of the total instances while 70% was set as the minimum confidence threshold [19]. Five UCI machine learning repositories datasets were tested in the experiments, i.e. Auto-Mpg (AM), Bupa Liver Disorders (BUPA), Pima Indians Diabetes (PID), Glass Identification Database (GID) and Iris Plants (IP). Brief information about the data is shown in Table 1.

Table 1. Brief information of total instance (TI), mode of data (MD), total attributes (TA), continuous attribute (Cont. Atrr.), discrete attribute (DA), categorical attribute (CA), missing values (MV), and decision class (DC) on datasets used

Name	TI	MD	TA	Cont. Attr.	DA	CA	MV	DC
AM	398	Mix Mode	8	4	3	1	6	Cont.
BUPA	345	Nominal	7	-	7	-	-	2
PID	768	Quantitative	8	8	-	-	-	2
GID	214	Quantitative	9	9	-	-	-	7
IP	150	Quantitative	4	4	-	-	-	3

The testing data were run through FGMA, BRQARM and RMRARM algorithms. Reducts generated from FsR attribute reduction method were used as the initial attributes set in the testing data of BQARM and RMRARM techniques while FGMA induced its reducts set with MMFF method. The implementation of FsR is in [8]. The research had also looked into the effect of number of iterations in frequent itemsets discovery towards the experimental results. Two sets of experiment settings were used, i. e. the maximum iterations and the 5-iteration [20] setting. Table 2 and 3 show the example of linguistic association rules from IP dataset and their respective confidence values generated from 100/100 training-testing group with RMRARM and BRQARM techniques correspondingly.

Table 2. Example of rules from IP dataset with RMRARM technique

Linguistic Association Rules	*Rule Confidence*
IF PL.Medium^PW.Medium THEN PW.Short	0.887834199
IF PL. Medium ^PW. Short THEN PW. Medium	0.904912136
IF PL. Short ^PW. Medium THEN PW. Short	1
IF PL. Short ^PW. Short THEN PW. Medium	0.9
IF PL. Medium ^PW. Medium THEN PW. Short	0.887834199

Table 3. Example of rules from IP dataset with BRQARM technique

Linguistic Association Rules	*Rule Confidence*
IF PL.ExtremeShort THEN PW.Short	1
IF PL. Short THEN PW. Short	1
IF PL.Long THEN PW.Long	0.941176471

3.1 Experimental Findings

Table 4 and 5 shows the results of the selected techniques against the proposed RMRARM technique. Generally, the RMRARM technique shows a competitive performance against the comparison techniques. From the accuracy perspective, RMRARM tops the list in PID, GID and WR dataset. The predictive ratio of RMRARM is generally higher than FGMA and BRQARM except in AM and IP datasets while BRQARM stated a higher performance than FGMA in three out of five sets of data. In terms of average rules confidence, BRQARM demonstrated slightly better results among all techniques followed by RMRARM and FGMA.

The average dimension of rules stated by RMRARM is the highest of all three techniques. The large number of rules generated from RMRARM in BUPA and PID datasets was due to the 5-iteration constraint. As a consequences of large rules set, RMRARM registered a high predictive ratio in both BUPA and PID datasets. In most cases, FGMA and BRQARM generated more general rules as compared to RMRARM. For example, the rules in table 2 has higher dimension (more specific) as compared to the rules in table 3. Thus, rules in table 2 reveal more information and indirectly having lower confidence value since fewer cases had fulfilled the conditions as oppose to rules in table 3. However, due to the high reduction power in FsR, the reducts set generated in the initial testing data for BQARM and RMRARM were very limited causing inability in these cases to generate frequent itemsets especially with RMRARM technique.

Table 4. The comparison of highest (H) and average (A) readings of PR and Conf

Data		PR			Conf.		
		FGMA	BRQARM	RMRARM	FGMA	BRQARM	RMRARM
AM	H	100.00	100.00	100.00	0.99	0.94	1.00
	A	73.03	90.30	76.97	0.88	0.88	0.87
BUPA	H	100.00	100.00	100.00	1.00	0.93	0.98
	A	82.59	78.36	100	0.86	0.81	0.88
PID	H	100.00	100.00	100.00	0.93	1.00	0.95
	A	66.65	37.56	92.50	0.84	0.85	0.87
GID	H	67.88	100.00	100.00	1.00	1.00	1.00
	A	35.70	42.96	59.32	0.80	0.83	0.82
IP	H	93.33	100.00	100.00	0.97	1.00	1.00
	A	72.38	86.21	57.61	0.87	0.94	0.93

Table 5. The comparison of DR and NR

Data	DR			NR		
	FGMA	BRQARM	RMRARM	FGMA	BRQARM	RMRARM
AM	1.82	2.00	2.49	3.73	3.99	3.32
BUPA	4.47	3.31	4.87	44.03	7.60	16863.18
PID	3.46	2.58	4.50	962.13	4.04	1917.89
GID	2.29	2.22	3.02	2.19	2.95	11.91
IP	1.84	2.01	2.91	5.26	4.23	3.88

Table 6 shows the results on datasets that generate maximum frequent itemsets as compared to the 5-iteration constraint by all the comparison methods. The predictive ratio and the rules confidence shows a slight increase in test cases with 5-iteration constraint while the number of rules generated in maximum iterations are lesser in contrast. A general rule shows higher predictive power while a specific rule may discover more associations from the data since it involves more items in its frequent set. Therefore, very much depends on the purpose of study when choosing the focus in mining the association rules.

Table 6. The comparison result on maximum iteration and 5-iteration

Data		PR		Conf.		DR		NR	
		Max Iter	5 Iter	Max Iter	5 Iter	Max Iter	5 Iter	Max Iter	5 Iter
FGMA	BUPA	36.32	82.59	0.84	0.86	4.4	4.47	14.34	44.03
	PID	57.81	66.65	0.84	0.84	3.73	3.46	11.46	962.13
RMRARM	BUPA	100.00	100.00	0.88	0.88	10.61	4.87	3130.99	16863.18
	PID	92.50	92.50	0.86	0.87	5.96	4.50	326.98	1917.89
	GID	58.69	59.32	0.82	0.82	3.06	3.02	7.48	11.91

4 Conclusion and Future Work

Linguistic terms can convey knowledge more naturally especially in association rules involving quantitative intervals. The rough-Apriori based RMRARM technique is comparatively capable in capturing the soft boundary intervals using the rough membership function. The experimental results showed that RMRARM technique is able to generate more specific rules as compared to other comparison techniques while maintaining its predictive ratio and confidence rate. However, the disadvantage is that it is unable to mine data with only one attribute involved. Thus, future research may look into setting a balance of reduction power, the rules prediction ratio and number of iteration in the frequent itemsets discovery while implementing RMRARM. Apart from that, the results show that by choosing a good discretization method, i.e. the Boolean reasoning method in quantitative association rules mining, the efficiency of the algorithm increases as compared to fuzzy association rules mining technique. Although this paper has pointed out the possibility of utilizing rough membership values in linguistic association rules mining, the appropriate parameters of minimum support, minimum confidence and the optimum iteration in frequent itemsets discovery will still need to be studied in detail.

Acknowledgement. We thank the anonymous reviewers for their valuable comments and suggestions that substantially improve this paper.

References

1. Srikant, R., Agrawal, R.: Mining Quantitative Association Rules in Large Relational Tables. In: Proc. The 1996 ACM SIGMOD International Conference on Management of Data, pp. 1–12. ACM Press, Montreal (1996)
2. Ishibuchi, H., Yamamoto, T., Nakashima, T.: Linguistic Modeling for Function Approximation Using Grid Partitions. In: Proc. The 10th IEEE International Conference on Fuzzy Systems, vol. 1, pp. 47–50. IEEE, Melbourne (2001)
3. Shu Yue, J., Tsang, E., Yeung, D., Shi, D.: Mining Fuzzy Association Rules with Weighted Items. In: Proc. IEEE International Conference on Systems, Man, and Cybernetics, Nashville, TN, vol. 3, pp. 1906–1911 (2000)

4. Pawlak, Z.: Rough Sets and Data Analysis. In: Proc. the 1996 Asian Fuzzy Systems Symposium, Soft Computing in Intelligent Systems and Information Processing, pp. 1–6. IEEE, Kenting (1996)
5. Ishibuchi, H., Nakashima, T., Yamamoto, T.: Fuzzy Association Rules for Handling Continuous Attributes. In: Proc. ISIE 2001 International Symposium on Industrial Electronics, vol. 1, pp. 118–121. IEEE, Pusan (2001)
6. Pawlak, Z.: Some Issues on Rough Sets. In: Peters, J.F., Skowron, A., Grzymała-Busse, J.W., Kostek, B.z., Świniarski, R.W., Szczuka, M.S. (eds.) Transactions on Rough Sets I. LNCS, vol. 3100, pp. 1–58. Springer, Heidelberg (2004)
7. Zhong, N., Skowron, A.: A Rough Set-Based Knowledge Discovery Process. International Journal of Applied Mathematics and Computer Science 11(3), 603–619 (2001)
8. Choo, Y.-H., Bakar, A.A., Hamdan, A.R.: The Fitness-Rough: A New Attribute Reduction Method Based on Statistical and Rough Set Theory. Intelligence Data Analysis 12(1), 73–87 (2008)
9. Ohrn, A.: Technical Reference Manual. Ph.D. Norwegian University of Science and Technology, Trondheim, Norway, pp.16-18 (2001)
10. Pawlak, Z., Skowron, A.: Rough Sets and Boolean Reasoning. International Journal of Information Sciences 177(1), 41–73 (2007)
11. Pawlak, Z., Skowron, A.: Rudiments of Rough Sets. Journal of Information Sciences 177(1), 3–27 (2007)
12. Yao, Y.: Two Views of the Theory of Rough Sets in Finite Universes. International Journal of Approximate Reasoning 15(4), 291–317 (1996)
13. Abu Bakar, A.: Propositional Satisfiability Method in Rough Classification Modeling for Data Mining. Ph.D. Universiti Putra Malaysia (2002)
14. Polkowski, L.: Rough Set Theory: An Introduction. Rough Sets Mathematical Foundations, pp. 5–6. Physica-Verlag, Heidelberg (2002)
15. Yao, Y.: A Comparative Study of Fuzzy Sets and Rough Sets. Journal of Information Sciences 109(1-4), 227–242 (1998)
16. Hong, T.-P., Lin, K.-Y., Wang, S.-L.: Fuzzy Data Mining for Interesting Generalized Association Rules. Fuzzy Sets and Systems 138(2), 255–269 (2003)
17. Kaya, M., Alhajj, R.: Mining Multi-Cross-Level Fuzzy Weighted Association Rules. In: Proc. Second IEEE International Conference on Intelligent Systems, vol. 1, pp. 225–230. IEEE, Los Alamitos (2004)
18. Hong, T.-P., Chen, J.-B.: Processing Individual Fuzzy Attributes for Fuzzy Rule Induction. Fuzzy Sets and Systems 112, 127–140 (2000)
19. Zhang, W.: Mining Fuzzy Quantitative Association Rules. In: Proc. 11th IEEE International Conference on Tools with Artificial Intelligent, pp. 99–102. IEEE, Chicago (1999)
20. He, Z., Xu, X., Huang, J.Z., Deng, S.: A Frequent Pattern Discovery Method for Outlier Detection. In: Li, Q., Wang, G., Feng, L. (eds.) WAIM 2004. LNCS, vol. 3129, pp. 726–732. Springer, Heidelberg (2004)

Mining Causal Knowledge from Diagnostic Knowledge

Xiangdong An[1,2] and Nick Cercone[1]

[1] Department of Computer Science and Engineering
York University, Toronto, ON M3J 1P3, Canada
xan@cs.yorku.ca, ncercone@yorku.ca
[2] Alpha Global IT Inc., Toronto, ON M3B 2W7, Canada
xiangdong.an@alpha-it.com

Abstract. Diagnostic knowledge is the basis of many non-Bayesian medical systems. To explore the advantages of their Bayesian counterparts, we need causal knowledge. This paper investigates how to mine causal knowledge from the diagnostic knowledge. Experiments indicate the proposed mining method works pretty well.

1 Introduction

In medical systems, the *diagnostic knowledge* or *rules* are those that govern the derivation of diseases from symptoms (laboratory test results), and the *causal knowledge* or *rules* are those contrary. We similarly call inference from symptoms to diseases *diagnostic* or *causal* (*predictive*) otherwise. It turns out many non-Bayesian medical systems work on diagnostic rules [1,2]. These rules may be induced from diagnostic knowledge [3]. In such systems, causal inference may not be supported. However, in healthcare we may need inference in both directions. For example, for evidence-based medicine [4] we need both diagnostic and causal inferences to evaluate evidence. Compared to other uncertain reasoning formalisms, Bayesian networks (BNs) are good in mathematically soundly combining inferences in both directions [5]. They are also good in showing the flow of information on dependency links. BNs can be specified by either diagnostic or causal or mixed knowledge, but those specified by causal knowledge tend to be sparse [6] and hence computationally efficient. Note to specify a dependency in a BN we only need knowledge (rules) in one direction. The inference in the other direction is automated by BNs based on Bayes' theorem. To explore the advantages of BNs, we may be motivated to construct the Bayesian counterparts of non-Bayesian medical systems, where the causal knowledge can be acquired in different ways: (1) we can learn it from medical records; (2) we can obtain it from medical experts; or (3) we find it from available diagnostic rules or knowledge bases. We may not be able to obtain sufficient medical records for every medical area of a general medical diagnostic system. Medical experts may not always be accessible or may not be comfortable working with uncertain concepts. Their knowledge could be very biased and needs a lot of adjustments for even a small system. Hence, it is beneficial to investigate how to extract causal knowledge from available diagnostic knowledge. It turns out diagnostic knowledge is not sufficient to derive causal knowledge from. In this paper, we discuss assumptions that need to be made to mine causal knowledge from diagnostic knowledge and how.

C. Tang et al. (Eds.): ADMA 2008, LNAI 5139, pp. 556–562, 2008.

The rest of the paper is organized as follows. In Section 2, we specifically discuss the advantages of medical BN systems. In Section 3, we present causal knowledge extraction method. In Section 4, we experimentally show the proposed mining method works well. Conclusions are made in Section 5.

2   Medical BN Systems

In the following discussion, we will use lowercase letters (e.g. x, y, z) for random variables, capital letters (e.g. X, Y, Z) for sets of variables, and boldfaced lowercase letters (e.g. **x, y, z**) for specific values taken by variables, and boldfaced capital letters (e.g. **X, Y, Z**) for value configurations assigned to sets of variables. We will use D_x or D_X to represent the space of x or X, which contains all values or configurations x or X can take. We will use short notation $P(\mathbf{x})$ for the probabilities $P(x = \mathbf{x})$, and $P(\mathbf{X})$ for $P(X = \mathbf{X})$, where $\mathbf{x} \in D_x$ and $\mathbf{X} \in D_X$.

Assume we use d to denote some disease concerned, which could take value *true* or *false*, and S to denote the set of symptoms (test results) related. Then the diagnostic knowledge regarding d and S can be represented by $P(d|S)$, which specifies the probability of $P(d = true)$ or $P(d = false)$ given each value configuration of S. Let $S = \{s_1, s_2, ..., s_m\}$. Table 1 illustrates $P(d = true|S)$, where $D_{s_1} = \{thickened, thinning, normal\}$, $D_{s_2} = \{low, high, normal\}$, ..., and $D_{s_m} = \{inverted, upright\}$.

Table 1. Illustration of $P(d = true|S)$

s_1	s_2	...	s_m	$P(d = true|S)$
thickened	low	...	inverted	0.96
thickened	low	...	upright	0.92
$\vdots$	$\vdots$	$\vdots$	$\vdots$	$\vdots$
thinning	high	...	inverted	0.72
thinning	high	...	upright	0.63
$\vdots$	$\vdots$	$\vdots$	$\vdots$	$\vdots$

With such diagnostic knowledge, a BN can be directly specified as in Figure 1 (a). In this BN, d is dependent on every symptom, and given d, every symptom is dependent of every other symptom. This makes the computational complexity of the inference grow exponentially in the number of variables in the domain. When applying the most popular and general junction tree inference [7] method to the BN, it would be compiled into a single clique junction tree. A clique in a junction tree corresponds to a maximal complete graph as shown in Figure 1 (b). Another problem with a BN specified such is that we cannot perform causal inference (i.e. the inference contrary to the arrow direction) properly due to the lack of $P(S) = P(s_1, s_2, ..., s_m)$. Without $P(S)$, we have difficulty to obtain $P(T|d)$ for any $T \subseteq S$ from $P(d|S)$. That is, a medical system built only on diagnostic knowledge may not be able to perform causal inference properly.

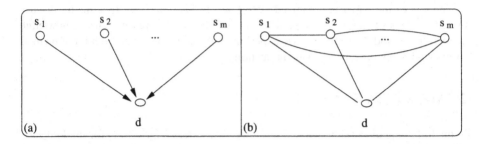

Fig. 1. A BN from diagnostic knowledge and its compilation: (a) The BN from diagnostic knowledge on relationship between disease d and symptoms $S = \{s_1, s_2, ..., s_m\}$; (b) The BN becomes a complete graph after compilation

How if we build a BN using causal knowledge? Figure 2 (a) shows the corresponding BN built from the causal knowledge $P(s_1|d)$, $P(s_2|d)$, ..., $P(s_m|d)$. Its junction tree is composed of a set of small cliques as shown in Figure 2 (b). An immediate observation is that we only need to maintain small probability distributions $P(d, s_1)$, $P(d, s_2)$, ..., $P(d, s_m)$ to perform inference. Compared to the inference by maintaining $P(d, s_1, s_2, ..., s_m)$ for the BN in Figure 1 (a), inference becomes much cheap here. Another advantage of building BNs from causal knowledge is that diagnostic knowledge $P(S)$ is generally more tenuous than causal knowledge [8]. For example, doctors usually have no idea on how many patients having headaches have flu though they do know how many patients with flu have headaches.

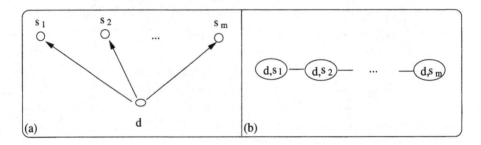

Fig. 2. A BN from causal knowledge and its compilation: (a) The BN from causal knowledge on relationship between disease d and symptoms $S = \{s_1, s_2, ..., s_m\}$; (b) The junction tree is composed of a set of small cliques

3   Causal Knowledge Mining

We prefer to build BNs with causal knowledge $P(s_1|d)$, $P(s_2|d)$, ..., $P(s_m|d)$. For our problem, we only have diagnostic knowledge $P(S) = P(d|s_1, s_2, ..., s_m)$, however. In this section, we discuss how to find causal knowledge from diagnostic one.

Since

$$P(s_i|d) = \frac{\sum_{S\setminus\{s_i\}} P(d|s_1, s_2, ..., s_m)P(s_1, s_2, ..., s_m)}{P(d)}(1 \leq i \leq m), \qquad (1)$$

we need probability distributions $P(s_1, s_2, ..., s_m)$ and $P(d)$ to specify $P(s_i|d)(1 \leq i \leq m)$ exactly. We have neither, however. Next we discuss if we can ignore one of them and based on what conditions the ignorance is valid.

Since

$$P(d, s_1, s_2, ..., s_m) = P(d|s_1, s_2, ..., s_m)P(s_1, s_2, ..., s_m),$$

and we can obtain $P(d)$ from $P(d, s_1, s_2, ..., s_m)$ by marginalizing out $s_1, s_2, ..., s_m$:

$$P(d) = \sum_S P(d, s_1, s_2, ..., s_m),$$

we can obtain $P(d)$ from $P(d|s_1, s_2, ..., s_m)$ and $P(s_1, s_2, ..., s_m)$. However, from $P(d)$ and $P(d|s_1, s_2, ..., s_m)$, we cannot obtain $P(s_1, s_2, ..., s_m)$. So, we choose to ignore $P(s_1, s_2, ..., s_m)$ if we have to ignore one of them. To validate the ignorance, we need Assumption 1.

Assumption 1. *Symptom distribution* $P(S) = P(s_1, s_2, ..., s_m)$ *is uniform.*

By Assumption 1, Equation 1 becomes

$$P(s_i|d) = \frac{\sum_{S\setminus\{s_i\}} P(d|s_1, s_2, ..., s_m)}{P(d)}(1 \leq i \leq m), \qquad (2)$$

where $P(d) = \sum_S P(d|s_1, s_2, ..., s_m)$. That is,

$$P(s_i|d) = \frac{\sum_{S\setminus\{s_i\}} P(d|s_1, s_2, ..., s_m)}{\sum_S P(d|s_1, s_2, ..., s_m)}(1 \leq i \leq m). \qquad (3)$$

Therefore, by Assumption 1, we can obtain all probability distributions $P(d)$, $P(s_1|d)$, $P(s_2|d)$, ..., $P(s_m|d)$ that are needed to specify the BN as shown in Figure 2 (a).

You may have noted that by modeling the relationship between a disease and its symptoms with a BN as shown in Figure 2 (a), another Assumption 2 is implied.

Assumption 2. *Given* d, s_1, s_2, ..., s_m *are independent of each other.*

BNs as shown in Figure 2 (a) are called naive BNs. Naive BNs have been proved successful in many medical applications (e.g. [9]), though assumption 2 may not necessarily hold in the real world. In the next section, we by experiments evaluate the causal knowledge mining method.

4   Experiment

The experiment is made based on the diagnostic knowledge of four cardiologic diseases. The four cardiological diseases are abdominal aortic aneurysm, aortic dissection, thoracic aortic aneurysm, and dilated cardiomyopathy. The diagnostic knowledge for each disease is presented in a table as shown in Table 1, which has been validated by medical experts. From the four tables of diagnostic knowledge we calculate four sets of causal knowledge and use them to construct four BNs, each modeling the relationship between one disease and its symptoms (lab test results). The four BNs can then be used to evaluate the probabilities of diseases given their symptoms. We would like our BNs to provide diagnoses which are consistent with the diagnostic knowledge tables. To verify this, we perform Bayesian inference with these BNs and obtain the probabilities of each disease on all different laboratory test results. We compare these probabilities with those provided in diagnostic knowledge tables. It turns out they are very consistent with each other.

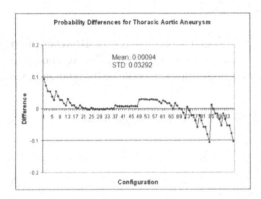 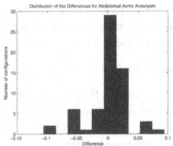

Fig. 3. Probability differences for thoracic aortic aneurysm

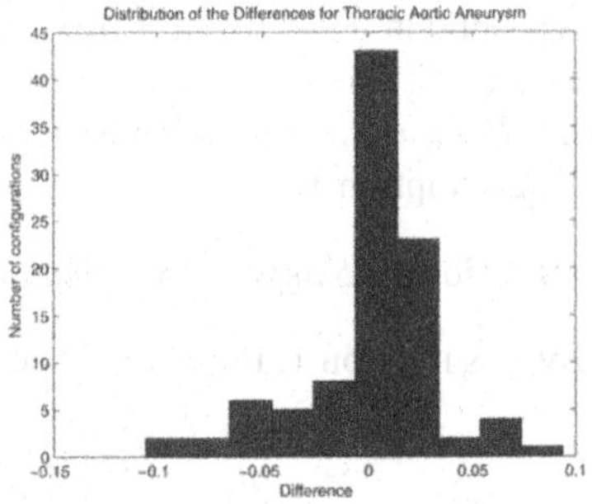

Fig. 4. Distribution of the probability differences for thoracic aortic aneurysm

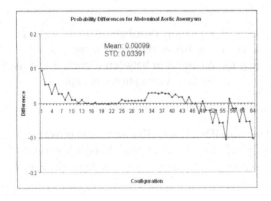

Fig. 5. Probability differences for abdominal aortic aneurysm

Fig. 6. Distribution of the probability differences for abdominal aortic aneurysm

Figure 3 shows the diagnosis differences on all different configurations of symptoms for thoracic aortic aneurysm. Almost all differences are within ±0.1 and most of them are close to 0. The mean and standard deviation are 0.00094 and 0.03292, respectively. Figure 4 specifically shows the distribution of these probability differences. As observed in Figure 3, most are located within ±0.025.

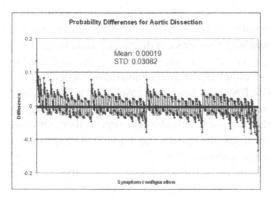

Fig. 7. Probability differences for aortic dissection

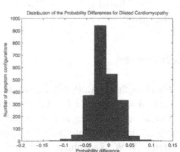

Fig. 8. Distribution of the probability differences for aortic dissection

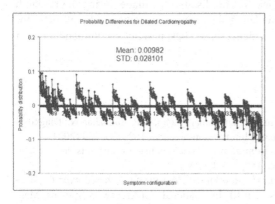

Fig. 9. Probability differences for dilated cardiomyopathy

Fig. 10. Distribution of the probability differences for dilated cardiomyopathy.

For the other three diseases, we get similar results, which are shown in Figures 5 and 6, 7 and 8, and 9 and 10, respectively. All means are less than 0.01 and all standard deviations are lower than 0.04. Their distribution figures indicate that an overwhelming majority of these differences is located within ±0.05. This indicates BNs from the mined causal knowledge work pretty consistently with the diagnostic knowledge tables.

With BNs, we do not have to get all test results to reason about the disease probabilities as with the diagnostic knowledge tables. That is, missing evidence is allowed, and we can infer with whatever evidence we have. Compared to other methods for uncertain reasoning, e.g. fuzzy rules based fuzzy logic, BNs can combine both causal and diagnostic inferences mathematically soundly. BNs can also show us how the information (influence) flows on dependency chains.

5   Conclusion

To explore the advantages of BN inference, in this paper we investigate how to mine causal knowledge from diagnostic knowledge. It turns out diagnostic knowledge is not sufficient to derive causal knowledge from. We provide two assumptions that need to be assumed to effectively extract causal knowledge from diagnostic knowledge for constructing naive BNs. Experiments show BNs built from the causal knowledge obtained from the proposed approach provide very consistent diagnoses as presented in diagnostic knowledge tables. This indicates the proposed method works very well on our cases in deriving causal knowledge from the diagnostic knowledge. Large scale experiments will be performed to further confirm the conclusion.

Besides medical areas, the proposed method can also be applied to non-medical areas such as equipment diagnosis.

Acknowledgment

We would like to thank William Melek for the discussions made during the research and diagnostic knowledge tables provided. This research is supported by NSERC for the project "finding best evidence for evidence-based best practice recommendations in health care".

References

1. Roychowdhury, A., Pratihar, D.K., Bose, N., Sankaranarayanan, K.P., Sudhahar, N.: Diagnosis of the disease-using a GA-fuzzy approach. Information Sciences 162, 105–120 (2004)
2. Tsumoto, S.: Mining diagnostic rules from clinical databases using rough sets and medical diagnostic model. Information Sciences 162, 65–80 (2004)
3. Melek, W.W., Sadeghian, A., Najjaran, H., Hoorfar, M.: A neurofuzzy-based expert system for disease diagnosis. In: Proceedings of IEEE International Conference on Systems, Man, and Cybernetics, pp. 3736–3741 (2005)
4. Eddy, D.M.: Evidence-based medicine: A unified approach. Health Affairs 24, 9–17 (2005)
5. Aradhye, H., Heger, A.S.: Signal validation using Bayesian belief networks and fuzzy logic. Fuzzy logic and probability applications: bridging the gap, 365–392 (2002)
6. D'Ambrosio, B.: Inference in Bayesian networks. AI Magazine 20, 21–36 (1999)
7. Jensen, F.V.: An introduction to Bayesian networks. UCL Press, London (1996)
8. Russell, S., Norvig, P.: Artificial Intelligence: A Modern Approach. Prentice Hall, New Jersey (1995)
9. Kukar, M., Grošelj, C.: Reliable diagnosis for coronary artery disease. In: Proceedings of the 15th IEEE Symposium on Computer-Based Medical Systems (CBMS 2002), Maribor, Slovenia, pp. 7–12 (2002)

Modified Particle Swarm Optimizer with Adaptive Dynamic Weights for Cancer Combinational Chemotherapy

Harish Chandra Soundararajan[1], Jagannathan Raman[2], and R. Muthucumaraswamy [3]

[1]Department of Electronics and Communication Engineering
[2] Department of Electrical and Electronics Engineering
[3] Department of Information Technology, Sri Venkateswara College of Engineering Pennalur, Sriperumbudur - 602105 :: Tamil Nadu, India
harish@svce.ac.in, jagan_raman567@yahoo.com,
msamy@svce.ac.in

Abstract. Cancer combinational chemotherapy is a complex treatment process that requires balancing the administration of anti-cancer drug to reduce tumor size with the adverse toxic side effects caused by these drugs. Methods of computational optimization like Genetic Algorithm (GA) and Canonical Particle Swarm Optimization (CPSO) have been used to strike the right balance. The purpose of this paper is to study how an alternative optimization technique - Modified Particle Swarm Optimizer (MPSO) - can be used for finding optimal chemotherapeutic treatments in an efficient manner. Comparison of its performance with the other existing algorithms of MPSO has been shown.

Keywords: Modified Particle Swarm Optimizer, Cancer chemotherapy, Adaptive dynamic weights, Computation optimization.

1 Introduction

Many decision-making processes involve searching through a large space of possible solutions. In the combinational chemotherapy optimization problem, the size of the solution space increases exponentially with the number of decision variables, the values of which need to satisfy certain feasibility criteria. Finding an optimal solution is a difficult task in such situations by using conventional optimization methods. It has been found that GA and CPSO show a good and robust performance on a class of non-linear, multi-constrained chemotherapy design problems [1] - [5]. However, the field of evolutionary computation is growing, and alternative techniques of particle swarm optimization (PSO) are being developed [6] - [8]. The attraction to PSO is that it is a population-based optimization technique that is based on the 'social-psychological tendency of individual particles' within the swarm to 'emulate the success of other individuals' [9]. The search behavior of a particle is governed by the experience of its neighbours, aimed at efficient search through complex structures that have unpredictable solutions spaces. Combinational chemotherapy exhibits properties as multimodality and disjoint

C. Tang et al. (Eds.): ADMA 2008, LNAI 5139, pp. 563–571, 2008.
© Springer-Verlag Berlin Heidelberg 2008

nature of feasible regions in the solution space. The purpose of this paper is to study the capabilities of MPSO [6] - [8] to solve the optimization problem of cancer combinational chemotherapy and to compare their efficiency.

2 Problem Background

Amongst the therapeutic methods to cure cancer, combinational chemotherapy is considered as the most complex methodology [10]. Hence it is very difficult to find effective chemotherapy treatments without a systematic approach. In order to arrive at such an approach, medical aspects of cancer treatment must be taken into account.

2.1 Medical Aspects of Chemotherapy

All the drugs used in cancer chemotherapy have narrow therapeutic indices. Therefore the concentration levels at which these drugs are administered to reduce the tumor size are close to those levels at which unacceptable toxic side-effects occur. Hence effective treatment schedule are obtained by balancing the beneficial and adverse effects of a combination of different drugs, administered in a well scheduled treatment period [2]. The beneficial effects of cancer chemotherapy correspond to treatment objectives that oncologists want to achieve by means of administering anti-cancer drugs. A cancer chemotherapy treatment may be either curative or palliative. Curative treatment attempts to eradicate the tumor; palliative treatments are applied only when a tumor is found to be incurable with the objective to maintain a reasonable quality of life as long as possible.Since most anti-cancer drugs are highly toxic and administered through the blood stream, they cause damage to sensitive tissues in many parts of the body. In order to limit this damage, toxicity constraints are placed on the amount of drug applied at any time interval. Constraints are also placed on the cumulative drug dosage over the treatment period, and on the damage caused to various sensitive tissues due to these drugs [10]. In addition to toxicity constraints, the tumor size must be maintained below a lethal level during the whole treatment period.

The goal of cancer chemotherapy therefore is to achieve the beneficial effects of chemotherapy treatment without violating any of the above mentioned constraints.

2.2 Problem Definition

To solve the optimization problem of cancer chemotherapy, a set of treatment schedules, which satisfies toxicity and tumor size constraints and at the same time yielding acceptable values of treatment objectives has to be found. Anti-cancer drugs are usually delivered according to a discrete dosage program in which there are n doses given at times $t_1, t_2, \ldots t_n$ [11]. In the case of combinational chemotherapy, each dose is a combination of d drugs defined by the concentration levels C_{ij}, $i \in (1,n)$, $j \in (1,d)$. The solution space Ω of the chemotherapy optimization problem is the set of control vectors $c = (C_{ij})$ representing the drug concentration profiles. But, not all of these profiles are used for chemotherapy treatment, since chemotherapy is constrained in a number of ways. Although the constraint sets of chemotherapeutic treatment vary for each drug and cancer type, they generally have the following form [5]:

1. Maximum instantaneous dose C_{max} for each drug acting as a single agent:

$$g_1(\mathbf{c}) = \{ C_{max\,j} - C_{ij} \geq 0, \ \forall\, i \in (1,n), \ \forall\, j \in (1,d) \} \tag{1}$$

2. Maximum cumulative C_{cum} dose for drug acting as a single agent:

$$g_2(\mathbf{c}) = \{ C_{cum\,j} - \sum_{i=1}^{n} C_{ij} \geq 0, \ \forall\, i \in (1,n), \ \forall\, j \in (1,d) \} \tag{2}$$

3. Maximum permissible size N_{max} of the tumor:

$$g_3(\mathbf{c}) = \{ N_{max} - N(t_i) \geq 0, \ \forall\, i \in (1,n) \} \tag{3}$$

4. Restriction on the toxic side-effects of multi-drug chemotherapy:

$$g_4(\mathbf{c}) = \{ C_{s\text{-}eff\,k} - \sum_{j=1}^{d} \eta_{kj}\, C_{ij} \geq 0, \ \forall\, i \in (1,n), \ \forall\, k \in (1,m) \} \tag{4}$$

The factors η_{kj} represent the risk of damaging the kth organ or tissue by administering the jth drug. Estimates of these factors for the drugs most commonly used in treatment of breast cancer can be found in [12, 13]. Tumor eradication is the primary objective of cancer combinational chemotherapy. Eradication of tumor is defined as the reduction of the tumor from an initial size of around 10^9 cancer cells to below 10^3 cancer cells. In order to simulate the response of cancer tumor to chemotherapy, the Gompertz growth model with a linear cell-loss effect is used [10]:

$$\frac{dN}{dt} = N(t).\left[\lambda \ln\left(\frac{\theta}{N(t)}\right) - \sum_{j=1}^{d} \kappa_j \sum_{i=1}^{n} C_{ij} \{ H(t - t_i) - H(t - t_{i+1}) \} \right] \tag{5}$$

where $N(t)$ represents the number of tumor cells at time t ; λ, Θ are the parameters of tumor growth, $H(t)$ is the Heaviside step function; κ_j are the quantities representing the efficacy of anti-cancer drugs, and C_{ij} denote the concentration levels of these drugs. One advantage of the Gompertz model from the computational optimization point of view is that the equation (5) yields an analytical solution after the substitution $u(t) = \ln(\theta / N(t))$ [14]. Since $u(t)$ increases when $N(t)$ decreases, the primary optimization objective of tumor eradication can be framed as follows [3]:

$$\underset{c}{\text{minimize}} \quad F(\mathbf{c}) = \sum_{i=1}^{n} N(t_i) \tag{6}$$

3 Methodology

This section explains how the optimization problem of cancer chemotherapy can be solved by the different algorithms of MPSO [6] - [8].

3.1 Modified Particle Swarm Optimizer (MPSO)

The MPSO algorithm is initialized with a population of particles which are considered to be solutions for the cancer combinational chemotherapy problem. These particles are flown through the hyperspace Ω of solutions to the chemotherapy optimization problem described in the previous section. The position of each particle c_i^{k+1} at iteration $k+1$ corresponds to a treatment regimen of anti-cancer drugs and is determined by the following formula:

$$c_i^{k+1} = c_i^k + v_i^k \qquad (7)$$

where v_i^k is a randomized velocity vector assigned to each particle in a swarm before the start of the algorithm. The velocity vector drives the optimization process towards the objective and reflects the 'socially exchanged' information. There exist different algorithms of the CPSO that regulate how this 'social' information is exchanged. The first algorithms – *individual best*, the second algorithm – *local best* and the third algorithm – *global best* [9]. Each particle in the swarm is attracted towards the position representing best chemotherapeutic treatments found by the particle itself, its neighbours, and/or the entire population. This is achieved by defining the velocity vector in (7) for each particle as:

$$v_i^k = \omega.v_i^{k-1} + b_1.r_1.(gbest - c_i^{k-1}) + b_2.r_2.(ibest - c_i^{k-1}) \qquad (8)$$

where, ω is the inertia coefficient; b_1 and b_2 are empirical coefficients used to improve PSO performance; r_1 and r_2 are random numbers in the range [0,1]; *ibest* and *gbest* are the best locations in Ω found by the particle i and the entire population respectively; v_i^{k-1} is the velocity value of particle i at the previous iteration of the algorithm, the initial velocity values are assigned at random. The PSO algorithm works by finding a new position for each particle using (7) and (8), evaluating them and updating the personal and global best values. There also exist three different models of MPSO that are demarcated based on the method by which inertia coefficient ω is updated for each iteration of the MPSO algorithm. All the three models use equation (7) for calculating and updating position. The difference in the three algorithms occurs in equation (8). The first model was proposed by Shi and Eberhart [15] and it uses the following formula to calculate ω (inertia coefficient):

$$\text{Model 1:} \quad \omega = (iter_{max} - iter_{cur})\left(\frac{\omega_{initial} - \omega_{final}}{iter_{max}}\right) + \omega_{final} \qquad (9)$$

where $\omega_{initial}$ and ω_{final} represent the initial and final inertia coefficient respectively at the start of a given run, $iter_{max}$ the maximum number of iterations in a offered run, and $iter_{cur}$ the current iteration number at the present time step. Then, a different version of dynamic inertia weight was proposed by Chatterjee and Siarry [7]. They presented a nonlinear function that modulates the inertia weight with time for improving the performance of the PSO algorithm. The main modification is the determination of the inertia weight as a nonlinear function of the current iteration number at each time step. The dynamic function of ω was modified as follows:

$$\text{Model 2:} \quad \omega = \left(\frac{iter_{max} - iter_{cur}}{iter_{max}}\right)^n (\omega_{initial} - \omega_{final}) + \omega_{final} \qquad (10)$$

More recently, a different version of dynamic inertia weight was proposed by Shu-Kai S.Fan, Ju-Ming Chang [8].They presented a novel nonlinear function regulating inertia weight adaptation with a dynamic mechanism for enhancing the performance of PSO algorithms. The principal modification is the determination of the inertia weight through a nonlinear function at each time step. The nonlinear function is given by:

Model 3: $$\omega = (d)^r \omega_{initial} \tag{11}$$

where d is the decrease rate ranging between 1.0 and 0.1, and r the dynamic adaptation parameter depending on the following rules for successive adjustment at each time step. For a minimization case, it follows [8]

$$\text{if } f(P_{gd\text{-}new}) < f(P_{gd\text{-}old}) \text{ then } r \leftarrow r\text{-}1;$$

$$\text{if } f(P_{gd\text{-}new}) > f(P_{gd\text{-}old}) \text{ then } r \leftarrow r\text{+}1;$$

where $P_{gd\text{-}new}$ and $P_{gd\text{-}old}$ denote the global best solutions at current and previous time steps, respectively. This mechanism is to ensure that particles fly more quickly toward the potential optimal solution, and then through decreasing inertia weight to perform local refinement around the neighborhood of the optimal solution.

4 Experiments

In this study we have compared three models (9), (10), (11) for the MPSO algorithm. Each of these models contain two algorithms one for global best MPSO and another for local best MPSO. The comparison has been done on the problem of multi-drug cancer combinational chemotherapy optimization addressed in [1] - [3], [5]. The optimization objective is to minimize the overall tumor burden $F(\mathbf{c})$ defined by (6) with the aim to eradicate the tumor. The initially declared swarm consists of 50 particles, these particles are the concentration value for each drug, in every dose in which the drug is administered (C_{ij}). The drug concentration values are declared in random based on the constraints in (1) - (4). Each particle in the swarm is also assigned a random initial velocity value in the range [0,2]. For the iterations performed after that, equation (7) and (8) carry out the updation of position and velocity v_i^k where k represents the iterations and i$\in$ (1,50). The following value are taken for the other parameters in (8) according to [16] - ω is assigned values according to (9), (10) and (11); $b_1=b_2=4$; r_1 and r_2 are randomly generated numbers in the range [0,1]. For the local best MPSO algorithm, the neighborhood size was chosen to be 20% of the population, i.e. each neighborhood contains 10 particles and is formed on the basis of the numerical indexes assigned to these particles. The programs implementing MPSO for all the three algorithms differentiated by (9) - (11) are written in MATLAB; these programs run until a predefined termination criterion is satisfied. Since it is really difficult for all the particles in the swarm to have the exact same value at the end of a run, a small threshold was chosen to find out when a solution was reached. Because of the randomized nature of algorithms under investigation, the programs implementing local and global best MPSO for all three algorithms were run 30 times each. In order to sharpen the comparison of performance, the same set of 30 random starting populations was used for each of the algorithms tested. This ensures that differences in performance between algorithms cannot be related to a relatively poor set of random starting values.

5 Results

During each trial run of the programs implementing MPSO for Model 1, 2 and 3, the following outcomes were recorded as [5]:

- the number of algorithms' iterations (referred to as generations) required to find a feasible (i.e. satisfying all the constraints (1)-(4) and having minimum fitness function value) solution;
- the minimum value of the fitness function found at each iteration of the algorithms;
- the best solution found at the end of a trial run.

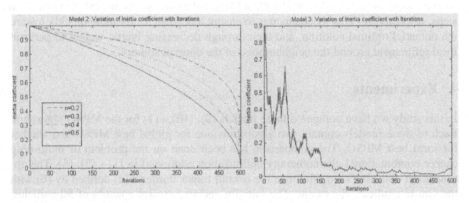

Fig. 1. Represents the variation of inertia coefficient (ω) with iterations for equation (10) for different n values (left) and equation (11) (right)

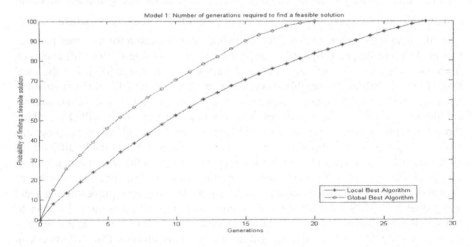

Fig. 2. Number of generations needed to find a feasible solution for Model 1

The figures 2, 3 and 4 below present the comparative results based on the first measure - the mean number of generations required to find a feasible solution. The data are represented in the format adopted in [17].

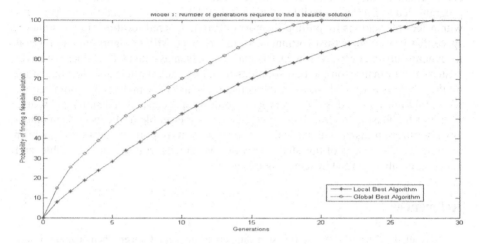

Fig. 3. Number of generations needed to find a feasible solution for Model 2

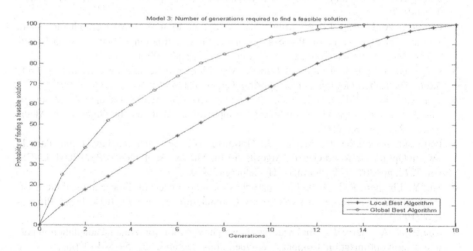

Fig. 4. Number of generations needed to find a feasible solution for Model 3

6 Discussions

Previous work [1] - [3], [5] has shown that GA and CPSO can be useful in solving the multi-constrained and multi-dimensional problem of cancer chemotherapy optimization. The present study has demonstrated that an alternative technique - Modified Particle Swarm Optimization - is able to achieve the same optimization objective in a new and faster method than [5]. The ability of the PSO algorithms to explore the solution space faster than GA has been reported in [16]. Our experimental results have shown that MPSO can explore the solution space faster than PSO. This work also shows that the MPSO algorithms, the global best MPSO in particular, optimize cancer chemotherapy treatments in a more robust manner – all trial runs of the MPSO programs led to finding a feasible solution. The PSO algorithms tend to keep particles within feasible regions by pulling them toward remembered locations in the solution space that proved their trustworthiness. In this respect, MPSO algorithm can rely on its dynamically changing inertia coefficient – the advantage that CPSO does not have. Historical information on the best solutions found by each particle and the population on the whole is a valuable asset in the context of cancer chemotherapy optimization, where multiple constraints and a very large solution space lead to a disjoint and sparse nature of the feasible region. Finding a solution to the problem of cancer chemotherapy optimization faster without losing its quality is an important and useful goal for oncologists. The results of this study show that MPSO algorithms can be a viable, and better, alternative to PSO in achieving this goal.

References

1. McCall, J., Petrovski, A.: A Decision Support System for Cancer Chemotherapy Using Genetic Algorithms. In: Proceedings of the International Conference on Computational Intelligence for Modelling, Control and Automation, vol. 1, pp. 65–70. IOS Press, Amsterdam (1999)
2. Petrovski, A., McCall, J.A.W.: Multi-objective optimisation of cancer chemotherapy using evolutionary algorithms. In: Proceedings of the First International Conference on Evolutionary Multi-Criterion Optimisation, Zurich, Switzerland (2001)
3. Petrovski, A.: An Application of Genetic Algorithms to Chemotherapy Treatment. Ph.D thesis, The Robert Gordon University, Aberdeen, U.K (1999)
4. Tan, K.C., Khor, E.F., Cai, J., Heng, C.M., Lee, T.H.: Automating the drug scheduling of cancer chemotherapy via evolutionary computation. Artificial Intelligence in Medicine 25(2), 169–185 (2002)
5. Petrovski, A., Sudha, B., McCall, J.: Optimising Cancer Chemotherapy Using Particle Swarm Optimisation and Genetic Algorithms. In: Yao, X., et al. (eds.) PPSN 2004. LNCS, vol. 3242, pp. 302–9743. Springer, Heidelberg (2004)
6. Shi, Y., Eberhart, R.C.: A modified particle swarm optimizer. In: Proceedings of the IEEE International Conference on Evolutionary Computation, pp. 69–73. IEEE Press, Piscataway (1998)
7. Chatterjee, A., Siarry, P.: Nonlinear inertia weight variation for dynamic adaptation in particle swarm optimization. Computers & Operations Research 33, 859–871 (2006)
8. Fan, S.-K.S., Chang, J.-M.: A Modified Particle Swarm Optimizer Using an Adaptive Dynamic Weight Scheme. HCI (12), 56–65 (2007)
9. Eberhart, R.: Computational Intelligence PC Tools, pp. 185–196. Academic Press Professionals (APP), London (1996)
10. Wheldon, T.: Mathematical models in cancer research. Adam Hilger, Bristol Philadelphia (1988)
11. Martin, R., Teo, K.: Optimal Control of Drug Administration in Cancer Chemotherapy. World Scientific, Singapore (1994)
12. Cassidy, J., McLeod, H.: Is it possible to design a logical development plan for an anticancer drug. Pharmaceutical Medicine 9, 95–103 (1995)

13. Dearnaley, D., et al.: Handbook of adult cancer chemotherapy schedules. The Medicine Group (Education) Ltd., Oxfordshire (1995)
14. Martin, R., Teo, K.: Optimal Control of Drug Administration in Cancer Chemotherapy. World Scientific, Singapore (1994)
15. Shi, Y., Eberhart, R.C.: Parameter selection in particle swarm optimization. In: Porto, V.W., Waagen, D. (eds.) EP 1998. LNCS, vol. 1447, pp. 591–600. Springer, Heidelberg (1998)
16. Trelea, I.: The particle swarm optimization: convergence analysis and parameter selection. Information Processing Letters 85, 317–325 (2003)
17. Hoos, H., Stutzle, T.: Local Search Algorithms for SAT: An Empirical Evaluation. J. Automated Reasoning, special Issue SAT 2000 (1999)

MPSQAR: Mining Quantitative Association Rules Preserving Semantics*

Chunqiu Zeng, Jie Zuo, Chuan Li, Kaikuo Xu, Shengqiao Ni, Liang Tang,
Yue Zhang, and Shaojie Qiao

Computer School of Sichuan University,
610065 Chengdu, China
{zengchunqiu,zuojie,lichuan}@cs.scu.edu.cn

Abstract. To avoid the loss of semantic information due to the partition of quantitative values, this paper proposes a novel algorithm, called MPSQAR, to handle the quantitative association rules mining. And the main contributions include: (1) propose a new method to normalize the quantitative values; (2) assign a weight for each attribute to reflect the values distribution; (3) extend the weight-based association model to tackle the quantitative values in association rules without partition; (4) propose a uniform method to mine the traditional binary association rules and quantitative association rules; (5) show the effectiveness and scalability of new method by experiments.

1 Introduction

The efficient discovery of quantitative association rules is considered as an interesting and important research problem. Previous researches in quantitative association rules mining mainly focus on applying binary association mining algorithms by partitioning the quantitative value into intervals [6,7, 9, 10, 12]. However, since each interval is mapped to a binary attribute relying on whether the attribute value falls into the range of interval, the quantitative semantic information of the original attribute disappears. Moreover, the generated rules just can reflect the co-occurrence relationship among bins of different attributes rather than among all the attributes directly [2]. Let T be a data set , $T(i)$ be the i-th transaction of T and $T(i, j)$ be the responding value of j-th item (or attribute) of the i-th transaction. Without partitioning, Min-apriori [2] processes the quantitative data by normalizing $T(i, j)$ into $T_n(i, j)$ with

$$T_n(i, j) = T(i, j) / \sum_{i=1}^{|T|} T(i, j) \tag{1}$$

where $|T|$ is the size of data set. And $T_n(i, j) \in [0,1]$.

For conventional binary association rule mining, traditional support (denoted by *Tsupport*) of an item set X is calculated as:

$$Tsupport \ (X) = \left|\{T(i) \mid 1 \le i \le |T| \land X \subseteq T(i)\}\right| / |T|. \tag{2}$$

* This work was supported by NSFC Grants (60773169 and 90409007), 11-th Five Years Key Programs for Sci. &Tech. Development of China under grant No. 2006BAI05A01.

C. Tang et al. (Eds.): ADMA 2008, LNAI 5139, pp. 572–580, 2008.

However, for Min-apriori in [2], after the normalization of the data set, the support of item set X is defined as follows:

$$support\ (X) = \sum_{i=1}^{|T|} min\ \{T_n(i, j) \mid j \in X\}.\tag{3}$$

In the rest of paper, $Nsupport(X)$ is used to denote the support of X, where $T_n(i, j)$ is normalized by Equation (1). In Equation (3), the support of X is defined as the sum of all the minimum $T_n(i, j)$ values of each transaction in data set. Obviously, the larger $T_n(i, j)$ makes a greater contribution to the support of X containing item j. Therefore, Min-apriori can keep the quantitative semantics during association rules mining.

Table 1. A data set contains 5 transactions and $I= \{A, B, C, D, E, F\}$

TID	A	B	C	D	E	F
TID_1	10	5	1	0	0	10
TID_2	2	5	1	0	0	0
TID_3	0	0	0	1	2	2
TID_4	1	5	1	0	0	0
TID_5	0	0	0	0	0	1

Table 2. Data set after normalization

TID	A	B	C	D	E	F
TID_1	0.77	0.33	0.33	0.0	0.0	0.77
TID_2	0.15	0.33	0.33	0.0	0.0	0.0
TID_3	0.0	0.0	0.0	1.0	1.0	0.15
TID_4	0.08	0.33	0.33	0.0	0.0	0.0
TID_5	0.0	0.0	0.0	0.0	0.0	0.08
Total	1.0	1.0	1.0	1.0	1.0	1.0

The data set in Table 1 can be normalized as shown in Table 2 with Equation (1). By Equation (3), for each item $i \in I$, $Nsupport(\{i\}) = 1.0$, thus the item set $\{i\}$ containing single item is always frequent. That does not show the truth that $\{D\}$ occurs rarely. This problem is called side effect. To address these problems, the rest of paper is organized as follows. Section 2 describes the new way to normalize the quantitative values. Section 3 introduces weight according to the variance of the values for each attribute. Section 4 presents the *MPSQAR* algorithm to mine quantitative association rules. Section 5 gives experiments to show the effective and scalable performance of *MPSQAR* algorithm. And in Section 6 a short conclusion is given.

2 Quantitative Values Normalization

In order to eliminate the side effect and unify both the binary and quantitative situations, we need the following new concepts.

Table 3. Data set with binary values

TID	A	B	C	D	E	F
TID_1	1	1	1	0	0	1
TID_2	1	1	1	0	0	0
TID_3	0	0	0	1	1	1
TID_4	1	1	1	0	0	0
TID_5	0	0	0	0	0	1

Definition 1. Given the j-th attribute in data set T, let v be the most possible nonzero value to occur for the attribute. Then v is called Expecting Value Filled, abbreviated as *EVF*. *EVF(j)* is estimated as follows:

$$EVF\ (j) = \sum_{i=1}^{|T|} T(i, j) \times \frac{1}{|\{T(i) \mid T(i, j) \neq 0, 1 \leq i \leq |T|\}|}. \tag{4}$$

Especially, Considering the Table 3 with all binary attributes, all *EVF* values are 1.

Definition 2. Let e be the value to normalize the values of j-th attribute in the data set. Then e is called Normalization Coefficient, abbreviated as NC, and defined as follows:

$$NC\ (j) = \frac{1}{|T| \times EVF\ (j)}. \tag{5}$$

According to Definition 2, $T(i, j)$ can be normalized into $T_n(i, j)$ in the following:

$$T_n(i, j) = T(i, j) \times NC(j). \tag{6}$$

In the rest of paper, *NCsupport(X)* is used to denote the support of X defined in Equation (3), where $T_n(i, j)$ is normalized by *NC*. So, data sets in Table 1 and Table 3 can be normalized as shown in Table 4 and Table 5 respectively.

Table 4. The normalization result of Table 1 by *NC*

Table 5. The normalization result of Table 3 by *NC*

TID	A	B	C	D	E	F
TID_1	0.46	0.2	0.2	0.0	0.0	0.46
TID_2	0.09	0.2	0.2	0.0	0.0	0.0
TID_3	0.0	0.0	0.0	0.2	0.2	0.09
TID_4	0.05	0.2	0.2	0.0	0.0	0.0
TID_5	0.0	0.0	0.0	0.0	0.0	0.05
Total	0.6	0.6	0.6	0.2	0.2	0.6

TID	A	B	C	D	E	F
TID_1	0.2	0.2	0.2	0.0	0.0	0.2
TID_2	0.2	0.2	0.2	0.0	0.0	0.0
TID_3	0.0	0.0	0.0	0.2	0.2	0.2
TID_4	0.2	0.2	0.2	0.0	0.0	0.0
TID_5	0.0	0.0	0.0	0.0	0.0	0.2
Total	0.6	0.6	0.6	0.2	0.2	0.6

Comparing Table 4 with Table 2, *NCsupport({A})=0.6*. Thus the side effect does not occur as Table 2 shows when the size of the item set is small. Given minimum support *minsupp=0.3*, then *Tsupport({A,F})=0.2*, so {A,F} is not frequent. While *NCsupport({A,F})=0.46*, so{A,F} is frequent. Especially, considering the binary values situation, according to Table 5, for any item set X, *NCsupport(X)=Tsupport(X)*.

Lemma 1. Given an item set X of a data set T. Assume that all the items in T are binary attributes. *Tsupport(X)=NCsupport(X)*. (Proof is omitted due to limited space.)

3   Incorporate Weight into Quantitative Association Rules

3.1   Introducing Weight

In previous sections, Equation (6) is used for normalization without side effect. It can unify the support definitions in both binary and quantitative situations. However, it does not consider the distribution of the values in each attribute. To introduce the weight of quantitative association rules, we give several observations.

Observation 1. In Table 1, the values of attribute A and attribute B are distributed quite differently. However, after normalizing the data by NC into Table 4, $NCsupport(\{A\})$ is same as $NCsupport(\{B\})$ although the distributions of A and B are quite different especially when the size of item set is not large enough.

Observation 2. In Table 1, attribute C always occurs with one or zero. So C is supposed to be a binary attribute. Comparing A with C in Table 4, it is obvious that $NCsupport(\{A\})$ is equal to $NCsupport(\{C\})$. So Equation (3) can not reflect the difference between A and C. And a reasonable result that $NCsupport(\{A\})$ is greater than $NCsupport(\{C\})$ is expected.

Based on the observations above, it is worthwhile to incorporate the distributions of different attributes into the way of calculating support.

Observation 3. In Table 1, attribute B always occurs with '5' or '0' in data set. Thus it should also be viewed as a binary attribute. As a result, that $NCsupport(\{B\})$ equals to $NCsupport(\{C\})$ is considered to be reasonable.

In order to reflect the distribution of each attribute described in observation 1 and 2, and keep the property in observation 3, a weight should be introduced for each attribute in the method of calculating support.

To be more convenient for discussion later, let $NAVA$ be an array which contains all the nonzero values for specific attribute in data set. And the $NAVA$ is abbreviated for Nonzero Attribute Value Array. In Table 1, $NAVA(1)=\{10,2,1\}$. Considering the Definition 1, it can be easily found that $EVF(j)$ is the mean value of $NAVA(j)$.

Definition 3. Let $NAVA(i, j)$ be the i-th value in the $NAVA(j)$, and $|NAVA(j)|$ be the size of $NAVA(j)$ array. Then the relative diversity value of $NAVA(j)$, is said to be the Variance Factor of the j-th attribute , abbreviated as VF, defined as:

$$VF(j) = \sum_{i=1}^{|NAVA(j)|} |NAVA(i, j) - EVF(j)| \times \frac{1}{|NAVA(j)| \times EVF(j)}. \qquad (7)$$

Considering that Equation (7) above, $VF(j)$ reflects the variance of the j-th attribute relative to $EVF(j)$ that is the expecting value of $NAVA(i, j)$ for the j-th attribute.

Lemma 2. Given a data set T, and $T(i, j) \geq 0$, then $VF(j) \in [0,2]$. If and only if each $NAVA(i, j)=EVF(j)$, $VF(j)=0$. (Proof is omitted, since it is straightforward)

By the Definition 3 and Lemma 2, given the specific j-th attribute, then the weight of the j-th attribute can be defined as follows:

$$weight(j) = 1 + VF(j)/2. \qquad (8)$$

Lemma 3. Given the specific j-th attribute, let $weight(j)$ be the weight of the j-th attribute as defines above. Then (1) $weight(j) \in [1,2]$. (2) And when each $NAVA(i, j)$ approaches $EVF(j)$, then $weight(j)$ approaches 1.

Proof. It follows from Lemma 2 clearly and immediately. Note that, the more the values of the j-th attribute vary, the greater the $weight(j)$ is. Especially, if the j-th item is a binary attribute, then it is inferred easily that $VF(j)=0$, therefore, $weight(j)=1$.

3.2 Modeling Weight

Weighted support and normalized weighted support for binary association rules are first proposed in [1]. In order to incorporate weights of quantitative attributes into association rules, the definition of support in Equation (3) should be revised.

Definition 4. Given an item set X from data set T and the j-th item attribute in the item set X, let *weight(j)* be the weight of the j-th attribute and let *Wsupport(X)* denote the weighted support described in the following.

$$Wsupport \ (X) = \frac{1}{|X|} \sum_{j \in X} weight \ (j) \times NCsupport \ (X) \cdot \tag{9}$$

Note that, as defines in [1, 2], let *minsupp* be a user specified minimum support, if *Wsupport(X)* $\geq$ *minsupp*, then X is a large (or frequent) item set. If the size of large X is k, then X is called large k-item set.

Lemma 4. Given a data set T, suppose all the items in T are binary attributes, and an item set X from data set T. Then *Tsupport(X)=NCsupport(X)=Wsupport(X)*. (proof is omitted)

As shows in Lemma 4, the definition of weighted support can handle the support of item set in both data sets with binary and quantitative attributes uniformly. Also it can tackle the quantitative attribute with the capability of reflecting the distribution of attribute values directly.

Given two item sets X and Y, and $X \cap Y = \varnothing$, an association rule r can be defined in the form: $X => Y$. Thus: (1) the support of r is: *support(r)* = *Wsupport(X∪Y)*; (2) the confidence of r is: *confidence(r)* = *NCsupport(X∪Y)* /*NCsupport(X)*.

Given *minsupp* be the minimum support and *minconf* be the minimum confidence, if *support(r)* $\geq$ *minsupp* and *confidence(r)* $\geq$ *minconf*, the rule r is an interesting rule.

4 Mining Association Rules with MPSQAR Algorithm

Min-apriori algorithm is proposed for handling quantitative association rules directly without partition [2]. Considering the weighted support of item set X defined in Definition 4, the apriori property does not make sense again. Note that although $\{C,F\} \subset \{A,C,F\}$, *Wsupport($\{A,C,F\}$)=0.258 > Wsupport($\{C,F\}$) =0.244*, $\{A,C,F\}$ is frequent while $\{C,F\}$ is not. In [1], *MINWAL(O)* and *MINWAL(W)* are proposed to tackle the weighted association rules with binary attributes. And the weight of each attribute is user specified, while this paper produces the weight of each attribute according to its distribution. Thus *MPSQAR* algorithm is proposed by revising the *MINWAL(O)* for the weighted quantitative association rules in this paper. Let X, Y be item set, *minsupp* be the minimum support, and $w(X) = \sum_{j \in X} weight(j) / |X|$, then *Wsupport(X)=w(X)×NCsupport(X)*. Let *MPW* be the maximum possible weight for any item set contains X, then define *MPW(X)* in mathematic form as *MPW(X)=* max$\{w(Y)|X \subseteq Y\}$. It is easy to draw that *NCsupport(X)* $\geq$ *NCsupport(Y)* when $X \subseteq Y$.

Lemma 5. If $NCsupport(X) < minsupp/MPW(X)$, then X cannot be the subset of any large item set.(Due to the limited space, the proof is omitted.)

Especially, according to Lemma 3, if $NCsupport(X) \leq minsupp/2$, X cannot be the subset of any large item set. To find the large item set, $MPSQAR$ employs large candidate k-1 item sets to produce candidate large k item sets. Let T be the data set, and T_n be the data set normalized from T, $Weights$ be set of item weights, C_i be the candidate large i-item sets and L_i be the large i-item sets, then the $MPSQAR$ algorithm is described as follows:

Algorithm. $MPSQAR$ (Mining Preserving Semantic Quantitative Association Rule)
Input: T: the data set; $minsupp$: the minimum support
Output: a list of large item set L

```
Begin
      Tₙ=normalize(T);
      Weights[]=calculateWeight(T);
      C₁=singleItem(Tₙ,minsup);
      L₁=check(C₁,minsup);
      for(i=1;|Cᵢ|>0;i++)
      Begin
         Cᵢ₊₁=join(Cᵢ);
         Cᵢ₊₁=prune(Cᵢ₊₁,minsup);
         Lᵢ₊₁=check(Cᵢ₊₁,minsup);
         L=L∪Lᵢ;
      End
      Return L;
End
```

All the methods in $MPSQAR$ are listed in the following:

normalize(T): use Equation (6) to normalize each value in T.
calculateWeight(T): according to Equation (8), get all the weights of all the attributes.
singleItem(T_n, $minsupp$): based on all the single item set, the single item set X will be pruned if $NCsupport(X) \leq minsupp/2$ or $NCsupport(X) \leq minsupp/MPW(X)$.
prune(C_{i+1}, $minsupp$): from candidate large $(i+1)$-item set, remove the item set X in following situations: (1)existing an i-item set which is a subset of X does not occur in C_i. (2) $NCsupport(X) \leq minsupp/2$. (3) $NCsupport(X) \leq minsupp/MPW(X)$.
join(C_i): similar to [1,3], return $(i+1)$-item sets.
check(C_{i+1}, $minsupp$): according to Equation(3), check data set T and the item set X which $Wsupport(X) \leq minsupp$ will be removed, return the large $(i+1)$-item sets.

5   Experiments and Performance Study

$MPSQAR$ is written in java. All the experiments are performed on HP Compaq 6510b with Intel(R) Core(TM)2 Duo CPU 1.8G HZ and 1G memory and Windows Vista.

$MPSQAR$ runs on both synthetic and real data sets. (1) For synthetic data set, the values of each attribute will be *0* with a probability generated randomly ranging from *0* to *1*. And the nonzero values of the attribute occur according to normal distribution whose mean and deviation are produced randomly. The range of nonzero values, the number of transactions and number of attributes are all user-specified. (2) For the real data set, we use the text data set called 19MclassTextWc from WEKA home page. In the data set, all the word count feature vectors have already extracted. So the patterns of the words occurrence can be mined.

To be more convenient, some notations are given: (a) *BI*: convert data set into binary data set depending on whether the value is greater than 0 firstly, then mine it with the apriori algorithm. (b) *MA*: mine data set with min-apriori algorithm [2]. (c) *QM*: normalize data set with *NC* and mine the data set without considering the weight of attribute. (d) *WQ*: mine the data set employing *MPSQAR* algorithm.

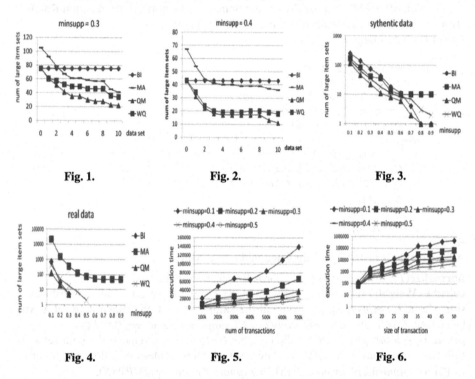

Fig. 1.   Fig. 2.   Fig. 3.

Fig. 4.   Fig. 5.   Fig. 6.

Step 1, with our data generator, *10* synthetic data sets containing 10k transactions and 10 attributes are generated. And the 10 data sets vary with the number of quantitative attributes in each data set. Especially, when the number of quantitative attributes is *0*, the data set can be viewed as a binary data set and when the number is *10*, all the attributes are quantitative. Given *minsupp=0.3* and *minsupp=0.4*, Variation in the number of large item sets on the synthetic data sets with changing number of quantitative attributes are shown in Fig.1 and Fig.2 respectively. As we see, when the number of quantitative attributes is *0*, *BI*, *QM* and *WQ* produce the same number of large item sets and that is in agreement with the Lemma 4, and the number for *MA* is greater than others due to its normalization way. For *BI*, there is no difference among different numbers of quantitative attributes, so *BI* cannot reflect the difference of quantitative attribute. Also, the number of large item sets for *WQ* is always greater than the one for *QM* due to the weight of attribute.

Step 2, given the synthetic data set containing all *10* quantitative attributes and the real data set containing *50* quantitative attributes extracting from the real text data, then the variation in the number of large item sets with different *minsupp* is shown in Fig.3 and Fig.4 respectively. As both figures shown, when the *minsupp* increases, the number of the large item set decreases. If the *minsupp* gets close to *1*, the number of large item sets for *BI*, *MA* and *WQ* approaches *0*. However, the number for *MA* stops decreasing due to its side effect.

Step 3, with the data generator, *7* data sets containing *50* attributes vary with different numbers of transactions from *100k* to *700k*. And execution time on these data sets is shown in Fig.5. Also, *9* data sets accommodating *100k* transactions vary with changing number of attributes from *10* to *50*. And execution time on these data sets is shown in Fig.6. From both figures, it shows that *MPSQAR* scales approximately linearly.

6 Conclusion and Future Work

Most existing work for quantitative association rules mining relies on partitioning quantitative values and employs binary mining algorithm to extract the association rules. And the result rules just reflect the association among these intervals of different items rather than the association among different items due to the semantic loss of the partition. To conquer the problem, this paper proposes the *MPSQAR* algorithm to mine the quantitative association rules directly by normalizing the quantitative values. *MPSQAR* also introduces a weight for each attribute according to the distribution of the attribute value and tackles the binary data and quantitative data uniformly without side effect existing in Min-apriori. The experiments show the efficiency and scalability of proposed algorithm. However, the modeled weight is sensitive to the noise of attribute values. More future work is needed to improve this feature.

References

1. Cai, C.H., Fu Ada, W.C., et al.: Mining Association Rules with Weighted Items. In: IEEE Int'l Database Engineering and Applications Symposium, Cardiff (1998)
2. Han, E.-H., Karypis, G., Kumar, V.: Min-apriori: An algorithm for finding association rules in data with continuous attributes. Technical report, Department of Computer Science, University of Minnesota, Minneapolis, MN (1997)
3. Agrawal, R., Imieliski, T., Swami, A.: Mining association rules between sets of items in large databases. In: Proceedings of ACM SIGMOD, pp. 207–216 (1993)
4. Agrawal, R., Srikant, R.: Fast algorithms for mining association rules in large databases. In: Proceedings of the 20th VLDB Conference, pp. 487–499 (1994)
5. Han, J., Pei, J., Yin, Y.: Mining frequent patterns without candidate generation. ACM SIGMOD (May 2000)
6. Miller, R.J., Yang, Y.: Association Rules over Interval Data. In: Proc 1997 ACM-SIGMOD Int Conf Management of Data, pp. 452–461 (1997)
7. Srikant, R., Agrawal, R.: Mining quantitative association rules in large relational tables. In: SIGMOD 1996 (1996)
8. Yi, D., Jianjiang, L., Zilin, S.: Mining Fuzzy Association Rules in Large Database (1999)

9. Ke, Y., Cheng, J., Ng, W.: MIC Framework: An Information-Theoretic Approach to Quantitative Association Rule Mining. In: ICDE 2006 (2006)
10. Aumann, Y., Lindell, Y.: A Statistic Theory for Quantitative Association Rules. Journal of Intelligent Information Systems(JIIS), 225–283 (2003)
11. Ruckert, U., Richater, L., Kramer, S.: Quantitative Association Rules Based on Half-Spaces: An Optimization Approach. In: Perner, P. (ed.) ICDM 2004. LNCS (LNAI), vol. 3275. Springer, Heidelberg (2004)
12. Born, S., Schmidt-Thieme, L.: Optimal Discretization of Quantitative Attributes for Association Rules (2004)

Using Support Vector Regression for Classification

Bo Huang, Zhihua Cai, Qiong Gu, and Changjun Chen

Faculty of Computer Science, China University of Geosciences
Wuhan, Hubei, P.R. China, 430074
huangbo929@gmail.com, zhcai@cug.edu.cn

Abstract. In this paper, a new method to solve the classified problems by using Support Vector Regression is introduced. Proposed method is called as SVR-C for short. In the method, through reconstructing the training set, each class through reconstructing the training set, each class value corresponding to a new training set, then use the SVR algorithm to train it and get a constructed model. And then, to a new instance, use the constructed model to train it and approximate the target class to the maximization of output value. Compared with M5P-C, SMO, J48, the effectiveness of our approach is tested on 16 publicly available datasets downloaded from the UCI. Comprehensive experiments are performed, and the results show that the SVR-C outperforms M5P-C and J48, and takes on comparative performance to SMO but has low standard-deviation. Moreover, our approach performs well on multi-class problems.

Keywords: Support Vector Regression, Model tree, SMO, J48, SVM, Classification.

1 Introduction

Support Vector Machines (SVM) were developed to solve the classification problem by Vapnik[1], and recently, SVM has been successfully extended to solve regression problems. SVM is gaining popularity due to many attractive features, such as mapping via the Kernel functions, absence of local minimal, sparseness of the solution and capacity control obtained by acting on the margin, using the Structure Risk Minimization (SRM) principle, which has been shown to be superior to the traditional Empirical Risk Minimization (ERM) principle employed in conventional learning algorithms like neural networks.

The traditional way to solve classification problem using SVM have many algorithms, which mainly use the Kernel function to map the data in a high dimension space and then construct an optimal hyperplane, but there are no one using regression way to solve the problem. Thus, in this paper, we try to use the Support Vector Regression (SVR) for classification. We wondered whether SVR could be used for classification. Surprisingly, the experimental results show that it performs very well. It's more accurate than the M5P-C[2][6], which use model tree for classification; J48[10], which is

C. Tang et al. (Eds.): ADMA 2008, LNAI 5139, pp. 581–588, 2008.

produced by Eibe Frank in a decision tree way; it also shows comparative performance to SMO[9], which is often used to solve SVM problems in an improved way.

This paper is organized as follows: In section 2, the SVR theory is reviewed and the new method is introduced. Experiment data and the results are reported in the next section. Following section briefly reviews our related work. Section 5 summarizes the results and concludes our paper.

2 A New Classification Method: SVR-C

E. FRANK[2] used the Model trees method for classification. It takes the form of a decision tree with linear regression functions instead of terminal class values at its leaves. During classification, the class whose model tree generates the greatest approximated probability values is chosen as the predicted class. As the linear regression is often restricted in local learning, and has the risk of over-learning; the SVR can be used to avoid the difficulties by using functions in the high dimensional feature space and optimization problem is transformed into dual convex quadratic programs; we wonder to use the SVR for classification. Like to E.FRANK constructed the Model trees[2], we employ the SVR to classification also use the approximated function value to approach the most likely class.

In this section, we first describe the SVR theory[3], and then give the SVR-C method which will be used for classification in our method, in the following we introduce the process of SVR-C and SVR-C procedure.

2.1 The SVR Theory

SVM can be applied not only to classification problems but also to the case of regression. Still it contains all the main features that characterize maximum margin[4] algorithm: a non-linear function is leaned by learning machine mapping into high dimensional feature space through the Kernel function induced.

In SVM regression, the input x (Instance) is first mapped into a m-dimensional feature space using some fixed mapping, and then a model is constructed in this feature space. Using mathematical notation, the model (in the feature space) $f(x,\omega)$ is given by: $f(x,\omega) = \sum_{j=1}^{m} \omega_j g_j(x) + b$. where $g_j(x), j = 1,...,m$ denotes a set of non-linear transformations, and b is the "bias" term. The data are often assumed to be zero mean (this can be achieved by preprocessing), so the bias term is dropped.

SVR performs in the high-dimension feature space using ε – insensitive loss and, at the same time, tries to reduce model complexity by minimizing $\|m\|^2$. This can be described by introducing (non-negative) slack variables ξ_i, $\xi_i^*, i = 1,...,n$, to measure the deviation of training samples outside ε -insensitive zone. Thus SVM regression is formulated as minimization of the following function:

$$\frac{1}{2}\|m\|^2 + C\sum_{i=1}^{n}(\xi_i + \xi_i^*)$$

$$s.t \begin{cases} y_i - f(x_i, \omega) \le \varepsilon + \xi_i^* \\ f(x_i, \omega) - y_i \le \varepsilon + \xi_i \\ \xi_i, \ \xi_i^* \ge 0, \ i = 1, \ldots, n \end{cases}$$

This optimization problem can transformed into the dual problem and its solution is given by:

$$f(x) = \sum_{i=1}^{n_{sv}} (\alpha_i - \alpha_i^*) K(x_i, x) \quad s.t \ 0 \le \alpha_i, \alpha_i^* \le C$$

Where n_{sv} is the number of Support Vectors (SVs) and the Kernel function:

$$K(x_i, x) = \sum_{j=1}^{m} g_j(x) g_j(x_i)$$

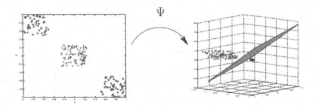

Fig. 1. Non-linear mapping of input examples into high dimensional feature space. (Classification case, however the same stands for regression as well).

2.2 The SVR-C Method

The method which we used for classification is called SVR-C for short. The key to SVR-C is constructing the training model for each class label. For a new instance, we use the constructed model to train it and approximate the target class to the maximization of output value.

Training starts by deriving several new datasets from the original dataset, one for each possible value of the class. In the next step the SVR inducer is employed to generate a model for each of the new datasets.

Take the dataset "Wine" for example. Which have 178 instances, 14 attributes and 3 classes. Firstly, we divided the dataset into 3 new datasets, which contains the same number of instances as the original, with the class value set to 1 or 0 depending on whether that instance has the appropriate class or not. Then, we employ the SVR algorithm to each new datasets and get 3 train models. For a new instance x, we use the 3 trained models to predict its target value, and the maximum one would be the most approximate to the class label. The process describes in figure 2:

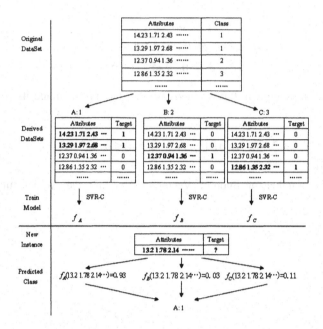

Fig. 2. The process of using Support Vector Machines for Classification

2.3 SVR-C Procedure

The procedure of the SVR-C can be described simply as follows:

Input: Training instance, newInsts	
Output: Training model, the class label	
BEGIN:	
1. getCapabilities();	// Can classifier handle the data?
2. makeCopies();	// Creates a given number of deep copies of the given classifier
3. insts.numClasses();	// A filter that creates a new dataset with a boolean attribute replacing a nominal attribute.
4. MakeIndicator();	
5. buildClassifier();	//Construct the classifier model
6. TrainModelt();	//Use the model train instance
7. GetTargetClass ;	//Get the class label
8. Input training set;	
9. **if**(getCapabilities()= =false)	
10. makeCopies(trainingSet)	// Copy the dataset
11. insts.numClasses(trainingSet)	// matching class attribute
12. **end if**	
13. MakeIndicator(SVR(trainingSet))	// SVR Constructor
14. buildClassifier(trainingSet)	
15. Instances newInsts;	// Give a new Instance: newInsts
16. TrainModelt(newInsts)	// Use the train models to train the newInsts
17. GetTargetClass(newInsts)	// Get the target class for the newInsts
END	

3 Experimental Method and Results

3.1 Data Preprocessed

We ran our experiments on 16 UCI datasets [8], which represent a wide range of domain and the data characteristics is listed in Table 1.

Table 1. Description of data sets used in the experiment. All these data sets are downloaded from the UCI collection in the format of arff.

NO.	DataSet	Instances	Attributes	Class	Missing	Numeric
1	banlance-scale	625	5	3	N	Y
2	bridges-version1	107	13	6	Y	Y
3	bridges-version2	107	13	6	Y	Y
4	colic	368	23	2	Y	Y
5	dermatology	366	35	6	N	Y
6	hayes-roth	132	5	3	N	Y
7	house-votes-84	435	17	2	Y	N
8	labor	57	17	2	Y	Y
9	promoters	106	58	2	N	N
10	solar-flare_1	323	13	2	N	Y
11	tic-tac-toe	958	10	2	N	N
12	trains	10	33	2	N	Y
13	vote	435	17	2	Y	N
14	weather.nominal	14	5	2	N	N
15	wine	178	14	3	N	Y
16	zoo	101	18	7	N	Y

Table 2. The detailed experimental results. Obtained with 10 times 10-fold cross validation, with a 95% confidence level. Each data is shown in the form of "percent-correct ± standard-deviation".

DataSet	SVR-C	M5P-C	SMO	J48
banlance-scale	89.76±2.26	86.29±2.53 v	90.04±2.29 *	64.14±4.16 v
bridges-version1	67.98±10.98	41.95±4.62 v	66.69±11.09 v	57.42±11.26 v
bridges-version2	66.80±11.21	41.95±4.62 v	66.94±10.80 *	56.46±10.69 v
colic	81.52±5.81	83.45±6.46 *	81.31±5.54 v	84.31±6.02 *
dermatology	95.66±3.23	96.50±2.78 v	95.04±2.67 v	94.10±3.34 v
hayes-roth	80.68±9.43	76.03±9.40 v	81.33±8.15 *	70.00±9.46 v
house-votes-84	95.63±2.76	95.61±2.77 v	95.81±2.89 *	96.57±2.56 *
labor	87.10±15.27	85.13±16.33 v	92.97±9.75 *	78.60±16.58 v
promoters	86.71±10.46	76.37±11.81 v	91.01±8.46 *	79.04±12.68 v
solar-flare_1	97.75±1.58	97.53±1.65 v	97.47±1.66 v	97.84±1.42 *
tic-tac-toe	98.33±1.28	94.43±2.70 v	98.33±1.28 v	85.28±3.18 v
trains	70.00±46.06	40.00±49.24 v	70.00±46.06 v	90.00±30.15 *
vote	95.63±2.76	95.22±2.62 v	95.79±2.91 *	96.27±2.79 *
weather.nominal	76.50±37.24	54.50±41.50 v	65.00±40.51 v	47.50±42.86 v
wine	99.21±1.97	97.13±3.44 v	98.76±2.73 v	93.20±5.90 v
zoo	93.36±6.25	92.51±7.06 v	96.24±5.04 *	92.61±7.33 v

3.2 Experiment

We conducted the experiments under the framework of Weka [7] to study the four methods, which are SVR-C(Using Support Vector Regression for classification, the SVR algorithm which we used is SMOreg developed by Smola and B. Scholkopf[3]), M5P-C[2][6] (Using Model trees for classification,), SMO[9](Sequential Minimal Optimization) and J48[10](Class for generating a pruned or unpruned C4.5 decision tree). The classification accuracy and standard-deviation of each classifier on each dataset was obtained via 1 run of 10-fold cross validation. Experiments with the various methodologies were carried out on the same training sets and evaluated on the same test sets. Particularly, the cross-validation folds are the same for all the experiments on each dataset. We compared them via two-tailed t-test with a 95% confidence level. Table 2 shows the detailed experimental results, "v", "*": statistically significant SVR-C improved or degraded to other algorithms.

3.3 Experimental Results

Seen from the experimental results, to SVR-C, compared with the other 3 methodologies, the statistical results were shown in table 3. The curves are shown in figure 3.

Table 3. The statistical data of experimental results

Items	SVR-C	M5P-C	SMO	J48
Mean accuracy	86.4±10.53	78.4±10.59	86.4±10.63	80.2±10.40
SVR-C Outperforms	———	14	8	11
Seven Multi-Class Mean accuracy	85±6.11	76±4.92	85±6.48	75±7.45

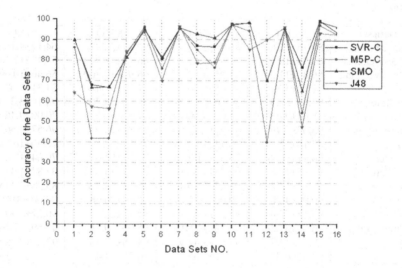

Fig. 3. The Curve of the experiment results

(1). SVR-C significantly outperforms M5P-C. In the 16 datasets we tested, SVR-C wins in 14 datasets, surprisingly loses in 2 datasets. SVR-C's average accuracy is 86.4%, much higher than that of M5P-C (78.4). This fact proves that, comparing with M5P-C, Support Vector Regression can be used for classification and performs well; and it can be seen that SVR-C can solve the difficulty of local restrictive learning to Model trees.

(2). SVR-C significantly outperforms J48. In the 16 datasets we tested, SVR-C takes priority in 11 datasets, only loses in 5 dataset, with the average accuracy is much higher than that of J48 (80.2%). This fact shows that, though decision tree methods often perform well to classification, SVR-C is a new efficient way to solve the classified problems.

(3). SVR-C shows comparative performance to SMO. In the 16 datasets, SVR-C wins in 8 datasets and loses in 8 datasets, with the same average accuracy to SMO, however, SVR-C has low standard –deviation. This fact suggests that SVR-C needs to be improved, on the other hand it shows that the mapped and kernel method are very useful way to solve many difficult problems.

(4). SVR-C performs better on multi-classifications. As the SVR-C method uses the way of function approximate, it doesn't need to consider the traditional way to reconstruct the instance. Moreover, it is efficient, which can be seen from Table 3, the mean accuracy of SVR-C method is 85%, which is outperformed than M5P-C and J48, and has lower standard –deviation than SMO.

4   Related Work

SVR-C is a new way of solving classified problems, though it performs well on the test datasets, we need to find the characteristic of the dataset which will be the best to fit for using SVR-C, so that we can get better application in practice.

The SVR-C is time-consuming, so investigating and improving its performance are other directions in our related work.

The traditional idea of solving multi-class problem is treating it as several two-way classification problems. However, SVR-C gives a new method to solve multi-class problem by function approximation to each new instance. How to find an appropriate function model to get better approximation to the label is another direction.

5   Conclusions

In this paper, we proposed a new method to classification: using Support Vector Regression for classifications. By deriving the original dataset, we get several new datasets which contains the same number of instances as the original, and then use the SVR algorithm to train the new datasets to get a function model. For a new instance, we use the train model to predict the target class, which is the maximum one of the outputs.

To SVR-C, we compared it with M5p-C, SMO and J48. We implement these methods using 16 datasets downloaded from the UCI on the platform of Weka. The experimental results show that SVR-C outperforms M5P-C and J48, and it shows comparative performance to SMO. This fact proves that SVR-C is a new and efficient way to solve classified problems.

Acknowledgments

This paper is supported by Civil aerospace pre-research project.

Many thanks to Eibe Frank , Y. Wang (etc.) for kindly providing us with the implementation of M5P-C.

References

1. Vapnik, V.: The Nature of Statistical Learning Theory, 2nd edn. Springer, New York (2001)
2. Frank, E., Wang, Y., Inglis, S., Holmes, G., I.H.: Using model trees for classification. Machine Learning 32, 63–76 (1998)
3. Smola, Scholkopf, B.: A Tutorial on Support Vector Regression. NeuroCOLT Technical. [C] Report NC-TR-98-030, Royal Holloway College, University of London, UK (1998)
4. Boser, B., Guyon, I., Vapnik: A training algorithm for optimal margin classifiers. In: Proceedings of the Fifth Annual Workshop on Computational Learning Theory. ACM Press, New York (1992)
5. Fan, R.-E., Chen, P.-H., Lin, C.-J.: Working Set Selection Using Second Order Information for Training Support Vector Machines. Journal of Machine Learning Research 6, 1889–1918 (2005)
6. Breiman, L., Friedman, J.H., Olshen, R.A., Stone, C.J.: Classification and regression trees. Wadsworth, Belmont (1984)
7. Ian, H., Frank: Data Mining: Practical machine learning tools and techniques, 2nd edn. Morgan Kaufmann, San Francisco (2005),
   http://prdownloads.sourceforge.net/weka/datasets-UCI.jar
8. UCI Repository of machine learning data-bases, Irvine, CA,
   http://www.ics.uci.edu/~mlearn/MLRepository.html
9. Platt, J.C.: Fast Training of Support Vector Machines using Sequential Minimal Optimization (1998), http://www.research.microsoft.com/_jplatt
10. Quinlan, R.: C4.5: Programs for Machine Learning. Morgan Kaufmann Publishers, San Mateo (1993)

Dynamic Growing Self-organizing Neural Network for Clustering

Daxin Tian[1], Yueou Ren[2], and Qiuju Li[2]

[1] School of Computer Science and Technology, Tianjin University, 300072, China
tiandaxin@gmail.com
[2] Department of Electronic Engineering, Armor Technique Institute of PLA, 130117, China
ryohaious@163.com, liqiuju608@sohu.com

Abstract. Neural Networks have been widely used in the field of intelligent information processing such as classification, clustering, prediction, and recognition. Unsupervised learning is the main method to collect and find features from large unlabeled data. In this paper a new unsupervised learning clustering neuron network—Dynamic Growing Self-organizing Neuron Network (DGSNN) is presented. It uses a new competitive learning rule—Improved Winner-Take-All (IWTA) and adds new neurons when it is necessary. The advantage of DGSNN is that it overcomes the usual problems of other clustering methods: dead units and prior knowledge of the number of clusters. In the experiments, DGSNN is applied to clustering tasks to check its ability and is compared with other clustering algorithms RPCL and WTA. The results show that DGSNN performs accurately and efficiently.

1 Introduction

Clustering is one of the most primitive mental activities of humans, used to handle the huge amount of information they receive every day. Processing every piece of information as a single entity would be impossible. Thus, humans tend to categorize entities (i.e., objects, persons, events) into clusters. Each cluster is then characterized by the common attributes of the entities it contains. Clustering is a major tool used in a number of applications, such as analyzing gene expression data [1,2], data mining [3-6], image processing [7-9], web mining, hypothesis generation, hypothesis testing, prediction based on groups and so on.

Unsupervised learning is the main learning method of different types of self-organizing neural networks. There are three basic types of neural networks presented: principal-component analysis (PCA)[7,8], self-organizing map (SOM)[1], and adaptive resonance theory (ART) networks [10]. PCA has been used extensively in many engineering and scientific applications, and it is the basis for principal-component regression (PCR). SOM developed by Kohonen is an unsupervised, competitive learning, clustering network, in which only one neuron is "on" at a time. ART, developed by Carpenter and Grossberg, overcomes stability/plasticity dilemma by accepting and adapting the stored prototype of a category only when the input is sufficiently similar to it.

C. Tang et al. (Eds.): ADMA 2008, LNAI 5139, pp. 589–595, 2008.
© Springer-Verlag Berlin Heidelberg 2008

A variation to the typical competitive learning algorithms is Rival Penalized Competitive Learning (RPCL)[2,8,11], which for each input not only the winner neuron is modified to adapt itself to the input, but also its rivals with a smaller learning rate. The main advantages of RPCL are: the heuristic is computationally efficient, it is no worse than other methods when high dimensional features, and it can be implemented in a distributed environment achieving even greater speed-up in generating indexing structure of feature vectors.

In long-term memory studying, dead units may arise if the number of output nodes is more than the number of clusters. Some methods have been presented in [9,12], to solve the problem, DGSNN grows (add neuron) when new cluster is finding. Growing networks are one way to work around these limitations of static networks. The first unsupervised growing neural network, the Growing Cell Structure (GCS), is based on the SOM [13]. Some other methods are Growing Neural Gas (GNG), Grow When Required (GWR), self-generating neural tree (SGNT), and self-generating neural networks (SGNNs) [13,14].

This paper introduces a dynamic growing self-organizing neural network—DGSNN for clustering. DGSNN uses competitive learning method and adds neurons whenever the network in its current state does not sufficiently match the input. In competitive learning an improved winner-take-all algorithm—IWTA is adopted, which is able to perform adaptive clustering efficiently and quickly leading to an approximation of clusters that are statistically adequate. The character of growing of DGSNN can prevent dead neurons from occurring.

The remainder of this paper is organized as follows. Section 2 presents the competitive learning algorithm IWTA and the architecture of DGSNN. In Section 3 the ability of DGSNN is shown through experiments and compared with other clustering methods. The article is concluded in Section 4.

2   The Dynamic Growing Self-organizing Neural Network

2.1   IWTA Algorithm

In the article we introduces a new competitive learning algorithm—Improved Winner-Take-All (IWTA), which extends the basic competitive learning algorithm—Winner-Tale-All (WTA). In WTA type learning, after an input sample is presented, only one neuron (the winner) in the competitive network will remain active (or switch on) after a number of iterations (or a single iteration, depending on which type of network is used) and its corresponding long-term memory will be updated.

The basic idea of IWTA is not only the winner is rewarded as in WTA but also all the losers are penalized in different rate. There are some similarities between IWTA and RPCL [2,8,11]. The principle underlying RPCL is that in each iteration, the cluster center for the winner's neuron is accentuated (rewarded) where at the weight for the second winner, or the rival, is attenuated (penalized), and the remaining neurons are unaffected. IWTA is similar to LTCL [12] too, but in IWTA the penalized rate is based on the dissimilarity level.

The IWTA is summarized as follows:

i Measure the dissimilarity between input vector x and weight vector $\mathbf{w}_i$ using Euclidean distance d_i.

ii Arrange the neurons according to d_i from small to big and the smallest is the winner. Determine the rewarding neuron and penalizing rate of other neurons as

$$\gamma_i = \begin{cases} 1, & \text{the winner} \\ -\beta\dfrac{d_i}{\vartheta}, & \text{others} \end{cases} \tag{1}$$

where β is the penalizing rate parameter, ϑ is the threshold of dissimilarity.

iii If the winner's dissimilarity measure $d < \vartheta$, then update the synaptic weight by unsupervised learning rule

$$\mathbf{w}_i(t+1) = \mathbf{w}_i(t) + \mu * \gamma_i[\mathbf{x}(t+1) - \mathbf{w}_i(t)] \tag{2}$$

where $\alpha \geq 0$ is the forgetting factor, i indicates ith neuron.
Else add a new neuron and set the synaptic weight $\mathbf{w} = \mathbf{x}$.

2.2 DGSNN

The behavior of the network can be described as follows. At first, a training vector $\mathbf{x}$ is presented to the network and each neuron receives this sample. Then the dissimilarity measure between $\mathbf{x}$ and each synaptic weight will be computed. After that, the competitive function will choose the winner neuron and compute the penalizing rate of other neurons. Last the learning rule part gets the result of competitive and updates the synaptic weights. The output is the winner neuron, which represents a cluster.

Now we summarize all operations of DGSNN into an algorithm:

Step0: Initialize learning rate parameter μ, penalizing rate parameter β, the threshold of dissimilarity ϑ;
Step1: Get the first input x and set $\mathbf{w}_0 = \mathbf{x}$ as the initial cluster center;
Step2: If the training is not over, randomly take a feature vector x from the feature sample set X and compute dissimilarity measure between x and each synaptic weight;
Step3: Decide the winner neuron j and test tolerance:If $(d_j >= \vartheta)$ add a new neuron and set synaptic weight $\mathbf{w} = \mathbf{x}$, goto Step2;
Step4: compute the penalizing rate (Eq.1);
Step5: Update the synaptic weight (Eq.2), goto Setp2.

DGSNN has the abilities of clustering unlabeled data, deciding the classification of an input data, and estimating the number of clusters. All the abilities will be showed in the next section.

3 Experimental Results

In order to show the capability of DGSNN to find the center of a cluster, an input space in a two dimensional space with predetermined number of clusters were generated with variance $\sigma = 0.5$, centered at (0,1.5), (0,-1.5), (1.5,0), (-1.5,0) and variance $\sigma = 0.05$, centered at (0,0.5), (0,-0.5), (0.5,0), (-0.5,0), see Fig.1 and Fig.2. Points are assigned to each center according to a Gaussian distribution. Since the dataset is generated randomly, there is an equal probability of picking points centered on any one of the four centers. A total of 50 points are associated with each center. The clusters in the dataset with variance $\sigma = 0.05$ are more distinct than the dataset with variance $\sigma = 0.5$. These will be referred to as tight and sparse clusters, respectively.

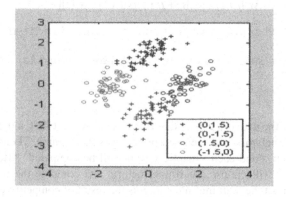

Fig. 1. Sparse Clusters (Variance=0.5)

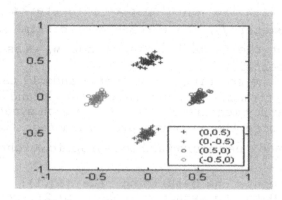

Fig. 2. Tight Clusters (Variance=0.05)

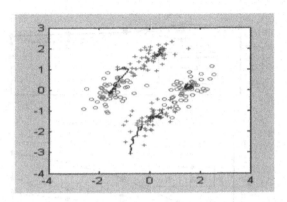

Fig. 3. Learning Progress of the Data Set of Fig.2

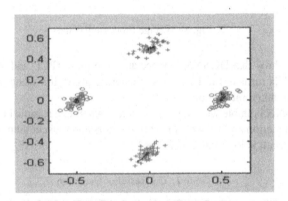

Fig. 4. Learning Progress of the Data Set of Fig.3

When the threshold of dissimilarity $\vartheta = 1.8$ for Fig.1 and $\vartheta = 0.28$ for Fig.2, the learning progress is reported in Fig.3 and 4.

At the end of learning, converged centers of the data set of Fig.1 arrive at (0.134536, 1.581388), (-1.544215, -0.105366), (0.724721, -0.694786), (1.641214, 0.133870), (-0.316027, -1.862309) and the data set of Fig.2 arrive at (0.005867, 0.504599), (-0.013072, -0.501574), (0.497693, 0.009718), (-0.504206, -0.022835).

We conduct experiments for DGSNN, RPCL, and WTA to compare their accuracy and efficiency in clustering. All of the experiments use the same 100 8-dimentional feature vectors which are separated into 5, 10, 15, 20, or 30 clusters. Each method is conducted 30 times with different iteration times. The average accuracy and average time used in accurate clustering are presented in Figs.5 and 6.

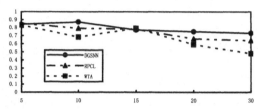

Fig. 5. Average Accuracy Rate

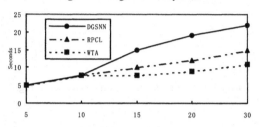

Fig. 6. Average Processing Time

The results show that DGSNN is more accurate than RPCL and WTA, but it is the slowest. DGSNN turns out to be a good clustering algorithm when accuracy and efficiency are both taken into account.

When DGSNN is stable we can use it to detect whether a sample belongs to a cluster. To show the detection ability, we choose five points and present them to stable DGSNN of Fig.2. The result is illustrated in Table 1.

Table 1. The Result of Detection

Sample points	(0.25,0.15)	(0.4,0.1)	(-0.36,0.15)	(0.21,0.7)	(-0.08,-0.41)
Belongs to	(0.5,0)	(0.5,0)	(-0.5,0)	(0,0.5)	(0,-0.5)
Experimental results	Right	Right	Right	Right	Right

4 Conclusions

This paper proposes a new clustering method (DGSNN) based on unsupervised learning neural network. DGSNN's learning algorithm (IWTA) improves the Winner-Take-All rule and the result is more accurate. The advantage of DGSNN is that it can perform clustering without requiring a prior knowledge about the number of clusters and prevent dead neurons through adding neurons whenever the current input is not matched sufficiently well by any of the current neurons. All the capabilities have been checked by experiments. The clustering ability of DGSNN has been compared with other two clustering algorithms RPCL and WTA. In the experiments, they are applied to the same clustering tasks and the results prove that DGSNN is perfect in accuracy and efficiency.

References

1. Ressom, H., Wang, D., Natarajan, P.: Adaptive Double Self-organizing Maps for Clustering Gene Expression Profiles. Neural Network 16, 633–640 (2003)
2. Nair, T.M., Zheng, C.L., Fink, J.L.: Rival Penalized Competitive Learning (RPCL): A Topology-determining Algorithm for Analyzing Gene Expression Data. Computational Biology and Chemistry 27, 565–574 (2003)
3. Chen, N., Chen, A., Zhou, L.X.: An Efficient Clustering Algorithm in Large Transaction Databases. Journal of Software 12(4), 475–484 (2001)
4. Song, L.P., Zheng, J.H.: Evaluation Method of the Corpus Segmentation Based on Clustering. Chinese Journal of Computers 27(2), 192–196 (2004)
5. Giuseppe, A., Ernesto, C., Girolamo, F., Silvano, V.: A Feature Extraction Unsupervised Neural Network for An Environmental Data Set. Neural Networks 16, 427–436 (2003)
6. Yang, Y.L., Guan, X.D., You, J.Y.: Mining The Page Clustering Based on the Content of Web Pages and the Site Topology. Journal of Software 13(3), 467–469 (2002)
7. Ezequiel, L.R., Jose, M.P., Jose, A.G.R.: Principal Components Analysis Competitive Learning. In: Mira, J., Álvarez, J.R. (eds.) IWANN 2003. LNCS, vol. 2686, pp. 318–325. Springer, Heidelberg (2003)
8. Liu, Z.Y., Chiu, K.C., Xu, L.: Local PCA for Line Detection And Thinning. In: Rangarajan, A., Figueiredo, M.A.T., Zerubia, J. (eds.) EMMCVPR 2003. LNCS, vol. 2683, pp. 21–34. Springer, Heidelberg (2003)
9. Kamimura, R.: Competitive Learning by Information Maximization: Eliminating Dead Neurons in Competitive Learning. In: Kaynak, O., Alpaydın, E., Oja, E., Xu, L. (eds.) ICANN 2003 and ICONIP 2003. LNCS, vol. 2714, pp. 99–106. Springer, Heidelberg (2003)
10. Fung, W.K., Liu, Y.H.: A Game-theoretic Adaptive Categorization Mechanism for ART-type Networks. In: Dorffner, G., Bischof, H., Hornik, K. (eds.) ICANN 2001. LNCS, vol. 2130, pp. 170–176. Springer, Heidelberg (2001)
11. Garcia-Bernal, M.A., Munoz-perez, J., Gomez-Ruiz, J.A., Ladron de, G.I.: A Competitive Neural Network Based on Dipoles. In: Mira, J., Álvarez, J.R. (eds.) IWANN 2003. LNCS, vol. 2686, pp. 398–405. Springer, Heidelberg (2003)
12. Andrew, L.: Analyses on the Generalized Lotto-type Competitive Learning. In: Leung, K.-S., Chan, L., Meng, H. (eds.) IDEAL 2000. LNCS, vol. 1983, pp. 9–16. Springer, Heidelberg (2000)
13. Marsland, S., Sphairo, J., Nehmzow, U.: A Self-organising Network That Grows When Required. Neural Networks 15, 1041–1058 (2002)
14. Hirotaka, I., Hiroyuki, N.: Efficiency of Self-generating Neural Networks Applied to Pattern Recognition. Mathematical and Computer Modelling 38, 1225–1232 (2003)

A Design of Reward Function Based on Knowledge in Multi-agent Learning

Bo Fan and Jiexin Pu

Electronic Information Engineering College, Henan University of Science & Technology,
471003 Luoyang, P.R. China
fanbo_box@hotmail.com

Abstract. The design of reward function is the key to build reinforcement learning system. With the analysis and research of the reinforcement learning and Markov games, an improved reward function is presented, which includes both the goal information based on task and learner's action information based on its domain knowledge. According with this reinforcement function, reinforcement learning integrates the external environment reward and the internal behavior reward so that learner can perform better. The results of the experiment illuminates the reward function involving domain knowledge is better than the traditional reward function in application.

1 Introduction

Markov games and reinforcement learning are main research methods to Multi-Agent System (MAS) [1~3]. Markov game can fit for dealing with MAS coordination and building the dynamic model of multi-agent's interaction. Reinforcement learning is an interactive learning. Q-learning [4], one of reinforcement learning, is the dynamic programming learning based on Markov Decision Process (MDP). Applied to multi-agent system, reinforcement learning is extended to Markov games. Although reinforcement learning is focused on widely by its convergence and biology relativity, it does not work well in practice, especially to application to robot.

Reinforcement learning does not provide the mapping of state and action. After choosing an action, an agent is signaled the effect but do not know which is the optimal. Therefore, the agent depends on the interacting with environment to collect states, actions, the transition of states and reward in order to get the optimal policy. However, in practice, the reward received from environment is not immediate, but delayed, so learning becomes more difficult within the time-limited. Currently, how to design the reinforcement function, which maybe the most difficult to reinforcement learning, is seldom discussed. M. J. Matalic [5] [6]designs the reinforcement function by reinforcing multiple goals and using progress estimators. Kousuk INOUE [7] presents reinforcement learning is accelerated by using experience information to distill the general rules. H. C. Calos [8] improves the performance of reinforcement learning by embedding the prior knowledge, which does not change data structure of learning. Richard Maclin [9] reviews external personnel's effect. He introduces the observer's suggestion to reduce training steps of Q-learning. L. P. Kaelbling [10] decomposes the learning task and combines the prior knowledge to direct reinforcement learning.

C. Tang et al. (Eds.): ADMA 2008, LNAI 5139, pp. 596–603, 2008.

Most research on reinforcement function is depended on application environment. Based on environment's property, learning system reduces complexity and introduces relative information to enrich reinforcement function so that the learner can obtain more knowledge about environment and itself to process reinforcement learning by. We have the same opinion. We design reinforcement function including two aspects: the information of goal state and the agent's action effect. The former is provided by environment, which is the interaction information between an agent and environment for accomplishing the special task, the latter is that the agent evaluates action effect, which depends on its domain knowledge of action ability. In this paper, the simulation game of Robot Soccer is applied.

2 Multi-agent Reinforcement Learning

In this section some basic principle of MDP is reviewed and then the formalisms of Markov games, which is an extension of MDPs. Q-learning algorithm is also presented, which is used to solve MDPs. Minmax-Q algorithm is proposed to solve Markov games.

2.1 MDP and Q-Learning Algorithm

Let us consider a single agent interacting with its environment via perception and action. On each interaction step the agent senses the current state s of the environment, and chooses an action to perform. The action alters the state s of the environment, and a scalar reinforcement signal r (a reward or penalty) is provided to the agent to indicate the desirability of the resulting state.

Formally, a MDP is represented by a 4-tuple <S, A, r, T>: S is a set of states, A is a set of actions, r is a scalar reinforcement function, r: $S \times A \to R$, T is a state transition function, T: $S \times A \to S$.

The goal of the agent in the most common formulation of the reinforcement learning problem is to learn an optimal policy of actions that maximizes an expected cumulative sum of the reinforcement signal for any starting state. The task of an agent with RL is thus to learn a policy π: $S \to A$ that maps the current state s into the desirable action a to be performed in s.

The action policy π should be learned through trial-and-error interaction of the agent with the environment, which means that the learner must explicitly explore its environment.

There is at least one optimal policy π^* that is stationary and deterministic. One strategy to learn the optimal policy π^* when the model (T and r) is not known in advance is to allow the agent to learn the evaluation function Q: $S \times A \to R$. Each Q(s, a) value (or action value for pair s, a) represents the expected cost incurred by the agent when taking action at state s and following an optimal policy thereafter.

Q-learning algorithm iteratively approximates Q, provided the system can be modeled as a MDP, the reinforcement function is bounded, and actions are chosen so that every state-action pair is visited an infinite number of times. Q-learning rules [4] are:

$$Q(s,a) \leftarrow Q(s,a) +$$
$$\alpha(r + \beta \max_{a'} Q(s',a') - Q(s,a)) \tag{1}$$

Where s is the current state, a is the action performed in s, r(s, a) is the reinforcement received after performing a in s, s' is the new state, β is a discount factor ($0 \le \beta < 1$) and α is the learning rate ($\alpha > 0$).

2.2 Markov Games and Minmax-Q Algorithm

Let us consider a specialization of Markov games, which consists of two agents performing actions in alternating turns, in a zero-sum game. Let A be the set of possible actions that the playing agent A can choose from, and O be the set of actions for the opponent player agent O. r(s, o, a) is the immediate reinforcement agent A receives for performing action $a \in A$ in state $s \in S$ when its opponent agent O performs action $o \in O$.

The goal of agent A is to learn an optimal policy of actions that maximizes its expected cumulative sum of discounted reinforcements. However, learning this policy is very difficult, since it depends critically on the actions the opponent performs. The solution to this problem is to evaluate each policy with respect to the opponent's strategy that makes it look the worst [1]. This idea is the core of Minmax-Q algorithm, which is essentially very similar to Q-learning algorithm with a minmax replacing the max function in the definition of the state value.

For deterministic action policies, the value of a state $s \in S$ in a MG is:

$$V(s) = \max_{a \in A} \min_{o \in O} Q(s,a,o) \tag{2}$$

And Minmax-Q learning rule is:

$$Q(s,a,o) \leftarrow Q(s,a,o) +$$
$$\alpha[r(s,a,o) + \beta V(s') - Q(s,a,o)] \tag{3}$$

where s is the current state, a is the action performed by agent A in s, o is the action performed by agent O in s, Q(s, a, o) is the expected discounted reinforcement for taking action a when Agent O performs o in state s, and continuing the optimal policy thereafter, r(s, o, a) is the reinforcement received by agent A, s' is the new state, β is a discount factor ($0 \le \beta < 1$) and α is the learning rate ($\alpha > 0$).

For non-deterministic action policies, a more general formulation of Minmax-Q has been formally defined elsewhere.

3   Reinforcement Function Based on Knowledge

Reinforcement learning systems learn a mapping from situations to actions by trial-and-error interactions with a dynamic environment. The goal of reinforcement learning is defined using the concept of a reinforcement function, which is the exact function of future reinforcements the agent seeks to maximize. In other words, there exists a mapping from state/action pairs to reinforcements; after performing an action in a given state the learner agent will receive some reinforcement (reward) in the form of a scalar value. The agent learns to perform actions that will maximize the sum of the reinforcements received when starting from some initial state and proceeding to a terminal state.

Perhaps, design of reinforcement is the most difficult aspect of setting up a reinforcement learning system. The action performed by the learner not only receives an immediate reward but also transits the environment to a new state. Therefore, the learning has to consider both the immediate reward and the future reinforcement caused by the current action. Nowadays, much of reinforcement learning work uses two types of reward: immediate, and very delayed. In reinforcement learning system, immediate reinforcement, when available, is the most effective. And delayed reinforcement requires introduction of sub-goal so that learning is performed within time-limited. Reinforcement learning is a feedback algorithm, so it is not good for long-term goal but more effective to the near goals. A learner can introduce medium-term goals and distributing task so as to accelerate the learning rate and increase the learning efficiency.

In traditional reinforcement learning, the agent-environment interaction can be modeled as a MDP, in which agent and environment are synchronized finite state automata. However, in real-world, the environment and agent states change asynchronously, in response to events. Events take various amounts of time to execute: the same event (as perceived by the agent) can vary in duration under different circumstances and have different consequences. Reinforcement learning gives the reward to what are caused by and in control of the agent.

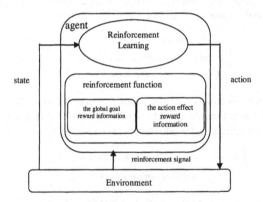

Fig. 1. Learning Model

Instead of encoding knowledge explicitly, reinforcement learning hides it in the reinforcement function which usually employs some ad hoc embedding of the semantics of the domain. We divide this reinforcement information involving domain knowledge into two types:

1. The global goal's reward;
2. The agent action effect's reward.

In each state, a learner agent chooses an appropriate action and performs it to environment, which is transited to a new state. On the one hand, the agent depends on the task to judge the environment and receives the global goal reward; on the other hand, based on the agent's domain knowledge about its action ability, it compares perform-ance effect and obtains the reward of action. The reinforcement function that we de-sign combines the global environment's reinforcement and the agent action's reinforcement. The reinforcement learning model with this reinforcement function is shown in Figure 1.

4 Experiments

4.1 Experimental Environment

We adopted the Robot Soccer to perform our experiments. Robot Soccer is a typical MAS: robots is the agents, the playground and ball are thought as environment.

State, actions of multi-agent learning are design as follows:

$S = \{threat, sub\text{-}threat, sub\text{-}good, good\}$;

Home agents' $A = \{Shoot, Attack, Defend, More\text{-}defend\}$;

Opponent agents' $O = \{Shoot, Attack, Defend, More\text{-}defend\}$

In traditional reinforcement learning, reinforcement function is usually developed that reward is +1 if home team scored; reward is -1 if opponent team scored. Instead of it, we design the reinforcement function including two kinds of information: game goal reinforcement and robot's action effect reinforcement.

In play, game goal reinforcement information is the reward received by score of both sides. The rewards signal r_s, is defined as:

$$r_s = \begin{cases} c, & our\ team\ scored \\ -c, & opponent\ team\ scored \\ 0, & otherwise \end{cases} \quad c > 0 \tag{4}$$

And, reinforcement information of the robot's action effect is that, after performing each action, the robot receives the reward signal r_a, which involves the robot's domain knowledge about each action and evaluates the action effect.

$$r_a = \begin{cases} d & action\ success \\ 0 & action\ unsuccesss \end{cases} \quad d > 0, \tag{5}$$

The combination reinforcement function considers the two kinds of reward and sums them with weighting their values constants appropriately.

$$R = \omega_s \cdot r_s + \omega_a \cdot r_a \tag{6}$$
$$\omega_s, \omega_a \geq 0, \quad (\omega_s + \omega_a) = 1$$

Thus, the robot agent evaluates its policy using comprehensive reinforcement. With learning continually, the agent improves its policy and increases its ability.

4.2 Experimental Result

We use SimuroSot, one of simulation match provided by FIRA [11] (see Figure 2), to conduct the experiments. In experiments, In order to evaluate the effectiveness of the reinforcement function presented in this paper, we compare its performance against traditional reinforcement function.

1   traditional reinforcement function:

$$R = \begin{cases} +1 & \text{hom} e \text{ } team \text{ } scored \\ -1 & opponent \text{ } team \text{ } scored \end{cases} \qquad (7)$$

2   reinforcement function based on knowledge:

$$R = \omega_s \cdot r_s + \omega_a \cdot r_a \qquad (8)$$

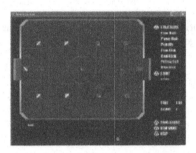

Fig. 2. The interface of SimuroSot platform

There are two group experiments. In experiment 1, the home team uses the conventional Q-learning. In experiment 2, the home team uses the Minmax-Q algorithm of Markov Games. The opponent team uses fix strategy. The team size is 1.

The parameters used in the algorithms were set at: $\beta = 0.9$, initial value of $\alpha = 1.0$, α decline $= 0.9$. In Q-learning, initial value of Q-table $= 0$. In Minmax-Q algorithm, initial value of Q-table $= 1$.

In experiment, we define that the appropriate policy is: $s_1 \rightarrow a_1, s_2 \rightarrow a_2, s_3 \rightarrow a_3, s_4 \rightarrow a_4$. For Q-learning algorithm, we save several Q-values, which are $Q(s_1, a_1)$, $Q(s_2, a_2)$, $Q(s_3, a_3)$, $Q(s_4, a_4)$. And for Minmax-Q algorithm, we save Q-values, which are $\underset{o \in O}{Min} Q(s_1, a_1, o)$, $\underset{o \in O}{Min} Q(s_2, a_2, o)$, $\underset{o \in O}{Min} Q(s_3, a_3, o)$ and $\underset{o \in O}{Min} Q(s_4, a_4, o)$.

During more than 1000 steps learning, we analyze their results. Q-learning with the two kinds of reinforcement function all can converge to appropriate policy, but the former needs long time. In Minmax-Q algorithm, it can get to appropriate policy with knowledge-base reinforcement function, while it does not learn appropriate policy with traditional reinforcement function even if spending too long time. We choose the same Minmax-Q value to observe.

The results of Q-learning are shown in Figure 3. The results of Minmax-Q are shown in Figure 4. Thereinto, Figure 3(a) and Figure 4(a) are respectively the learning with traditional reinforcement function; Figure 3(b) and Figure 4(b) are respectively the learning with knowledge-base reinforcement function. Obviously, we can observe that learning with traditional reinforcement function has worse convergence and still has many unstable factors at end of experiment, while the learning with knowledge-base reinforcement function converges rapidly and it gets to stable value about half

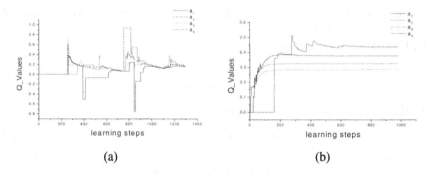

Fig. 3 (a). Q-learning algorithm with the traditional reinforcement function; **(b).** Q-learning algorithm with the knowledge-base reinforcement function

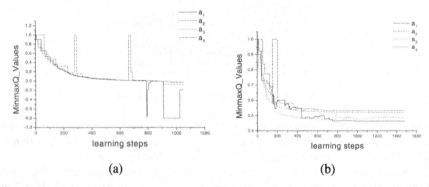

Fig. 4. (a). Minmax-Q algorithm with the traditional reinforcement function; **(b).** Minmax-Q algorithm with the knowledge-base reinforcement function

time of experiment. Therefore, with the external knowledge (environment information) and internal knowledge (action effect information), multi-agent learning has better performance and effectivity.

5 Summary

When Multi-agent learning is applied to real environment, it is very important to design the reinforcement function that is appropriate to environment and learner. We think that the learning agent must take advantage of the information including environment and itself domain knowledge to integrate the comprehensive reinforcement information. This paper presents the reinforcement function based on knowledge, with which the learner not only pays more attention to environment transition but also evaluates its action performance each step. Therefore, the reinforcement information of multi-agent learning becomes more abundant and comprehensive, so that the leaning can converge rapidly and become more stable. From experiment, it is obviously that multi-agent learning with knowledge-base reinforcement function has better performance than traditional reinforcement. However, we should point out, how to design the reinforcement must depend on the application background of multi-agent learning system. Different task, different action effect and different environments are the key factors to influence multi-agent learning. Hence, differ from traditional reinforcement function; the reinforcement function is build by the characteristic based on real environment and learner action.

References

1. Littman, M.L.: Value-function reinforcement learning in Markov games. Journal of Cognitive Systems Research 2, 55–66 (2001)
2. Boutilier, C.: Planning, Learning and Coordination in Multi-agent Decision Processes. In: Shoham, Y. (ed.) Proceedings of the Sixth Conference on Theoretical Aspects of Rationality and Knowledge, pp. 195–210. Morgan Kaufmann, San Francisco (1996)
3. Bowling, M., Veloso, M.: Existence of Multiagent Equilibria with Limited Agents. J of Artificial Intelligence Research 22(2), 353–384 (2004)
4. Watkons, C.J.C.H., Dayan, P.: Q-leanign. Machine Learning 8(3), 279–292 (1992)
5. Matalic, M.J.: Reward Functions for Accelerated Learning. In: Proc. Int. Conf. on Machine learning, pp. 181–189 (1994)
6. Mataric, M.J.: Learning in behavior-based multi-robot systems: policies, models, and other agents. Journal of Cognitive Systems Research 2, 81–93 (2001)
7. Inoue, K., Ota, J., Katayama, T., Arai, T.: Acceleration of Reinforcement Learning by A Mobile Robot Using Generalized Rules. In: Proc. IEEE Int. Conf. Intelligent Robots and Systems, pp. 885–890 (2000)
8. Calos, H.C.: Embedding a Priori Knowledge in Reinforcement Learning. Journal of Intelligent and Robotics Systems 21, 51–71 (1998)
9. Maclin, R., Shavlik, J.W.: Creating Advice-Taking Reinforcement Learners. Machine Learning 22, 251–281 (1996)
10. Smart, W.D., Kaelbling, L.P.: Effective reinforcement learning for mobile robots. In: Proceedings of the IEEE International Conference on Robotics and Automation (2002), http://www.ai.mit.edu/people/lpk/papers/icra2002.pdf
11. http://www.fira.net

A Learning Method of Detecting Anomalous Pedestrian

Yue Liu[1], Jun Zhang[2], and Zhijing Liu[2]

[1] Communication Engineering Department, Beijing Electronic Science Technology Institute,
100070, Beijing, China
[2] School of Computer Science and Technology, Xidian University, 710071 Xi'an, China
yue_china2005@yahoo.com.cn
zhang72jun@163.com
Liuzhijing@vip.163.com

Abstract. Abnormal behavior detecting is one of the hottest but most difficult subjects in Monitoring System. It is hard to define "abnormal" in different scenarios. In this paper firstly the classification of motion is conducted, and then conclusions are made under specific circumstances. In order to indicate a pedestrian's movements, a complex number notation based on centroid is proposed. And according to the different sorts of movements, a set of standard image contours are made. Different behavior matrices based on spatio-temporal are acquired through Hidden Markov Models (HMM). A Procrustes shape analysis method is presented in order to get the similarity degree of two contours. Finally Fuzzy Associative Memory (FAM) is proposed to infer behavior classification of a walker. Thus anomalous pedestrians can be detected in the given condition. FAM can detect irregularities and implement initiative analysis of body behavior.

Keywords: FAM, HMM, Behavior Classification, Procrustes, Centroid.

1 Introduction

For public security intelligent video surveillance is becoming more and more important, especially after the 9.11 event. Abnormal behavior recognition is one of the most significant purposes of such systems [1]. As an active research topic in computer vision, visual surveillance in dynamic scenes attempts to detect, track and recognize certain objects from image sequences, and more generally to understand and describe object behaviors. The aim is to develop intelligent surveillance to replace the traditional passive video surveillance which has proved to be ineffective when the number of cameras exceeds the capability of human operators to monitor [2]. In short, the goal of visual surveillance is not only to put cameras to take place of human eyes, but also to accomplish the entire surveillance task as automatically as possible.

All of the visual surveillances are evidence of a great and growing interest in detecting moving walker, which can find crimes, accidents, terrorist attacks etc. The prerequisites for effective automatic detect using a camera includes the following steps: motion detection, objects tracking, behavior understanding. What we do in this paper is a model-free method with prior knowledge which denotes the entire body,

C. Tang et al. (Eds.): ADMA 2008, LNAI 5139, pp. 604–611, 2008.

and it belongs to the work of the behavior understanding. Our paper therefore offers three main contributions:

- We propose an approach for inferring and generalizing anomaly from just contour, even if those particular motions have never been seen before.
- We present a Fuzzy Associative Memory method which allows efficiently classification movement.
- We present a method which robust, compact and effective represent pedestrian. The method is a complex number notation based on centroid.

The paper is organized as follows. In Section 2 we briefly review some related work. Then, in Section 3 we present the similarity comparison method based on Procrustes, and in Section 4 describe a method of getting different sorts of movement variety matrix using HMM. In Section 5 we present movement classify using FAM. Experimental results and conclusions are drawn in Section 6.

2   Related Work

Automatic recognition of human actions is a challenge, since human actions are hard to describe under different situations. It is not easy to define which actions are abnormal. Some attempts to automatically detect and predict abnormal behaviors have already been performed. One of the pioneers is Ghallab [3], who has proposed a method of model temporal scenarios whose occurrences need to be recognized on-line. He suggested a description of behaviors, which had a set of events and temporal constraints. The algorithm implements propagation of temporal constraints with an incremental path consistency algorithm derived from Mackword [4].

A more recent work is carried out by Mecocci [5], who introduces architecture of an automatic real-time video surveillance system. The proposed system automatically adapts to different scenarios without human intervention, and applies self-learning techniques to automatically learn typical behavior of targets in each specific environment. Oren Boiman [6] tried to compose a newly observed image region or a new video segment using chunks of data extracted from previous visual examples.

Recent researches on the major existing methods for abnormal detecting are reviewed. They are Model-based method, Statistical method, Physical-parameter-based method and spatio-temporal motion-based method [2]. In theory models are sufficient for recognition of people by their gait. However accurately recovering models from a walking video is still an unsolved problem and the computational cost is quite high. Statistical methods are relatively robust to noise and change of time interval in input image sequences. Compared with model-based approaches, the computational cost of is low. Physical-parameter-based methods are intuitive and understandable, and independent on viewing angles. However they depend greatly on the vision techniques used to recover the required parameters and the parameters used for recognition may be not effective enough across a large population. Spatio-temporal motion-based methods are able to capture both spatial and temporal information of gait motion better. Their advantages are low computational complexity and a simple implementation. However they are susceptible to noise.

Despite the considerable achievements on the field accomplished in the recent years, there are still some challenges to overcome. The optimal abnormal behavior detecting should allow the detection of suspicious events with a minimal description of the scene context, perform the detection without the need of dataset, and comprise the real-time constraints of a surveillance system [7].

To achieve this goal, we developed a method of FAM to classify movements and detect anomalism, which is described and evaluated in this paper.

3 Similarity Comparison

In order to robust, compact and effective represent pedestrian, a complex number notation based on human centroid is proposed. Furthermore we compare similarity of two contour using Procrustes Mean Shape Distance (PMSD).

3.1 Represent Body Contour

An important cue in determining underlying motion of a walking figure is the temporal changes in the walker's silhouette shape [8]. The method proposed here provides a simple, real-time, robust way of detecting contour points on the edge of the target. The centroid (x_c, y_c) of the human blob is determined using the following:

$$x_c = \frac{1}{N_b} \sum_{i=1}^{N_b} x_i \qquad y_c = \frac{1}{N_b} \sum_{i=1}^{N_b} y_i \tag{1}$$

Where (x_i, y_i) represents the points on the contour and there are a total of N_b points on the contour. Let the centroid be the origin of the 2-D shape space. Then we can unwrap each shape anticlockwise into a set of boundary pixel points sampled along its outer-contour in a common complex coordinate system [10]. That is, each shape can be described as a vector of ordered complex numbers with N_b elements.

$$Z = [z_1, z_2, \ldots\ldots, z_i, \ldots\ldots z_{N_B}]^T \tag{2}$$

Where $z_i = x_i + j * y_i$. The silhouette shape representation is illustrated in Fig 1, where the black dot indicates the shape centroid, and the two axes Re and Im represent the real and imaginary part of a complex number, respectively.

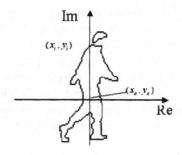

Fig. 1. Silhouette shape representation

3.2 Procrustes Shape Analyses

Procrustes shape analysis [10] is a popular method in directional statistics, and it is intended to cope with 2-D shapes. A shape in 2-D space can be described by (2) called a configuration. For two shapes, z_1 and z_2, their configurations are equal through a combination of translation, scaling, and rotation.

$$\begin{cases} z_1 = \alpha 1_k + \beta z_2, \alpha, \beta \in C \\ \beta = |\beta| e^{i\angle\beta} \end{cases} \tag{3}$$

Where $\alpha 1_k$ translates z_2, and $|\beta|$ and $\angle\beta$ scale and rotate z_2 respectively, we may consider they represent the same shape [11]. It is convenient to define the centered configuration $U = [u_1, u_2, \ldots \ldots u_k]^T$, $u_i = z_i - \overline{z}$, $\overline{z} = \sum_{i=1}^{k} z_i / k$. The full Procrustes distance $d_F(u_1, u_2)$ between two configurations can be defined as:

$$d_F(u_1, u_2) = 1 - \frac{|u_1 * u_2|^2}{\|u_1\|^2 \|u_2\|^2} \qquad \left\| \frac{u_1}{\|u_1\|} - \alpha 1_k - \beta \frac{u_2}{\|u_2\|} \right\|^2 \text{ (Which minimizes)} \tag{4}$$

The superscript * represents the complex conjugation transpose and $0 \le d_F \le 1$. The Procrustes distance allows us to compare two shapes independent of position, scale, and rotation.

3.3 Similarity Measure

To measure similarity between two gait sequences, we make use of the PMSD in the following way.

1) Compute the two gait sequences which are the capture image $\hat{u}_1$ and the standard image $\hat{u}_2$. 2) Find the Procrustes distance between the two mean shapes.

$$d(\hat{u}_1, \hat{u}_2) = 1 - \frac{|\hat{u}_1 * \hat{u}_2|^2}{\|\hat{u}_1\|^2 \|\hat{u}_2\|^2} \tag{5}$$

The smaller the above distance measure is, the more similar the two gaits are.

4   Motion Sequence

Gait changes both in spatial and temporal information. We model some usual actions.

4.1 Standard Sequence

We can divide human beings' different actions into a set of standard image sequences [6], such as walk, side walk, crouching, jump, uphill, downhill and tussling etc. We use a set of continuous frame to express a cycle of canonical behavior, distill people's

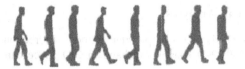

Fig. 2. A process of walking

contours, and establish libraries for them. In order to express our method, a sample of walk is selected in this paper. Fig 2 shows a set of image sequence of a walking man.

4.2   HMM Model

HMM is widely used to forecast the potential sequence of an event according to its samples [12]. It is very efficient in learning and matching behavior models. Three base questions on HMM include evaluation, decoding and learning. The decoding means to work out the most possible state sequence for the present model and observation sequence. And the Viterbi Arithmetic can settle this problem. In this paper we will find the probability of each status in one motion sequence using Viterbi.

Describe the HMM using the model which has five factors and expresse as $\lambda_i = (N_i, M_i, \Pi_i, A_i, B_i)$. The N_i represents ith motion states, M_i is the deputy of the pictures' total number in i^* motion base, and the Π_i is the probability of choosing i^* certain motion base, the A_i is the transfer probability, the B_i represents the image distributing in each base. The question is to get a correct state sequence $S^i = q_1^i, q_2^i, ... q_r^i$, for the observation sequence $O^i = o_1^i, o_2^i, ... o_r^i$ and the model λ, so as to S^i is the best explain of the observation sequence O^i. As for decoding, we put forward the Viterbi arithmetic, the details are as follow.

$$\delta_t(i) = \max_{q_1, q_2, \cdots q_{t-1}} P[q_1, q_2, ... q_{t-1}, q_t = i, O_1, O_2, ... O_t \mid \lambda_i] \tag{6}$$

N is the amount of states and the T is the length of the sequence. The sequence we looking for is the state sequence that the biggest $\delta_T(i)$ represents in the time point T. Initialize at first.

$$\delta_1(i) = \pi_i b_i(O_1), 1 \le i \le N \qquad \varphi_1(i) = 0, 1 \le i \le N \tag{7}$$

Recursion by the formula:

$$\begin{cases} \delta_t(j) = \max_{1 \le j \le N}[\delta_{t-1}(i)a_{ij}]b_j(O_t), 2 \le t \le T, 1 \le j \le N \\ \varphi_t(j) = \arg\max_{1 \le j \le N}[\delta_{t-1}(i)a_{ij}], 2 \le t \le T, 1 \le j \le N \end{cases} \tag{8}$$

Then, we can work out the end.

$$P^* = \max_{1 \le j \le N}[\delta_T(i)] \qquad q_T^* = \arg\max_{1 \le j \le N}[\delta_T(i)] \tag{9}$$

And the sequence S^i we looking for is.

$$q_t^* = \varphi_{t+1}(q_{t+1}^*), t = T - 1, T - 2, ... 1 \tag{10}$$

Thus we can get the walk matrix:

$$M_1 = [q_1^i, q_2^i, ... q_r^i]^T = \begin{pmatrix} b_{11}^1 & \cdots & b_{1m}^1 \\ \vdots & \ddots & \vdots \\ b_{r1}^1 & \cdots & b_{rm}^1 \end{pmatrix} \tag{11}$$

Follow this way we can get side walk, crouching, jump, uphill, downhill and tussling matrices as $M_2, ..., M_n$.

5 Motion Classification

By combining associative memory and fuzzy logic, Kosko devised FAM, which encodes the fuzzy output set Y with the fuzzy input set X. The numerical framework of FAM allows us to adaptively add and modify fuzzy rules. As shown in Fig 3 associative neural networks are simple nets, in which the weights, denoted by W, are determined by the fuzzy Hebb rule matrix or the "correlation-minimum encoding" scheme. Each association is a pair of vectors connecting X and Y. The weight or correlation matrix W maps the input X to the associated output Y by a max–min composition operation "$\circ$"

$$Y = X \circ W \tag{12}$$

In general, a FAM system encodes and processes a set of rules in parallel. Each input to the system will activate each encoded rule to a different degree. The proposed FAM network is composed of three layers: X, R and Y, as shown in Fig 3 A node in the X-layer represents a fuzzy set in the antecedent part of a fuzzy rule. A node in the Y-layer represents the membership of different motion. Fuzzy inference is then invoked between the X-layer and the R-layer by the max–min composition operation. Finally, the inferred results obtained by each rule are aggregated to produce a final result for the Y-layer. The aggregation is given by adding the associative relationships between the R–layer and the Y-layer.

The X-layer is membership function layer which turns the input values into membership. That is the similarity degree between the capture images and the standard gait of all libraries.

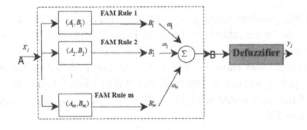

Fig. 3. FAM system architecture

In the R -layer each node represents one rule. These acquired rules based on learning algorithms. In this layer each input vector of similarity degree and the motion matrix using fuzzy vector-matrix multiplication.

$$A_i \circ M_i = B_i', B_i = \max(B_i') \tag{13}$$

Where, $A = (a_1, ...a_r), B = (b_1, ...b_m)$, M is a fuzzy n-by-p matrix (a point in $I^{r \times m}$)

$$b_j = \max_{1 \le i \le r} \min(a_i, m_{i,j}) \tag{14}$$

The Y -layer is output, which is a result layer. In the multi-input single-output system, the initial value weight ω_i is the membership of rules. And then use iteration algorithm, the output layer function:

$$y = \sum_{i=1}^{z} \omega_i B_i \tag{15}$$

In our system [13], there are four separate modules—fuzzification, FAM, translation, and defuzzification. In addition, a training module that modifies FAM weights to improve system performance is also included. The outline of the proposed system is shown in Fig 4. If additional data sets containing different relationships are available, the training module can also learn these different pairs from the data sets.

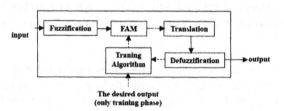

Fig. 4. The proposed model

6 Evaluation and Conclusion

In order to verify the result of FAM to abnormal behavior, we do some researches.

I In order to ensure the integrality of the contour, after we have got the person's contour by using Background Deduction and Time Difference Method, we use Region Inosculating combined with the Theory of Morphologic Erosion and Expansion [14] to run.

II To solve the problem when people enter or leave the scene the contour is not full, we cut off the frames about the process. Detect the motion while the target entered the scene completely.

III The experiment was carried out on a PC running at 1.7GHz. Taking a speed of about 15 frames per second can be achieved, which is efficient for real time surveillance.

IV The FAM model is tested with over 120 data. The recognition results on testing data are more than 70%.

V In our test system, we defined as "regular behavior" motions include walking, jogging, uphill and downhill etc. While other behaviors, such as crouching, jumping, side walking, tussling are identified as anomalistic ones. At the same time the sequence of video is judged abnormal. Security alarm system will automatically alarm.

We have described an approach to detect the motion of people using fuzzy associative memory network. On the basis of the results, we could build an intelligent security system. In some special scenes, after capturing motive target by camera, we can trace it and give an alarm aiming at the suspicious action. If we do this, we could save money and manpower, and the more important is that we could prevent from crime. Thus, computer can be not only people's eyes, but also an assistant, who can understand people and describe the action of motive target.

References

1. Chen, Y., Liang, G., Lee, K.K., Xu, Y.: Abnormal behavior detection by multi-SVM-based Bayesian network. In: Proc. int. conf. Information Acquisition, pp. 298–303 (2007)
2. Hu, W., Tan, T., Wang, L., Maybank, S.: A survey on visual surveillance of object motion and behaviors. IEEE Trans. System, Man, And Cybernetics 34(3), 334–352 (2004)
3. Ghallab, M.: On Chronicles: Representation, On-line Recognition and Learning. In: 5th Int. Conf. on Principles of Knowledge Representation and Reasoning, Cambridge, pp. 597–606 (1996)
4. Mackworth, A.K., Freuder, E.C.: The Complexity of Some Polynomial Network Consistency Algorithms for Satisfaction Problems. Artificial Intelligence 25, 65–74 (1985)
5. Mecocci, A., Pannozzo, M., Fumarola, A.: Automatic Detection of Anomalous Behavioural Events for Advanced Real-Time Video Surveillance. In: Int. Symposium on Computational Intelligence for Measurement Systems and Applications, Lugano, pp. 187–192 (2003)
6. Boiman, O., Irani, M.: Detecting irregularities in images and in video. In: Proc. IEEE Int. conf. Computer Vision, pp. 462–469 (2005)
7. Duque, D., Santos, H., Cortez, P.: Prediction of abnormal Behaviors for intelligent video surveillance system. In: Proc. IEEE Int. conf. Computational Intelligence and Data Mining, pp. 362–367 (2007)
8. Fujiyoshi, H., Lipton, A.: Real-time human motion analysis by image skeletonization. In: Proc. IEEE Workshop on Applications of Computer Vision, Princeton, NJ, pp. 15–21 (1998)
9. Takagi, T., Sugeno, M.: Fuzzy identification of systems and its applications to modeling and control. IEEE Trans. Syst., Man, Cybern. SMC-15(1), 116–132 (1985)
10. Wang, L., Tan, T., Hu, W., Ning, H.: Automatic Gait Recognition Based on Statistical Shape Analysis. IEEE Trans. Image Processing 12(93), 1120–1131 (2003)
11. Boyd, J.: Video phase-locked loops in gait recognition. In: Proc. Int. Conf. Computer Vision (2001)
12. Birney, E.: Hidden Markov Models in Biological sequence analysis. IBM Journal of Research and Development 45(3/4) (2001)
13. Ralescu, A.L. (ed.): Applied Research in Fuzzy Technology: Three Years of Research at the Laboratory for International Fuzzy Engineering (LIFE), Yokohama, Japan, pp. 295–369. Kluwer, Norwell (1994)
14. Gonzalez, R.C., Woods, R.E.: Digital Image Processing. Publishing House of Electronics Industry (2002)

Moment+: Mining Closed Frequent Itemsets over Data Stream*

Haifeng Li and Hong Chen

School of Information, Renmin University of China
Key Laboratory of Data Engineering and Knowledge Engineering, MOE
Beijing 100872, China
mydlhf@126.com, chong@ruc.edu.cn

Abstract. Closed frequent itemsets(*CFI*) mining uses less memory to store the entire information of frequent itemsets thus is much suitable for mining stream. In this paper, we discuss recent *CFI* mining methods over stream and presents an improved algorithm *Moment+* based on the existent one *Moment*. *Moment+* focuses on the problem of mining *CFI* over data stream sliding window and proposes a new structure Extended Closed Enumeration Tree(*ECET*) to store the *CFIs* and nodes' *BPN* which is introduced to reduce the search space, with which new mining method is designed to mine more rapidly with little memory cost sacrifice. The experimental results show that this method is effective and efficient.

1   Introduction

The concept closed itemset was first proposed in [4] in 1999. An itemset is closed if none of its super-itemsets have the same weight with it, and a closed frequent itemset(*CFI*) is both closed and frequent. The importance of *CFI* mining rests on not only the requiring of the complete and compressed information of *FIs* but also the more meaning of association rules extraction from CFI[7]. Many researches on *CFI* mining over traditional database have been proposed such as CLOSET[5], CLOSET+[6] and CHARM[8]. Extended works also focus on the Closed Cube mining[3] and Closed Graph mining[9].

Recently, some *CFI* mining approaches over stream sliding window were presented include *Moment*[1] and *CFI-Stream*[2]. In [1], Chi et al proposed a *CFI* mining over sliding window of stream and used *CET* (Closed Enumeration Tree) to maintain the main information of itemsets. Each node in *CET* represents an itemset and is with different type. When the window slides, new transactions arrive and old transactions disappear, then nodes are inserted, updated and deleted according to their type. In *Moment*, the exploration and node type check spend

---

* This research is partly supported by the National Science Foundation of China(60673138,60603046), Key Program of Science Technology Research of MOE(106006), Program for New Century Excellent Talents in University and Chinese National Programs for Science and Technology Development(2005BA112A02).

C. Tang et al. (Eds.): ADMA 2008, LNAI 5139, pp. 612–619, 2008.

much computation time when the minimum support is low. In [2], Jiang and Gruenwald proposed a novel approach *CFI-Stream* in which a *DIU* (DIrect Update) tree is introduced to maintain only closed itemsets. Furthermore, series of theorems are presented to acquire the pruning conditions. *CFI-Stream* achieves a much condensed memory usage and running time cost than *Moment* when the minimum support is low.

In this paper, a new conception *BPN* is proposed to address the computation bottleneck of *Moment*, thus an Extended Closed Enumeration Tree (*ECET*) is employed to store the *CFI* nodes and some other information. Moreover, an improved algorithm named *Moment+* is proposed based on *ECET* to accelerate the computation speed.

The rest of this paper is organized as follows: In Section 2 we present the preliminaries of *CFI* mining and define the mining problem. Section 3 describes the detail of *Moment+* algorithm. Section 4 evaluates the performance of *Moment+* with experimental results. Finally, Section 5 concludes this paper.

2   Preliminaries and Problem Statement

2.1   Preliminaries

Given a set of distinct items $I = \{i_1, i_2, \cdots, i_n\}$ where $|I| = n$ denotes the number of I, a subset $X \subset I$ is called an itemset, suppose $|X| = k$, we call X a k-itemset. For two itemsets $\alpha = \{a_1, a_2, \cdots, a_s\}$ and $\beta = \{b_1, b_2, \cdots, b_t\}$, if $\exists c_1, c_2, \cdots, c_s$ satisfy $1 \le c_1 < c_2 < \cdots < c_s \le t$ and $a_1 \subseteq b_{c_1}$, $a_2 \subseteq b_{c_2}$, $\cdots$, $a_s \subseteq b_{c_s}$, we call α a subset of β and β a superset of α, denoted as $\alpha \subseteq \beta$ (if $\alpha \ne \beta$, then denoted as $\alpha \subset \beta$).

A database $D = \{T_1, T_2, \cdots, T_v\}$ is a collection wherein each transaction is a subset of I. Each transaction $T_i (i = 1 \cdots v)$ is related with an id, i.e. the id of T_i is i. The complete support (*CS*) of an itemset α is the number of transactions which include α, which is also called α's weight and denoted as $support_c(\alpha) = \{|T| | T \in D \wedge \alpha \subseteq T\}$; the relative support (*RS*) of an itemset α is the ratio of *CS* with respect to $|D|$, denoted as $support_r(\alpha) = \frac{support_c(\alpha)}{|D|}$. Given a minimum support $\lambda (0 \le \lambda \le 1)$, a FI is the itemset satisfies $support_r(\alpha) \ge \lambda \times |D|$. Let T be the subsets of D and X be the subsets of I, the concept of closed itemset is based on two following functions f and g: $f(T) = \{i \in I | \forall t \in T, i \in t\}$ which returns the set of itemsets included in all transactions belonging to T, and $g(X) = \{t \in D | \forall i \in X, i \in t\}$ which returns the set of transactions containing item set X. An itemset is said to be closed[2] iff $C(X)=f(g(X))=X$.

We also assume that there is a lexicographical order denoted as $\prec$ among distinct items in I, and thus an itemset in D can be reordered and represented with a sequence, then two itemsets can be compared according to the lexicographical order. For example, we have 3 distinct items $\{1\}$, $\{2\}$ and $\{3\}$, $\{1\}$ is lexicographical smaller than $\{2\}$ and $\{2\}$ is smaller than $\{3\}$, denoted as $\{1\} \prec \{2\} \prec \{3\}$. Giving two itemsets $\{1, 2, 3\}$ and $\{2, 3\}$, then we have $\{1, 2, 3\} \prec \{2, 3\}$.

2.2   Problem Definition

The problem is to mine *CFI* in the recent N transactions in a data stream. Fig.1 is an example with $I = \{1,2,3,4\}$, window size $N=4$ and minimum support $\lambda = 0.5$.

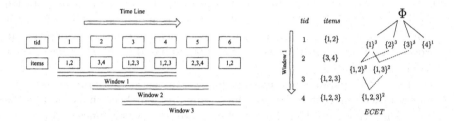

Fig. 1. A runing example of sliding window   **Fig. 2.** The initial ECET

3   *Moment+* Method

In this section, we introduce an in-memory structure to store *CFI*s, moreover, the tree building and maintenance are described.

3.1   Extended Closed Enumeration Tree

In *Moment*, the computational bottleneck lies on 1) the closure checking process when deciding node type, 2) the sliding window scanning process to generate new child node when a node becomes frequent or promising in addition function, or to delete old child node when a node becomes infrequent or unpromising. In this paper, we design an extended closed enumeration tree(called *ECET*) to focus on improving the computational efficiency. In *ECET*, we use n_α denote a node of itemset α. Giving the minimum support λ, then n_α is also divided into four types as described in [1]: infrequent node, unpromising node, intermediate node and closed node, and intermediate node and closed node are called promising node.

Definition 1. *Given a node* n_α, *for a node collection, in which each node* n_β *satisfies* $\alpha \subset \beta \wedge \alpha \succ \beta$, *we define the node* n_β *with the maximum CS and the minimum lexicographic order as the backward parent node(BPN) of* n_α.

Property 1. A node n_α has an unique *BPN*.

Property 2. Infrequent or intermediate node n_α has no *BPN*; Unpromising node n_α always has *BPN*.

In *ECET*, each node is a 4-tuples $< bp, iss, cps, wt >$, where *iss* is the itemset α, *cps* is a pointer collection to its children, *wt* is the *CS*, and *bp* points its

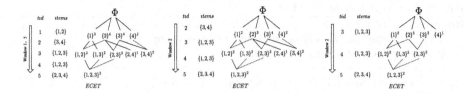

Fig. 3. $\{2,3,4\}$ is added   **Fig. 4.** $\{1,2\}$ is deleted   **Fig. 5.** $\{1,2,3\}$ is deleted

backward parent node, *BPN* has two advantages: One is to decide node type, another is to reduce the search space when a node changes type.

Fig.2 shows the *ECET* of the first window. The value at the right-top corner is the *CS*, and the dashed line point the backward parent node. $\{4\}$ is infrequent; $\{2\}$ and $\{1,3\}$ are unpromising nodes because they have the equal *CS* with their *BPNs*; $\{1\}$ is intermediate node because it has the equal *CS* with its child node $\{1,2\}$ even though it has no *BPN*; and $\{3\},\{1,2\}$ and $\{1,2,3\}$ are closed nodes.

3.2   *ECET* Building

Adding a New Transaction. When new transaction is added, if the node type does not change, we update the node information, i.e., the *CS* and *BPN* with little cost, otherwise new nodes are generated. We describe operations for different type nodes in detail in *Algorithm 1*.

Lemma 1. *An unpromising node n_α has no multiple equal CS's BPN.*

Proof. Suppose unpromising node n_α has nodes n_β and n_γ s.t. $n_\beta.iss \prec n_\gamma.iss$ and $n_\beta.wt = n_\gamma.wt$, i.e. $n_\alpha.wt = n_\beta.wt = n_\gamma.wt$, so $n_{\beta\cup\gamma}$ exists and its *CS* equals to the *CS* of n_γ, that means $n_{\gamma-\alpha}$ is also an unpromising node, so n_γ does not exist. Proof done.

Lemma 2. *When an unpromising node n_α turns promising, If n_α's children has BPN, it must be one of the children of n_α's BPN.*

Proof. We use S_n denote the collection wherein each transaction comprises *n.iss*. Because n_α is unpromising, we use n_δ to denote $n_\alpha.bp$, then $n_\alpha.wt = n_\delta.wt \wedge n_\alpha.iss \succ n_\delta.iss \wedge n_\alpha.iss \subset n_\delta.iss$, i.e., $S_{n_\alpha} = S_{n_\delta}$. Given n_α's child n_β, then $S_{n_\beta} \subseteq S_{n_\alpha}$ and $n_\beta.iss \succ n_\alpha.iss \wedge n_\alpha.iss \subset n_\beta.iss$, so there exists a child $n_{\delta\cup\beta}$ of n_δ s.t. $n_{\delta\cup\beta}.iss \prec n_\beta.iss$, because $S_{n_{\delta\cup\beta}} \subseteq S_{n_\delta}$ and n_δ is with the maximal *CS* as the n_α's *BPN*, then $n_{\delta\cup\beta}$ is also with the maximal *CS* in all the nodes that include n_β and lexicographically smaller than n_β, from *Lemma 1*, we can see that $n_{\delta\cup\beta}$ is n_β's *BPN*. Proof done.

A node n_α is ignored if it is not relevant to addition(*line 1-2*). For each n_α's child n_β, we will not generate its child node until n_β turns promising. Given each n_β's frequent sibling n_γ, there are two instances to perform(*line 4-8*): First, if $n_\beta.bp$ exists, from *Lemma 2* we will traverse from $n_\beta.bp$ to search the minimal length

---

Algorithm 1. Addition Function

Require: n_α: $ECET$ node; N_{new}: added transaction; tid: id of transaction N_{new}; N_{old}: deleted transaction; D: sliding window; λ: minimum support;

1: **if** n_α is not relevant to addition **then**
2:     return;
3: **for** each child node n_β(relevant to addition) of n_α **do**
4:     **if** n_β is newly promising **then**
5:         **for** each right frequent sibling node n_γ(relevant to addition) of n_β **do**
6:             create a new child node $n_{\beta\cup\gamma}$ for n_β;
7:             compute $n_{\beta\cup\gamma}.wt$ and $n_{\beta\cup\gamma}.bp$;
8:             update $n_\eta.bp(n_\eta.iss \subset n_{\beta\cup\gamma}.iss \wedge |n_\eta.iss| = |n_{\beta\cup\gamma}.iss| - 1)$;
9:     **else if** n_β keeps promising **then**
10:       **for** each right frequent sibling node(relevant to addition) n_γ for n_β **do**
11:          **if** $n_{\beta\cup\gamma}$ does not exist **then**
12:             create a new child node $n_{\beta\cup\gamma}$ for n_β;
13:             compute $n_{\beta\cup\gamma}.wt$ and $n_{\beta\cup\gamma}.bp$;
14:          **else**
15:             update $n_{\beta\cup\gamma}.wt$;
16:             update $n_\eta.bp(n_\eta.iss \subset n_{\beta\cup\gamma}.iss \wedge |n_\eta.iss| = |n_{\beta\cup\gamma}.iss| - 1)$;
17: **for** each child node n_β of n_α **do**
18:     Call Addition(n_β,N_{new},tid,N_{old},D,λ);
19: decide if n_α is closed;

---

node n_δ with $n_{\beta\cup\gamma}.iss \subset n_\delta.iss$. If n_δ exists and $!(n_\delta \subseteq N_{new})$, we compute as $n_{\beta\cup\gamma}.wt = n_\delta.wt + 1$ and $n_{\beta\cup\gamma}.bp = n_\delta$; if n_δ exists and $n_\delta \subseteq N_{new}$, we compute as $n_{\beta\cup\gamma}.wt = n_\delta.wt$ and $n_{\beta\cup\gamma}.bp = n_\delta$; if n_δ does not exist, we compute as $n_{\beta\cup\gamma}.wt = 1$ and $n_{\beta\cup\gamma}.bp = null$; Second, if $n_\beta.bp = null$, we will scan the sliding window to compute the n_β's child's CS $n_{\beta\cup\gamma}.wt$ and set as $n_{\beta\cup\gamma}.bp = null$. On the other hand, if n_β is already promising(*line 9-16*), we will update its children's CS if n_β's child $n_{\beta\cup\gamma}$ exists(*line 14-15*), whereas generate new child $n_{\beta\cup\gamma}$ for n_β and compute its CS by scanning the sliding window(*line 11-14*). After a child node $n_{\beta\cup\gamma}$ is generated or updated, we need to update all nodes' BPN i.e. $n_\eta.bp$ that n_η satisfies $n_\eta.iss \subset n_{\beta\cup\gamma}.iss \wedge |n_\eta.iss| = |n_{\beta\cup\gamma}.iss| - 1$(*line 8 and 16*). We separate three situations to discuss the updating strategy: First, if n_η exists, n_η has no BPN and $n_\eta.iss$ is lexicographical bigger than $n_{\beta\cup\gamma}.iss$, i.e., $n_\eta \neq null \wedge n_\eta.bp = null \wedge n_\eta.iss \succ n_{\beta\cup\gamma}.iss$, then we set as $n_\eta.bp = n_{\beta\cup\gamma}$; Second, if n_η exists, n_η's BPN exists, say n_ξ, and $n_\xi.ws < n_{\beta\cup\gamma}.ws$ or if $n_\xi.ws = n_{\beta\cup\gamma}.ws$ and $n_{\beta\cup\gamma}.iss \prec n_\xi.iss$, $n_\eta.bp$ is updated from n_ξ to $n_{\beta\cup\gamma}$; Third, if all above conditions are not satisfied, we perform nothing. Finally, we call addition on each child node n_β of n_α(*line 17-18*) and decide if n_α is closed(*line 19*).

We add a new transaction $\{2,3,4\}$ into the sliding window and get the $ECET$ as shown in Fig.3. $\{2\}$ turns promising, so we generate $\{2\}$'s children $\{2,3\}$ and $\{2,4\}$; because $\{2\}$ has BPN $\{1,2\}$, so we traverse from $\{1,2\}$ and find $\{1,2,3\}$ that contains $\{2,3\}$ thus set $\{2,3\}$'s CS to $\{1,2,3\}$'s CS plus 1 and set $\{2,3\}$'s BPN as $\{1,2,3\}$, find no node contains $\{2,4\}$ thus set $\{2,4\}$'s CS to 1 and set $\{2,4\}$'s BPN as null. we further update $\{3\}$'s BPN from $\{1,3\}$ to $\{2,3\}$ because

---

Algorithm 2. Deletion Function

Require: n_α: *ECET* node; N_{old}: deleted transaction; *tid*: id of transaction N_{old}; N_{new}: added transaction; D: sliding window; λ: minimum support;

1: **if** n_α is not relevant to deletion **then**
2:     return;
3: **for** each child n_β(relevant to deletion) of n_α **do**
4:     **if** n_β keeps promising **then**
5:         **for** each right sibling n_γ(relevant to deletion) of n_β **do**
6:             **if** n_γ is newly infrequent **then**
7:                 remove $n_{\beta\cup\gamma}$ and its descendant from closedcollection;
8:                 prune $n_{\beta\cup\gamma}$ and its descendant from *ECET*;
9:             **else**
10:                 update $n_{\beta\cup\gamma}.wt$;
11:     **else**
12:         **if** n_β is newly infrequent **then**
13:             **for** each left promising sibling n_γ(not relevant to deletion) of n_β **do**
14:                 remove $n_{\gamma\cup\beta}$ and its descendant from closedcollection;
15:                 prune $n_{\gamma\cup\beta}$ and its descendant from *ECET*;
16:         remove n_β's descendant from closedcollection;
17:         prune n_β's descendant from *ECET*;
18: **for** each child n_β(relevant to deletion) of n_α **do**
19:     CALL Deletion($n_\beta,N_{old},tid,N_{new},D,\lambda$);
20: **for** each child n_β(relevant to deletion) of n_α **do**
21:     update $n_\beta.bp$;
22: decide if n_α is closed;

$\{2,3\}$'s *CS* is bigger than $\{1,3\}$'s. On the other hand, because $\{3\}$ is not newly promising, we scan the sliding window to compute the *CS* of new node $\{3,4\}$. After adding $\{2,3,4\}$, $\{2\}$ turns closed, $\{2,3\}$ and $\{3,4\}$ are new and closed nodes.

Deleting an Existing Transaction. After adding a new transaction, we need to delete an existing transaction. Here we use the traditional strategy to delete the earliest transaction in sliding window. In most cases only updating for related nodes is performed; after a node turns unpromising or infrequent, we will prune brunches. The deletion function is described in *Algorithm 2*.

A node n_α is ignored if it is not relevant to deletion(*line 1-2*). For each child n_β of n_α, if n_β keeps promising(*line 4-10*), we will find all n_β's right sibling n_γ, if n_γ is newly infrequent, we prune $n_{\beta\cup\gamma}$ and its descendant from *ECET* and delete from closed linked list if any of them are closed(*line 6-9*), whereas we only update $n_{\beta\cup\gamma}.wt$(*line 9-10*); on the other hand, if n_β is newly unpromising(*line 11-17*), we will prune its descendant(*line 15-17*), in particular, if n_β is newly infrequent, we will find all its left sibling n_γ and prune $n_{\gamma\cup\beta}$ and its descendant(*line 13-15*). Then we call deletion on each child node n_β of n_α and update $n_\beta.bp$(*line 18-21*); finally, we decide if n_α is closed(*line 22*). When we update $n_\beta.bp$, there are four condition for discussion: First, when $n_\beta.bp$ is null, we keep it null; Second, when n_β turns infrequent, we set as $n_\beta.bp = null$; Third, if $n_\beta.bp$ is not null and not relevant to deletion, we keep it unchanged; Fourth, if $n_\beta.bp$ is not null and relevant to deletion, we will scan all its left frequent sibling n_δ to find a node $n_{\delta\cup\beta}$ satisfies $n_{\delta\cup\beta}.wt > n_\beta.bp.wt$ or $n_{\delta\cup\beta}.wt = n_\beta.bp.wt \wedge n_{\delta\cup\beta}.iss \prec n_\beta.bp.iss$, if $n_{\delta\cup\beta}$ exists, we set as $n_\beta.bp = n_{\delta\cup\beta}$.

In Fig.4, we delete the first transaction $\{1, 2\}$ from sliding window, because no nodes become unpromising or infrequent, we only update the related node's *CS*. We further delete the second transaction $\{3, 4\}$ in Fig.5. $\{4\}$ turns infrequent, so $\{2, 4\}$ and $\{3, 4\}$ are pruned and $\{4\}$'s *BPN* turns null.

4   Experimental Results

We use *Moment*[1] and *CFI-Stream*[2] as the evaluation algorithms, both of them perform *CFI* mining over stream's sliding window. All experiments are implemented with C++, compiled with Visual C++ in Windows XP and executed on a Pentium IV 3.2GHz PC with 512MB main memory. We use the real-life click stream dataset *KDDCUP2000* (http://www.ecn.purdue.edu/KDDCUP) to evaluate these algorithms, *KDDCUP2000* contains 515,597 transactions with 1657 distinct items, the maximal transaction size is 164 and the average transaction size is 6.5.

We compare the performance among three algorithms and thus set a fixed sliding window's size $|W| = 100,000$. Fig.6 presents the running time cost of *Moment+* in comparison with *Moment* and *CFI-Stream* at different minimum supports $\lambda(0.01 < \lambda < 0.1)$. The figure reflects the uniform changing trends of mining results of the three algorithms. But *Moment+* spends much less time than the other two algorithms even though when the minimum support is small.

We then compare the computation time of three algorithms when the minimum support is fixed, i.e., $\lambda = 0.05$ in different sliding windows' size$(50K < \lambda < 250K)$. Fig.7 presents the running time cost. As can be seen, when the size of sliding window increases, *Moment+* keeps its low computation cost and *Moment* costs a little more, and *CFI-Stream* costs much more because it stores all closed itemsets without minimum support constraint.

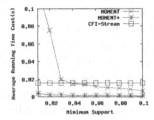
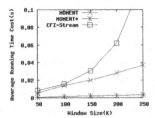

Fig. 6. Running time cost for different minimum support

Fig. 7. Running time cost for different window size

Because *Moment+* uses the similar framework with *Moment* in mining, the added item is the *BPN* pointer, on the other hand, the sum of id and the type of node is deleted, the experimental results also show that *Moment+*'s maximal memory cost is almost the same with *Moment*'s, so we ignore the presentation of memory evaluation.

5 Conclusions

In this paper we make a research on *CFI* mining over stream's sliding window, in allusion to the properties that sliding window can be adjusted according to the memory's size, we focus on caring more about running time cost thus a new algorithm *Moment+* is proposed. In *Moment+*, a new conception *BPN* is presented to address the computation bottleneck of *Moment*, then an extended tree *ECET* makes use of *BPN* is introduced to store data synopsis; base on *ECET* a maintaining process includes transaction addition and deletion is presented to improve the running time cost; Extensive experiments show that *Moment+* is effective and efficient.

References

1. Chi, Y., Wang, H., Yu, P., Muntz, R.: MOMENT: Maintaining Closed Frequent Itemsets over a Stream Sliding Window. In: Proceeding of IEEE ICDM the International Conference on Data Mining (2004)
2. Jiang, N., Gruenwald, L.: CFI-Stream: Mining Closed Frequent Itemsets in Data Streams. In: Proceeding of ACM SIGKDD the International Conference on Knowledge Discovery and Data Mining (2006)
3. Li, C., Cong, G., Tung, A.K.H., Wang, S.: Incremental Maintenance of Quotient Cube for Median. In: Proceeding of ACM SIGKDD the International Conference on Knowledge Discovery and Data Mining (2004)
4. Pasquier, N., Bastide, Y., Taouil, R., Lakhal, L.: Discovering frequent closed itemsets for association rules. In: Proceedings of ICDT the International Conference on Database Theory (1999)
5. Pei, J., Han, J., Mao, R.: Closet: An efficient algorithm for mining frequent closed itemsets. In: ACM SIGMOD the Internatial Workshop on Data Mining and Knowledge Discovery (2000)
6. Wang, J., Han, J., Pei, J.: CLOSET+: Searching for the Best Strategies for Mining Frequent Closed Itemsets. In: Proceeding of ACM SIGKDD the International Conference on Knowledge Discovery and Data Mining (2003)
7. Zaki, M.J.: Generating non-redundant association rules. In: Proceeding of ACM SIGKDD the International Conference on Knowledge Discovery and Data Mining (2000)
8. Zaki, M.J., Hsiao, C.: Charm: An efficient algorithm for closed itemset mining. In: Proceedings of SDM the SIAM International Conference on Data Mining (2002)
9. Zheng, Z., Wang, J., Zhou, L.: Out-of-Core Coherent Closed Quasi-Clique Mining from Large Dense Graph Databases. ACM Transactions on Database Systems (2007)

CDPM: Finding and Evaluating Community Structure in Social Networks[*]

Li Wan[1,2], Jianxin Liao[1,2], and Xiaomin Zhu[1,2],

[1] State Key Laboratory of Networking and Switching Technology,
Beijing University of Posts and Telecommunications, Beijing, China 100876
[2] EBUPT Information Technology Co., Ltd, Beijing, China 100083
{wanli,liaojianxin,zhuxiaomin}@ebupt.com

Abstract. In this paper we proposed a CDPM (Clique Directed Percolation Method) algorithm, which clusters tightly cohesive cliques as cluster atoms and merge the cluster atoms into communities under the direction of a proposed object function, namely Structure Silhouette Coefficient (SSC). SSC could measure the quality of community divisions which allows communities share actors. Experiments demonstrate our algorithm can divide social networks into communities at a higher quality than compared algorithms.

Keywords: community detection, percolation, clique.

1 Introduction

Finding communities in social networks is recently a challenge problem in both computer science and social network analysis communities. It's considered as a graph clustering problem in computer science community. Although there is not a critical definition of community structure, most of the existed literatures define that the density of intra cluster edges is larger than that of inter cluster edges. There are two types of communities, one is disjointed community, which not allowed an actor to appear in two different communities. The other type is overlapping community, which allowed communities to share actors. Approaches of finding community fall into two classes, divisive [1] and agglomerative [2, 3]. The divisive algorithm is a top-down process which split the graph into communities by removing edges with different strategies. Agglomerative algorithm is a bottom-up process which assigned actors into communities according to different similarity metrics.

However, in real world, communities often overlap each other. For example, an actor in social network may often belong to many communities, such as family, college

---

[*] This work was jointly supported by: (1) National Science Fund for Distinguished Young Scholars (No. 60525110); (2) National 973 Program (No. 2007CB307100, 2007CB307103); (3) Program for New Century Excellent Talents in University (No. NCET-04-0111); (4) Development Fund Project for Electronic and Information Industry (Mobile Service and Application System Based on 3G).

C. Tang et al. (Eds.): ADMA 2008, LNAI 5139, pp. 620–627, 2008.

and friend communities. Palla [2, 3] proposed a k-clique percolation method (CPM) to find overlapping communities in social networks, and induced the percolation point of clique percolation in random graphs. Ref. [4] proposed an extending algorithm of GN to find overlapping communities.

In this paper, authors cluster the graph using a proposed method CDPM (clique directed percolation method). Not as CPM [2], our algorithm considers a directed percolation method of maximal cliques, and qualifies the overlapping community divisions by a proposed Structure Silhouette Coefficient.

In this paper, we tackle the problem of overlapping community detection and make the following contributions:

1. We proposed an algorithm CDPM to find overlapping community in graphs. The proposed algorithm generates all maximal cliques in given graphs, and assigned them in different cluster atoms through a directed percolation method.
2. We proposed a Structure Silhouette Coefficient to qualify community divisions, which conduct the merging of cluster atoms. CDPM outputs the division with highest Structure Silhouette Coefficient.
3. Experiments demonstrate that CDPM performs well than the compared algorithm under both F-measure and VAD (vertex average degree).

The remainder of this paper is organized as follows: after the Related Work Section, the problem is formulated in Section 3. Section 4 details the CDPM algorithms. Section 5 describes experiments. Conclusion and future work are contained in Section 6.

2 Related Work

Ref. [2, 3, 5] proposes a k-clique percolation method (CPM) to find overlapping communities, and the method is implemented in CFinder [6]. It defines a model of rolling a k-clique template. Thus, the k-clique percolation clusters of a graph are all those sub-graphs that can be fully explored but cannot be left by rolling a k-clique template in them. Ref. [5] theoretically deduces the critical point of k-clique percolation on a random graph. But CPM doesn't propose object function to quantitatively qualify the clustering results.

Ref. [4] proposed CONGA algorithm to find overlapping communities by extending GN algorithm. It proposed split betweenness $c_B(v)$ and pair betweenness $c_B(e)$ which decide when and how to split vertices. Although not as CPM, CONGA qualify clustering results by Q function proposed in GN, CONGA also inherit the time complexity $O(m^3)$ in the worst case, the time of running CONGA on large graph is unacceptable.

Li et al. [7] form overlapping clusters using both the structure of the network and the content of vertices and edges. There are two phase in the algorithm, the first one finds densely connected "community cores", the "community cores" are defined as densely overlapped cliques. In the second phase, further triangles and edges whose content (assessed using keywords) is similar to that of the core are attached to the community cores.

3 Preliminary

3.1 Basic Definitions

Definition 1. Clique r-Adjacent and Maximal-Adjacent

Two maximal clique with size L and S respectively are r-adjacent, if they share O vertices, and $\dfrac{(S-1)}{(L+S-O)} \geq r$, where $L \geq S$ and $0 \leq r \leq 1$. If $O = S - 1$, the two cliques are maximal-adjacent.

Definition 2. Directed Percolation

Suppose two cliques are r-adjacent or maximal-adjacent, the percolation direction is constraint from the larger one to the smaller one. If the two cliques have the same sizes, the percolation could occur in any direction. The cliques not smaller than any r-adjacent and maximal-adjacent are the sources of percolation.

Definition 3. Galois Lattice

Consider a triple (A, C, M) where A and C are finite non-empty sets and $M \subseteq A \times C$ is a binary relation. The relation M can be used to define a mapping f: $B \rightarrow f(B)$ from P(A) to P(C) (P(A) denotes the power sets of A):

$$f(B) = \{c \in C \mid (a,c) \in M, a \in B\}$$

M can be used to define another mapping g: $D \rightarrow g(D)$ from P(C) to P(A):

$$g(D) = \{a \in A \mid (a,c) \in M, \forall c \in D\}$$

Let S(A)={f(A1), f(A2),...}, the collection of images of f, and S(C) = {g(C1), g(C2),...}, the subsets that make up S(C) form a lattice under inclusion, as do the subsets that make up S(A). These two lattices are dual inverse, and they can be represented in a single lattice $S(C) \times S(A)$. A dual lattice of this sort is called Galois.

Lemma 1. Minimum edge connectivity

Let n-graph Q = (V, E) be a r-quasi-clique ($0.5 \leq r \leq 1$, $n \geq 2$). The edge connectivity of Q cannot be smaller than $\left\lfloor \dfrac{n}{2} \right\rfloor$, namely, $\kappa(Q) \geq \left\lfloor \dfrac{n}{2} \right\rfloor$

The proof of the lemma is detailed in [8].

3.2 Problem Definition

In this paper, the ultimate goal is to find the overlapping community in a given graph, and we formulate the problem of finding overlapping community as follows:

Given a graph G = (V, E), the goal of the overlapping community finding problem is to find a cluster graph CG = (V_c, E_c), in which vertices denote clusters and if the actors in two clusters have interactions in G, there exist an edge between corresponding cluster vertices in CG, such CG maximizes the Structure Silhouette Coefficient (see section 4.1).

4 Community Detection

4.1 Structure Silhouette Coefficient

Dealing with attribute data, the Silhouette Coefficient [9] is a measurement, which qualifies the clustering quality independent of the number of clusters. It compares for every data object the distance to the assigned cluster center with the distance to the second-closest cluster center. Formally, $s = \frac{1}{n}\sum_{i=1}^{n}\frac{b(i)-a(i)}{\max\{b(i),a(i)\}}$, where a(i) is the distance from data object i to the center of the cluster, to which it was assigned, and b(i) is the distance to the second-closest cluster center. This definition of Silhouette Coefficient is not applicable to a graph clustering problem, since the goal of a graph cluster analysis is to discover clusters which are as distinctive as possible from connected clusters. The key point of proposed Structure Silhouette Coefficient is to determine the center of a sub-graph.

According to Def. 3.3 all the maximal cliques of a graph could be organized in a Galois lattice (V, C, M), V is the set of vertices, C is the set of all maximal cliques and M is a binary relation in $V \times C$, the level 0 of Galois lattice contains the vertices in the graph. Each point in level 1 corresponds to a maximal clique, the points in level n contain the vertices belongs to $n-1$ overlapped cliques. Intuitively the center of a sub-graph is the vertex from which the shortest paths to all the other vertices in the sub-graph have nearly the same length. So we define the center of a cluster atom as the vertex which is at the deepest level of the Galois lattice, compared with the other vertices in the cluster atom.

So we could formally define Structure Silhouette Coefficient as follows: (*Structure Silhouette Coefficient*) Given a graph G = (V, E) and cluster graph CG = (V_c, E_c), the Structure Silhouette Coefficient (SSC) is $s = \frac{1}{|V|}\sum_{i\in V}\frac{b(i)-a(i)}{\max\{b(i),a(i)\}}$, where a is the cluster to which i was assigned. a(i) is the graph distance to the center of a and b(i) is the average graph distance to all neighboring clusters of a in CG.

4.2 CDPM Algorithm

CDPM is an agglomerative algorithm to find overlapping communities. The input of CDPM is a simple graph G, the output is an overlapping community division. It's listed as follows.

CDPM Algorithm
1: INPUT: G(V, E), r (see definition 3.2)
2: OUTPUT: overlapping communities in graph G(V, E)
3: \\ FIRST PHASE: Generating maximal cliques
4: Init() \\Reading graph and Index the vertices
5: TriangleSet = FindTriangles(G)
6:MaximalCliques = GenerateMaximalCliques(TriangleSet)
7: \\ SECONDE PHASE: Finding cluster atoms
8:CliqueRlinkeGraph=ConstructCRLGraph(MaximalCliques,r)
9:ClusterAtoms=DirectedPercolation(CliqueRlinkedGraph)
10:initClusterGraph=ConstructCG(ClusterAtoms)
11:\\ THIRD PHASE: Maximizing SSC
12:GaloisLattice=ConstructLattice(CliqueRlinkedGraph)
13:finalClusterGraph=mergeAtoms(initClusterGraph,GaloisLattice)
14:OutputCommunity(finalClusterGraph)
15:\\finalClusterGraph maximize Structure Silhouette Coefficient

The first phase generates all maximal cliques, the related algorithms are detailed in our previous work [10]. In the second phase, CDPM cluster the maximal cliques into cluster atoms. A cluster atom is a directed percolation cluster in the clique r-linked graph (i.e. vertices denote cliques, if two cliques are r-adjacent or maximal adjacent, there exist and edge between them). The cluster atoms are initiated by percolation sources, and the vertices in clique r-link graph are added to corresponding cluster atoms following percolation rule (see Def. 3.2). In the third phase, CDPM construct Galois lattice from the clique r-linked graph, then merge cluster atoms by mergeAtoms. It keeps on merging vertices in cluster graph until there is only one vertex left. Before every mergence, mergeAtoms iterate every edge of cluster graph and calculate the SSC supposing that the two vertices connected by this edge is merged, then really merge the end points of the edge that get the maximum supposing SSC. The output of mergeAtoms is the cluster graph with the highest SSC.

5   Experiments

In this section, we compare CDPM with CPM[1] [6] and GN [1] algorithms, to assess the efficiency and clustering quality of the algorithms.

5.1   Experimental Evaluation

We test all algorithms on real-world datasets. We use *F-measure* and *vertex average degree (VAD)* to numerically measure how well each algorithm can find the community structure from a graph.

F-measure is calculated as follows:

- *Recall*: the fraction of vertex pairs belonging to the same community which are also in the same cluster.

---

[1] CPM is implemented in CFinder (version-2.0-beta3).

- *Precision*: the fraction of vertex pairs in the same cluster which are also in the same community.

- F-measure:$=\dfrac{2\times recall\times precision}{recall+precision}$

Besides the common measure of clustering algorithms (i.e. F-measure), there is no widely accepted alternative measure for the overlapping cluster divisions, but a promising candidate is the average degree measure [11]. Vertex average degree (VAD) is defined as:

- $vad(S)=\dfrac{2\sum\limits_{C\in S}\mid E(C)\mid}{\sum\limits_{C\in S}\mid C\mid}$, where S denotes a set of clusters, E(C) denotes the

set of edges in cluster C. The justification of VAD is discussed in [11].

We run our experiment on a 1.8 GHz Pentium IV with 1.0 GB of memory running Windows2003 platform.

The results of algorithms running on these datasets which define the community could be measured by F-measure, and they are listed in table 1. The other datasets doesn't define the community, and we could only measure them by VAD, results are listed in table 2. All the results of CDPM listed in the two tables are got by setting r = 0.5, the empirical study shows that when r=0.5 we get best results.

"Karate-club" is a classic studied social network in social network analysis [12], it describes the interactions between the members of a karate club at an American university. There are two known communities in the dataset.

"Dolphin" is a social network of bottlenose dolphins of Doubtful Sound [13], there are two known communities in the social network.

"College football" [14] is a network based on games between teams that belong to 15 disjoint real-world communities as illustrated in Fig. 3. This network has many intercommunity edges.

Table 1. Results of real-world datasets defined communities under F-measure and VAD

dataset		recall	Precision	F-measure	VAD
karate club	GN	0.48	0.96	0.64	3.18
	CPM	0.71	0.52	0.60	4.22
	CDPM	0.73	0.96	0.82	4.21
dolphin	GN	0.92	0.44	0.60	4.09
	CPM	0.36	0.89	0.52	5.08
	CDPM	0.91	0.54	0.68	4.67
College football	GN	0.82	0.48	0.60	5.87
	CPM	0.73	0.44	0.54	5.56
	CDPM	0.90	0.51	0.66	6.00

As shown in table 1, CDPM performs well by F-measure, it beats both GN and CPM on all data sets. CPM has the lowest F-measure value, because it doesn't consider the vertices not contained in k-cliques, so its recall and precision is relatively lower than the other two algorithms. But CPM performs better by VAD, because the k-clique clusters don't consider the one-degree vertices, so they have higher edge density of intra cluster.

"Co-authorship" is a collaboration network. It's delivered with CFinder software as a demo file [6]. The communities are not known in the network. The datasets "Call-graph01" to "Call-graph04" are call graphs of a telecom career in China. The size of these graphs are listed in table 2, we could conclude that CDPM and CPM are both scalable to large graphs (GN could not get results on these large graphs in acceptable time), but CDPM performs well under the VAD measure.

Table 2. Results of real-world datasets don't define communities under VAD measure

Data sets	Co-authorship	Call-graph01	Call-graph02	Call-graph03	Call-graph04
Vertices	16662	512024	503275	540342	539299
Edges	22446	1021861	900329	1030489	1014800
CDPM	2.81	3.87	4.71	4.13	3.94
CPM	2.73	3.56	4.33	4.02	3.94

5.2 Computational Complexity

Our algorithm inherit the complexity of the algorithm newClim[11], It runs with time $O(d^2 * N * S)$ delay and in $O(n + m)$ space, where D, N, S denote the maximum degree of G, the number of maximal cliques, the size of the maximum clique respectively, and d is the number of triangles contain a vertex with degree D, $d = C*T$ where C and T denote the clustering coefficient of the vertex with degree D and the maximum number of triangles can be constructed that contain the vertex with degree D (i.e. $T = D*(D - 1)/2$) respectively. The computational complexity of directed percolation and cluster atoms mergence is $O(n^2)$ and $O(m*n)$ respectively. So the complexity of CDPM is $O(d^2 * N * S)$.

6 Conclusion and Future Work

We proposed an algorithm to find overlapping communities in social networks based on a clique directed percolation method. Our algorithm performs well on real-world datasets under both F-measure and VAD measure. We organized all maximal cliques in a graph in two patterns, i.e. clique r-linked graph and Galois lattice. The first pattern presents the overlapping topological structure among cliques, and we can easily cluster the cliques into cluster atoms by a directed percolation method on this r-linked graph. The Galois lattice pattern let us numerically measure the role of a vertex in cluster atoms, and we define the center vertex of a cluster atom according to its position in the Galois lattice. Based on the definition of cluster atom center, we proposed Structure Silhouette Coefficient, which could evaluate the quality of community division. The optimal community division should maximize the value of Structure Silhouette Coefficient.

How to visualize the community division to help analyzers comprehending clustered results is an interesting topic for future work.

References

[1] Newman, M.E.J., Girvan, M.: Finding and evaluating community structure in networks. Phys. Rev. E 69(026113), 56–68 (2004)

[2] Palla, G., Derényi, I., Farkas, I., Vicsek, T.: Uncovering the overlapping community structure of complex networks in nature and society. Nature 435, 814–818 (2005)

[3] Derényi, I., Palla, G., Vicsek, T.: Clique Percolation in Random Networks. PRL 94 (160202), 76–85 (2005)

[4] Gregory, S.: An Algorithm to Find Overlapping Community Structure in Networks. In: Knowledge Discovery in Databases: PKDD 2007. LNCS, vol. 4213, pp. 593–600 (2007)

[5] Palla, G., Barabási, A.-L., Vicsek, T.: Quantifying social group evolution. Nature, 446–664 (2007)

[6] Adamcsek, B., Palla, G., Farkas, I., Derényi, I., Vicsek, T.: CFinder: locating cliques and overlapping modules in biological networks. Bioinformatics 22, 1021–1023 (2006)

[7] Li, X., Liu, B., Yu, P.S.: Discovering overlapping communities of named entities. In: Fürnkranz, J., Scheffer, T., Spiliopoulou, M. (eds.) PKDD 2006. LNCS (LNAI), vol. 4213, pp. 593–600. Springer, Heidelberg (2006)

[8] Zeng, Z., Wang, J., Zhou, L., Karypis, G.: Out-of-Core Coherent Closed Quasi-Clique. Mining from Large Dense Graph Databases. ACM Transactions on Database Systems 13(2), Article 13 (2007)

[9] Kaufman, L., Rousseeuw, P.: Finding Groups in Data: An Introduction to Cluster Analysis. Wiley, New York (1990)

[10] Li, W., Bin, W., Nan, D., Qi, Y.: A New Algorithm for Enumerating All Maximal Cliques in Complex Network. In: Li, X., Zaïane, O.R., Li, Z. (eds.) ADMA 2006. LNCS (LNAI), vol. 4093, pp. 606–617. Springer, Heidelberg (2006)

[11] Baumes, J., Goldberg, M., Magdon-Ismail, M.: Efficient identification of overlapping communities. In: Kantor, P., Muresan, G., Roberts, F., Zeng, D.D., Wang, F.-Y., Chen, H., Merkle, R.C. (eds.) ISI 2005. LNCS, vol. 3495, pp. 27–36. Springer, Heidelberg (2005)

[12] Zachary, W.W.: An information flow model for conflict and fission in small groups. Journal of Anthropological Research 33, 452–473 (1977)

[13] Lusseau, D., Schneider, K., Boisseau, O.J., Haase, P., Slooten, E., Dawson, S.M.: The bottlenose dolphin community of Doubtful Sound features a large proportion of long-lasting associations. Behavioral Ecology and Sociobiology 54, 396–405 (2003)

[14] Girvan, M., Newman, M.E.J.: Community structure in social and biological networks. Proc. Natl. Acad. Sci. USA 99, 7821–7826 (2002)

Using Matrix Model to Find Association Rule Core for Diverse Compound Critiques

Li Yu

School of Information, Renmin University of China, Beijing 100872, P. R. China
Key Laboratory of Data Engineering and Knowledge Engineering
(Renmin University of China), MOE, Beijing 100872, P. R. China
{buaayuli,yang}@ruc.edu.cn

Abstract. Dynamic critiquing approach is capable of automatically identifying useful compound critiques during each recommendation cycle, relative to the remaining cases. In current method, it is often too similar compound critiques are produced and presented to user. They limit the scope of the feedback options for the user. In this paper, a novel rule matrix model is proposed to find minimal association rule core for enhancing diverse compound critiques. All association rules generated though a frequent itemset are shown in elements of rule matrix, and minimal association rule core can be quickly determined though base elements in matrix. Association rule core is used to produce dynamic compound critiques. An example given better illustrates our method.

Keywords: Recommender Systems, Association Rules, Compound Critique.

1 Introduction

E-commerce web sites, such as Shopping.com or Expedia.com, offer large catalogues of different products. It provides a challenge for user about how to quickly get his preferable production. One solution to this information overload problem is the use of recommender systems, which help user to decide what should buy [1]. Conversational case-based recommender systems take the user through an iterative recommendation process, alternatively suggesting new products and soliciting feedback in order to guide the search for an ideal product. There are various kinds of recommender systems, such as rating-based, preference-based etc [2]. In this paper we are specifically interested in recommender systems based on critiquing that a user indicates his preference over a feature by critique it. Dynamic critiquing approach is capable of automatically identifying useful compound critiques during each recommendation cycle, relative to the remaining cases.

As pointed in previous work, there exists a key limitation in dynamic critique although good advantage over unit critique is shown [2, 3]. That is, in many recommendation cycles the compound critiques presented to users are very similar to each other. Generally, similar compound critiques often result into longer session time. Also similar critiques are hard to acquire wide preference. So, for dynamic compound critique, it is very important to generate diverse compound critiques, where differences

C. Tang et al. (Eds.): ADMA 2008, LNAI 5139, pp. 628–635, 2008.

between compound critiques are maximize. In this paper, the question is focused. A novel rule matrix model is proposed to quickly find association rule core for generating diverse compound critique.

In the next section, dynamic compound critique is first introduced. In section 3, association rule and its redundant question are described. In section 4, a novel rule matrix model used to generate association rule core for dynamic compound critique is proposed in detail. In section 5, an example is given. Conclusion and future research is made finally.

2 Dynamic Compound Critiques

2.1 Example-Critiquing with Suggestions

In conversation recommender systems, each recommendation session will be commenced by an initial user query and this will result in the retrieval of the most similar case available for the first recommendation cycle [3, 4]. If the user accepts this case, the recommendation session will end. Otherwise, the user will critique this case. In general, there are two kinds of critique. One is unit critique where single-feature is critiqued by user. Another is compound critique where multi-features are combined to been critiqued together [2]. For example, the critique "a different manufacture & smaller monitor & cheaper" shows critique for manufacture, monitor and price together.

	Current Case	Cased c from CB	Critique Pattern
Manufacture	Compaq	Sony	$\neq$
Monitor	14''	12''	$<$
Memory	512	512	$=$
Hard Disk	120	60	$<$
Processor	Pentium 4	Pentium 5	$>$
Speed	1500	1200	$<$
Price	2000	3000	$>$

Fig. 1. Generating a Critique Pattern [2]

The key to exploiting compound critiques is to recognize useful recurring subsets of critiques within the potentially large collection of critique patterns (the pattern-base). For example, we might find that 50% of the remaining cases have a smaller screen-size but a larger hard-disk size than the current case; that is, 50% of the critique patterns contain the sub-pattern {[*Monitor* <], [*Hard-Disk* >]}. Association rule is a good method for recognize and collate these recurring critique patterns within the pattern-base. In this method, each critique pattern corresponds to the shopping basket for a single customer, and the individual critiques correspond to the items in this basket. When association rule be used to discover compound critique, there include two key processes:

STEP 1: *Generating Critique Patterns.* This step is to generate a set of so-called critique patterns from the remaining cases, as shown in Fig.1.

STEP 2: *Mining Compound Critiques.* After critique patterns is build, association rule be used to produce the compound critiques. According to well-known Apriori algorithm, all frequent itemsets should been identified firstly, and then compound critique can be produced along with a measure of its support.

$$Support(A \rightarrow B) = \frac{\# \ of \ critique \ pattern \ containing \ A \ and \ B}{total \ \# \ critique \ pattern}$$

Unfortunately, using the above method, it is often that many similar compound critiques are produced. When these similar compound critiques are presented to user, they limit the scope of the feedback options for the user. For example, in Fig.2(A), three compound critique could been presented to user. It is easy to find that the three critiques refer to lower price and two of the critiques refer to lower resolution.

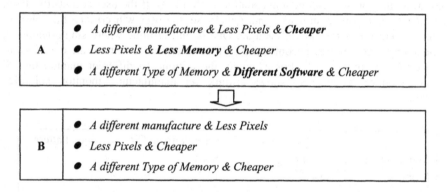

Fig. 2. Transferring Compound Critiques toward Diverse

2.2 Our Idea for Enhancing Diverse Compound Critique

In order to maximize difference among compound critiques, redundant information must be deleted according to association relation between different sub-itemsets. For example, in Fig.2, the critique rule "*A different manufacture & Less Pixels →* *Cheaper*" which shows that critique "*A different manufacture & Less Pixels*" has same critique information as critique "*A different manufacture & Less Pixels &* *Cheaper*" because "*A different manufacture & Less Pixels*" is strongly related to "*Cheaper*". So, the critique "*A different manufacture & Less Pixels & Cheaper*" can be substituted with "*A different manufacture & Less Pixels*". Similarity, for other two compound critiques as shown in Fig.2(A), compound critiques in Fig.2(B) only include independent critiques by deleting redundant critique.

In above method, it is most important step to produce minimal critique association rule base (or called as association rule core). By using these critique rules, reduced compound critiques can be generated. So, in this paper, mining minimal association rules core is focused, and a novel matrix model is presented to generate rule core.

3 Association Rule and Redundant Information

An *association rule* is a condition of the form r: $X \rightarrow Y$, where X and Y are two sets of items, $X?Y=\Phi$. $X\Phi Y$ is called as attribute (Item) sets of rule r, noted as *attr*(r), where X is condition attribute set, noted as $X= antc(r)$, and Y is consequence attribute (Item) set, noted as $Y= cons(r)$.

Definition. For association rule r_1 and r_2, if information in rule r_1 includes the information in r_2, then rule r_2 can be inferred though rule r_1, noted as $r_1 \rightarrow r_2$. If there are $r_1 \rightarrow r_2$ and $r_2 \rightarrow r_1$, then association rule r_1 and r_2 are equivalent, noted as $r_1 \leftrightarrow r_2$.

Definition. For two association rule sets R_1 and R_2, if for any $r_2 \in R_2$, there exists rule $r_1 \in R_1$, and $r_1 \rightarrow r_2$, then rule sets R_2 can be inferred though rule set R_1, noted as $R_1 \rightarrow R_2$.

A challenge question in association rule is to improve association rules relevance and usefulness by extracting as few rules as possible without losing information by deleting redundant rules.. In the following, a rule matrix model is proposed to deleting redundant rule.

4 Using Association Rule Matrix Model to Generate Rule Core

4.1 Association Rule Matrix Model

According the above theorem [5], we can get two basic inference rules.

Inference 1. For itemset A, B, C, D, (AB) = (CD), $supp(C) < supp(A)$ and r: $A \rightarrow B$ is association rule, then r': $C \rightarrow D$ is an association rule, such as $r \rightarrow r'$.

Inference 2. For itemset A, B, C, D, (CD) (AB), $supp(C)=supp(A)$ and r: $A \rightarrow B$ is association rule, then r': $C \rightarrow D$ is an association rule, such as $r \rightarrow r'$.

According the two above inferences, there hold the following,

Rule le set $GR_i^j (I)$ $_i$ consisted of rules generated though i items of itemset I, and pattern number of supporting its condition itemset is j.can be produced as following

$$GR_i^j (I) = \{r \in GR(I) // attr(r) |= i, supp = j\}$$

Where G(r) as rule set, where all rules are inferred by rule r; Q(r) as rule set, where all rules are equivalent to rule r; GR(I) as rule set, where all rules are generated though itemset I.

Obviously, rules in $GR_{|I|}^{j}(I)$ $_I$ are equivalent, and is called as *Basic Equivalent Rule Set* of itemset I. So, rule set $GR_i (I)$ $_i$ generated though i items of itemset I.can be represented,

$$GR_i (I) = \bigcup_{j \geq min\ supp} R_i^j$$

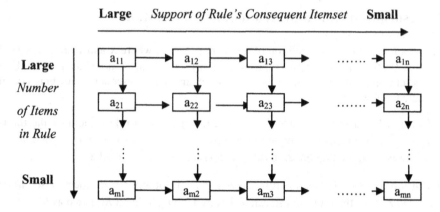

Fig. 3. Association Rule Matrix for a Maximal Frequent Itemset

Based sed on GR_i $(I$ $)$, rule set $GR(I)$, including rules generated though itemset I, can be generated. That is,

$$GR(I) = \bigcup_{i=2}^{|I|} R_i(I)$$

Further more, all rule can generated as following,

$$GR = \bigcup_{I \in IMFS} R(I)$$

According to above method, all rules generated by one maximal frequent itemset could be shown in rule matrix $R = GR$ (I), as shown in Fig.3. In R, rules in same row have equal number of items, and rules in the same column have equal support of consequent itemset. That is,

$$R = GR(I) = (a_{ij})_{m \times n} \quad (i = 1, 2, .., m; \, j = 1, 2, ..., n)_,$$

Where

$$a_{ij} = GR_{m_0-i}^{n_0-j}, \quad m_0 = |I| + 1, \quad n_0 = \max_{r \in GR(I)} supp(attr(r)) + 1,$$

$$m = |I| - 1, \quad n = \max_{r \in GR(I)} supp(attr(r)) - min\,supp - 1$$

4.2 Using Rule Matrix Model to Derive Minimal Association Rule Core

Based on two above basic inferences in 4.1, for rule matrix in Fig.3, there have the following conclusions, as shown in Fig.4.

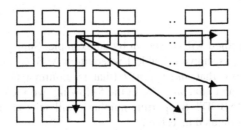

Fig. 4. Inferring Relation between Elements in Rule Matrix

(1) $a_{ij} \rightarrow a_{(i+1)j}$, $a_{ij} \rightarrow a_{i(j+1)}$;
(2) if $i<k$, then $a_{ij} \rightarrow a_{kj}$; if $j<l$, then $a_{ij} \rightarrow a_{il}$;
(3) for any a_{ij}, $a_{kl} \in R$, ($i<k$, $j<l$), there exist $a_{ij} \rightarrow a_{kl}$.

Definition. For $a_{ij} \in R$, if there not exist element $a'_{ij} \in R$, such that $a'_{ij} \rightarrow a_{ij}$, then a_{ij} is called as *Base Element* in rule matrix. The set including all base elements in a rule matrix is *Base Set (BS)*.

In fact, there exist a lot of null elements where no rule exists. It is easy to know that null elements lie in left-above part and right-down part of rule matrix, as shown in Fig.5 For any base element $a_{ij} \in BS$, all rules included in a_{ij} can be present as Rule(a_{ij}), so all rules included in based set (*BS*) can be computed as

$$Rule(BS) = \bigcup_{a_i \in BS} Rule(a_i)$$

It is easy to know that, all rules in rule matrix might be derived though *Rule(BS)* which does not include redundant rule information. We call it as *core* of rule matrix R.

$$Core(R) = Rule(BS)$$

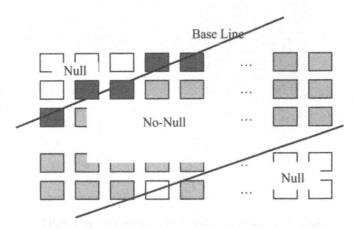

Fig. 5. Distribution of Null and No-Null Elements in Rule Matrix

5 An Example

In this section, our method will be shown by an example. Supposing that there a critique pattern database, as shown in Table 1 where item A, B, C and D means four unit critiques. Let's suppose that *minsupp*=0.4 (that is, minimal number of transaction records is equal to 2) and *minconf*=2/3. In the following, we focus the rule generated by frequent itemset "ABCD". Supporting number of all subsets of maximal frequent itemset "ABCD" is computed in Table 2.

Table 1. An Simple Critique Pattern Base

OID	Items
1	A C D
2	B C E
3	A B C E
4	A B E
5	A B C E

Table 2. # of Subset of "ABCD"

Supp(I)=4	*Supp*(I)=3	*Supp*(I)=2
A, B	AB, AC	ABC
C, E	AE, BC	ACE
BE	CE, BCE	
	ABE	

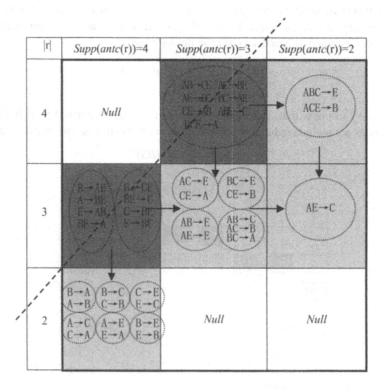

Fig. 6. Association Rule Matrix of Frequent Itemset "ABCD"

After computing, rule matrix generated by maximal frequent itemset "ABCD" is shown in Fig.6. It includes 39 rules. In this matrix, a11, a32 and a33 are null element, indicating that there is no corresponding rule. And element a12 and a21 are base elements, represented in red.

According to our proposed method, 15 rules in base elements a12 and a21 can substitute for 39 rules in matrix. So, we can produce condensed compound critiques only by using 15 rules, not 39 rules.

6 Conclusions

Conversational recommender systems help prospective buyers quickly navigate to suitable products by facilitating the incremental construction of a more accurate picture of their requirements through a series of recommendation interactions. Dynamic critiquing approach is capable of automatically identifying useful compound critiques during each recommendation cycle, relative to the remaining cases. But too similar compound critiques limit the scope of the feedback options for the user.

In this paper, a novel rule matrix model is proposed to find minimal association rule core for enhancing diverse compound critiques. All association rules are shown in elements of rule matrix, and minimal association rule core can be quickly determined though base elements. Association rule core is used to produce dynamic compound critiques. An example is used to effectively illustrate our method.

The success of a compound critiquing recommender depends on recommendation efficiency, recommendation and critique quality, and system usability. In the future, empirical evaluations and analysis need to make for verifying our method by surveying.

Acknowledgement

This research was partly supported by Open Foundation of Key Laboratory of Data Engineering & Knowledge Engineering, Ministry of Education P. R China; partly by Open Foundation of Key Laboratory of Information Management and Information Economics, Ministry of Information Industry P. R. China under grants F0607-31 and partly by Research Foundation of Renmin Univ. of China.

References

1. Schafer, J.B., Konstan, J., Riedl, J.: Recommender Systems in E-Commerce. In: EC 1999: Proceedings of the First ACM Conference on Electronic Commerce, Denver, CO, pp. 158–166 (1999)
2. McCarthy, K., Reilly, J., Smyth, B.: On the Generation of Diverse CompoundCritiques. In: The 15th Artificial Intelligence and Cognitive Science (AICS) Conference, Mayo, Ireland (2004)
3. Reilly, J., McCarthy, K., McGinty, L., Smyth, B.: Dynamic Critiquing. In: Proceedings of the 7th European Conference on Case-Based Reasoning, Madrid, Spain (2004)
4. Rafter, R., Smyth, B.: Towards Conversational Collaborative Recommendation. Artificial Intelligence Review 24(3-4), 301–318 (2005)
5. Cristofor, L., Simovici, D.: Generating an information cover for association rules. University of Massachusets (2002)
6. Toivonen, H., Klemettinen, M., Ronkainen, P., Hätönen, K., Mannila, H.: Pruning and-grouping discovered association rules. In: MLnet Workshop on Statistics, Machine Learning,and Discovery in Databases, Crete, Greece (April 1995)

Link-Contexts for Ranking

Jessica Gronski

University of California Santa Cruz
jgronski@soe.ucsc.edu

Abstract. Anchor text has been shown to be effective in ranking[6] and a variety of information retrieval tasks on web pages. Some authors have expanded on anchor text by using the words around the anchor tag, a *link-context*, but each with a different definition of link-context. This lack of consensus begs the question: What is a good link-context?

The two experiments in this paper address the question by comparing the results of using different link-contexts for the problem of ranking. Specifically, we concatenate the link-contexts of links pointing to a web page to create a *link-context document* used to rank that web page. By comparing the ranking order resulting from using different link-contexts, we found that smaller contexts are effective at ranking relevant urls highly.

1 Introduction

In their 2001 paper on anchor text, Craswell et al.[6] show that ranking based on anchor text is twice as effective as ranking based on document content. This finding spurred many researchers to leverage anchor text for various information retrieval tasks on web pages including ranking, summarizing, categorization, and clustering [13,5,4,2,3].

As descriptive words often appear around the hyperlink rather than between anchor tags, many researchers have expanded the words past anchor text to a 'context' around the link. These *link-contexts* have been defined as sentences [8], windows [4], and HTML DOM trees [13,2] around the anchor text. Given these competing definitions of link-context, this paper investigates which definition performs best for the task of ranking.

Specifically, the two experiments in this paper explore how defining link-context as either windows, sentences, or HTML trees effect ranking quality. The link-contexts of links pointing to a single page are concatenated to create a *link-context document* for that page. Each link-context document is then ranked by the BM25 algorithm[17] and the order evaluated by various ranking metrics.

The results of the Syskill/Webert[15] experiment indicate that smaller link-contexts tend have better precision and NDCG[11] at low recall and thresholds while larger link-contexts have better precision and NDCG at higher recall and threshold levels. The results of the followup experiment on the AOL collection [14] generally indicate that small link-contexts have the lower mean click-through url ranks which corroborates the earlier conclusion that smaller link-contexts are effective at low thresholds.

C. Tang et al. (Eds.): ADMA 2008, LNAI 5139, pp. 636–643, 2008.

This paper proceeds by describing related works (§2), an experiment overview (§3), the experiment results (§4), and concludes with future work (§5).

2   Related Work

The inspiration for this paper was Craswell et al.[6] where link-context was defined as anchor text and their resulting documents were found to be more effective than page source in ranking documents. Prior to Craswell et al. a couple of papers highlighted the effectiveness of anchor text as a feature for ranking web pages[3,7]. Anchor text has been used for a variety of information retrieval tasks since McBrian's WWWW indexing worm[12], including topical web crawling [13,5], and subject classification [4,2].

The name "link-context" comes from Pant's paper on topical web crawling[13] but appeared in earlier papers under different names. Link-contexts have been defined as sentences containing the anchor tag[8], a fixed window before and after the anchor tag [4], the enclosing HTML DOM tree [2,13,5], and the enclosing ad-hoc tag (paragraph, list item, table entry, title, or heading)[18].

Of the papers that use a link-context some justified their definition of link-context. Chakrabarti et al. [4] justified using a window of 50 bytes for classifying pages by looking at the incidence rate of the word 'yahoo' within 100 bytes of hyperlinks to 'http://www.yahoo.com'.

The context of an anchor is important to topical web crawlers because it determines which hyperlink to follow, hence a number of papers in the area experiment with different link-contexts. Notably, Chakrabarti et al. [5] trained a classifier to crawl websites for topic relevant links. Windows of up to five HTML DOM text elements around a hyperlink were part of the feature set, because larger windows only marginally increased their accuracy. Pant[13] experimented with defining link-context as windows of words or HTML DOM trees containing the hyperlink to decide which hyperlink to follow and found parent trees to be most effective.

The results of the Chakrabarti and Pant papers are not immediately applicable to the task of ranking for two reasons. First, the evaluation metrics for topical web crawling do not directly apply to the task of ranking web pages. Second, in topical web crawling one link-context is used per target page, whereas in ranking algorithms, as presented by Craswell, use many link-contexts to create a single document.

3   Experiment

The experiments reproduce the original Craswell et al.[6] experiment by ranking each document's relevance to a query by both the page content and the content of the anchor text in hyperlinks pointing to the page. In addition, we define several link-contexts and compare the effectiveness of link-context documents in ranking web pages. The two experiments in this paper use the following framework and differ only in the source of the data and the evaluation metrics.

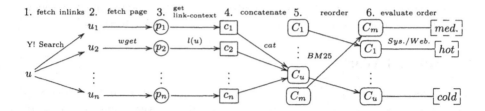

Fig. 1. Creating the link-context document

Briefly, as illustrated by fig. 1, for every url u in a given subject, the experiment found the link-context document defined by link-context l using the following approach:

1. Use the Yahoo! Search API[1] to find the urls of pages linking to u.
2. Fetch pages of in-linking urls from the internet.
3. Parse pages for the link-context l around the hyperlink to u ($l(u)$).
4. Concatenate link-contexts to create the link-context document.

Given all the link-context documents for urls in a subject the experiment then:

5. Use the BM25 algorithm to rank the link-context documents.
6. Evaluate the success of the ranking against the Syskill-Webert ranking of the pages or the AOL click-through data (fig. 1 illustrates the former).

3.1   Data

Syskill/Webert Experiment. The data for the first experiment comes from the Syskill/Webert (SW) data[15] available through the UCI KDD archive [10] and was created in 1997 for the purpose of predicting user ratings of web pages with respect to a given topic. Each user was given an 'index' page with links to websites on a single subject. After visiting each link the user was intercepted with a screen asking the user to rate the visited page by adding it to a 'hot' list, a 'lukewarm' list (medium) or a 'cold' list[15]. While the user rating is not an explicit ranking order for the pages, it provides a partial order. One subject in the SW dataset, Bands, was dropped for lack of in-links to the SW pages.

The link-contexts for the SW pages were found by querying the Yahoo! Search API. While the Yahoo! Search API did not find any pages linking to a couple SW pages, 90% of pages were viable for this experiment. In total 253 SW pages were used in the project and 7,277 pages were used to construct in-link documents.

One potential criticism of the data used for this experiment is that the SW data was collected in 1997 while the in-link pages were collected in 2008. However, as there is no reason to believe that this time gap between data will effect any link-context unequally, the data still permits a relative comparison between link-contexts.

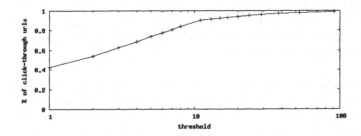

Fig. 2. Percent of click-through urls in the AOL User Data with AOL rank lower than the threshold

AOL User Data Experiment As the data in the first experiment was collected in 1997, we use a more current data source, the 2006 AOL User Session Collection[14], for the second experiment. The data contains user queries and, if a search result was chosen, the base domain of the clicked hyperlink and the rank of the result.

Of the queries in which a user clicked a url, over 90% had a rank of 11 or less and 97.5% had a rank of 50 or less, fig. 2. For this reason we choose the first 50 pages returned by the Yahoo! search API for a query as the candidate pages to rank using link contexts.

Of the 19,442,629 click-through queries in the AOL dataset, we randomly chose queries discarding those where no click-through event occurred or if the click-through url was not found in the first 50 results returned by the Yahoo! Search API. In total 100 click-through queries were collected and used as subjects for this experiment.

The link-context documents for these first 50 results are, as in the first experiment, constructed using the Yahoo! Search API. In total there are 100 queries, with 5,000 primary pages and 250,000 secondary pages (used to construct link-context documents).

3.2 Ranking Algorithm

The ranking algorithm used in the original Craswell et al.[6] paper is BM25[17] and to allow for direct comparison with the Craswell et al. paper, both experiments in this paper also use BM25 for ranking. To this end, the Xapian package[19] was used to index and query the documents generated by different context definitions.

3.3 Link-Context Definitions

Both the main and auxiliary experiments employ three kinds of link-contexts found in the literature: windows of words [4], HTML DOM trees[2,13], and sentence[8] link-contexts.

Window Contexts. A window link-context grabs the n words before and after the hyperlink pointing to the target web page. Words are defined as whitespace-separated strings of letters in HTML DOM text elements. The value of n in this experiment ranges from one to five.

Tree Contexts. The tree-based link-contexts are defined by the HTML DOM tree structure and all text elements found in the tree are included in the context. Trees rooted at the parent, grandparent, and great-grandparent elements of the target anchor tag are candidate link-contexts. Not all HTML pages come well-formed but by using HTML Tidy[16], we extracted a reasonable approximation of the HTML tree intended.

Sentence Context. We also consider a syntactic link-context, defined as the sentence in which the hyperlink appears. A sentence is defined as the words between punctuation marks (./?/!). Though not all anchor tags appear within well-formed sentences, we accept paragraph tags, cell tags, and list tags as sentence boundaries if they appear closer than punctuation.

3.4   Performance Metrics

Syskill/Webert Experiment. The metrics used to compare different link-contexts in ranking web pages are precision, recall, and NDCG[11]. The performance of each link-context is graphed in a 11-point precision-recall graph and the NDCG is graphed for thresholds up to ten. When calculating precision and recall only 'hot' documents are considered relevant. For NDCG the rating of hot/medium/cold documents are treated as the rating 2/1/0, respectively.

AOL Experiment. The experiment using the AOL data has the same candidate link-contexts but uses the rank of the click-through result as the performance metric of the results. Specifically the mean rank of the click-through result over all queries is the metric for evaluating this experiment.

4   Results

4.1   Syskill/Webert Experiment

Initially we compared window, sentence and tree contexts separately and then compared the most viable contexts from the initial experiments to draw overall conclusions. For brevity, the results of the intermediate results are published in an extended paper[9] and here we present the overall comparison and examine whether we reproduce the original Craswell et al. experiment.

This experiment was not a successful reproduction of the Craswell et al. experiment[6] in that the anchor text doesn't generally outperform page source. Except at recall levels of 10%, anchor text's precision was worse than the page source, fig. 3(a). In the NDCG graph, fig. 3(b), anchor text performs worse than the page source after a threshold of two.

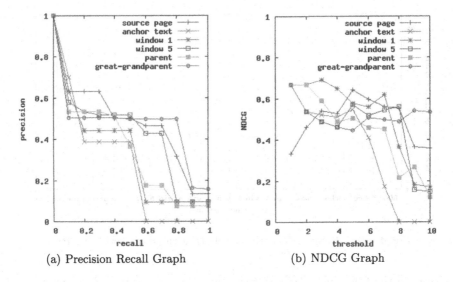

(a) Precision Recall Graph   (b) NDCG Graph

Fig. 3. Overall Comparison

The poor performance of anchor text at low levels may be due to the time difference between when the pages were rated and when the link-contexts were collected(§3.1). This may not only indicate a shift in page relevance but also fewer anchor texts pointing to the page if it is no longer online.

For an overall comparison the results for the anchor text, page source, window of size 1, window of size 5, parent and great-grandparent link-contexts are included because they performed best in their class of link-context[9]. Figure 3(a) and 3(b) highlight a general trend that small contexts, anchor text, windows of size 1, and parent link-contexts perform well at low thresholds and recall while large contexts tend to dominate at higher thresholds and recall.

The precision of the anchor text, page source, window of size 5, and great-grandparent link-contexts beat out the others at higher levels of recall. The NDCG levels of window 1 link-context equal or exceed other link-contexts until a threshold of 5 when the source page exceeds it, (excepting at threshold 7 where window 1 is again the highest). Finally, at thresholds above nine the great-grandparent context's NDCG is greatest.

4.2 AOL User Data Experiment

Since small contexts are good at pushing the most relevant pages to the top (high NDCG at low thresholds §4.1) and click-through pages are quite relevant, we expect small contexts to have the lowest mean click-through rank. Also, because the data collection time and the validation data time are current, we expect to see better performance from link-contexts than the page source.

The average rank of the click-through domain using the link-context documents and BM25 ranking is displayed in figure 4. Though all link-contexts are

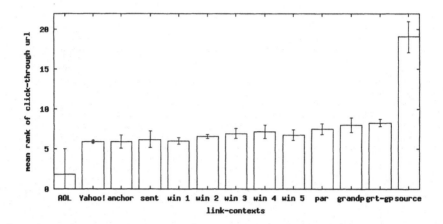

Fig. 4. Mean Rank of Click-through URL with (standard) Error Bars

beaten by the full-scale search engines, small link-contexts such as windows of size 1 are highly competitive. The sentence and anchor link-contexts have mean ranks comparable to Yahoo!'s but with greater standard error. Contrary to our hypothesis the larger context window of size 5 did better than those of size 3 and 4. Though all three contexts are within one another's error range, this weakens our hypothesis and requires further investigation. Though the BM25 ranking combined with link-context documents perform worse than search engines it is remarkable how well it performs without a complicated feature set. Finally, the experiment does reproduce the results in the Craswell experiment as the source page performs worse than all link-context documents.

5   Conclusion and Future Work

This pilot study is a step toward answering the question of which link-context to use. The first experiment implies that if one cares about the first pages returned then a small context is preferable and if overall quality of results is more important than a larger one is better. The second experiment generally corroborates the first by showing that small link contexts have low mean click-through urls ranks. Particularly, using link-contexts defined by windows of size 1 was effective in bringing click-through url to the top of the list. While these small link-contexts are not better than established search engines, they may be highly effective features in a search engine.

Future work includes using a linear regression to explore the merit of using a linear combination link-contexts. Also, because of the effect of size on ranking it may be interesting to train the algorithm for different NDCG thresholds. Finally, in future experiments increasing the variety of link-context definitions, for example taking larger windows or the whole page as a link context, may prove fruitful.

References

1. Yahoo! search web services, http://developer.yahoo.com/search/
2. Attardi, G., Gullı, A., Sebastiani, F.: Automatic web page categorization by link and context analysis. In: Hutchison, C., Lanzarone, G. (eds.) THAI 1999, Varese, IT, pp. 105–119 (1999)
3. Brin, S., Page, L.: The anatomy of a large-scale hypertextual web search engine. Computer Networks and ISDN Systems 30(1–7), 107–117 (1998)
4. Chakrabarti, S., Dom, B., Gibson, D., Kleinberg, J., Raghavan, P., Rajagopalan, S.: Automatic resource list compilation by analyzing hyperlink structure and associated text. In: WWW7 (1998)
5. Chakrabarti, S., Punera, K., Subramanyam, M.: Accelerated focused crawling through online relevance feedback. In: WWW 2002. ACM, New York (2002)
6. Craswell, N., Hawking, D., Robertson, S.: Effective site finding using link anchor information. In: SIGIR 2001, pp. 250–257. ACM Press, New York (2001)
7. Cutler, M., Deng, H., Maniccam, S.S., Meng, W.: A new study on using HTML structures to improve retrieval. In: Tools with Artificial Intelligence, pp. 406–409 (1999)
8. Delort, J., Meunier, B.B., Rifqi, M.: Enhanced web document summarization using hyperlinks (2003)
9. Gronski, J.: Link-contexts for ranking. Technical report (2008), http://www.soe.ucsc.edu/~jgronski/papers/ADMAext.pdf
10. Hettich, S., Bay, S.D.: The UCI KDD archive (1999), http://kdd.ics.uci.edu
11. Järvelin, K., Kekäläinen, J.: Cumulated gain-based evaluation of IR techniques. ACM Trans. Inf. Syst. 20(4), 422–446 (2002)
12. Mcbryan, O.A.: GENVL and WWWW: Tools for taming the web. In: Nierstarsz, O. (ed.) WWW1, CERN, Geneva (1994)
13. Pant, G.: Deriving link-context from html tag tree. In: DMKD 2003, pp. 49–55. ACM, New York (2003)
14. Pass, G., Chowdhury, A., Torgeson, C.: A picture of search. In: InfoScale 2006. ACM Press, New York (2006)
15. Pazzani, M.J., Muramatsu, J., Billsus, D.: Syskill webert: Identifying interesting web sites. In: AAAI/IAAI, vol. 1, pp. 54–61 (1996)
16. Raggett, D.: Clean up your web pages with hp's HTML tidy. Comput. Netw. ISDN Syst. 30(1-7), 730–732 (1998)
17. Robertson, S.E., Walker, S., Hancock-Beaulieu, M., Gull, A., Lau, M.: Okapi at trec. In: Text Retrieval Conference, pp. 21–30 (1992)
18. Slattery, S., Craven, M.: Combining statistical and relational methods for learning in hypertext domains. In: Page, D. (ed.) ILP 1998. LNCS, vol. 1446, pp. 38–52. Springer, Heidelberg (1998)
19. Xapian. Xapian, http://www.xapian.org/

DC-Tree: An Algorithm for Skyline Query on Data Streams

Jing Yang [1], Bo Qu [1], Cui-Ping Li [2], and Hong Chen [2]

[1] Information School, Renmin University of China
Beijing 100872, China
{jingyang,qubo}@ruc.edu.cn
[2] Key Lab of Data Engineering and Knowledge Engineering of MOE
Beijing 100872, China
{cpli,chong}@ruc.edu.cn

Abstract. Skyline query asks for a set of interesting points that are non-dominated by any other points from a potentially large set of data points and has become research hotspot in database field. Users usually respect fast and incremental output of the skyline objects in reality. Now many algorithms about skyline query have been developed, but they focus on static dataset, not on dynamic dataset. For instance, data stream is a kind of the dynamic datasets. Stream data are usually in large amounts and high speed; moreover, the data arrive unlimitedly and consecutively. Also, the data are variable thus they are difficult to predict. Therefore, it is a grim challenge for us to process skyline query on stream data. Real-time control and strong control management are required to capture the characteristic of data stream, because they must settle data updating rapidly. To this challenge, this paper proposes a new algorithm: DC-Tree. It can do skyline query on the sliding window over the data stream efficiently. The experiment results show that the algorithm is both efficient and effective.

1 Introduction

The points $x = (x_1, x_2, ..., x_d)$ and $y = (y_1, y_2, ..., y_d)$ in the two D-dimension space, if $x_i \leq y_i$ which $1 \leq i \leq d$, we call that x dominates y. Given a set of objects $p_1, p_2, ..., p_N$, the operator returns all objects p_i which is not dominated by another object p_j. More formally, the skyline is defined as those points which are not dominated by any other points. A point dominates another point if it is as good or better in all dimensions and better in at least one dimension, as shown in Figure 1.

Skyline query gives important value to multi-criteria decision making applications. For example, a stockholder goes to buy stocks, and he wants to know the optima trade off on stock A up to now. But the Standard of "Quality Stocks" is that the successful bidder price is low, and the dicker volume is high. Unlike static information, this stock information updates continually. So it is better to sign in a skyline query and output query results incessantly. The query relies on two standards: the successful

---

[1] This research is partly supported by the National Science Foundation of China (60673138, 60603046), Key Program of Science Technology Research of MOE (106006), and Program for New Century Excellent Talents in University.

C. Tang et al. (Eds.): ADMA 2008, LNAI 5139, pp. 644–651, 2008.

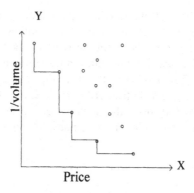

Fig. 1. The Skyline of the Stock Exchange

bidder price is low, the dicker volume is high. In this paper, the smaller value is the better value, so 1/volume represents the better, as shown in Figure 1.

Skyline query and its transmutation [1,2,3,4], have been extensively studied and numerous algorithms have been proposed. In [1,2,5]we can find some algorithms for main memory processing. And the algorithms which are related to database application can also be found in [6,7,8,9,10].

However, the above mentioned algorithms are not used in online computation, because the online computation faces quickly updated data. And in many applications, quick data updating often happens. For example, in the model of the sliding window over data stream, it needs to delete old data and insert new data followed the new data incessantly coming. Although Xue-min Lin and someone else proposed an algorithm of skyline computation over data stream in [12], the data structure is complex, and cannot be used in the contemporary data stream system easily. According to personalized survey, there are few people doing investigation on this aspect.

This paper proposes a skyline query algorithm toward the sliding window over data stream. The rest of the paper is organized as follows. Section 2 reviews previous related background knowledge of algorithms for skyline computation. Section 3 proposes the kernel algorithm. Finally, section 4 evaluates the accuracy of the DC-Tree experimentally, comparing it under a variety of settings.

2   Related Work

2.1 Data Stream and the Siding Window

According to the exist model of the data, the process of the data can be classified into static data process and fluxional data process. Fluxional data process the online, continual, high-speed data stream, the model of the object which the system process is very different from the typical static data process. Because of the limitation of the memory space, these data can`t be stored to the memory absolutely as often as not, at the same time, it should process these data stream incessancy and have no delay so as to acquire the real-time results. When we process the continually arriving data stream,

there is not always interest in all the arriving data, but only interest in the recent partial data which require the introduction of the sliding window model [11].

At present, there are many kinds of sliding window model that can be used, but
here we just introduce the one that this paper refers to: consolidate N tuples as the
volume of window.(Fig. 2:N=10).When the data a, b, c,...in the data stream arrive
continually, according to the alphabetical order, it needs to delete the oldest data from
the window(such as a, b) and insert the newest arriving number(such as l, m), the
tuples which are used for computation in the window are no more than 10.

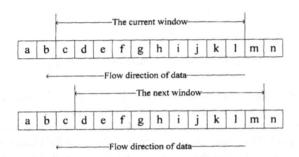

Fig. 2. The Sliding Window Model of the Stationary Volume

2.2 DC Algorithm

DC algorithm is used to compute the skyline on a given set of data points. The algorithm firstly divides the data points into several blocks, and then computes each block
of skyline. Finally they merge the skyline of these blocks, and find the last skyline.
The basic DC Algorithm followed: **1)** Compute the median (m_1) of all the data points
in one dimension (d_p), according to the median divide all the data points into two data
points (P_1,P_2),the value of all the data points in block P_1 on the d_p dimension is better
than m_1 (small), P_2 contains all other points. **2)** Compute the skyline S_1 in block P_1
and the skyline S_2 in block P_2 distinguishingly. The way is to implement this algorithm as a whole recursively in two blocks of P_1, P_2. For example, P1 and P_2 will
continue to be divided. Recursively implement the block operations, until a block
contains only one point (or meets a critical setting value). At this time, to compute the
skyline of each block is very easy. **3)** Recursively merge all the skyline of the blocks,
and at last merge S_1 and S_2 to ultimate skyline. Merging method is to remove those
points from S_2 which are dominated by the points in S_1 (the points in S_1 cannot be
dominated by the point S_2, because at least in d_p dimension, the points in S_1 is superior than every point in S_2).

Because each time the algorithm partitions in one dimension, it depends on the median of all the points in this dimension, so once new data appear or delete certain data,
all operations (partition and merge) will start again, such efficiency is far from satisfying the data flowed on the high-speed data updates. The method we mentioned
below is to avoid this problem skilfully.

3 DC-Tree Algorithm

In this Section, we present a new skyline algorithm based on a divide and conquer paradigm, and this new DC algorithm images the data into the points in the D-dimension (n is the query dimension) space, divides the space into 2^d equal pieces of block according to the dimension, computes the skyline of each block and then merges every block into the final skyline. We first introduce the most basic case of two-dimension, the algorithm is as follow: d=2, and set these two dimensions as X, Y the maximal value as M_x and M_y:

1) Divide all the points on the space into four equal pieces P_1,P_2,P_3,P_4 ,according to $M_x/2$, $M_y/2$.
2) Compute the skyline on each space respectively: S_1, S_2, S_3 and S_4. The method is to continue the implementation of the algorithm recursively on each block. For instance, continue the block operations to P_1, P_2, P_3, P_4 until a block contains only one point (or meets a set threshold). This time can quickly calculate the skyline of each block.
3) Merge the skyline of all the block recursively, with the final S_1, S_2, S_3 and S_4 to be the ultimate skyline.

The biggest advantage of these equal installments is to retain the structure of the block: a tree, we call it DC-Tree. Each father node splits to four children nodes, leaf nodes record of all the points, each father node only records the skyline point of this block (merge the skyline points of the four children nodes).

3.1 Skyline Query

All the points in the root node of DC-Tree are the final skyline points.

3.2 Update

All the points in the root node of DC-Tree are the final skyline points.
Insert: (The sliding window will insert a new data T)

1) Find out the leaf node which it belongs to: find out the leaf node P according to the value of T on the two skyline query dimension X, Y.
2) If the points included by P more than the setting threshold when we insert this point, we will ramify the point P. And then T returns to the new leaf node P_t .
3) Compute the affection of this point towards the skyline: If T is dominated by the other points in the leaf node P_t ,then T will not affect the final skyline, the update end; If T is not dominated by the other points in P_t ,T will become the skyline point in P_t ,then we need to record the point T in the father node, continue to consider the influence on skyline that T nodes in his father node, if have no affection, the update end, or else continue until up to the root node.

Delete: (Data T deletes from the sliding window) T belongs to the leaf node P_t .

1) If T is not the skyline point of P_t , delete T from the tree directly, end the update.
2) If T is the skyline point of P_t , delete T, and then recalculate the skyline of P_t , update the recording point of the father node, continue updating until to the root node.

3) If the points are contained by P_t and the other brother node is less than the threshold after deleting T, delete the four leaf node, and then merge the inside points to the father nodes, at this time, the father node of P_t will become the leaf node, record all the points in the four leaf nodes which are deleted.

Algorithm INSERT DC-TREE (Node, Data, Scope, Count)
Input: Node: a data structure which stands for the region holding the points.
   Data: the point that will be inserted into the data structure.
   Scope: the boundary of the region
   Count: record the degree of the recursion
Output: An Index tree for the data in data stream
   the number we assume to end the recursion
1.   **if** (Count == THRESHOLD)   **return**;
2.   **if** (Count == THRESHOLD – 1) the last layer
3.   put Data in Node;   in the last layer, we don't need to divide the region
4.   position = Com_position(Data);   record the position of the Data
5.   datastream.place[num—]=position;
6.   **else** not the last layer
7.   **for** point = the first point in the Node to the last **do**
8.   **if** (Data control) pointErase point;
9.   **if** (point control Data)
10.   record the position of point in the Node in the point;
11.   **break**;
12.   **if** ((reach the end of the Node) put the Data in the Node;
      compute which child point the Data should be in
13.   temp_place = compute_place(Data, Scope);
14.   construct a new child node Child_Node;
15.   node.childpos[temp_place] = Child_Node;
16.   Count—;
17.   **INSERT DC-TREE** (Child_Node, Data, Scope, Count);

Algorithm DELETE DC-TREE (Position)
Input: Position: the variable which points out the position of
   the point in the leaf node.
1.   **if** (count == THRESHOLD – 1) the last layer
2.   point = get(Position);
3.   erase(Position);   delete the point in the leaf node
4.   **if** (getNode(Position)< MINNUM)
5.   Node = getNode(Position);
6.   Merge(Node, Node.parent);
7.   eraseNode(Node);
8.   **PARENT_ERASE** (Position.node.parent, point);
Algorithm PARENT_ERASE (Node_position, Point)
Input: Node_position: the memory position of the parent node
   Point: the point must be deleted
1.   **if**(Count == -1) **return**;   reach the root
2.   Node = * Node_position;
3.   **if**(find(Point) == Node.lengh) **return**;
4.   Set =**RECALCULATE**(Node, find(Point));
5.   **for** (data = each point in the set)
6.   **for** (point = each point in the node)
7.   **if** (point control data) **break**;
8.   **if**(reach the end of the Node) put the Data in the Node;
9.   **if** (getNode(Position)< MINNUM)
10.   Node = getNode(Position);
11.   Merge(Node, Node.parent);
12.   eraseNode(Node);
13.   Position =Node.parent;
14.   parent_erase (Position, Point);

3.3 For Example

We set the threshold q (equal to 2) which will induce splitting. The sliding window can accommodate ten data, at this moment it has nine points (a,b,…,h,i) and the counterpart DC-Tree (as in Figure 3).

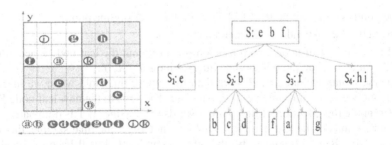

Fig. 3. The Distribution and the Tree Structure of the Points

And then insert new data j to the window, find the position of j in the tree (on left of Fig. 4), because j isn`t the skyline point of this block, so it`ll not impact the final results, delete it directly, then insert end.

At the same time, the old data a should be deleted from the sliding window, because a is not the skyline point in this block, so it will not affect the results of the skyline, delete it directly (on right of Fig. 4).

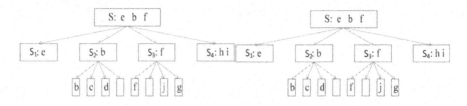

Fig. 4. Insert the Point j and Delete the Point a

And then new data k enter the window, the block of k has only two points h and i before it, at this time k is added into the block so that the points in this block outreach the threshold q=2, so it must continue to branch, the new data k are the new skyline points of the block, so at the same time, the record of the remained skyline points are in the father node (on left of Fig. 5).

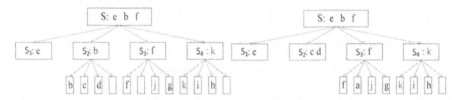

Fig. 5. Modify the Skyline Points and Delete Points, Merge the Child to the Father

At last, the old data b should be deleted from the sliding window, and when the point b is deleted, the nodes in the block equal to the threshold, then delete the block and combine all the points to the father node. Continue to update, the final results (on right of Fig. 5).

4 Experimental Results

We experimented that the algorithms are in high availability when being queried and updated, and also in high expansibility. All datasets were running on a Pentium 4,CPU 2.40GHZ DELL PC equipped with 256MB of main memory and a 40GB hard drive, under the Windows XP Professional Edition operating system. Our algorithm was implemented in C++ on a client machine.

We firstly experimented the skyline query efficiency by using synthetic and static data. We generated correlated, independent and anti-correlated dataset having 10000 tuples with the dimensionality varying from 2 to 5 to compare our algorithm with the DC[6] and the algorithm in paper[12](we call it BBS algorithm),the results as in Figure 6 for independent, correlated and anti-correlated dataset, the X axis denotes the dimension of the generated data, Y axis denotes the time of getting the query results .we can see the DC-Tree algorithm has relative high effect towards static datasets all the same. It takes a little longer time than BBS, but much better than DC.

At last we compare our algorithm with the DC[6] algorithm and the algorithm in paper [12](we call it BBS algorithm) on data stream, the method is to compare the

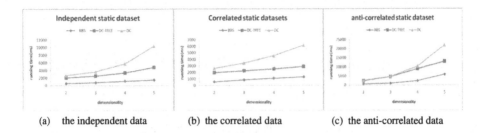

(a)   the independent data   (b) the correlated data   (c) the anti-correlated data

Fig. 6. Varying Dimensionality in Static Data Set

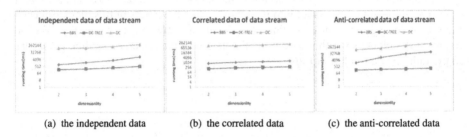

(a) the independent data   (b) the correlated data   (c) the anti-correlated data

Fig. 7. Varying Dimensionality in Dynamic Data Set

time of the processing 1000 data with these three algorithms, which means the average delay of 1000 times data updating. The result as Figure 7 is for independent, correlated and anti-correlated dataset. DC-Tree in these pictures shows the high effect of updating in data stream substantially.

5 Conclusions

The application of the skyline query becomes broader and broader, but the present algorithm can not support the skyline query on data stream effectively, because these algorithms can not support the quick and effective data updating. Towards the skyline query in sliding window of data stream, this paper proposes a kind of algorithm: DC-Tree. It supports the effective data updating and it can output the fast and incremental skyline objects in reality. At last, we propose some improvement measures. And the results of experiment show that the DC-Tree is both efficient and correct. A further interesting issue would be applied to modify this algorithm so that it can be practiced in the SubSkyline [13] and Skyline Cube [14] computation and storage on data stream.

References

1. Bentley, J.L., Kung, H.T., Schkolnick, M., Thompson, C.D.: On the average number of maxima in a set of vectors and applications. J. ACM 25(4), 536–543 (1978)
2. Kung, H.T., Luccio, F., Preparata, F.P.: On finding the maxima of a set of vectors. J. ACM 22(4), 469–476 (1975)

3. McLain, D.H.: Drawing contours from arbitrary data points. Computer J. 17, 318–324 (1974)
4. Steuer, R.: Multiple Criteria Optimization. Wiley, New York (1986)
5. Kapoor, S.: Dynamic maintenance of maxima of 2-d point sets. SIAM J. Comput (2000)
6. Borzsonyi, S., Kossmann, D., Stocker, K.: The Skyline Operator. In: Proc. 17th Intern. Conf. On Data Engineering, Heidelberg, Germany (April 2001)
7. Chomicki, J., Godfrey, P., Gryz, J., Liang, D.: Skyline with presorting. In: Proceedings of the IEEE International Conference on Data Engineering. IEEE Computer Society Press, Los Alamitos (2003)
8. Kossmann, D., Ramsak, F., Rost, S.: Shooting stars in the sky: An online algorithm for skyline queries. In: Proceedings of the International Conference on Very Large Data Bases (2002)
9. Papadias, D., Tao, Y., Fu, G., Seeger, B.: An optimal and progressive algorithm for skyline queries. In: Proceedings of ACM SIGMOD, pp. 467–478 (2003)
10. Tan, K.-L., Eng, P.-K., Ooi, B.C.: Efficient progressive skyline computation. In: Proceedings of VLDB, pp. 301–310 (2001)
11. Babcock, B., Babu, S., Datar, M., Motawani, R., Widom, J.: Models and issues in data stream systems. In: Popa, L. (ed.) Proc. of the 21st ACM Symp. on Principles of Database Systems, pp. 1–16. ACM Press, Wisconsin (2002)
12. Lin, X., Yuan, Y., Wang, W., Lu, H.: Stabbing the Sky: Efficient Skyline Computation over Sliding Windows. In: Proc. 21st IEEE Int'l Conf. Data Eng (ICDE 2005), pp. 502–513 (2005)
13. Tao, Y., Xiao, X., Pei, J.: SUBSKY: Efficient Computation of Skylines in Subspaces. In: Proceedings of the 22nd International Conference on Data Engineering (ICDE 2006), Atlanta, GA, USA, April 3-7 (2006)
14. Yuan, Y., Lin, X., Liu, Q., Wang, W., Yu, J.X., Zhang, Q.: Efficient computation of the skyline cube. In: Proceedings of the 31st international conference on very large databases, pp. 241–252. ACM, USA (2005)

Sequential Pattern Mining for Protein Function Prediction[*]

Miao Wang, Xue-qun Shang, and Zhan-huai Li

School of Computer Science and Engineering, Northwestern Polytechnical University,
Xi'an, China, 710072
riyushui@gmail.com

Abstract. The prediction of protein sequence function is one of the problems arising in the recent progress in bioinformatics. Traditional methods have its limits. We present a novel method of protein sequence function prediction based on sequential pattern mining. First, we use our designed sequential pattern mining algorithms to mine known function sequence dataset. Then, we build a classifier using the patterns generated to predict function of protein sequences. Experiments confirm the effectiveness of our method.

Keywords: protein function prediction, frequent pattern mining, frequent closed pattern, frequent pattern classifier.

1 Introduction

One of the problems arising in the analysis of biological sequences is the prediction of sequence function. Protein is one of the base substances of organism. Therefore, protein sequence function prediction is more important in the post-genomic era.

Several methods have been proposed for dealing with this problem. One widely used class of algorithms employs global string alignment[1]. Using edit operations(e.g. mutations, insertions, deletions) and their associated costs, they transform one sequence to another. What is sought is a minimum-cost consensus sequence that highlights the regions of similarity among the input sequences. However, alignment algorithms have several inherent drawbacks. First, the computation is very expensive. It is known to be an NP-hard problem[2]. Second, alignment of entire sequences can reveal only global similarities; if the sequences under comparison are distantly related, it is quite impossible to produce the substantial alignment.

One way to overcome the difficulty that alignment algorithms met is to focus on the discovery of patters shared by the training sequences. Some pattern-discovery algorithms[3] have been appearing in the past few years. Most of the proposed approaches proceed by enumerating the solution space, so the efficiency is not very well.

---

[*] Supported by Graduated Innovation Lab of Northwestern Polytechnical University(Grant Nos. 06044 and 07042).

C. Tang et al. (Eds.): ADMA 2008, LNAI 5139, pp. 652–658, 2008.

Sequential pattern mining is another way to find the patterns, which discovers frequent subsequences as patterns in a sequence database. It is an important data mining problem applications. The sequential pattern mining problem was first introduced by Agrawal and Srikant[4]. Recently, many previous studies contributed to the efficient mining of sequential patterns. Agrawal and Srikant proposed the GSP[4] algorithm based on Apriori idea. However, the Apriori idea has its drawback. Han et al. proposed the pattern-growth algorithm PrefixSpan[5], which can find frequent patterns efficiently. Zaki proposed the SPADE[6] algorithm based on vertical data format. The efficiency of these algorithms is not well when dealing with bio-dataset. Traditional algorithms for sequential pattern mining have limits when dealing with biological datasets. Wang et al. proposed Two-phase[7] algorithm based on dealing with bio-dataset. However, Two-phase algorithm may miss some important patterns.

In this discussion, we present a novel method of protein sequence function prediction based on sequential pattern mining. First, we use JPS[8] to discover the frequent patterns. Second, the JCPS[9] algorithm mines frequent closed patterns to reduce the redundant patterns. Third, we build a classifier using the patterns generated by mining known function dataset to predict function of protein sequences.

The remainder of the paper is organized as follows: In Section 2, the Joined frequent Pattern Segment approach for protein sequence mining, JPS and the closed pattern mining method, JCPS, are illustrated. In Section 3, we build a classifier based on closed frequent patterns. Through the experimental results and performance analysis, we improve the accuracy of our classifier. Our study is concluded in Section 4.

2   Pattern Mining Problem Definition and Algorithms

In this section, the joined pattern segment-based sequential pattern mining algorithm, JPS and the joined pattern segment-based closed sequential pattern mining algorithm, JCPS, are illustrated.

2.1   JPS Algorithm

As outlined in Section 1, traditional algorithms for sequential pattern mining have limits when dealing with biological datasets. Biology sequence has its own characters. Based on these characters, we developed Joined frequent Pattern Segment approach, JPS[8], for mining protein sequences. First, the joined frequent pattern segments are generated. Then, longer frequent patters can be obtained by combining the above segments. The detail of JPS can be found in [8].

Using JPS, we can get frequent patterns efficiently. However, JPS may produce redundant patterns. For example, we can get pattern (abacda) in two ways. One is to combine (ab) to (ac), then combine (abac) to (da). The other is to combine (ab) to (acda). Both of them can get the same pattern. How to reduce these redundant patterns will be illustrated in the next part.

2.2 JCPS Algorithm

In the last part, we illustrated the JPS algorithm. Because JPS may produce some redundant patterns, we proposed the JCPS[9] algorithm, which can mine the closed patterns. First, the joined closed frequent pattern segments are produced. Then, longer closed frequent patterns can be obtained by combining the above segments, at the same time deleting the unclosed patterns. The detail of JCPS can be found in [9].

The purpose of producing closed patterns is to use them to construct a classifier for protein function prediction. So using non-redundant patterns can improve the accuracy of classification.

3   Protein Sequence Function Prediction Based on Frequent Patterns

In this section, the problem of sequential function prediction method is defined. Then we propose a novel ways to predict protein sequential function based on sequential closed patterns of each protein function dataset. Based on the characters of protein sequence and experimental data, we design a new marking function to improve the accuracy of prediction.

3.1   Problem Definition

Let D={$d_1,d_2,\ldots,d_m$}be the whole dataset. $d_k (1 \le k \le m)$ is one of the function dataset of D. Let I_k be the set of all items in d_k, and Y_k be the class label of d_k. A frequent pattern rule is an implication of the form $X \rightarrow d_k$, where $X \subseteq I_k$. A rule $X \rightarrow d_k$ holds in d_k with support s if s% of cases in d_k that contain X.

Our frequent pattern is different from the association rule in classification by association rule mining. The later method deals with the whole dataset which contains all different function sub-dataset, in order to improve the accuracy of classification, it must have the confidence for each rule. Both support and confidence are absolute data. In our method, we produce frequent pattern rules in each function dataset, only use support to measure each rule, which is relative data. Using relative data for classification can get less effect of each function dataset and more accuracy of classification.

3.2   Classification by Frequent Patterns

[10] analyzed some famous algorithms of classification by association rules, the result shows that it doesn't exist an algorithm can classify well all the datasets. The character of dataset is important. So we propose some different ways for classification, the best method can be got by experiment.

3.2.1   Best First Rule

The frequent patterns for classification are closed patterns obtained by JCPS. Using all patterns is not well. We use the first best pattern for classification. The ordering is defined as follow:

1. **Support:** A rule r_1 has priority over a rule r_2 if $sup(r_1) > sup(r_2)$.
2. **Size of antecedent:** A rule r_1 has priority over a rule r_2 if $sup(r_1) = sup(r_2)$ and $|r_1| > |r_2|$.
3. **Rule position:** A rule r_1 has priority over a rule r_2 if $sup(r_1) = sup(r_2)$, $|r_1| = |r_2|$ and r_1 is generated earlier than r_2.

In order to get the accuracy rate of above method, through the experiment data we can obtain the data, and by analyzing it to improve our method. All experiments were conducted on a 2.6GHz Intel(R) Pentium(R) 4 CPU PC with 512M main memory, running Microsoft XP SP2, the experiment of developing algorithms is Microsoft Visual C++ 6.0 SP6. The datasets are ten protein sequence families, which can be downloaded by PIR(http://pir.georgetown.edu/pirwww/). The dataset is PIRSF000130, PIRSF000132, PIRSF000135, PIRSF000136, PIRSF000141, PIRSF000142, PIRSF000146, PIRSF000160, PIRSF000170 and PIRSF000180, respectively.

Table 1 shows the minimum support and minimum length of frequent patterns obtain by JCPS in each protein family. The second column of Table 2 shows the accuracy rate of each family(original parameter) by best first rule. From the accuracy rate, the whole rate isn't well. So we improved our method in the next part.

Table 1. Support and length of each family

Family ID	Original Parameter		Changed Parameter	
	Minimum Support Rate	Minimum Length	Minimum Support Rate	Minimum Length
PIRSF000130	0.7	5	0.7	4
PIRSF000132	0.6	4	0.6	4
PIRSF000135	0.6	5	0.6	4
PIRSF000136	0.6	5	0.7	3
PIRSF000141	0.5	4	0.6	4
PIRSF000142	0.5	5	0.5	3
PIRSF000146	0.5	3	0.5	3
PIRSF000160	0.6	5	0.6	5
PIRSF000170	0.6	4	0.6	4
PIRSF000180	0.6	4	0.6	4

3.2.2 Best K Rules

The reason the accuracy rate is low by best first rule may be the character of bio-data. As we know, all organisms are evolved by the original ones. So different organism may have the same conserved information, especially ones in the same species. If the best rule is the conserved information, the accuracy rate must be affected. We choose 5 patterns to construct the classifier. Why choosing 5 can be seen in [11].

The ordering is defined as the same of the best first method order. The marking function is chosen by the sum of suitable patterns. The reason why not use average is

Table 2. Accuracy of each method

Family ID	Best Rule	Best 5 Rules			
		Accuracy Rate by Sum of Support		Accuracy Rate by Average of Support	Accuracy Rate by Support*Length
		Original Parameter	Changed Parameter	Original Parameter	
PIRSF000130	0.89	0.93	0.93	0.93	0.98
PIRSF000132	0.85	0.98	0.60	0.60	0.96
PIRSF000135	0.96	1.00	1.00	1.00	0.96
PIRSF000136	0.80	0.91	0.96	0.96	0.96
PIRSF000141	0.68	0.78	0.85	0.85	1.00
PIRSF000142	0.59	0.59	0.60	0.60	0.70
PIRSF000146	0.74	1.00	0.85	0.85	0.85
PIRSF000160	0.92	1.00	1.00	1.00	1.00
PIRSF000170	0.95	0.97	0.97	0.97	0.97
PIRSF000180	1.00	0.94	1.00	1.00	0.96
Average Rate	0.84	0.91	0.88	0.88	0.94

different family may have different support. If the pattern with higher support is chosen wrongly, the accuracy would be affected seriously. The following experiment can prove our choice. The third column and fifth column of Table 2 shows sum marking is better than average marking by using the same data of original parameter.

From the third column of Table 2, we see the accuracy of PIRSF000141 and PIRSF000142 is not well. So we changed the support and length of generated by JCPS, as is shown in Table 1. The fourth column of Table 2 is the changed accuracy rate, which shows the whole accuracy rate is lower, although the rates of these families are higher. The reason is the existence of conservation information. The length of pattern also affects the accuracy. We improved our ordering method, which considers not only the support of pattern, but also the length of it. The ordering is defined as follow:

1. A rule r_1 has priority over a rule r_2 if $\sup(r_1)*|r_1|>\sup(r_2)*|r_2|$.
2. A rule r_1 has priority over a rule r_2 if $\sup(r_1)*|r_1|=\sup(r_2)*|r_2|$ and $\sup(r_1)>\sup(r_2)$.
3. A rule r_1 has priority over a rule r_2 if $\sup(r_1)*|r_1|=\sup(r_2)*|r_2|$, $\sup(r_1)=\sup(r_2)$ and $|r_1|>|r_2|$.

4.   A rule r_1 has priority over a rule r_2 if $\sup(r_1)*|r_1|=\sup(r_2)*|r_2|$, $\sup(r_1)=\sup(r_2)$, $|r_1|=|r_2|$ and r_1 is generated earlier than r_2.

The last column of Table 2 shows the accuracy rate obtained by above method. We see the accuracy rate is higher than foregoing methods. It also proved the character of protein or other biology sequence, the conservation information affects function classification seriously.

4   Conclusions

We have performed a systematic study on bio-sequence function classification methods. Instead of traditional methods, we proposed a new prediction model using sequential frequent patterns. Compared it to other methods, our method has more efficiency. Based on the character of protein sequence, author proposed two bio-sequential pattern mining algorithms: JPS and JCPS. The former can get the patterns having more biology characters, the later can reduce the redundant patterns. Based on JCPS, we design the protein sequence function classifier. By experiments, we constructed more classifier, through the experimental data, we improved our classification method to get the better accuracy rate. We also proved the character of conservation in biology.

There are many interesting issues that need to be studied further, including the improvement of ordering method and marking method. Using sequence to predict protein function is limited. One protein may have several functions, different condition may get different function. In the next step, we will use protein to protein interaction(PPI) map to predict protein function.

References

1. Neville-Manning, C.G., Sethi, K.S., Wu, D., Brutlag, D.L.: Enumerating and ranking discrete motifs. In: Proceedings of Intelligent Systems for Molecular Biology, pp. 202–209. AAAI Press, Menlo Park (1997)
2. Wang, L., Jiang, T.: On the complexity of multiple sequence alignment. J. Comput. Biol. 1, 337–348 (1994)
3. Suyama, M., Nishioka, T., Jun'ichi, O.: Searching for common sequence patterns among distantly related proteins. Protein Eng. 8, 1075–1080 (1995)
4. Agrawal, R., Srikant, R.: Mining Sequential Patterns: Generalizations and Performance Improvements. In: Apers, P.M.G., Bouzeghoub, M., Gardarin, G. (eds.) EDBT 1996. LNCS, vol. 1057, pp. 3–17. Springer, Heidelberg (1996)
5. Jian, P., Jiawei, H.: Mining Sequential Patterns by Pattern-growth: The PrefixSpan Approach. IEEE Transactions on Knowledge and Data Engineering 6(10), 1–17 (2004)
6. Zaki, M.: SPADE: An Efficient Algorithm for Mining Frequent Sequences. Machine Learning 40, 31–60 (2001)
7. Wang, K., Xu, Y., Yu, J.X.: Scalable Sequential Pattern Mining for Biological Sequences. In: CIKM 2004, Washington, DC, USA, November 13 (2004)

8. Wang, M., Shang, X.-q., Xue, H.: Joined Pattern Segment-based Sequential Pattern Mining Algorithm for Biological Datasets (in Chinese). Computer Engineering and Applications 44, 190–193 (2008)

9. Wang, M., Shang, X.-q., Xue, H.: Joined Pattern Segment-based Closed Sequential Pattern Mining Algorithm (in Chinese). Computer Engineering and Applications 44, 148–151 (2008)

10. Coenen, F., Leng, P.: An Evaluation of Approaches to Classification Rule Selection. In: Proceedings of the 4th IEEE International Conference on Data Mining (ICDM 2004), Brighton, UK, pp. 359–362. IEEE Computer Society, Los Alamitos (2004)

11. Yin, X., Han, J.: CPAR: Classification based on Predictive Association Rules. In: Proc. SIAM Int. Conf. on Data Mining (SDM 2003), San Francisco, CA, pp. 331–335 (2003)

Improving Web Search by Categorization, Clustering, and Personalization

Dengya Zhu and Heinz Dreher

CBS and DEBII, Curtin University of Technology, GPO Box U1987, Perth, WA Australia
dengya.zhu@postgrad.curtin.edu.au,
h.dreher@curtin.edu.au

Abstract. This research combines Web snippet[1] categorization, clustering and personalization techniques to recommend relevant results to users. RIB – Recommender Intelligent Browser which categorizes Web snippets using socially constructed Web directory such as the Open Directory Project (ODP) is to be developed. By comparing the similarities between the semantics of each ODP category represented by the category-documents and the Web snippets, the Web snippets are organized into a hierarchy. Meanwhile, the Web snippets are clustered to boost the quality of the categorization. Based on an automatically formed user profile which takes into consideration desktop computer information and concept drift, the proposed search strategy recommends relevant search results to users. This research also intends to verify text categorization, clustering, and feature selection algorithms in the context where only Web snippets are available.

Keywords: text categorization, clustering, personalization, Web searching, Web snippets.

1 Introduction

The low quality of Web search [1] in terms of *recall* and *precision* stems from

1) the synonymous and polysemous characteristics of natural languages [2];
2) information overload on the Web [3, 4];
3) the imperfection of the information retrieval models so far developed; and
4) the lack of consideration of personal search interests and preferences [5, 6].

Text categorization [7] and clustering [8] are predominant approaches used to address problems of large amounts of information, and the challenges resulting from the polysemous characteristics of natural languages. Text categorization, or supervised learning, is the automatic assigning of predefined categories to free documents [9], while document clustering, or unsupervised learning, tries to discover groups in a document set such that similar documents are grouped together. For text categorization, the main issue is that it is expensive to obtain sufficient human edited training data. The main challenge for clustering algorithms is that the automatically formed cluster hierarchy may mismatch the human mental model [4, 10]. Furthermore, when

---

[1] A Web snippet, returned from search engines, contains only the title of a Web page and an optional very short (less than 30 words) description of the page.

C. Tang et al. (Eds.): ADMA 2008, LNAI 5139, pp. 659–666, 2008.
© Springer-Verlag Berlin Heidelberg 2008

only Web snippets, which are not as informative as full text document, are available, the developed algorithms for text categorization/clustering have not been sufficiently verified. This lack of 'informativeness' also makes it difficult to judge the relevance of these snippets of information, while relevance judgment is at the core of information retrieval [11].

Personalization is regarded as a promising approach to improve the relevance of Web search results because it concerns not only retrieval based on literally relevant information, but also a user's information consumption patterns, searching strategies, and applications used [12]. There are two main issues for personalized searching: concept drift [13, 14]; and privacy protection [15].

To approach the above issues, *RIB* – Recommender Intelligent Browser is proposed. The main purpose of *RIB* is to combine text categorization and clustering techniques to address synonymy, polysemy, and information overload problems by re-ranking, hierarchically organizing, and ontologically filtering returned Web snippets; to personalize Web search results by means of building a user profile based on a reference ontology - "a shared taxonomy of entities" [16] - created from a Web directory (such as the ODP); and taking search concept drift into consideration. *RIB* will recommend to users the re-ranked relevant results according to the user profile.

The contribution of this paper is twofold. First, a new approach to boost the quality of Web snippet categorization is proposed. The approach first estimates the *inter-similarities* between the Web snippets and the semantic of categories of an ontology; and then estimates the *intra-similarities* among the Web snippets to form some clusters which are used to boost the quality of categorization. Second, *RIB*, a novel Web information retrieval approach aims at recommending refined results to users based on automatically learned user profiles and ontologically filtering search results. *RIB* is to be developed and its performance in terms of *precision* is expected to comparable with or superior in some way to the results of *Windows Live Search API*.

2 Related Work

Text Categorization. Text categorization automatically assigns predefined categories to free documents [9]. Klas and Fuhr [17] use tf-idf weighting scheme [18] and probabilistic retrieval model to classify Web documents under the hierarchical structure of *Yahoo! Web Directory*. The texts of all documents belonging to a category are concatenated to form a so-called megadocument. To classify a document, the first n best terms (according to their idf values) are selected as a query vector. [19] proposes to disambiguate single-term queries by clustering and categorizing Web search results based on the meanings of WordNet for the queries.

The ODP categories are also used to classify Web snippets [10, 20]. The semantic aspects of the ODP categories are extracted, and category-documents are formed based on the extracted semantic characteristics of the categories. A special search browser is being developed to obtain Web snippets by utilizing *Yahoo! Search Web Service API*. Similarities between vectors represent Web snippets and the category-documents are compared. A majority voting strategy is used to assign a Web snippet to the proper category without overlapping. One weakness of the research is while the *precision* is improved, there is a decrease in *recall*.

Web Snippet Clustering. One of the early works on Web snippet clustering is *Scatter/Gather* [21] which uses a partitional algorithm named Fractionation. It is found in the research that search results clustering can significantly improve similarity search ranking. *Grouper* [22] is another example of early work on clustering Web search results. Zeng et al. [23] propose the Web snippets clustering problem can be dealt with as a salient phrase ranking problem. The Web documents are assigned to relevant salient phrases to form candidate clusters, which are then merged to form the final clusters.

Personalization. Pitkow et al. [12] use the information space of the ODP to represent their user model. Again using the ODP, [1] creates a user profile according to a reference ontology in which each concept has a weight reflecting the user's interest in that concept. URLs visited by a user are periodically analyzed and then classified into concepts in the reference ontology. Chirita et al. [5] also suggest using the ODP metadata and combining a complex distance function with Google *PageRank* to achieve a high quality personalized Web search. Godoy and Amandi [6] propose an incremental, unsupervised Web Document Conceptual Clustering algorithm to set up user profiles. They use kNN to determine the similarities between concepts in user profiles and Web pages.

3   Conceptual Framework of RIB

RIB intends to investigate how does the use of Web snippet categorization and personalization enhance the relevance of Web search results by comparing three sets of search results:

1) the results directly obtained from meta-search engines [24, 25];
2) the results categorized without considering the clustered results; and
3) the categorized results refined with clustered results.

We also want to check to what degree the combination of categorization and clustering boosts the performance (in terms of *recall, precision*, and *F1*) of Web snippet categorization. We compare the categorized results of Support Vector Machines, k-Nearest Neighbors , and naïve Bayesian, with and without combining the results clustered by LSI [2], k-means [8], and Expectation Maximization clustering algorithms. The conceptual framework of *RIB* is illustrated in Fig.1. Obviously, *RIB* is not going to simply put all the algorithms together that will do nothing better except dramatically increase the computational complexity. The algorithms are mentioned here because one purpose of this research is to evaluate the effectiveness of the algorithms for Web snippets.

Meta Search Engine. The Meta-search engine obtains search results directly *from Yahoo! Search Web Service API* or *Windows Live Search API* after an application ID is applied. Both search APIs allow developers to retrieve from their Web databases directly. For non-commercial licenses, the maximum number of results per query for Yahoo! is 100; and Microsoft API can return up to 1000 results. In this research, *Windows Live Search API* is employed because it provides full-size result sets the same as all the popular search engines, providing an opportunity to make a real-word comparison between *RIB* and Microsoft Live Search.

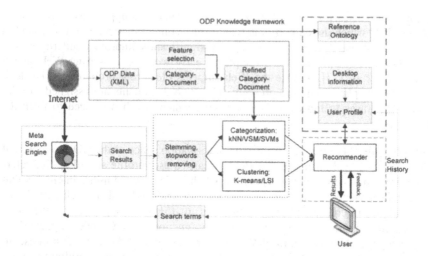

Fig. 1. The conceptual framework of Recommender Intelligent Browser

The Category-Document Extraction and Feature Selection. The ODP is selected as a predefined knowledge hierarchy because it is the largest and most comprehensive Web hierarchy edited by humans. A category-document is created based on these two files [10]. The category-document set extracted from the ODP is refined by feature selection algorithms [7, 26] such as χ^2, Mutual Information, Odds Ratio, and Information Gain [7]. Data from *structure.rdf* is used to map the ODP knowledge hierarchy to a reference ontology, which will represent users' search preferences.

Categorization/Clustering Algorithms. Lucene [27] is used to calculate similarities between documents and queries. A modified k majority voting algorithm has already been developed by Zhu [10] and can be used in this research. Naïve Bayesian, and k-means clustering algorithms are developed using the C# programming language.

Categorization creates some groups with distinct topics. The number of groups is to be used as k for the k-means algorithms because how to decide k is always a nontrivial problem for k-means algorithms [8].

User Profile Creation. Desktop computer information, indexed by *Google Desktop Search SDK*, is used to initialize the user profile. For each of the indexed documents, the similarities sim (d_j, c_i) between a document d_j in a personal computer and a category-document representing a category c_i in the ODP are estimated by Lucene. When a Web page is visited, the time factor is considered [28]. The impact of concept drift will be a weighting factor which represents user search preferences [28]. Let w_i be the weight of concept c_i in the profile, and the width of slide time window is 400, then,

$$w_i = u(t) \times w_i, \quad u(t) = \begin{cases} 0.95 & current - most\ current\ 200\ searches \\ 0.75 & recent - past\ 201 - 400\ searches \\ 0.30 & historical - searches\ earlier\ than\ 400 \end{cases}$$

Recommender. Search results returned from the meta-search engine are categorized into the ODP knowledge hierarchy. Suppose the Web snippets are categorized into category c_i, and its corresponding category weight in the user profile is w_i ($i = 1, 2, \ldots N$). According to the descending order of w_i, the corresponding category is recommended to users in the same order. Users can adjust the number of categories to be recommended.

4 Combination of Inter- and Intra-similarities

Fig. 2. illustrates how the *inter-similarity* and *intra-similarity* are combined to boost the effectiveness of Web snippet categorization. In Figure 2 (a), there are five categories labeled as C1 to C5 and five Web snippets labeled from S1 to S5. The five snippets are to be categorized under these five categories. According to the cosine similarities between the category-document and the Web snippets, and suppose one snippet can only be classified into one category, S1 and S2 are categorized under category C3; S3 is categorized under category C4; and S4 and S5 are categorized under category C1. Suppose the topic of interest is C3, when that category is selected, Web snippets S1 and S2 will be presented to the user.

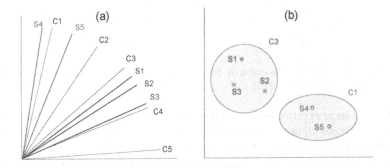

Fig. 2. Illustration of inter- and intra-similarities of Web snippets [29]

However, as can be seen from (b) in Fig. 2, the snippets S1, S2 and S3 are also similar to each other and will thus form a cluster. It is reasonable to assign category C3 to S3 as well. Therefore, to increase *recall*, one snippet should be allowed to assign more than one categories. That is, when category C3 is selected, snippets S1, S2 and S3 should all be presented; not only S1 and S2. When C4 is selected, because S3 and S2 are not in a cluster, only snippet S3 is to be presented.

5 Experimental Results

Our early stage experimental data [10] reveal that Web snippet categorization under the ODP can improve the relevance of Web search. The experiment uses five ambiguous search-terms to obtain search results from *Yahoo! Search Web Service API*, the similarity between the Web search results and the ODP category-documents are calculated by Lucene. A majority voting algorithm is used to make a final categorization decision. For each search-term, 50 search results are taken into consideration. One unique information need is specified for each of these search-terms and one search result is classified to one ODP category. The relevance of Web search results and the supposed information needs are judged by five human experts. Their judgments are summarized to make the final binary relevance judgment decisions. Because the Web search results are often categorized into more than one of the ODP categories, when estimating *precision* and *recall*, two categories with most relevant results are selected. The standard 11 points *precision-recall* curves of the results of Yahoo! API, and our categorized results are shown in Fig. 3.

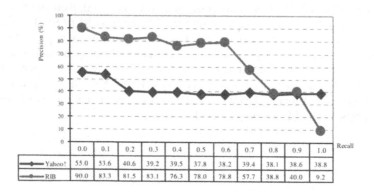

	0.0	0.1	0.2	0.3	0.4	0.5	0.6	0.7	0.8	0.9	1.0	Recall
Yahoo!	55.0	53.6	40.6	39.2	39.5	37.8	38.2	39.4	38.1	38.6	38.8	
RIB	90.0	83.3	81.5	83.1	76.3	78.0	78.8	57.7	38.8	40.0	9.2	

Fig. 3. Average recall-precision curve of Yahoo! search results and the categorized results of RIB over the five search-terms [10]

This early stage experimental result demonstrates that according to the standard 11 points *precision-recall* curve, an average 23.5% *precision* improvement is achieved.

The limitations of this early stage experiment are:

1) the ODP categories are not merged, there are 59,000 category-documents corresponding to the huge ODP categories;
2) document terms are only stemmed; no feature selection algorithms are applied. The computational efficiency therefore has scope for improvement.

6 Future Work

The next goal is to implement *RIB* which is expected to address the problems discussed in the introduction (section 1). Allowance to assign more than one categories to one search result can also improve *recall* of categorized results.

RIB will obtain 100 Web search results for each of 50 selected search-terms to get 5000 search results. Around 50 human experts will be employed, they will be divided into five groups, and each group will have 500 Web results to judge. In addition to relevance judgment, human experts this time will also decide which ODP category a result is to be assigned, and consequently give sufficient training and test data for our experiments to verify and evaluate the developed categorization, clustering, and feature selection algorithms in the context where only Web snippets are available. The effectiveness of personalization and search concept drift process will also be verified.

7 Conclusion

The purpose of this research is to improve the relevance of Web searching by recommend to users with personalized results. A new Web search system, *RIB*, which combines Web snippet categorization, clustering, and personalization was proposed. *RIB* intended to boost the Web snippet categorization by exploring not only inter-similarities between Web snippets and category-documents formed by extracting semantic characteristics of ODP categories; but also the intra-similarities among the returned Web snippets by grouping similar documents into clusters. Users search concept drift problem was addressed by adjusting the weighting factor which represents the users' search preferences in user profiles. Experimental results so far were inspiring; a 23.5% *precision* improvement was achieved when Web search results were categorized under the ODP categorization scheme; and a further boost of Web searching is expected with the implementation of *RIB*.

References

1. Gauch, S., Chaffee, J., Pretschner, A.: Ontology-based personalized search and browsing. Web intelligence and Agent System 1, 219–234 (2003)
2. Deerwester, S., Dumais, S.T., Furnas, G.W., Landauer, T.K., Harshman, R.: Indexing by latent semantic indexing. J. Am. Soc. Inf. Sci. 41, 391–407 (1990)
3. Montebello, M.: Information Overload–An IR Problem? In: Proceedings of String Processing and Information Retrieval: A South American Symposium, pp. 65–74. IEEE Computer Society, Los Alamitos (1998)
4. Zhu, D., Dreher, H.: IR Issues for Digital Ecosystems Users. In: Proceedings of the Second IEEE Digital Ecosystems and Technologies Conference, pp. 586–591. IEEE, Los Alamitos (2008)
5. Chirita, P.-A., Nejdl, W., Paiu, R., Kohlschütter, C.: Using ODP Metadata to Personalize Search. In: Proceedings of the 28th Annual International ACM SIGIR Conference on Research and Development in Information Retrieval, pp. 178–185. ACM Press, New York (2005)
6. Godoy, D., Amandi, A.: Modeling user interests by conceptual clustering. Inform. Syst. 31, 247–265 (2006)
7. Sebastiani, F.: Machine Learning in Automated Text Categorization. ACM Comput. Surv. 34, 1–47 (2002)
8. Jain, A.K., Murty, M.N., Flynn, P.J.: Data Clustering: A Review. ACM Comput. Surv. 31, 264–323 (1999)
9. Yang, Y.: An Evaluation of Statistical Approaches to Text Categorization. Inform. Retrieval 1, 69–90 (1999)
10. Zhu, D.: Improving the Relevance of Search Results via Search-term Disambiguation and Ontological Filtering. School of Information Systems, Curtin Business School, Master. Curtin University of Technology, Perth, pp. 235 (2007)
11. Mizzaro, S.: Relevance: The Whole History. J. Am. Soc. Inf. Sci. 48, 810–832 (1997)

12. Pitkow, J., Schütze, H., Cass, T., Cooley, R., Turnbull, D., Edmonds, A., Adar, E., Breuel, T.: Personalized Search: A contextual computing approach may prove a breakthrough in personalized search efficiency. Commun. ACM 45, 50–55 (2002)
13. Tsymbal, A.: The problem of concept drift: definitions and related work. Technical report, Trinity College Dublin (2004)
14. Webb, G.I., Pazzani, M.J., Billsus, D.: Machine Learning for User Modeling. User Model User-Adap. 11, 19–29 (2001)
15. Shen, X., Tan, B., Zhai, C.: Privacy Protection in Personalization Search. ACM SIGIR Forum 41, 4–17 (2007)
16. Smith, B.: Ontology. In: Floridi, L. (ed.) Blackwell Guide to the Philosophy of Computing and Information, pp. 155–166. Blackwell, Oxford (2004)
17. Klas, C.-P., Fuhr, N.: A New Effective Approach for Categorizing Web Documents. In: Proceedings of the 22nd Annual Colloquium of the British Computer Society Information Retrieval Specialist Group (BCSIGSG 2000) (2000)
18. Salton, G., Buckley, C.: Term-Weighting Approaches in Automatic Text Retrieval. Inform. Process. Manag. 24, 513–523 (1988)
19. Hemayati, R., Meng, W., Yu, C.: Semantic-based Grouping of Search Engine Results Using WordNet. In: Dong, G., Lin, X., Wang, W., Yang, Y., Yu, J.X. (eds.) APWeb/WAIM 2007. LNCS, vol. 4505, pp. 678–686. Springer, Heidelberg (2007)
20. Zhu, D., Dreher, H.: An Integrating Text Retrieval Framework for Digital Ecosystems Paradigm. In: Proceedings of the Inaugural IEEE Digital Ecosystems and Technologies Conference, pp. 367–372. IEEE, Los Alamitos (2007)
21. Hearst, M.A., Pedersen, J.O.: Reexamining the Cluster Hypothesis: Scatter/Gather on Retrieval Results. In: Proceedings of the 19th annual international ACM/SIGIR conference on Research and development in information retrieval, pp. 76–84. ACM Press, New York (1996)
22. Zamir, O., Etzioni, O.: Grouper: A Dynamic Clustering Interface to Web Search Results. In: Proceedings of the Eighth International World Wide Web Conference (WWW8), pp. 283–296. Elsevier, Amsterdam (1999)
23. Zeng, H.-J., He, Q.-C., Chen, Z., Ma, W.-Y., Ma, J.: Learning to Cluster Web Search Results. In: Proceedings of the 27th Annual International ACM SIGIR Conference on Research and Development in Information Retrieval, pp. 210–217. ACM Press, New York (2004)
24. Arasu, A., Cho, J., Garcia-Molina, H., Paepcke, A., Raghavan, S.: Searching the Web. ACM Trans. Inter. Tech. 1, 2–43 (2001)
25. Meng, W., Yu, C., Liu, K.-L.: Building Efficient and Effective Metasearch Engines. ACM Comput. Surv. 34, 48–89 (2000)
26. Mladenic, D., Grobelnik, M.: Feature selection on hierarchy of web documents. Decis. Support Syst. 35, 45–87 (2003)
27. Gospodnetić, O., Hatcher, E.: Lucene In Action. Manning Publications, Greenwich (2005)
28. Zhu, D., Dreher, H.: Personalized Information Retrieval in Digital Ecosystems. In: Proceedings of the Second IEEE Digital Ecosystems and Technologies Conference, pp. 580–585. IEEE, Los Alamitos (2008)
29. Zhu, D.: RIB: A Personalized Ontology-based Categorization/Clustering Approach to Improve the Relevance of Web Search Results. In: Proceedings of Curtin Business School Doctorial Colloquium. Curtin University of Technology, Perth (2007)

JSNVA: A Java Straight-Line Drawing Framework for Network Visual Analysis

Qi Ye, Bin Wu, and Bai Wang

Beijing Key Laboratory of Intelligent Telecommunications Software and Multimedia
Beijing University of Posts and Telecommunications, Beijing, China, 100876
jack_hill@263.net, wubin@bupt.edu.cn, wangbai@bupt.edu.cn

Abstract. Although information visualization technologies are indispensable in complex data analysis, wide-spread tools still need to be developed, as successful information visualization applications often require domain-specific customization. In this paper we introduce a software framework JSNVA for network visual analysis in different applications. JSNVA has a clear architecture and supports a more systematic way of implementing different straight-line graph drawing algorithms which show different networks on different views. JSNVA can be used as a front-end for visualization and a back-end for analysis in applications, and it can be customized for different applications. To evaluate JSNVA, we will give its applications in different graph mining tasks. Through visual analyzing these networks by different interactive visualization techniques and algorithms, we can get their underlying structure intuitively and quickly.

1 Introduction

To gain insight into today's large data resources, data mining extracts interesting patterns. To generate knowledge from patterns and benefit from human cognitive abilities, meaningful visualization of patterns are crucial [1]. Graph drawing is a conventional technique for the visualization of relation information. Perhaps the first general approach to graph visualization framework is proposed by Kamada and Kawai [2]. There are some famous tools for graph visualization, such as Pajek [3]. There are also some famous open source visualization frameworks for drawing graphs, such as prefuse [4] and JUNG (http://jung.sourceforge.net). However, the tools and frameworks mentioned above are all large programs and their structure is hard to comprehend, introducing new function into existing frameworks without recoding becomes very difficult.

In order to explore the link relations in real-world networks explicitly, we propose JSNVA (Java Straight-line Drawing Network Visual Analysis framework), a lightweight framework for network visual analysis. The goal of JSNVA is to give simple and elegant solutions to analyze real-world networks vividly and intuitively, so we both focus on drawing graphs and analysis. To evaluate its function, we apply JSNVA to analyze real-world networks in different large scale data sets and we can get their underlying structure intuitively and quickly.

This paper is organized as follows: first, we outline graph based visual analysis and related frameworks in section 2. Afterwards, we discuss the design of our framework, which especially includes the architecture of JSNVA and the function of each module

C. Tang et al. (Eds.): ADMA 2008, LNAI 5139, pp. 667–674, 2008.

in section 3. In section 4, we will give the applications by applying JSNVA to analyze different real-world networks.

2   Design of the Framework

2.1   Straight-Line Drawing

A drawing Γ of a graph G maps a distinct point of the plane and each edge (u, v) of G to a simple Jordan curve with endpoints u and v. Γ is a straight-line drawing if each edge is a straight-line segment. In this case the drawing problem reduces to the problem of positioning the vertices by determining a mapping $L : V \rightarrow R$. There are many famous algorithms are based on the string-line drawing [5,6], especially the ones used for drawing large networks. In recent years, many algorithms for drawing large networks automatically are proposed [7] and most of them use straight-line drawing convention. Considering straight-line drawing convention is widely used in drawing real-world networks and well studied, we implement our domain-independent framework with strict straight-line drawing convention.

2.2   Architecture

A framework is a set of cooperating classes that make up a reusable design for a specific class of software [8]. JSNVA is written in Java programming language using Java2D graphics, and it provides a clear framework for graph based visual analysis. JSNVA draws from pioneering work on drawing graphs and existing system like JUNG, prefuse. To make JSNVA more flexible, reusable and understandable, we apply some design patterns in it and divide the framework into different modules based on their functions. JSNVA is mainly composed of the following modules: Graph, Layout, Render, Engine, Algorithm and GraphPaint.

Graph Module. The Graph module implements the underlying data structure of the graph to be drawn or analyzed. The graph data structure can store attributes by different attribute keys. JSNVA provides both a directed graph interface and an undirected graph interface for abstract graphs. These graph interfaces enable us to handle general graph structures, so that we are not restricted to special graph structures such as general tree or rooted tree structures. In the same time, we can use the graph structures to analyze real-world network efficiently as a general graph library independent of other modules.

Layout Module. The Layout module is the core module of JSNVA which determines the positions of vertices under geometric constraints. In this module, developer can implement different layout algorithms strictly and don't need to connect them together, for which can be done in the Engine module. Layout module supplies different drawings algorithms to map the vertices' positions of abstract graph to the panel and store the positions of vertices in the graph structure. JSNVA implements many general layout algorithms, including forced directed layout [5,6], radical layout [9] etc.

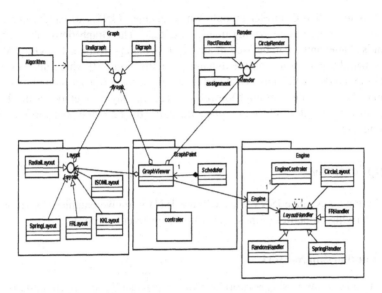

Fig. 1. The architecture of JSNVA

Engine Module. The Engine module uses the LayoutHandlers to determine the positions of vertices under geometric constraints. It plays the same role as the Layout module, but its function is more powerful and flexible. The Engine interface uses the different LayoutHandlers which use the Chain of Responsibility pattern [8] to map the positions of vertices based on the positions mapped by previous handler. As a reasonable initial layout can produce adequate graph drawings, we divide the layout process of the Engine into two steps. In the first step, the Engine will place the vertices initially through the initial handler chain. Then, in the second step, the Engine will place the vertices repeatedly for visualization.

Render Module. The vertices and edges are drawn by Render module. This module separate visual components from their rendering methods, allowing dynamic determination of visual appearances. Changing the appearance of vertices and edges just requires overriding the paint methods in the module. In the Render module there is a submodule called Assignment module which is used to set visual attributes of the graph structure, such as size, colors, labels and font etc.

Algorithm Module. The Algorithm module focuses on implementing the algorithms from graph theory. This module only use the basic graph structure in the Graph module, and it is still under development. We have implemented some basic algorithms on graph theory, such as Dijkstra algorithm, Kruskal algorithm and Prim algorithm etc. We have also implemented some community detecting algorithms, such as maximal clique detecting algorithm, GN algorithm [10], K-clique-community detecting algorithm [11].

GraphPaint Module. The GraphPaint module is the top one of the framework, and it use other modules to draw a network on a panel. In the GraphPaint module there is a submodule called Controler module which enables JSNVA to handle interactive events, such as mouse event, saving images event etc. The GraphViewer is a subclass of Swing's JPanel and it can be used in any Java Swing application. The GraphViewer uses a Scheduler pattern to provide dynamic visualization [12] which updates visual properties and redraws the network at certain time intervals. At each step of displaying the graph, the Scheduler in GraphViewer will call the layout method in the Engine interface or the Layout interface to replace the network and redraw the vertices on the panel dynamically.

3   Applications

In this section, to evaluate JSNVA, we will use JSNVA to give graphical representation of the underlying properties of these networks for different purposes.

3.1   Co-authorship Network

Here we build a co-authorship network to investigate kinship patterns, community structure in it. We get the published papers written by the students and faculty at Beijing University of Posts and Telecommunications from 1998 to 2004, which are indexed by SCI, EI and ISTP. There are about 1990 papers in the data set. We extract authors' names from the files and put the first name before the surname manually and connect all the authors in each paper together. In the co-authorship network, the size of the giant component is 1453, filling 87.4% of the total volume. In the following parts of this paper, we only focus on characters of the giant component. We also get the clustering coefficient of the network is 0.712 and average length of shortest paths between vertices is 5.15. All these algorithms are implemented in the Algorithm Module.

Community Detecting. Detecting the relations among communities is also crucial to the understanding of structural and functional properties of networks, and it is a useful way to handle information overload to get an overview of the network. There are two kinds of famous community detecting algorithms to find the clusters in network. One method is to divide the network into different separated sets of communities, and the other method is trying to detect sets of overlapping communities.

Separated Communities. Here we set the collaboration times between authors as the weights of edges, then use the algorithm provided by Newman [13] in the Algorithm module to detecting community structures in the weighted giant component, which is implemented in the Algorithm module. Through the algorithm, we get 34 communities in the component and all of them are in different colors. The thickness of edges in Fig. 2 indicates the collaboration times between authors and the size of vertices shows the productivity of authors.

We choose "focus+detail" views to get an overview of the giant component firstly by using the FR algorithm in the Layout module [5]. After that we choose the largest community which is in the red circle in Fig. 2 (A) to show the detailed view. Fig. 2 (B) shows the largest community in the giant component. To avoid the graph image

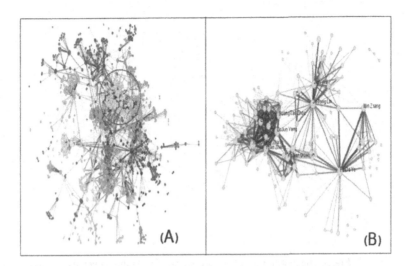

Fig. 2. (A) Communities in the giant component (B) The largest community in the giant component

confused by authors' names, we label some famous authors in the community. We find some of the authors labeled are professors in the school of Telecommunication Engineering, while others are in the school of Science. PeiDa Ye is an academician from Chinese Academy of Sciences and JinTong Lin used to be a student of professor PeiDa Ye. Both of them are in the Optical Communication Center in the school. Bo-Jun Yang and XiaoGuang Zhang et al. are professors in the Science school. Although the authors are from different schools, they are in the same research field of Optical Communication.

Overlapping Communities. To uncover the stable communities, we will filter the unstable links in it and link these communities together to show their research fields. First, we set a threshold of 3 to filter the co-authorship network. After that, We use the k-clique-community detecting algorithm [11] in the Algorithm module to connect these highly overlapping cliques in this network. At last, we find 29 4-clique-communities in the stable network. We find out the most frequent school name in each community to describe it.

As shown in Fig. 3, the green vertices represent authors from the school of Telecommunication Engineering; the yellow ones are from the Science school; the red ones are from the school of Computer Science; the cyan ones are from the school of Electrical Engineering; the purple ones are from the school of Information Engineering. Through Fig. 3, we find most of communities are from the school of Telecommunication Engineering which indicates the main research interest of the university is related to telecommunication. We can find that the authors from the school of Science are closely connected with the authors from the school of Telecommunication Engineering because they are all have a main common research interest in Optical Communication.

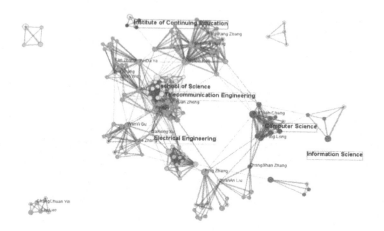

Fig. 3. The institutions of these communities at the university

3.2   Co-citation Network

In this application, we use JSNVA to detect different research areas in article co-citation network. We use two sets of bibliographic record to build the co-citation networks from different data sources. One data set we used in is from the data set of CiteSpace [14]. This data set are the bibliographic record on Medical Informatics from 1994 to 2004. The other data set used contains 3308532 articles and their citations in the field of life sciences in a Chinese digital library data base from 1997 to 2007. Among these articles in the Chinese digital library, there are 1585640 articles that contains keywords and 1689756 articles that contains citation information. We build the article co-citation networks by connecting the co-cited articles together in each paper. Finally, we can get a weighted graph, the weights of edges show how many times two articles are co-cited together. The weighted network reflect inherent characteristics of their content similarity.

Research Fields. Here, we use the K-Clique-Community detecting algorithm to find the clustering areas in the co-citation network. We get 5-clique-communities in the stable network by filtering the unstable links whose weights are less than 4. At last we get the network shown in Fig. 4 (A). As we can not get keywords in each cited articles to describe the characteristics of these communities, we use the keywords in the citing articles to describe the common characters of the clusters. By finding the most important keywords to summarize the characteristics of these communities, we use the $TF \times IDF$ measure which is widely used in information retrieval to detect the important terms.

As shown in Fig. 4 (A), we can find clearly that: The most important term in community 1 which is the largest in yellow is "Physician Order Entry". We find its meaning in Wikipedia, which is "Computerized physician order entry, or CPOE, is a process of electronic entry of physician instructions for the treatment of patients". It is usually used to reduce medication-related errors, such as adverse drug events. The community

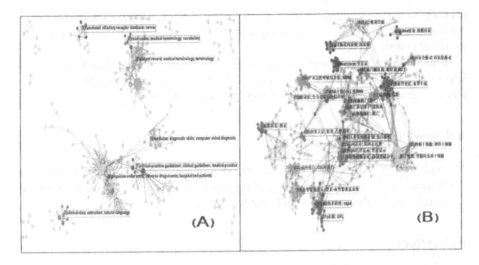

Fig. 4. (A) The 4-Clique-Communities in the Medical Informatics Co-citation Network (B) The 5-Clique-Communities in the Life Sciences Co-citation Network of Chinese digital library

2 and 6 are mainly about medical terminology, which are neighboring. Two of the most frequent terms in community 3 are about diagnosis, so we judge that it is mainly about computer-aided diagnosis. We can also find that community 4 is mainly about mining data from clinical-data. We speculate that community is mainly about clinical-practice guidelines and community 5 is about the computer systems used for medical.

We choose the high cited articles in the Chinese digital library data set to form a co-citation network of Life Sciences. By using the same method, we can get 5-clique-communities in the co-citation network of the Chinese digital library data set. As shown in Fig. 4 (B), Community 5 in yellow is the largest community in the network, and it is related with the topic of stem cell; community 13 is linked with community 5, and it is also on the topic of stem cell; community 3 and 17 are adjacent , and they are related with the topic of gastric cancer and tumor etc.

4 Conclusions and Future Work

In this paper we have introduced JSNVA, a lightweight network visual analysis framework for analyzing real-world networks visually. First, we show the architecture of JSNVA and the function of each module. Second, to evaluate JSNVA, we present two applications to show its flexibility and performance. In the first application, we try to analyze the statistical and clustering features of a co-authorship network. By using "focus+detail" views, we show an overview of the relations between different communities and the detailed relations between authors in the largest community. After finding the clustering and labeling the institute names in different stable communities, we can get an overview of the different research fields of the university and their relations. In the second application, we try to find different research areas of two large co-citation networks in these bibliographic data sets. By using JSNVA, we can explore real-world networks more intuitively and naturally and this framework can be widely used as a front-end in different applications.

In the future, we intend to implement more powerful layout algorithms to show even larger networks, and provide more general algorithms for different applications. We intend to devote it to open source community in the future.

Acknowledgement

The authors gratefully acknowledge the supports of the National Science Foundation of China under Grants No 60402011, and the National Eleven Five-Year Scientific and Technical Support Plans under Grant 2006BAH03B05.

References

1. Assent, I., Krieger, R., Müler, E., Seidl, T.: Visa: Visual subspace clustering analysis. ACM SIGKDD Explorations Special Issue on Visual Analytics 9(2), 5–12 (2007)
2. Kamada, T., Kawai, S.: A general framework for visualizing abstract objects and relations. ACM Transactions of Graphics 10(1), 1–39 (1991)
3. Batagelj, V., Mrvar, A.: Pajek–analysis and visualization of large networks. In: Proceedings of International Symposium on Graph Drawing, pp. 477–478 (2001)
4. Heer, J., Card, S.K., Landay, J.A.: prefuse: a toolkit for interactive information visualization. In: Proceedings of the SIGCHI, pp. 421–430 (2005)
5. Fruchterman, T., Reingold, E.: Graph drawing by force-directed placement. Software Practice and Experience 21, 1129–1164 (1991)
6. Kamada, T., Kawai, S.: An algorithm for drawing general undirected graphs. Information Processing Letters 31(5), 7–15 (1989)
7. Gajer, P., Goodrich, M.T., Kobourov, S.G.: A multi-dimensional approach to force-directed layouts of large graphs. In: Graph Drawing, pp. 211–221 (2001)
8. Gamma, E., Helm, R., Johnson, R., Vlissides, J.: Design Patterns: Elements of Resuable Object-Oriented Software. Addison-Wesley, Reading (1995)
9. Yee, K.P., Fisher, D., Dhamija, R., Hearst, M.: Animated exploration of dynamic graphs with radial layout. In: Proceedings of the Information Visualization (2001)
10. Girvan, M., Newman, M.E.J.: Community structure in social and biological networks. PNAS (12), 7821–7826 (2002)
11. Palla, G., Derényi, I., Farkas, I., Vicsek, T.: Uncovering the overlapping community structure of complex networks in nature and society. Nature 435, 814–817 (2005)
12. Heer, J., Agrawala, M.: Software design patterns for information visualization. IEEE Transactions on Visualization and Computer Graphics 12(5), 853–860 (2006)
13. Newman, M.E.J.: Analysis of weighted networks. Physical Review E 056131 (2004)
14. Chen, C.: Citespace II: Detecting and visualizing emerging trends and transient patterns in scientific literature. J. Am. Soc. Inf. Sci. Technol. 57(3), 359–377 (2006)

Recognition of Data Records in Semi-structured Web-Pages Using Ontology and χ^2 Statistical Distribution

Amin Keshavarzi[1], Amir Masoud Rahmani[2], Mehran Mohsenzadeh[3], and Reza Keshavarzi[4]

[1] Islamic azad univ.Marvdasht branch, Iran
keshavarzi@miau.ac.ir
[2] Islamic azad univ.Science and research branch, Tehran, Iran
rahmani@sr.iau.ac.ir
[3] Islamic azad univ.Science and research branch,Tehran, Iran
mohsenzadeh@sr.iau.ac.ir
[4] University of isfahan, Iran
r.keshavarzi85@gmail.com

Abstract. Information extraction (IE) has been emerged as a novel discipline in computer science. In IE, intelligent algorithms are employed to extract the required data, and structure them so that they are appropriate for query. In most IE systems, a web-page structure, e.g. HTML tags are used to recognize the looked-for information. In this article, an algorithm is developed to recognize the main region of web-pages containing the looked-for information, by means of an ontology, a web-page structure and goodness-of-fit χ^2 test. After recognizing the main region, the existing records of the region are recognized, and then each record is put in a text file.

Keywords: semi-structured, DOM tree, ontology, information extraction, wrapper, χ^2 Statistical Distribution.

1 Introduction

Systems which are competent to extract required information out of web pages and suggest them to the user in an appropriate format is called information extraction (IE) in literature. IE deals with documents with a vast range of formats. The documents could be categorized in three classes; non-structured, semi-structured, and structured documents. Most web pages are semi-structured with HTML format. Semi-structured documents consist of tree-like structured tags, plus free text sentences [8]. A product description page, as shown in Fig. 1, provides an example of a semi-structured page.

As displayed in Fig. 1, a semi-structured page consists of regions such as advertisement bar, search panel, etc. These regions are often unnecessary and users do not pay attention to them. In Fig. 1, the useful information of the web-page is enclosed by the gray box. In different systems, there are two methods to extract the main information on a web-page. In some systems [8], the unnecessary regions are deleted one by one, so that the main region is finally recognized. Another method uses intelligent algorithms to recognize the main region from the other ones [2,3,5,6].

C. Tang et al. (Eds.): ADMA 2008, LNAI 5139, pp. 675–682, 2008.

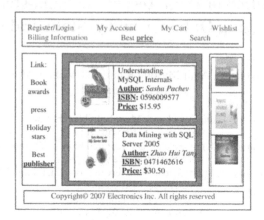

Fig. 1. A Semi-Structured Web-Page

Programs that perform the task of IE are referred to as extractors or wrappers, wrapper induction or information extraction systems are software tools that are designed to generate wrappers [4]. IE systems use some methods to generate wrappers. In most information extraction methods, the web-page structure (e.g. HTML tags), are of great importance. In systems using web-page structure, the main region of the web-page including invaluable data is recognized by means of different algorithms. In this study, the ontology technology is called to develop a system which applies goodness-of-fit χ^2 test to recognize the main region of the semi-structured web-page, and then specifies the number of data records in the region by means of a path matching algorithm and finally separates them.

In the following, we will review the related literature in Section 2. Section 3 presents our suggested architecture, and Section 4 compares our system with former ones with a focus on our achievements. The closing section comments on conclusion.

2   Related Work

Most IE methods work based on web-page structure. In these techniques, the data records including looked-for data are of great significance and several algorithms are developed to recognize them. In NET [5], first a web-page tag tree is built to recognize data records, and then by means of a post-ordered traverse and matching sub- trees, using the tree edit distance method and visual cues, the data records are recognized. This method is capable in recognizing nested records too.

In Odaies [8], the table tree of the web-page is filtered by means of an ontology in some steps, and finally after the deletion of unnecessary regions, the main region of the web-page is recognized. This system employs one template for each filter and these templates are created using a Domain Knowledge Engine (DKE) including the ontology.

In MDR[6], to recognize the data records, first the web-page tag tree is formed, next the data region and finally the very data records of the data region are recognized. To recognize the data region of the generalized node, the neighbor nodes which have the same parent are recognized and a set of two or more similar generalized nodes with the same parent are recognized as a region. To exclude non-data records of generalized nodes, a string matching technique is used for each generalized node.

In STAVIES [2], a method is presented that uses the web-page structure to extract information. Here, parts of a web-page containing the relevant information are identified, and then they are extracted by means of a hierarchical clustering technique. In this system, the texts in a tree of a web-page are clustered according to the number of parents and ancestors, and then a level of the hierarchical clustering is recognized as the main region. Next step involves using a new level in hierarchical clustering to separate and recognize the data records in the main region.

In [3], to recognize the main region, some web pages are compared. Since several regions of these pages are identical, and the great difference is centered around the main region, the relevant sub-trees of the main region are recognized.

3 System Architecture

Our system, OntDRR(Ontology based Data Record Recognition), uses an ontology, and $\chi 2$ statistical distribution for recognition of the main region of a web-page, and also the number of existing records in the region and then extracts them. It works based on the web-page structure (DOM tree [7]). The system architecture is illustrated in Fig. 2. As shown in the figure, the web-pages are given to the system as input, and at the end for each existing record, one text file is generated. For simplicity of record separation, one text file is generated for each record. This system would be applicable for a large number of domains. All system components are fixed, with the exception of ontology which varies for each specific domain.

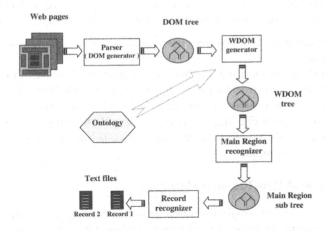

Fig. 2. Architecture of Our Developed System (OntDRR)

3.1 Ontology

An ontology includes general terms and concepts (senses) used for describing and representing an area of knowledge [9]. Here the ontology is employed to enhance the

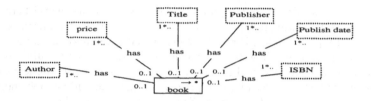

Fig. 3. Conceptual Model of Book Ontology

precision and recall. Furthermore, for each domain, its specific ontology is considered. For example, if the system concerns web pages related to books, the book ontology is used. Fig. 3 illustrates a part of conceptual model of book ontology.

3.2 Generating DOM Tree

Using a parser, first the DOM tree of a web page is built so that in the following steps the related algorithms could be implemented. In building DOM tree, tags such as SCRIPTS, COMMENT, etc. which bear no useful text information, are ignored to raise algorithm precision. With respect to the nested structure of web-pages, a tree could be created for each HTML page. A sample of such tree corresponding to a web-page, previously represented in Fig. 1, is shown in Fig. 4(a).

3.3 Generating WDOM Tree

Definition 1. Weight of leaf nodes in DOM tree: The weight of one leaf node is equal to the number of keywords (attributes) related to domain that are in the node.

Weight of non-leaf nodes in DOM tree: The weight of one non-leaf node is the sum of weight of children.

Relying on the definition 1 the weight of different nodes of the DOM tree is calculated, and then the Weighted Document Object Model (WDOM) is created. For example, considering the number of underlined keywords on the web-page, shown in Fig. 1, and DOM tree on Fig. 4(a), the corresponding WDOM tree can be illustrated in Fig. 4(b). The figures written on nodes imply the nodes' weights that are calculated based on discussed definitions.

3.4 Recognition of Main Region of Web-Page

Main region is a contiguous region in web page that contains the information to be extracted. The following observations will help us recognize the main region.

Observation 1. In the main region of web-page, the domain specific attributes are observed, and compared with other regions, their frequency tends to be higher.

Observation 2. In the main region of semi-structured web pages, there are at least two records with identical structure and content.

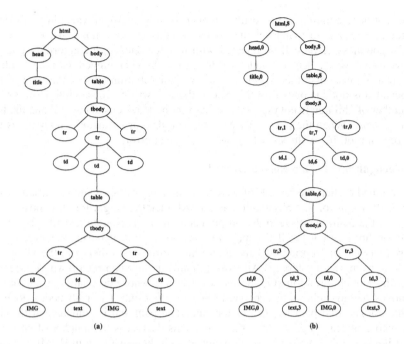

Fig. 4. a) DOM Tree corresponding to web page on Fig. 1 **b)** WDOM Tree corresponding to DOM Tree on Fig. 4(a)

Observation 1 helps us recognize the sub-tree of main region of web-page on WDOM. Doing so, using statistical methods are encouraged. As of Observation 2, in the sub-tree of main region, it is estimated to have at least two sub-branches with nearly the same weight. In other words, the weight of children in the main region root can be identically distributed. The best statistical criteria to recognize the root of main region of a web page is goodness-of-fit χ^2 test.

As shown in formula (1), Pearson χ^2 statistic is used in χ^2 goodness-of-fit test[1]. In this formula, e_i is the expected frequency of i-th , o_i is the observed frequency of i-th , and V_k is Pearson χ^2 statistic.

$$V_k = \sum_{i=1}^{k} \frac{(o_i - e_i)^2}{e_i} \tag{1}$$

In other methods for the main region recognition, introduced in Section 2, only web-page structure is under focus. In works such as[2], [5] and [6] only web-page structure, i.e. tag tree or DOM tree is considered, and the web-page content is ignored. In our developed method, in addition to the web-page structure, its content is also considered. In other words, the main region is recognized conceptually. The procedure starts from the tree root, and χ^2 test is performed level by level until the sub-tree root of the main region is found. First the tree root is considered as the current node. If the number of children of this node is more than one, χ^2 test will be performed on the current node children. If the result is higher than the expected value in χ^2 distribution table, it means in that level the nodes' weights (w_i) are not expected and the model's goodness of fit will be rejected with α value. Hence, the algorithm goes to the lower level with a heaviest node, and the procedure is continued until the result of the χ^2 test is lower than the expected value in χ^2 distribution table. Otherwise, if the number of this node is one, a level lower in the tree will be considered. However, if the number of children is not one, then the current node is considered null and the tree traverse stops. When the tree traverse is stopped, the current node is returned as the main region root. In goodness-of-fit χ^2 test, α is type I error.

3.5 Recognition of Main Region Records

As mentioned earlier, the records of web-page main region have similar structure and content. By means of this observation and a path matching algorithm it is possible to recognize the main region records and put each one in a separate text file. To do so, this algorithm is used: (1) If the main region root is null, it means the structure of web-page is not appropriate and the algorithm terminates, otherwise, the algorithm carries on from second step, (2) All existing paths in the main region whose origin is one of the root children found in the former step, and whose destination is one of text leaf nodes having value, are generated from left to right. The path nodes do have weight; (3) The first path is taken as the candidate path and is compared with other paths whose origin node weight is the same. This decreases the number of comparisons. Likewise, other paths which are matched with the same path in HTML tags and nodes' weight are searched; (4) If another path is not found, the path is ignored. The reason lies in the fact that at the first and end of main region, usually there are paths that do not belong to any record and if a path belongs to a record, it should be repeated equal to the number of records (at least twice) in the main region. As such, the next path will be taken and algorithm shall be repeated. If there is one or more than one matching for one path, then the count of candidate records equals the count of matching plus one. Therefore, the texts between the candidate path and the first matched path would be regarded as the first record, the texts between the first and second matching would be considered as the second record, etc.

4 Evaluation and Results

Here the developed system is evaluated and compared with MDR [6] system. Table 1 illustrates the results. In this experiment, web-pages are selected from 15 web sites on various domains, e.g. digital camera, books, laptops, etc. By processing web pages and extracting items, we generate the ontology manually.

We use the standard measures of precision and recall to evaluate the results from different systems. To calculate the recall, formula 2 is used, and formula 3 is used to calculate precision.

$$recall = \frac{TP}{TP + FN} \tag{2}$$

$$precision = \frac{TP}{TP + FP} \tag{3}$$

Table 1. Comparison between OntDRR and MDR

Site (.com)	Records Count	OntDRR Found	OntDRR Corr.	OntDRR Remarks	MDR Found	MDR Corr.	MDR Remarks	RECALL % OntDRR	RECALL % MDR	PRECISION % OntDRR	PRECISION % MDR
Shopping.yahoo	15	15	15		15	15		100	100	100	100
authorhouse	10	10	10		10	10		100	100	100	100
cokesbury	20	20	20		26	20	in 4 reg	100	100	100	76.9
bookpool	10	2	0	all_in_1*	17	10	in 2 reg	0	100	0	58.8
bookshopofindia	10	10	10		24	10	in 5 reg	100	100	100	41.7
abebooks	4	4	4		4	4	in 2 reg	100	100	100	100
artbook	10	3	3	*	9	9	in 3 reg	30	90	100	100
amazon	14	14	14		14	0	in 2 reg	100	0	100	0
nikon	11	11	11		0	0		100	0	100	0
jstore	7	3	3		0	0		42.9	0	100	0
akçart	12	12	12		0	0		100	0	100	0
Jvc	4	4	4		12	3	in 4 reg	100	75	100	25
sangestersbook	7	11	1	split*	6	6	in 3 reg	14.3	85.7	9.1	100
byubookstore	5	5	5		5	5		100	100	100	100
skyxlaptopstore	2	6	0	split*	2	2		0	100	0	100
TOTAL	141	130	112		144	94		72.5	70	80.6	60.2

In the above formula, TP is the number of records that exist in the main region and are recognized correctly, and FN is the number of records that exist in the main region and are not recognized, and FP is the number of records that do not exist in the main region but are recognized as records.

Before further discussing the experimental results, we first explain the problem descriptions used in the table 1:

All_ in_1: It means that all data records are identified as *1* data record.

split : This means that correct data records are split into smaller ones, i.e., a data record is not found as one but a few.

*: The main region is recognized correctly but data records are not recognized correctly.

in n reg: The data records are recognized as n data region.

As shown in Table 1, recall/precision of our developed system is higher than that of MDR system. The reason is obvious. MDR recognizes the data records only based on the web-page structure, while in our suggested algorithm the content of web-pages is considered too.

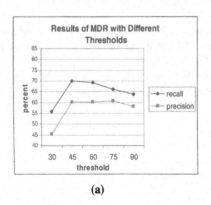

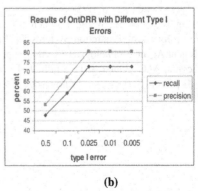

(a)   (b)

Fig. 5. a) Results of MDR with Different Thresholds **b)** Results of OntDRR with Different Type I Errors

The results of MDR system with different thresholds are shown in Fig. 5(a). As shown in the Figure, the best result is related to the threshold of 45%. The results of OntDRR system with different type I errors are also shown in Fig. 5(b). As it shows the best precision and recall are connected with 0.025.

5 Conclusion and Future Work

The web IE systems are currently expanding to let users access the needed information in a quick and accurate way. In most of these systems, first the web page main region is found and then the information is extracted. The more exact this region is identified, the higher is the final precision of the system. To enhance the system precision, an ontology is employed to follow the process conceptually. The goodness-of-fit χ^2 test is also used in recognizing the main region of the web page, and then data records of the main region are recognized by means of a matching algorithm. This algorithm can be used as a component of a conceptual-based IE system.

References

1. Casella, G., Berger, R.L.: Statistical Inference, 2nd edn. Duxbury Press (2001)
2. Papadakis, N.K., Skoutas, D., Raftopoulos, K.: STAVIES: A System for Information Extraction from Unknown Web Data Source through Automatic Web Wrapper Generation Using Clustering Techniques. IEEE Transaction on Knowledge and Data Engineering 17(12), 1638–1652 (2005)
3. Ye, S., Chua, T.S.: Learning Object Models from Semistructured Web Documents. IEEE Transaction on Knowledge and Data Engineering 18(3), 334–349 (2006)
4. Chang, C.H., Gigis, M.R.: A Survey of Web Information Extraction Systems. IEEE Transaction on Knowledge and Data Engineering 18(10), 1411–1428 (2006)
5. Liu, B., Zhai, Y.: NET—A System for Extracting Web Data from Flat and Nested Data Records. In: Proc. Sixth Int'l Conf. Web Information Systems Eng, pp. 487–495 (2005)
6. Liu, B., Grossman, R., Zhai, Y.: Mining Data Records in Web Pages. In: Proc. Int'l Conf. Knowledge Discovery in Databases and Data Mining (KDD), pp. 601–606 (2003)
7. http://www.w3.org/DOM/
8. Zhang, N., Chen, H., Wang, Y., Chen, S.J., Xiong, M.F.: Odaies: Ontology-driven Adaptive Web Information Extarction Systems. In: Proc. IEEE/WIC International Conference on Intelligent Agent Technology (IAT 2003), pp. 454–460 (2003)
9. Daconta, M.C., Obrst, L.J., Smith, K.T.: The Semantic Web: A Guide to the Future of XML, Web Service, and Knowledge Management. Wiley publishing, Inc., Chichester (2003)

Organizing Structured Deep Web by Clustering Query Interfaces Link Graph

Pengpeng Zhao, Li Huang, Wei Fang, and Zhiming Cui

Jiangsu Key Laboratory of Computer Information Processing Technology,
Soochow University, Suzhou 215006, China
szzmcui@suda.edu.cn

Abstract. There are a lot of pages on internet that are generated dynamically by the back-end database and the traditional searching engines can't reach these pages, which are called Deep Web. These sources are structured and provide structured query interfaces and results. Organizing structured Deep Web sources by their domain can let users browse these valuable resources and is one of the critical steps toward the large-scale Deep Web information integration. We propose a new strategy that automatically and accurately classifies Deep Web sources based on the form link graph, which can be easily constructed from web forms, and apply Fuzzy partition technique which is proved to be better suited for the features of Deep Web. Experiments using real Deep Web data show that our approach provides an effective and scalable solution for organizing Deep Web sources.

Keywords: Deep Web, Form Link Graph, Fuzzy Partition.

1 Introduction

Exploring the huge amount of online databases is a hotspot which researchers pay more attention to, the research on Deep Web is rather prevalent. The initial concept of Deep Web is proposed by Dr. Jill Ellsworth in 1994, it is the web page whose content can't be discovered by general search engine [1]. Deep Web contains a great deal of available information, whose value is far more than that of static web in the Surface Web. The structured query interfaces are usually served as the only entry points of Deep Web. However, searching for the right Web database in the Deep Web can be very challenging, because huge irrelevant information may impact information retrieving effect seriously. Since Deep Web is large scale, dynamic and heterogeneous, manual search manner can't satisfy the requirement of user's needs at all. Hence, only realizing efficient classification management on Deep Web, can it make us retrieve information more conveniently.

Heterogeneity and autonomy of Deep Web source have brought several challenges in large-scale data integration. Firstly, it needs a scalable solution which could process and organize the query interfaces automatically for users' query demands. Second, query interfaces' schemas are not uniform and content is hidden to users and hard to retrieve, so we need a strategy to extract relevant

C. Tang et al. (Eds.): ADMA 2008, LNAI 5139, pp. 683–690, 2008.

domain schema information automatically. In addition, heterogeneity of Deep Web makes many attributes crossing several domains, so there may be some uncertainty in schema matching.

To identify relevant forms as belonging to a domain, there are two general methods of Form classification on query interface: Pre-query and Post-query. Post-query is based on keywords, which uses probe queries and the retrieval results to identify content belonging to a domain to accomplish classification. Keyword-based query interfaces are easy to fill out automatically, but they have little information relevant to domain. And it is hard to apply to structured multi-attribute interfaces, because it can't fill out structured query form automatically. On the other hand, Pre-query relies on visible features of forms, and classifying or clustering is based on attribute features of forms. Deep Web interfaces have some indicative features and well-defined structures. There are some differences in structures and attributes among interface forms, but many similar aspects are still existed among the query interfaces of the same or similar domains. It brings us an effective method that making use of attribute features of forms to classify heterogeneous source.

In this paper we describe a new framework-Form Graph Clustering (FGC) for organizing Deep Web sources by using Pre-query method and Fuzzy Clustering Method (FCM). As far as we know, our work is the first to take such data model to Deep Web research, and our approach is scalable and accurate. Form Section 2 to Section 4, we discuss the frame realization. An extensive experiment, using real Web data, is discussed in Section 5. The results prove that our approach is beneficial to large-scale Deep Web integration.

2   Form Link Graph Definition

Since the heterogeneity and autonomy of Deep Web, the whole Deep Web could be formally expressed to be a graph model with heterogeneous multiple relationships. The node in the graph denotes query interface form, the line denotes the relation between relevant query interfaces, and relative weight is used to denote the similarity between them. The form link graph model could be expressed abstractly to be an undirected graph $G = (V, E)$, which is composed of nodes denoted by V and lines denoted by E, the line is an undirected.

We depict the form set as a weighted undirected graph. The weight of line in the graph could be measured by matching degree between schemas of two attribute sets. Traditional schema matching technique is based on binary value logic and exact data tools, which can't describe some uncertain situations. In fact, the Web is an uncertainty circumstance, but traditional data integration system didn't consider uncertain factors. With the Fuzzy set theory proposed by Zedeh [2], it supplies theory foundation for uncertain matching, people could use probability to depict uncertain events and make uncertain calculations. Given two query interface forms' attribute sets, which are denoted as $F_s = \{(l_1, v_1), \ldots, (l_n, v_n)\}$, and $F_t = \{(l_1', v_1'), \ldots, (l_m', v_m')\}$. Create the matching relation between Fs and Ft based on probability in the form of triple (F_s, F_t, ω), ω denotes the probability (i.e. match degree) between F_s and F_t, which is a relative weight between two form nodes. It has improved the traditional method that only using 0 or 1 to denote the relation between two schemas.

According to above description, we may analyze of Deep Web source clustering in real uncertain circumstance objectively. Thus, the Deep Web query interface form link graph could be expressed as $G = (V, E, W)$, $V = \{F_1, \ldots, F_n\}$, $W = \{\omega_1, \ldots, \omega_m\}$, F_i denotes query interface form, and $omega_j$ denotes relative weight between two forms.

3   Form Link Graph Construction

Because of the heterogeneity and autonomy of Deep Web, vast Web source refer to multiple domains. In a special domain, similar forms are on the same topic. It could be depicted to a construction process of a Web graph model abstractly, and then we could mine the relevant features on the Web, discover and exploit multiple domain topics hidden in the Deep Web.

3.1   Form Features Extraction

Query interface forms are served as the effective way for our research on Deep Web classification. Large differences and heterogeneity exist among interface form schemas with respect to different domains. However, form schemas in similar domains are rather singular, there are some similarity among relevant forms, so they provide us abundant structured features and content information.

The interface forms which returned by Form-Focused crawler may contain some irrelevant interfaces in other domains. They bring much inconvenience to information retrieval. For example, in Fig.1, the two forms were retrieved by the Form-Focused Crawler to find rental car search forms, but neither belongs to the target rental car database domain-one is a hotel search form and the other is a airfare search form.

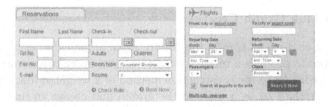

Fig. 1. Searchable forms obtained among car rental related Web pages

To locate and retrieve multiple domain sources effectively, we cluster the structured query interfaces. It contains multiple attributes, including some meta-data and special data with respect to some domain. Generally, a query interface is a web form in HTML. Form controllers could be classified into three kinds:

INPUT controller, SELECT controller and TEXTAREA controller. Query interface could be formally defined as $F = \{a_1, \ldots, a_n\}$, a_i denotes the controller attribute on forms. Each controller has corresponding describing Label, and each controller has one or more than one value. Usually, a controller and its relevant label constitute an attribute. The Label could be treated as an attribute name, and the form controller could be treated as attribute value. So a query interface could be formally described as $F = \{(L_1, V_1), \ldots, (L_n, V_n)\}$, L_i denotes label value, and $V_i = \{E_j, \ldots, E_k\}$ denotes one or more than one controller corresponding to a label.

Query interface extraction only focuses on relevant semantic information, including label extraction and form controller extraction. Form controller extraction contains controller name and controller value, including INPUT, SELECT and TEXTAREA in $< Form >$. Other appearance attributes are eliminated.

Query interface feature set is a multiple dimension space. We construct large amount of features to be feature spaces on Labels and Values. Firstly, extracted labels and values are constituted respectively to be Label Space (LS) and Value Space (VS); Second, constitute a corresponding feature vector for each form feature set in LS and VS; Finally, constitute three similarity matrics: LableMatrix, ValueMatrix and LableValueMatrix by comparing similarity among vectors. During the process of label comparison, use the same feature terms' quantity to evaluate, and make standardization.

$$\text{Sim}_L(F_1, F_2) = \frac{sw}{len} \tag{1}$$

where sw denotes the quantity of same Labels between F_1 and F_2, len denotes the length of F_1's vector, the division of the two could standardize the similarity.

Value and Label&Value's similarity comparison could use vector similarity function. $Sim_{LV}(F_1, F_2)$ is similar to $Sim_V(F_1, F_2)$.

$$\text{Sim}_V(F_1, F_2) = \frac{\sum_{k=1}^{n} W_{1k} \times W_{2k}}{\sqrt{(\sum_{k=1}^{n} W_{1k}^2) \cdot (\sum_{k=1}^{n} W_{2k}^2)}} \tag{2}$$

3.2   Form Link Graph Creation

Merge the above three matrics in the feature space organically, weighted sum up the similarities to produce a relative weight between every two associated query interfaces. According to the construction method of a weighted link graph, make each query interface to be a node in the graph, and create an undirected line between every two similar query interface nodes, so the similarity between the nodes could be treated as a weight of the line.

$$\omega = \omega_1 * \text{Sim}_L(F_1, F_2) + \omega_2 * \text{Sim}_V(F_1, F_2) + \omega_3 * \text{Sim}_{LV}(F_1, F_2) \tag{3}$$

where ω_i denotes the weight distributed to every similarity, and one of them may not equal to each other, $\omega_i \in [0, 1]$. We will discuss how to choose proper ω_i in the experiment.

To make sure the superiority of our approach's capability, we set a threshold for creation of line. If the weight is more than or equal to the threshold, then line could be created. The form set could be denoted as a triple (F_s, F_t, ω), F_s and F_t denote two relative forms, ω denotes the weight between two relative forms. At last, depict the query interface link graph formally in the form of adjacency list.

4   Form Link Graph Clustering

On the basic of proper feature space, constitution of feature matrics provides a data source for the form link graph partition. Strict feature choice and filtration make form partition more precise, and Graph Mining technique is introduced to provide a new approach for domain topic discovery, which improve the traditional method.

Traditional partition method distributes every object into a certain class strictly whose membership is either 0 or 1. This strict partition doesn't reflect uncertain membership between object and class exactly. Ruspini has firstly proposed analytic Fuzzy clustering algorithm [3], and Bezdek has introduced weight exponent in the membership function in the extended Fuzzy clustering algorithm, and introduce information entropy into target function of C-means algorithm [4]. This Fuzzy theory also could be applied to form link graph clustering.

FCM algorithm distributes n vectors x_i into c fuzzy clusters, and calculates each cluster center to minimize target function. FCM target function could be defined as:

$$J_m(u,v) = \sum_{k=1}^{n} \sum_{i=1}^{c} (u_{ik})^m d(x_k, v_i) \tag{4}$$

where $\sum_{i=1}^{c} u_{ik} = 1, u_{ik} \in (0,1), \forall k, d(x_k, v_i) = ||x_k - v_i||^2, m$ denotes fuzzy weight exponent, $1 < m < +\infty$. In order to minimize the target function, clustering center and membership could be expressed as following:

$$v_i = \frac{\sum_{k=1}^{n} u_{ik}^m x_k}{\sum_{k=1}^{n} u_{ik}^m} \qquad (i = 1, 2, \ldots, c) \tag{5}$$

$$u_{ik} = \frac{1}{\sum_{j=1}^{c} (\frac{d_{ik}}{d_{jk}})^{1/(m-1)}} \qquad (i = 1, 2, \ldots, c; k = 1, 2, \ldots, n) \tag{6}$$

FCM has a virtue of simple calculation and high speed, and has an intuitionistic geometry value. In addition, entropy $\sum_{k=1}^{n} \sum_{i=1}^{c} u_{ik} log(u_{ik})$ is introduced into target function, create a Fuzzy Clustering algorithm on the basic of maximum entropy, and introduce a Lagrange multiplier λ [5]. Target function is depicted formally:

$$J = \sum_{k=1}^{n} \sum_{i=1}^{c} u_{ik}^m d_{ik} + \lambda^{-1} \sum_{k=1}^{n} \sum_{i=1}^{c} u_{ik} log(u_{ik}) \tag{7}$$

We extract feature vector set from query interfaces, and use the above FCM algorithm cluster the vector set by domain. According to the principle that forms in similar domain have similar Labels and content, and the quantity of Label in the same domain tends to stabilization along with the increment of form quantity. There are also many differences of Labels and content among different domains. Input the form link graph in the form of adjacency list, and standardize the weight of lines. Finally, some cluster of forms can be got by using FCM. We identify the robust capability of FCM in the Deep Web source clustering based on a query interface form link graph, and get a better cluster effect.

5   Experiment Evaluation

In this section, we discuss and verify the validity of the new FGC approach through strict experiment. We verify the rationality of form link graph model, then identify the practicability of FCM algorithm in the form link graph clustering.

5.1   Experiment Setup

Database Domains. In order to evaluate the validity of our solution of clustering Deep Web source based on a query interfaces link graph, we selected 524 Deep Web query interface forms from the UIUC Web Integration Repository, referring to eight domains (see in Table1). These forms are based on multiple attributes, apparently, the more similar terms between forms, the more similar they are.

Table 1. Deep Web query interface forms set

Domain	Airfare	Automobile	Book	CarRental	Hotel	Job	Movie	Music
#ofForms	47	105	69	25	46	53	118	79

After obtaining a plentiful dataset, we extract form features by rules. Then execute schema matching calculation based on probability for the similarity between forms' attributes. At last, get a large experimental dataset.

Performance Metrics. We introduce Entropy and F-measure to evaluate the capability of our experiment. Apparently, the less Entropy value is, the smaller out-of-order probability the dataset has. That is to say, the more regular and sequential the dataset attributes are, the better clustering effect is. The F-measure provides a combined measure of Recall and Precision. Generally speaking, the higher value of F-measure, the better effect of clustering.

5.2   Effectiveness of FGC

Our FGC method's validity depends on the construction of data model and how the clustering method realizes partition on the data model. In order to identify FGC validity, we make a strict experiment by using FCM method, based on the above rules, evaluate experiment results, and compared with K-means and DBSCAN, according to measure of Entropy and F-measure.

Table 2. Evaluation of Deep Web source clustering results

Algorithm	FCM		K-means		DBSCAN	
Domain	Entropy	F-measure	Entropy	F-measure	Entropy	F-measure
Airfare	0.21	0.91	0.23	0.88	0.21	0.90
Automobile	0.25	0.87	0.30	0.84	0.24	0.88
Book	0.19	0.89	0.21	0.87	0.18	0.88
CarRental	0.16	0.92	0.34	0.83	0.37	0.81
Hotel	0.15	0.93	0.19	0.92	0.23	0.85
Job	0.20	0.90	0.24	0.89	0.31	0.87
Movie	0.54	0.77	0.58	0.74	0.61	0.76
Music	0.56	0.79	0.63	0.72	0.64	0.70

Experiment results show that, using FCM algorithm to cluster Deep Web source by query interface features could get a better effect. F-measure of our solution is high, varying form 0.77 to 0.93, which is a little better than K-means and DBSCAN. And we also find that F-measures are varying in a small range among different domains (see Table 2). This is because every domain has different structured characteristics, the number of special features with respect to domain is more or less, some of which is homogeneous, but some are very heterogeneous. In a word, our solution provide an effective and general mechanism to automatically clustering online databases, and produce an considerable practical value for real research and practice.

6   Related Work

Reasonable organization of Deep Web source contributes an immeasurable benefit to Deep Web information retrieval and large-scale data integration. More and more researchers pay attentions to Deep Web source organization. Many classifying and clustering methods have been applied to Deep Web research. Plentiful multiple features in the query interface help researchers organize huge amount of hidden information behind query interface easily. B.He proposed a hierarchy classification approach of Deep Web sources in terms of query interface schema information. A kind of effective classification approach towards widely used e-commerce Web databases by clustering manner are proposed by Q.Peng [6]. H.He proposed WISE integration approach to realize query interfaces integrate automatically [7]. And many schema mapping and matching approaches are produced. X.Dong proposed a schema matching approach based on probability to solve uncertainty problem in schema mapping [8].

7 Conclusion

This paper proposes a new frame for Deep Web source organization automatically. Through analyze the form features of Deep Web query interface, extract relevant semantic features, and consider the uncertain factors in schema matching to construct a form link graph. Finally, apply FCM algorithm to cluster the form link graph. Experiment indicates that, this strategy receives a good effect.

In short, the FGC method supplies an efficient way for Deep Web source organization researches, and make the information retrieval approach more effective and convenient. The researches on Deep Web are continuing and further. Combing ontologies will help us further improve the clustering capability on Deep Web source, which need us pay more attention to.

Acknowledgments. This work is partially supported by NSFC(No.60673092); the Key Project of Chinese Ministry of Education(No.205059); The "Six Talent Peak" Project of Jiangsu Province, China(No.06-E-037); Specialized Fund Project for the Software and IC of Jiangsu Province, China(No.[2006]221-41) and the Higher Education Graduate Research Innovation Program of Jiangsu Province, China(No.cx07b-122z).

References

1. Bergman, M.K.: The deep web: surfacing hidden value. Journal of electronic publishing 7(1), 8912–8914 (2002)
2. Zadeh, L.A.: Fuzzy sets. Information and Control 8(3), 338–353 (1965)
3. Bezdek, J.C.: Cluster validity with fuzzy sets. Cybernet 3(3), 58–73 (1974)
4. He, B., Tao, T., Chang, K.C.: Clustering structured Web sources: a schema-based, model-differentiation Approach. EDBT, 536–546 (2004)
5. Li, R.P., Mukaidon, M.: A maximum entropy approach to fuzzy clustering. In: Proc. Of the 4th IEEE Int'l Conf. on Fuzzy System, pp. 2227–2232. IEEE, Yokohama (1995)
6. Peng, Q., Meng, W., He, H., Yu, C.T.: WISE-cluster: clustering e-commerce search engines automatically. In: Proceedings of the 6th ACM International Workshop on Web Information and Data Management, Washington, pp. 104–111 (2004)
7. He, H., Meng, W., Yu, C.T., Wu, Z.: Automatic integration of Web search interfaces with WISE-Integrator. VLDB Journal 13(3), 256–273 (2004)
8. Dong, X., Halevy, A., Yu, C.: Data Integration with Uncertainties. In: VLDB (2007)
9. Ru, Y., Horowitz, E.: Indexing the invisible Web: a survey. Online Information Review 29(3), 249–265 (2005)
10. Barbosa, L., Freire, J., Silva, A.: Organizing Hidden-Web Databases by Clustering Visible Web Documents. In: ICDE (2007)
11. Barbosa, L., Freire, J.: Combining Classifiers to Identify Online Databases. In: WWW (2007)

CBP: A New Efficient Method for Mining Multilevel and Generalized Frequent Itemsets

Yu Xing Mao and Bai Le Shi

Department of Computer and Information Technology, Fudan University,
Shanghai 200433, China
{myuxing,bshi}@fudan.edu.cn

Abstract. The taxonomy(is-a hierarchy) data exists widely in retail, geography, biology and financial area, so mining the multilevel and generalized association rules is one of the most important research task in data mining. Unlike the traditional algorithm, which is based on Apriori method, we propose a new CBP (correlation based partition) based method, to mine the multilevel and generalized frequent itemsets. This method uses the item's correlation as measurement to partition the transaction database from top to bottom. It can shorten the time of mining multilevel and generalized frequent itemsets by reducing the scanning scope of the transaction database. The experiments on the real-life financial transaction database show that the CBP based algorithms outperform the well-known Apriori based algorithms.

Keywords: Generalized frequent itemsets, Generalized association rules, Correlation, Cluster.

1 Introduction

Association rule mining [1] is one of important tasks in data mining. Over the last decade, many efficient algorithms [2],[3] have been proposed. Unlike the single level data, the taxonomy data reference to the items such as the "wheat bread" belongs to "bread", and "bread" belongs to "food". The research of mining multilevel and generalized association rules usually has two directions. One direction is to generate the association rules called generalized association rules (GAR) from all the items including the generalized items. It was first introduced by R. Srikant and R. Agrawal [4]. Another direction is to generate the association rules only on the same level of taxonomy data from top to bottom. It was first introduced by Jiawei Han and Yongjian Fu [5]. Recently, cluster based method applied in some algorithms [6] for mining generalized frequent itemsets and achieved good performance. But the major limitation of these algorithms is that they divide the transaction database into static cluster table by the different length of items in transactions and it still spends a lot of time on scanning the whole transaction database for many times.

In this paper, we present a new efficient and flexible CBP method. It partitions the transaction database into several smaller transaction databases level by level using the

C. Tang et al. (Eds.): ADMA 2008, LNAI 5139, pp. 691–698, 2008.

correlation of items and makes the algorithms more efficient by reducing the time of scanning the transaction database. The paper is organized as follows. Section 2 is problem statements. In section 3, the CBP theory and method is proposed. In section 4, we give the implement of CBP_GAR and CBP_MAR. In Section 5, we compared our algorithms with the well-known algorithms. The study is concluded in the last section, along with some future work.

2 Problem Statement

Besides the taxonomy data in retail data, the financial transaction data we studied also has the taxonomy structure in Figure 1. The transaction code, which has 4 bits, has the naming convention. The 0*** represents the first digit of transaction code, which means the personal transaction. The 01** represents the first two digits of transaction code, which means the personal transactions of credit card. The 015** represents the first three digits of the transaction code, which means the personal transaction of credit card query. The leaf node 0154 represents the complete transaction code, which means the personal transaction of query the balance of a credit card.

Suppose transaction database $D=\{t_1,t_2,...,t_n\}$, t_i is any single transaction, and itemsets $I=\{ I_1,I_2,...,I_m \}$, I_a is a subset of I. Figure2 is an transaction database according to Figure1.

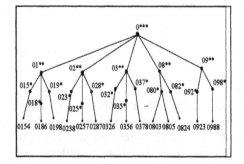

	Business Trancaction DB		
Tran ID	Trancaction Code	Tran ID	Trancaction Code
T1	{0153, 0283, 0303, 0512, 0883}	T6	{0153, 0287, 0357, 0901}
T2	{0123, 0257, 0301, 0503, 0622}	T7	{0146, 0311, 0583}
T3	{0198, 0287, 0526, 0805, 0901}	T8	{0197, 0287, 0326, 0612, 0901}
T4	{0186, 0238, 0508, 0923}	T9	{0132, 0238, 0303, 0401, 0923}
T5	{0186, 0238, 0303, 0501, 0923}	T10	{0154, 0238, 0303, 0501, 0723}

Fig. 1. A multilevel financial transaction tree   **Fig. 2.** A financial transaction database

Definition 1 Multilevel Taxonomy Tree (T). We use the DAG=(V, E) to depict. V is the set of all item nodes, E is the set of all edges, and V_0 represents the root node, each node represents an item. For any simple path $P=(v_0,v_1,...,v_n)$, then:

(1) v_{n-1} is the *parent* item of v_n, noted *parent(v_n)*. In contrast, v_n is the *child* item of v_{n-1}, noted *child(v_{n-1})*.

(2) v_0, ...,v_{n-1} are the *ancestor* items of v_n, noted *ancestor(v_n)*. In contrast, v_1,...,v_n are the *descendant* items of v_0 , noted *descendant(v_0)*.

(3) The item without child item is called *leaf* item, the node except root and leaf items are called *interim* or *generalized* items.

(4) The *subtree* x noted as: G ' =(V ' ,E '), V ' is the set of x and their descendants, E ' is the set of edges between x and all the items of its descendants.

Definition 2. The *support* (A) equals to $|D_A|/|D|$, where $|D_A|$ is the number of transactions containing pattern A in D. The *confidence* (A=>B) equals to P(B|A), which means the probability that pattern B occurs when pattern A occurs in D.

Definition 3. Pattern A is *frequent* in D if $|D_A|/|D|$ is greater than σ, where σ is the *minimum support threshold*. A rule A=>B is *strong* if P(B|A) is greater than φ, where φ is the *minimum confidence threshold*. In this paper, we use the uniform σ_{minsup} and φ_{mincon} for the whole taxonomy tree.

Definition 4 Association Rules in Taxonomy

(1) *Generalized association rules* (GAR): {A => B | A,B∈T, A∩B= Φ,

and($\neg\exists item_1 \in A$, $\neg\exists item_2 \in B$, ancestor($item_1$)=$item_2$ or ancestor ($item_2$)=$item_1$) ,

and ($\exists item_1 \in A$, $\exists item_2 \in B$, depth($item_1$)≠depth($item_2$)}

(2) *Multilevel association rules* (MAR):{A => B | A, B∈T, A∩B= Φ, B≠Φ, and

($\forall item_1 \in A$, $\forall item_2 \in B$, depth($item_1$)= depth($item_2$)}

3   Item Correlation Theory

3.1   The Definition of Items' Correlation

Definition 5 Leaf item-leaf item correlation. If leaf items A and B (A, B∈T) never occur together (or support(A, B)<σ_{minsup}) in any transaction, then we call A and B are *weakly related*.

Definition 6 Generalized itemsets(g-i)-generalized itemsets(g-j) correlation. if g-i and g-j never occur together (or supp(g-i, g-j)< σ_{minsup}) in transaction database D, then we call g-i and g-j are weakly related.

Definition 7 The value of correlation between 2 generalized-items

$$cor(g_i, g_j) = \frac{|D_{g_i} \cap D_{g_j}|}{|D_{g_i} \cup D_{g_j}|} = \frac{|D_{g_i} \cap D_{g_j}|}{|D_{g_i}| + |D_{g_j}| - |D_{g_i} \cap D_{g_j}|} \tag{1}$$

The value of correlation between 2-generalized items implies the degree of overlapping, and closely related with their support. It is easily we get that:

$$cor(g_i, g_j) = \begin{cases} = 0, non-related \\ < \sigma_{min\,sup}, weakly-related \\ \geq \sigma_{min\,sup}, related \end{cases} \qquad (2)$$

Definition 8. A set of correlated generalized itemsets are called a *item-cluster*.

Definition 9. The value of correlation between 2 item-clusters we use the idea of a hierarchical clustering algorithm for categorical attributes [7]:

$$COR(C_i, C_j) = \frac{links[C_i, C_j]}{(n_i + n_j)^{1+2f(\theta)} - n_i^{1+2f(\theta)} - n_j^{1+2f(\theta)}} \qquad (3)$$

The links$[C_i, C_j]$ means the sum of all the element correlation of cluster C_i and C_j,

$$links[C_i, C_j] = \sum_{p_q \in C_i, p_r \in C_j} cor(p_q, p_r) \qquad (4)$$

To deal with outlier, we set $f(\theta)=(1-\theta)/(1+\theta)$.

3.2 Property of Items' Correlation

Theorem 1. If generalized itemsets g-i and g-j are weakly related. Then any descendants of subtree rooted with g-i and g-j are weakly related.

Theorem 2. If the generalized itemsets g-i and g-j are weakly related. Then g-i and g-j cannot form frequent itemsets.

Corollary 1. If generalized itemsets g-i and g-j are weakly related. Then any descendant of subtree rooted with g-i and g-j cannot form frequent itemsets.

3.3 The Main Idea of CBP Method

Step 1 Locating. The partition work usually starts from the second level of the taxonomy transaction tree. (And it can start from any level).

Step 2 Preprunning. For each generalized item of second level, the 1-itemsets are generated firstly, and then we delete all the descendant of the items from the transaction database, which are not frequent.

Step 3 Clustering. For the frequent itemsets of second level, we use the formula (1) and (3) to calculate the correlation of items or clusters and use hierarchical clustering method to get several clusters of itemsets $C_1, C_2, C_3, ..., C_k$.

Step 4 Partitioning and pruning. According to the result of the clustering, we partition the transaction database D into several smaller transaction databases $D_1, D_2, D_3, ..., D_k$ and pruning each D_i with only items in C_i left.

Through repeating the step 1 to step 4 from the second level to the upper leaf level of the multilevel transaction tree, the original or the partitioned transaction databases are partitioned into some smaller transaction databases.

4 Algorithms Based on CBP Method

4.1 Algorithm CBP_MAR-Mining the Multilevel Frequent Itemsets

Input: D(1)- The original transaction database; MinSupport- Minimum support for all the levels; MinCluster- The supposed cluster number; θ-The adjusting parameter of cluster algorithm;

Output: LL(l)-The multilevel frequent itemsets of level l.

```
1) Push D(1) into Dstack; l=1; push l into FStack;
2) do {Pop up D from DStack; Pop up l from FStack;
3)       if (l=MaxLevel){Pop up L(l-1,1) from KStack;
4)         Get_frequent_1-itemset L(l,1);
5)           if (!L(l,1).isEmpty) {
6)             Apriori_gen L(l,k) until L(l,k-1) is empty}}
7)       else {if (l=1) {L(l-1,1) is null}
8)             else {Pop up L(l-1,1) from KStack}
9)        Get_frequent_1-itemset L(l,1);
10)       if (!L(l,1).isEmpty){
11)         Apriori_gen L(l,k) until L(l,k-1) is empty;
12)           if (!L(l,2).isEmpty){Compute COR(C_i,C_j); CBP(T,COR(C_i,C_j))}
13)           else {Prune D, push it into DStack; Push L(l,1) into KStack;
Push l+1 into FStack}}}}
14) while (!DStack.isEmpty());
15) LL(l)=∪_kL(l,k);
```

4.2 Algorithm CBP_GAR-Mining the Generalized Frequent Itemsets

Input: D(1)-The original transaction database; MinSupport-Minimum support for all the levels; MinCluster-The supposed cluster number; θ-The adjusting parameter of cluster algorithm; Ancestor Level-The level of ancestor that will be add to D(1); StartPartitionLevel-The level at which partitioning begins; EndPartitionLevel-The level at which partitioning stops.

Output: L-The generalized frequent itemsets.

```
1)  Push D(1) into Dstack; ℓ=1; push ℓ into FStack;
2)  do {Pop up D from Dstack; Pop up ℓ from FStack;
3)      if (ℓ=1) {L(ℓ-1,1) is null}
4)      else {Pop up L(ℓ-1,1) from KStack}
5)        Get_frequent_1-itemset(L(ℓ,1));
6)      if (ℓ< StartPartitionLevel){Prune D; push it into Dstack; Push
L(ℓ,1) into KStack; Push ℓ+1 into FStack}
7)          else {if(ℓ>=StartPartitionLevel&& ℓ<=EndPartitionLevel) {
8)          if (!L(ℓ,1).isEmpty) {Apriori_gen L(ℓ,2);
9)              if (!L(ℓ,2).isEmpty){Compute COR(Cᵢ,Cⱼ); CBP(D,COR(Cᵢ,Cⱼ))}
10)             else {Prune D, push it into Dstack; Push L(ℓ,1) into KStack;
Push ℓ+1 into FStack}}
11)             else {D=Add_ancestor(D,AncestorLevel);
12)               Apriori_gen L(k) until L(k-1) is empty}}}}
13) while (!Dstack.isEmpty());
14) L=∪ₖL(k);
```

4.3 Algorithm CBP-Partitioning the Transaction Database

Input: D- The transaction database; COR(Cᵢ,Cⱼ)- The correlation of item-cluster i and j.

Output: Dstack-the stack keeps transaction database; Kstack-the stack keeps frequent itemsets; Fstack-the stack keeps level flag.

```
1)  Init item-Cluster with only one item of L(ℓ,1);
2)  if (item-Cluster.size()>MinCluster) {
3)      Init links(Cᵢ,Cⱼ ) from COR(Cᵢ,Cⱼ);
4)      while (item-Cluster.size()>MinCluster) {
5)          if successfully get two nearest Clusters{
6)              Merge them into one item-Cluster;
7)                if (item-Cluster.size()>MinCluster){
8)                    Re_compute links(Cᵢ,Cⱼ)}}
```

9)   **else** break}}

10) **for** every item-Cluster {Prune and partition D by item-cluster; push
it into Dstack; Prune and partition L(ℓ,1) by item-cluster; push it into
KStack; Push ℓ+1 into FStack}

5 Performance Study

To evaluate the efficiency of our CBP algorithm, we implement it by using the JAVA.
The database is a real-life financial transaction database about 250k transactions, 200
items and the depth of taxonomy is 4.

Our experiments have two groups. In group one, we verify whether CBP_MAR is
more efficient than the ML_series. In group two, we test whether CBP_GAR is more
efficient than the Apriori_series. The result of Figure3 shows that CBP_MAR run
faster than the ML_series by 22% to 73% with only less than 7% loss ratio of frequent
itemsets. The result of Figure4 shows that CBP_MAR run faster than the ML_series by
71% to 75% with only less than 8% loss ratio. The result of Figure5 shows that

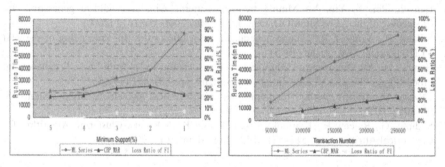

Fig. 3. Performance study by minimum support   **Fig. 4.** Performance study by database size

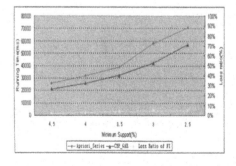
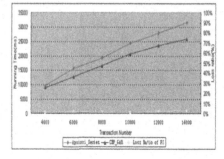

Fig. 5. Performance study by minimum support   **Fig. 6.** performance study by database size

CBP_GAR run faster than the Apriori_series by 18% to 28% with only lower than 5% frequent itemsets lost. The result of Figure6 shows that CBP_GAR run faster than Apriori_series by 14% to 18% with less than 3% frequent itemsets lost.

6   Conclusions and Future Work

The CBP method improves the efficiency of mining the frequent itemsets in taxonomy data by reducing the scanning scope of the transaction database. Of course, there still some improvements in our CBP method, such as the loss of frequent itemsets and it will be addressed in our future research.

References

1. Agrawal, R., Imielinski, T., Swami, Swami, A.: Mining association rules between sets of items in large databases. In: Proceeding of the ACM SIGMOD, pp. 207–216. Washington, D.C (1993)
2. Agrawal, R., Srikant, R.: Fast Algorithms for mining association rules. In: Proceeding of the 20th VLDB, Santiago, Chile (September 1994)
3. Han, J., Pei, J., Yin, Y.: Mining frequent patterns without candidate generation. In: Proceeding of the ACM SIGMOD, Dallas, TX, May 2000, pp. 1–12 (2000)
4. Srikant, R., Agrawal, R.: Mining generalized association rules. In: Proceeding of the 21st VLDB, Zurich, Switzerland (1995)
5. Han, J., Fu, Y.: Discovery of Multiple Level Association Rules from Large Databases. In: Proceeding of the 21st VLDB, Zurich, Switzerland, pp. 420–431 (1995)
6. CBAR: An efficient method for mining association rules. Knowledge-based systems 18, 99–105 (2005)
7. Sudipto, G., Rajeev, R., Kyuseok, S. (eds.): ROCK: A Robust Clustering Algorithm for Categorical Attributes, pp. 512–521. IEEE, Los Alamitos (1999)

Supporting Customer Retention through Real-Time Monitoring of Individual Web Usage

Peter I. Hofgesang and Jan Peter Patist

VU University Amsterdam, Department of Computer Science
De Boelelaan 1081A, 1081 HV Amsterdam, The Netherlands
{hpi,jpp}@few.vu.nl

Abstract. Customer retention is crucial for any company relying on a regular client base. One way to approach this problem is to analyse actual user behaviour and take proper actions based on the outcome. Identifying increased or decreased customer activity on time may help on keeping customers active or on retaining defecting customers. Activity statistics can also be used to target and activate passive customers. Web servers of online services track user interaction seamlessly. We use this data, and provide methods, to detect changes real-time in online individual activity and to give measures of conformity of current, changed activities to past behaviour. We confirm our approach by an extensive evaluation based both on synthetic and real-world activity data. Our real-world dataset includes 5,000 customers of an online investment bank collected over 3 years. Our methods can be used, but are not limited to, trigger actions for customer retention on any web usage data with sound user identification.

1   Introduction

Imagine a client of an online service (e.g. an online retail shop or an internet bank) decreasing his activity – measured, for example, by the number of daily visits to the site of the service – in a continuous or abrupt manner (Figure 1-c). This drop in activity may be a sign of customer defection, thus early detection, that may trigger proper marketing actions, is a requisite for retaining the client. Yet another scenario, on the contrary, is an increased activity (Figure 1-a) which may mark a rising interest in certain services. Detected change and proper actions in this case may uphold interest. To sum up, our first goal is to detect changes incrementally, as new data flow in, in individual user activity.

Let us assume that we are able to detect changes and estimate their change points with certain accuracies. Can we take actions solely on this kind of information? What if we take the decreasing activity of the previous example (Figure 1-c) and place it into context by including past activity? As we see in Figure 2 this particular user had highly fluctuating activity over time: up hills followed by downhill activities. Raising an alarm, in this case, on client defection would most likely be false. Both decreased and increased (thus changed) activities should be put in context in order to interpret them. Our second goal is to provide a manner to measure conformity of the current behaviour to the

C. Tang et al. (Eds.): ADMA 2008, LNAI 5139, pp. 699–708, 2008.

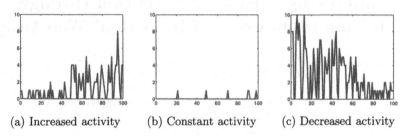

(a) Increased activity   (b) Constant activity   (c) Decreased activity

Fig. 1. Example of change in activity (horizontal axes represent days, while vertical axes show activity frequencies). Subfigure (a) shows a clear increase in activity, (c) depicts a dropping activity, while (b) represents a constant (infrequent) activity.

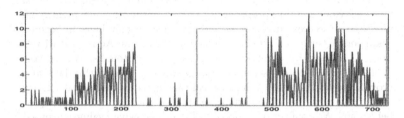

Fig. 2. Example of changing individual activity over time. Rectangles mark the samples for Figure 1-a,b, and c consecutively: interpretation of changes requires context.

past–in other words, to measure the likelihood of current activities based on the past. The combined information about the change point, direction of the change and the likelihood together can be used to decide on taking certain marketing actions. However, the discussion of alerts and concrete actions are out of the scope of this paper.

The contribution this work makes is the identification and description of an important problem, online change detection in individual user activity, and the methods that provide its solution. We justify our methods on activity data of 5,000 customers of an online investment bank collected over 3 years as well as on synthetically generated data.

The remainder of the paper is organised as follows. Section 2 provides related work. Section 3 describes the problems at hand and sets our main goals for this work. Section 4 presents our proposed online individual change detection method and provides details on our "change conformity" measure. We present our experimental setup in Section 5 and describe our empirical findings in Section 6. Finally, Section 7 concludes.

2   Related Work

Change detection. Early work on change detection stems from the domain of statistics with the development of sequential hypothesis testing [1] and the cumulative sum test [2]. For an overview of abrupt change detection algorithms from a statistical perspective, see [3]. This reference covers the above methods and methods such as Bayesian change detection, generalized likelihood ratio test, etc. A possible disadvantage of these methods is the assumption of a known underlying family of distribution. Another disadvantage is that not all methods are fully incremental, and computational problems can arise when the data rate is very high. Change detection is often used as a tool to adjust the current model to the changing distribution. [4] uses a variable size sliding window to cope with change. The window size is increased when new data comes in and decreased when the window can be split into two parts of which the means are significantly different. In [5], the error of a classifier system is monitored. It is assumed that the error is binomially distributed. Two levels are defined that trigger the learning of new concepts, and one which triggers rebuilding. Unfortunately, if true class labels are not provided for the system, it cannot be used at all. A change detection method based on wavelet footprints is proposed in [6]. When the data are transformed into footprints, non-zero coefficients at the times of the changes are created. This fact is used to find the time and magnitude of change using a lazy and an absolute method. In [7], martingales are used to detect change. Although martingales are built on univariate data, the framework can be used for change detection in higher dimensional data. Martingales can be calculated incrementally and require no reference distribution or window. The two-sample framework in [8] uses non-parametric two-sample tests on sliding windows to detect change. It is shown that these test statistics can be maintained efficiently. In [9] the sequential hypothesis testing method [1] is adopted and investigated for the scenario of a violation of the independence assumption. The method resulted in time and space efficient algorithms and is not dependent on window assumptions and has shorter delays than window-based solutions.

Web usage change detection and monitoring. Baron and Spiliopoulou [10] present PAM, a technique to monitor the changes of a rule base over time. Ganti et al. [11] describe a dynamic environment to exploit systematic evolution of blocks of data. They introduce the data span dimension that enables the user to select the most recently collected blocks (most recent window). Mazeroff et al. [12] model sequences of system calls by probabilistic suffix tree and probabilistic suffix automaton for real-time data monitoring, to detect malicious application behaviour.

Time Series Segmentation. The main difference between change detection and segmentation algorithms is that the later minimizes the error dependent only on the discovered segments, whereas change detection focuses on maximizing the detection rate, minimizing the false alarm rate and the detection latency. As a consequence segmentation algorithms are globally, while change detection algorithms are locally oriented. Ihler et al. [13] described a framework for finding and extracting anomalous events in human behaviour measurements, based on a time varying Poisson model. Their method is evaluated on traffic and building access data, over non-statistical thresholding methods. For an overview of traditional and online segmentation algorithms we refer to [14].

3   Problem Definition

The source of information for our experiments is the web usage data that are generated by web servers and aggregated in so-called web access log files. The raw log data need to be pre-processed and transformed into individual user sessions (see e.g. [15]). Since our methods need highly reliable individual identification (e.g. in case of login enforced web sites), in the rest of the paper we assume that this condition is satisfied. We transform the sessionised data into activity frequencies, for each individual, by counting the number of sessions in a given period of time (based on the time stamp of the first page of each session). We formulate the notation of activity data as follows:

Notation 1. *Let us denote our observed activity data set as $A = \{A_1, \ldots, A_N\}$ generated by N individuals, where A_i is the activity data of the ith user, $1 \leq i \leq N$. Each A_i consists of a sequence of frequency counters for a given period of time, $A_i = (a_i^{t_1}, \ldots, a_i^{t_j}, \ldots, a_i^{t_n})$, where $a_i^{t_j} \in \{\mathbb{N}, 0\}$ and t_j is the jth time period.*

Note, that (1) our dataset is incremental and so t_n refers to the last observed data point; (2) t_1 reflects a global starting point in our notation and individuals may have different starting points in their activities.

We gave motivation to our work briefly in Section 1. Here we decompose the task in hand to specific goals and provide their descriptions:

1. **Change detection in individual user activity.** The goal of this task is to identify (estimate) a set of C_i time points for each individual (i), in real time, such as the C_i points split the user activity data into more or less homogeneous segments.
2. **Aggregate past behaviour.** Here we maintain simple statistics, the mean activity and the length of each segment, for each individual over the past segments along with statistics over the current segment.
3. **Measure conformity.** We need a measure to compare aggregated past behaviour to the current behaviour to decide on whether the current behaviour is typical or a-typical to the actual user. Conformity should be expressed in percentages.
4. **Alerting.** The estimated change points together with information about the change conformity can be used to trigger automatic actions. However the discussion of alerting is not part of our current work.

We provide efficient solutions to these problems in Section 4. In practice, these solutions need to be both memory and computationally efficient, to support their application on a large number of customers and to facilitate real-time processing.

4   Change Detection

4.1   Modelling the Individual Activity Data

We model the users activity, a sequence of positive integers, by a piecewise constant distribution function. For that, we assume the data is a sequence of segments filled with independent, identically distributed (i.i.d.) data. The likelihood of an observed frequency (a^i) can be formulated as:

$$P^\lambda_{(r,s)}(a^i)|r \leq i \leq s,$$

where indices r, s define the segment and mark two change points. We assume that the frequencies between two change points are distributed according to a mixture of a Poisson distribution and an outlier distribution. The Poisson distribution is defined as $P^\lambda_{(k,l)}(a^i, \lambda) = \frac{\lambda^{a^i} \exp^{-\lambda}}{a^i!}$. Where λ is the Poisson parameter and is estimated by $\frac{(1+\sum_{i=1}^n a^i)}{(1+n)}$. The outlier distribution is equal to the uniform distribution.

4.2   Online Change Detection Algorithm

The online change detection algorithm successively applies the log likelihood ratio test. If the ratio exceeds a user defined threshold, an alarm is signalled and the actual change point is estimated. The online algorithm is then re-initialised from the point after the estimated change point in the data stream.

The log likelihood ratio is the log ratio of the likelihood of two hypotheses. The zero hypothesis (H_0) assume that no change has occurred, whereas the alternative hypothesis (H_1) assumes a change at time t. Assuming i.i.d. segments, the log likelihood ratio is defined by

$$LLR = \log \frac{\sup_t P_{H_{11}}(a^1, \ldots, a^t) P_{H_{12}}(a^{t+1}, \ldots, a^n)}{P_{H_0}(a^1, \ldots a^n)} + \gamma.$$

γ is a penalty term to circumvent overfitting; it is set to compensate for the gain obtained by splitting a sequence when no change occurred and its value is set to $\log n$. $P_{H_{11}}$, $P_{H_{12}}$, and P_{H_0} are mixtures of a Poisson distribution and an outlier distribution defined as follows.

$$P(a^1, \ldots, a^m) = \prod_i^m \alpha \cdot \text{Poisson}(a^i, \lambda) + (1 - \alpha) \cdot \beta,$$

where λ is estimated by $\frac{(1+\sum_{i=1}^m a^i)}{(m+1)}$, and α and β are user given constants defining a uniform distribution over the outlier values. The probability distributions $P_{H_{11}}$ and $P_{H_{12}}$ are estimated on $a^1, \ldots, a^t$ and $a^{t+1}, \ldots, a^m$ respectively by splitting the sequence $a^1, \ldots, a^m$ at the maximum likelihood split t; and λ's are calculated on the corresponding segments.

To bound the time complexity of our algorithm we constrain the maximum likelihood split t to lie within a smaller subset (S), instead of considering potentially the whole data stream. We defined S to contain the n last points. Although, S can be defined in other ways – e.g. to select elements with indices given by the Fibonacci numbers or by an exponential sequence – and while in theory the choice of definition affects the power and delay of change detection, in practice we did not experience significant differences.

Due to the fixed size of S the time complexity of the algorithm is constant. The algorithm can be efficiently implemented by maintaining the following statistics: $T = (f_{it}, \sum f_{it}, \lambda_t)$, where f_i denotes an observed frequency, $\sum f_{it}$ the sum of these frequencies and λ_t the mean over the last t points. A triple T is stored for every point t belonging to the last n-points. These statistics are updated incrementally. The likelihood of possible splits can be efficiently calculated. In practice, the number of different values for a^i is very small, and calculating $P_\lambda(a^i, \lambda)$ is an inexpensive operation. The log likelihood of a segment can be efficiently calculated by the dot product of $F \cdot \log P_\lambda(a^i, \lambda)$, where F holds the frequencies of a^i.

4.3 Measuring Change "conformity"

The historical activity of an individual is defined by a sequence of segments – identified by the change detection algorithm – and summarized by their means (μ) and lengths (n). The distance between the current and the summarised historical activity can be decomposed by summing up the pairwise subdistances between the current and each historical activity segments. The pairwise segment distances are weighted by the length of the particular historical segment. The distance measure can be defined as

$$d(H, s_c) = d(\{s_i | s_i \in H\}, s_c) = \sum_{s_i \in H} w_{s_i} \cdot d(s_i, s_c), \quad w_{s_i} = \frac{n_{s_i}}{\sum_{i=1}^{|H|} n_{s_i}},$$

where s_c is the current segment and H the set of historical, summarized activities. The distance of two segments is equal to the squashed symmetric Kullback-Leibler divergence:

$$d(s_1, s_2) = d((\mu_1, n_1), (\mu_2, n_2)) = \tanh(\alpha \cdot (KL(\mu_1, \mu_2) + KL(\mu_2, \mu_1))).$$

The symmetric divergence is squashed to bound the distance and resized by a constant α. The Kullback-Leibler divergence is estimated using the estimated Poisson distributions (P_{μ_1} and P_{μ_2}) of the two segments. P_{μ_1} and P_{μ_2} are determined by the Poisson parameters, μ_1 and μ_2, which are estimated by the means of the segments, s_1 and s_2. The KL-divergence is the expected log likelihood ratio over $\mathbb{N}^+$:

$$KL(\mu_1, \mu_2) = \sum_{i=1}^{\infty} P_{\mu_1}(a = i) \log \frac{P_{\mu_1}(a = i)}{P_{\mu_2}(a = i)}$$

5 Experimental Setup

In this section we describe our offline activity data labelling and synthetic activity data generation processes. We use the labelling process to provide "true" change detection labels to evaluate our online algorithm; while the synthetic data generator provides artificial user activity data for repeatability and to supplement our results.

5.1   Offline Labelling of Activity Data

In this section we describe an offline algorithm to automatically obtain homogeneous segments on activity data. The algorithm provides high quality segmentation but, due to its complexity, it is not suitable for real-time data processing. We use the segment boundaries, as change point labels, in our experiments (Section 6).

The offline segmentation algorithm derives segments by optimizing the log likelihood of the piecewise constant distribution function. We define the log likelihood, LL, of a segment sequence as:

$$LL(f_{i1}, \dots, f_{ik}) = \sum_{i}^{N} \log P_{(m,n)}(f_{ik})|m \leq i < n,$$

$$P_{(m,n)}(f_{ik}) = \alpha \frac{\lambda^k \exp^{-\lambda}}{k!} + (1 - \alpha)\beta$$

The above formula is maximal when the segments are of size 1, thus every point is a segment. To circumvent overfitting a penalty is added and set to $\log n$, where n is the sequence length. In case the sequence is modelled by a k-piecewise constant function the error is $k \log(n)$. Furthermore, it is assumed that segments are of a minimum length and the least likely observation is not used for calculating the likelihood.

The optimal segmentation problem can be solved by dynamic programming. Dynamic programming saves considerable amount of computation over a naive brute force method by exploiting the optimality of the subproblems. The complexity of finding the optimal model, with respect to the data, is $O(kn^2)$, where n is the sequence length and k is the number of segments. Our experiments include reasonably short sequences and a relatively small number of individuals thus allow the application of this technique. However, as the length of the sequences and the number of individuals grow, the complexity may go beyond control at a certain point, rendering the procedure inapplicable even in an offline setup.

To reduce the computational complexity of dynamic programming, we preselect a number of potential splitting points by sampling. To do so, first we randomly select (relatively short) subsequences of the activity data and identify their best splitting. Then for each point in the original activity data we count the number of times it occurred as the best split on the subsequences. Finally, the set of potential splitting points is identified by the most frequent k points and then dynamic programming is used to find the optimal m ($m < k$) splitting points within this set. The application of this methodology greatly simplifies the problem ($k << n$) and thus highly improves efficiency – without a considerable loss of accuracy.

5.2   Synthetic Data Generation

We generate synthetic activity data based on piecewise constant functions, i.e. the user activity history is a sequence of homogeneous segments. The number of split points, thus the boundaries of the segments, follows a mixture of two Poisson distributions. The position of the splitting points is sampled uniformly. The segment distribution is a mixture of two components, the majority distribution, with additive noise from an outlier distribution, and a zero mean distribution.

The mean of the outlier distribution is set by the user, the majority distribution is sampled from a gamma distribution and the zero mean distribution is a Poisson distribution with zero mean. The majority distribution is constrained to differ sufficiently from neighbouring segments achieved by rejecting samples by the Mann-Whitney (MW) two sample test of random samples from the segment distributions.

6   Evaluation

Our experiments included results on server-side web access log data of an investment bank collected over a 3-years period (REALWORLD) and on synthetically generated activity data (SYNTHETIC). The REALWORLD dataset consists of 5,000 randomly chosen customers with 3,278,798 sessions in total. Both individuals and their sessions are identified reliably, since clients had to identify themselves in order to be able to reach the secured internal pages. The SYNTHETIC dataset includes activity data of 5,000 artificial individuals over a "3-years" period with 1,731,339 sessions in total. We applied the data generator with the following settings (as referred to the description in Section 5.2): we set the prior of the outlier distribution to 0.01, the distribution a Poisson distribution with a mean twice as large as the segment mean, the prior of the zero mean distribution to 0.01, the distribution of the mean of the segments to $Gamma(1, 0.5)$ and we set 0.5 detection probability for the MW test.

We applied our offline labelling algorithm on the REALWORLD dataset. The algorithm identified 2,647 change points in total. In case of SYNTHETIC, the data generation process set a total number of 8,818 change points. We used these change points ("true" change points) to evaluate the performance of the online change detection algorithm on both datasets.

Evaluation criteria. For each and every true change point we check whether there is a detected change point in the following δ time periods. In case of a match we calculate the distance between the true and detected change points, the number of time periods elapsed, and mark the true change point detected. If there is no detected change point within δ, the true change point goes undetected. Any additional points detected within or outside the δ neighbourhood would count as false alarms. We set δ to 30 in case of both datasets[1]. We set the parameters of the online change detection algorithm to $\alpha = 0.95$ and $\beta = \frac{1}{60}$. Furthermore, the subset of potential change points (S) was set to the 20 most recent data points.

---

[1] Since majority of the clients are weekly or monthly visitors our method needed a larger time window to detect most of the changes.

Given this setup, the accuracy[2] of change detection on REALWORLD was 71.63% with an average detection latency of 7.03 days and the total number of false alarms was 9,931, which translates to less than one (0.66) false alarm per client per year. We achieved a slightly better accuracy, 76.45%, on SYNTHETIC, with an average detection latency of 10.23 days and 13,386 false alarms in total (0.89 false alarms per user per year).

For each change we calculated its conformity based on our conformity measure. Here we present two examples: Figure 3-a shows a change that highly conforms with past activities ($d = 22.59\%$), thus we most likely would not report it; while Figure 3-b depicts a change that does not conform with past activities ($d = 85.23\%$).

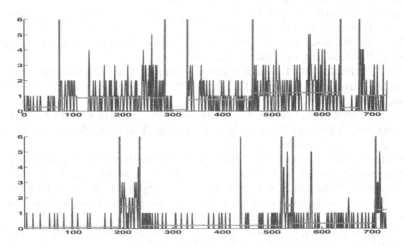

Fig. 3. Examples of (a) highly conform (top) and (b) highly non-conform (bottom) changes, $d = 22.59\%$ and $d = 85.23\%$ consecutively. In the examples we compared the last segments to the past activities. Axes depict frequencies (vertical) and time periods in days (horizontal), thick vertical line show detected segment boundaries and thick horizontal lines represent segment means.

7   Conclusion

We identified and described an important problem: online change detection in individual user activity. We divided it into specific subtasks – real-time change detection and measuring change conformity – and provided methods to solve them efficiently. We justified our methods on activity data of 5,000 customers of an online investment bank collected over 3 years, as well as on synthetically generated data. Our online change detection method achieved 71.63% accuracy

---

[2] Note, that we are not aware of any approach that would solve the problems described in our paper and therefore could serve as a baseline for comparison. Furthermore, our goal was to provide efficient, reasonable solutions to the aforementioned real-world problems and not to improve an existing state-of-the-art method.

with an average detection latency of 7.03 days on the real-world dataset; and 76.45% accuracy on the synthetic data with an average detection latency of 10.23 days. The false alarm rate was 0.66 and 0.89 per user per year, consecutively, on the real-world and on the synthetic datasets. Detected change points, together with information on the directions of the changes and change conformities, can be used in many real-world problems including decision support for marketing actions to retain online customers.

References

1. Wald, A.: Sequential analysis. Wiley, New York (1947)
2. Page, E.: On problems in which a change in a parameter occurs at an unknown point. Biometrika 44, 248–252 (1957)
3. Basseville, M., Nikiforov, I.V.: Detection of Abrupt Changes - Theory and Application. Prentice-Hall, Inc., Englewood Cliffs (1993)
4. Bifet, A., Gavaldà, R.: Learning from time-changing data with adaptive windowing. In: Jonker, W., Petković, M. (eds.) SDM 2007. LNCS, vol. 4721. Springer, Heidelberg (2007)
5. Gama, J., Medas, P., Castillo, G., Rodrigues, P.P.: Learning with drift detection. In: Bazzan, A.L.C., Labidi, S. (eds.) SBIA 2004. LNCS (LNAI), vol. 3171, pp. 286–295. Springer, Heidelberg (2004)
6. Sharifzadeh, M., Azmoodeh, F., Shahabi, C.: Change detection in time series data using wavelet footprints. In: Bauzer Medeiros, C., Egenhofer, M.J., Bertino, E. (eds.) SSTD 2005. LNCS, vol. 3633, pp. 127–144. Springer, Heidelberg (2005)
7. Ho, S.S.: A martingale framework for concept change detection in time-varying data streams. In: ICML, pp. 321–327 (2005)
8. Kifer, A., Ben-David, S., Gehrke, J.: Detecting change in data streams. In: VLDB, pp. 180–191. Morgan Kaufmann, San Francisco (2004)
9. Muthukrishnan, S., van den Berg, E., Wu, Y.: Sequential change detection on data streams. In: ICDMW, pp. 551–550. IEEE Computer Society, Los Alamitos (2007)
10. Spiliopoulou, M., Baron, S.: Monitoring the evolution of web usage patterns. In: Berendt, B., Hotho, A., Mladenič, D., van Someren, M., Spiliopoulou, M., Stumme, G. (eds.) EWMF 2003. LNCS (LNAI), vol. 3209, pp. 181–200. Springer, Heidelberg (2004)
11. Ganti, V., Gehrke, J., Ramakrishnan, R.: DEMON: Mining and monitoring evolving data. Knowledge and Data Engineering 13, 50–63 (2001)
12. Mazeroff, G., Cerqueira, V.D., Gregor, J., Thomason, M.: Probabilistic trees and automata for application behavior modeling. In: Proceedings of 41st ACM Southeast Regional Conference (2003)
13. Ihler, A., Hutchins, J., Smyth, P.: Adaptive event detection with time-varying poisson processes. In: SIGKDD, pp. 207–216. ACM, New York (2006)
14. Keogh, E.J., Chu, S., Hart, D., Pazzani, M.J.: An online algorithm for segmenting time series. In: ICDM, pp. 289–296. IEEE Computer Society, Los Alamitos (2001)
15. Cooley, R., Mobasher, B., Srivastava, J.: Data preparation for mining world wide web browsing patterns. Knowledge and Information Systems 1, 5–32 (1999)

A Comparative Study of Correlation Measurements for Searching Similar Tags[*]

Kaikuo Xu[1], Yu Chen[1], Yexi Jiang[1], Rong Tang[1,2],
Yintian Liu[2], and Jie Gong[1]

[1] School of Computer Science, SiChuan University, ChengDu, 610065, China
[2] Chengdu University of Information Technology, ChengDu, 610225, China

Abstract. In recent years, folksonomy becomes a hot topic in many research fields such as complex systems, information retrieval, and recommending systems. It is essential to study the semantic relationships among tags in folksonomy applications. The main contributions of this paper includes: (a) proposes a general framework for the analysis of the semantic relationships among tags based on their co-occurrence. (b)investigates eight correlation measurements from various fields; then applying these measurements to searching similar tags for a given tag on datasets from del.icio.us. (c) conducts a comparative study on both accuracy and time performance of the eight measurements. From the comparison, a best overall correlation measurement is concluded for similar tags searching in the applications of folksonomy.

1 Introduction

Taxonomy, a traditional top-down classification method, is considered not sufficient to solve web classification problems [1]. When taxonomy is used for web classification, domain experts construct a hierarchical classification structure and the features of a certain class are normally identified. By this means, documents can be classified according to the expert-constructed hierarchy. However, there are three main problems to use this method: (1) The hierarchy and the features may not fully reflect the real classification of the documents since the experts' domain knowledge are limited; (2) The updates of the hierarchy may not describe the increasing on timely since the growth of web pages is too fast; (3) The classification may not stand for all web users' mind since it is just the opinion of the experts who are a small fraction of users. Folksonomy [2,3,4], also known as 'collaborative tagging', is introduced to alleviate all problems mentioned above. In collaborative tagging, web users are exposed to a web page and freely associate tags with it. Users are also exposed to tags previously entered by themselves and other users. The collective tagging activity creates a dynamic correspondence between a web page and a set of tags, i.e. an emergent categorization in terms of tags shared by a community of web users. Tags stand for the

---

[*] Supported by the 11th Five Years Key Programs for Sci. &Tech. Development of China under grant No. 2006BAI05A01, the National Science Foundation under grant No 60773169, the Software Innovation Project of Sichuan Youth under Grant No 2007AA0155 and the Development Foundation of Chengdu Univeristy of Information Technology(KYTZ200811).

C. Tang et al. (Eds.): ADMA 2008, LNAI 5139, pp.709–716, 2008.

users' true opinion to classify the web pages. From the description above, it is clear that tag is the core concept of folksonomy and the classification is conducted through tags of all users. Thus to study the semantic relationships among tags is the key for applications of folksonomy.

A general framework to analyze the semantic relationships among tags based on their co-occurrence is proposed in this paper. In the framework, the whole analysis process is partitioned into eight steps. The task of each step is identified and the difficulties in each step are discussed in detail. The task to search similar tags for a given tag is left for further research. The definition of 'similar tags' is given, and eight correlation measurements from applications of various fields are investigated. The comparisons among correlation measurements are conducted over the datasets from del.icio.us on both the accuracy and time performance. The experiment results are analyzed and a remark on all the eight correlation measurements is given.

The rest of the paper is organized as follows. Section 2 describes the general framework to analyze the semantic relationship among tags. Section 3 investigates the correlation measurements to search similar tags for a given tag, and section 4 demonstrates the experimental evaluation. At last, Section 5 concludes the paper.

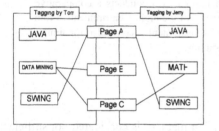

Tag	Page	User_count
java	A	2
swing	A	2
data mining	B	1
data mining	C	1
math	C	1

Fig. 1. An example of tagging in folksonomy   **Fig. 2.** An example of tagging in folksonomy

2 A General Framework for Tag Analysis

According to the observation, co-occurrence between tags is widespread in folksonomy systems. Figure 1 shows such an example. On the purpose of understanding user count, Figure 1 is transformed into Figure 2,which contains an attribute 'user_count'. Let's formulate the notions first. Let the tag set be T, the number of pages that tag A annotates be *La*, the number of pages tag B annotates be *Lb*, the number of common pages both tag A and tag B annotate be *Lab* and the number of web pages be *N*.

Definition 1 (Similarity between Tags). Let A and B be two Tags and Lab be the number of shared web pages of A and B. Let the threshold be δ, δ>= 1 .if Lab > δ the A and B is called similar tags. 'similarity' is used to describe the degree how they are similar to each other. 'similarity' between A and B is denoted as s(A,B).

Definition 2 (User Count). The number of users who use tag A to annotate Page P is defined as the **user count** of A to P.

A process for tags' analyzing based on the co-occurrence among tags is described below. The analysis process consists of eight steps and the output of each former step is the input of its latter step.

Step 1. Preprocessing. The main goals of this step are to: (a) Eliminate system tags. System tags are provided to users by folksonomy systems to complete some special tasks. For example, when users want to import bookmarks from other Social Bookmarking Service (SBS) providers to del.icio.us, the folksonomy system adds tag 'imported' to these bookmarks. These tags are collected to build a dictionary. Then tags matching any tag in the dictionary will be eliminated. (b) Eliminate meaningless tags. Users' mistakes or the system's mistakes produce meaningless tags. For example, a ' ' is taken as a meaningless tag. One solution to identify these meaningless tags can be the outlier checking algorithm.

Step 2. Classification. This step is to classify tags into three classes[5]: (a) Personal tags. These tags are used by only one user but assigned to more than one pages. The tags may be understood as personal vocabulary. Thus, they are useful for individual retrieval but useless for the rest users of the community. (b) Unpopular tags. These tags are assigned to different resources by different users but only once or several times. These tags can be treated as unpopular tags when they are only used by a small fraction of users quite occasionally. (c) Popular tags. These tags are assigned to various resources by different users frequently and they can be taken as global tags which are generally used by many users.

Step 3. Natural language processing. This step deals with tags under the class label 'Personal tags' and 'Unpopular tags'. Since these tags do not appear frequently, the traditional natural language processing methods are considered to be sufficient to solve the problem. The simplest way is to directly get insight into these tags by 'http://wordnet.princeton.edu/'.

Step 4. Frequent pattern mining. This step uses the mature frequent pattern mining techniques like *fpgrowth* to capture the co-occurrence between tags. The most difficult problem in this step is how to specify the threshold δ to judge whether a pattern is a frequent pattern. Obviously the deficiency of the support-confidence framework [6] still exists. Therefore, the result of this step needs further investigation in the future.

Step 5. Similar tag searching. This step searches the similar tags for a given tag. The correlation analysis is applied on the result of frequent pattern mining in our research. Since there are many correlation measurements on both statistics and data mining, the problem that needs to be solved is how to choose a 'better' measurement.

Step 6. Core-based clustering. Given a tag and its similar tags, the similar tags are clustered into groups in this step. Tags in each group should be the same 'close' to the given tag semantically. The given tag is taken as the 'core'. Both the hierarchical clustering and the density-based clustering are considered as candidate methods.

Step 7. Similar tag searching (multi-tag). This step searches the similar tags for a given tag group. The co-occurrence is used here and correlation analysis will takes effect in this step too. However, it is very difficult to reach a satisfy precision by existing methods because of two major reasons: (a) the occurrence of tag groups is rare; (b) it is not easy to judge what users mean only from a given tag group.

Step 8. Tag network building. The hierarchical structure implies a 'containing' relationship among class labels in taxonomy: the web pages that higher level class labels annotate contains the web pages that the lower level class labels annotate. However, the case is different for tags. Based on our observation, large number of tags normally annotates the same web pages. But these tags themselves usually annotate many unique web pages. The ultimate relationship among tags is likely to be a network, and each tag is a node in the network. It still needs further investigation whether this thought can be implemented.

The rest of the paper concentrates on step 5.

3   Similarity Measurements for Comparison

In this section, eight similarity measurements are discussed and compared in order to obtain the better measurements. These eight measurements are: Augmented Expected Mutual Information [7], Simrank[8], Pythagorean Theorem [9], Pessimistic Similarity [10],Cosine similarity [11], adjusted Cosine similarity [11], Pearson coefficient [11], and TF/IDF [12]. These measurements are divided into two groups: measurements with user count and without user count.

3.1   Measurements without User Count

Augmented Expected Mutual Information (AEMI). The concept of mutual information [13] is from the information theory. Given two objects, the mutual information measures how much the knowledge to one object reduces the uncertainty about the other. In the context of correlation analysis, it can be a common correlation metric. The augmented expected mutual information [7] is adopted in our study, as shown in formula 1.

$$\text{AEMI(A,B)} = \text{MI(A,B)} + \text{MI}(\overline{A}, \overline{B}) - \text{MI}(A, \overline{B}) - \text{MI}(\overline{A}, B) \quad (1)$$

Simrank. The formula proposed in [8] is an intuitive formula, and also the simplest one among the four, as shown in formula 2. Here, C is a constant between 0 and 1 and it shows less confidence on the similarity between A and B than the confidence between A and itself. In this paper, $C = 0.8$.

$$\begin{cases} s(A,A) = 1 / La \\ s(A,B) = C*Lab/(La*Lb) \text{ if } A \mathrel{!=} B \end{cases} \quad (2)$$

Pythagorean Theorem (PT). *Pythagorean Theorem* is a classic theorem in Euclidean geometry. It describes the relationship among the three sides of a right triangle, as "The square on the hypotenuse is equal to the sum of the squares on the other two sides". Let *Lab* be the length of one leg, and (La - Lab) + (Lb - Lab) be the length of the other legs respectively; then the length of the hypotenuse is $\sqrt{Lab^2 + (La + Lb - 2*Lab)^2}$. The formula to measure the similarity between two tags is shown in formula 3. According to formula 3, s(A,B) increases along the increasing of Lab and decreases along the increasing of La and/or Lb.

$$s(A,B) = \frac{Lab}{\sqrt{Lab^2 + (La + Lb - 2*Lab)^2}} = \frac{1}{\sqrt{1+(\frac{La}{Lab}+\frac{Lb}{Lab}-2)^2}} \qquad (3)$$

Pessimistic Similarity (PS). Pessimistic prune is a prune strategy adopted by C4.5 [10]. In our method, the pessimistic confidence on 'A is the same to B' is taken as the similarity between A and B. Let's consider a proposition P 'tag A is similar to tag B', for which La + Lb - Lab = K and the observed error rate is f. For this proposition there are K training instances to support. The observed error rate is simply the number of pages annotated by only one tag divided by K, i.e.(La + Lb -2 * Lab)/K. A random variable is also considered standing for the true error rate: a random variable X with zero mean lies within a range 2z with a confidence of Pr[-z <=X<=z] = c. According to Normal distribution, there is a corresponding z once c is specified. For example, Pr[-1.65 <= X <= 1.65] = 0.9. From the notation above, we can obtain $X = \frac{f-e}{\sqrt{e(1-e)/K}}$, where f is the error rate and e is the mean. According to the formula above, the range of true error rate e for rule R can be found based on the observed error rate f and the number of supporting instances K. Let the confidence range value be z, the confidence value corresponding to z be cf, the number of supporting instances count (La+Lb-Lab) be K, and the observed error rate be f. Then the upper bound on the estimated error e is $U_{cf}(f,K)$[10]. The pessimistic confidence value sim(A,B) for the rule 'A is the same to B' can be defined as formula 4. The pessimistic confidence value shows the confidence level on "tag A is similar to tag B". This can be also explained as "how much tag A is similar to tag B", i.e. the value of the similarity. In this paper, the confidence is set as c = 80%, then z = 1.28.

$$s(A,B) = 1 - U_{cf}(f,K) \qquad (4)$$

3.2 Measurements with User Count

In this section, the set of pages that tag i annotates is denoted as I_i, and the number of users who have annotated page j by tag i is denote as $C_{i,j}$.

$$s(A, B) = \frac{\sum_{j\in I_A} C_{A,j} * C_{B,j}}{\sqrt{\sum_{k\in I_A} C_{A,k}^2}\sqrt{\sum_{k\in I_B} C_{B,k}^2}} \qquad (5)$$

Cosine Similarity (CS). In information retrieval, the similarity between two documents is often measured by treating each document as a vector of word frequencies and computing the cosine of the angle formed by the two frequency vectors. This formalism can also be adopted to calculate the similarity between tags, where tags take the role of documents, pages take the role of words, and usercount take the role of word frequencies. Then the similarity is defined as formula 5.

Adjusted Cosine Similarity (ACS). The adjusted cosine similarity is derived from cosine similarity, which is commonly used in collaborative filtering. However, this formula can not be applied directly to compute the similarity between tags since negative result may be obtained for $C_{i,j}$ - $\overline{C_i}$. Therefore, data are preprocessed as follows. For a single tag, all the pages with user counts less than the average user count are eliminated. This maintains the pages that the tag primarily annotates.

$$s(A, B) = \frac{\sum_{j\in I_A}(C_{A,j} - \overline{C_A}) * (C_{B,j} - \overline{C_B})}{\sqrt{\sum_{k\in I_A}(C_{A,k} - \overline{C_A})^2}\sqrt{\sum_{k\in I_B}(C_{B,k} - \overline{C_B})^2}} \qquad (6)$$

Pearson Coefficient (PC): The Pearson's product-moment correlation coefficient is a measurement for the degrees of two objects linearly related. The correlation between tag A and tag B is shown in formula 7. Here the summations over i are over the urls to which both tag A and B are linked. For very small common annotations, this similarity metric returns inaccurate results. This needs to be solved by methods such as 'default voting' or 'minimum common votes'. The results of a given tag are pruned beforehand. Therefore, it is unnecessary to specify a minimum number of common annotations in order to calculate a valid similarity actually.

$$s(A, B) = \frac{\sum_{j\in I_A}(C_{A,j} - \overline{C_A}) * (C_{B,j} - \overline{C_B})}{\sqrt{\sum_{i\in I_A}(C_{A,i} - \overline{C_A})^2}\sqrt{\sum_{i}(C_{B,i} - \overline{C_B})^2}} \qquad (7)$$

IDF/TF: The IDF/TF method is a classic method in document classification. In this paper, it is applied to compute the similarity between Tags as in paper [10]. Let $TF_{i,j}$ be the ratio of tag i in all tags annotating page j, IDF_i be the rareness of tag i,

$$TF_{i,j} = C_{i,j} / \sum_i C_{i,j} \qquad (8)$$

$$IDF_i = \log(C_{i,j} / \sum_i C_{i,j}) \qquad (9)$$

Then the degree $rel_{i,j}$ of relation between tag i and page j is defined as formula 10.

$$rel_{i,j} = \sum_j \sum_i C_{i,j} / \sum_j C_{i,j} \qquad (10)$$

$$s(A, B) = \sum_j C_{A,j} * rel_{B,j} \qquad (11)$$

At last, the similarity sim(A,B) of tag B from the view point of tag A is defined as formula 11. Here, sim(A,B) is not necessarily the same as sim(B,A) for formula 11. This requires more computations than other seven measurements.

4 Experiments

The real data sets from del.icio.us from Nov 30 to Dec 15 are collected. There are 234023 unique tags and 749971 unique web pages. Though web2.0 data provide valuable resource for data mining, there are no public benchmark data for research yet. Therefore, in our work, three human evaluators are asked to judge the performance of each formula. 30 tags are randomly selected as the given tags. Top-N similar tags can be obtained for each given tag A. For each tag T_i in the Top-N results, evaluators give a score to T_i as formula 12. Since our problem is actually a ranking problem, the classical evaluation method adopted in Information Retrieval is also used to solve our problem. Precision (P) at top N results is used as a measurement to evaluate the performance, as shown in formula 13.

$$score(T_i) = \begin{cases} 2 \text{ if } T_i \text{ is similar to } A \\ 1 \text{ if } T_i \text{ is somewhat similar to } A \\ 0 \text{ if } T_i \text{ is not similar to } A \end{cases} \quad (12)$$

$$P@N = \sum_{i=1}^{N} score(T_i) / (2*N) \quad (13)$$

All experiments are conducted on an INTEL core 2DuoProcessorE2160 with 2G memory, running UBUNTU OS. Table 1 shows the performance of eight measurements. There are two numbers in each cell. The first number is the average precision from the three evaluators and the second one in parentheses is the standard deviation. PC performs the worst among the eight measurements, which is the only one not in support of the counter evidence. This phenomenon indicates the necessity of the usage of counter evidence for similar tags' searching. CS is of the best performance among all eight measurements. Although ACS and IDF/TF are more complex than CS, their performance is worse than CS. The experiment result also shows that IDF/TF performs even worse than Simrank and PT although it takes user_count into account, while Simrank and PT are two measurements that do not use user_count. The performances of both AEMI and PS are out of our expectation: they are surpassed by Simrank and PT, the two simplest measurements in this paper. As we know, the performances of Simrank and PT are really good by considering their simplicity.

Table 1. P@N of eight measurements& CPU time(s)

Measurement	N = 10	N = 20	N = 30	Rank	CPU time
AEMI	0.508(0.046)	0.567(0.042)	0.570(0.037)	7	10.31
Simrank	0.679(0.148)	0.643(0.122)	0.615(0.106)	4	0.68
PT	0.688(0.054)	0.609(0.035)	0.581(0.039)	3	1.84
PS	0.555(0.119)	0.538(0.104)	0.534(0.085)	6	4.01
CS	0.749(0.068)	0.662(0.071)	0.619(0.072)	1	9.52
ACS	0.710(0.075)	0.641(0.074)	0.603(0.076)	2	15.84
PC	0.526(0.130)	0.576(0.106)	0.561(0.093)	8	11.34
IDF/TF	0.665(0.045)	0.608(0.044)	0.577(0.045)	5	713.31

Table 1 also shows CPU time consumed by eight measurements, respectively. The CPU time for IDF/TF is one/two orders of magnitude longer than those of the other measurements. Due to its relatively bad performance, it is considered not suitable for similar tags' searching. Since the CPU time consumed by either Simarank or PT is extremely small, they are considered as the candidate measurements for the similar tags' searching. Although the CPU time consumed by CS is one order of magnitude longer than the former two, it is still considered as the candidate measurement for the searching as well. In real applications, many techniques, such as high performance clustering, parallel computing, etc, can be applied to improve the speed although it is very difficult to improve P@N. Considering these two factors, CS is considered the best overall measurement for similar tags' searching in this paper.

5 Conclusions

A framework to analyze the relationship among tags is proposed and discussed. The former five steps of the framework are under research and the latter three steps are in our vision for the whole project. To search similar tags for a given tag becomes the focus of this paper. The steps before this task in the framework are dealt with in a pessimistic way. Eight measurements are investigated in a whole. Experiments are conducted on datasets from del.icio.us. Both the accuracy and CPU time consumed by each measurement are compared from one another. Cosine Similarity is considered as the best overall measurement due to its high accuracy and relatively low CPU consumption. Simrank and Pythagorean Theorem are considered good as well because of their extremely low CPU consumption and relatively high accuracy.

References

[1] Shirky, C.: Ontology is overrated: Categories, links, and tags. Clay Shirky's Writings About the Internet Website (2005)
[2] del.icio.us, http://del.icio.us/
[3] Cattuto, C., Loreto, V., Pietronero, L.: Semiotic dynamics and collaborative tagging. Proceedings of the National Academy of Sciences United States of America 104, 1461 (2007)
[4] Cattuto, C., Loreto, V., Servedio, V.D.: A yule-simon process with memory. Europhysics Letters 76(2), 208–214 (2006)
[5] Lux, M., Granitzer, M., Kern, R.: Aspects of Broad Folksonomies. In: 18th International Conference on Database and Expert Systems Applications (2007)
[6] Brin, S., Motwani, R., Silverstein, C.: Beyond Market Baskets: Generalizing Association Rules to Correlations. In: Proceedings ACM SIGMOD International Conference on Management of Data, Tucson, Arizona, USA, May 13-15 (1997)
[7] Chan, P.K.: A non-invasive learning approach to building web user profiles. In: KDD 1999 Workshop on Web Usage Analysis and User Profiling (1999)
[8] Jeh, G., Widom, J.: SimRank: A measure of structural-context similarity. In: Proc. 8th ACM SIGKDD Intl. Conf. on Knowledge Discovery and Data Mining (July 2002)
[9] Pythagorean Theorem, http://mathworld.wolfram.com/PythagoreanTheorem.html
[10] Quinlan, J.R.: C4.5: Programs for Machine Learning. Morgan Kaufmann, San Francisco (1993)
[11] Deshpande, M., Karypis, G.: Item-based top-n recommendation algorithms. ACM Trans. Inf. Syst. 22(1), 143–177 (2004)
[12] Thorsten, J.: Probabilistic Analysis of the Rocchio Algorithm with TFIDF for Text Categorization. In: Proceedings of 14th International Conference on Machine Learning (1996)
[13] Rosenfeld, R.: A maximum entropy approach to adaptive statistical language modeling. Computer,speech, and language 10 (1996)

Structure of Query Modification Process: Branchings

Nikolai Buzikashvili

Institute of System Analysis, Russian Academy of Sciences
9 prospect 60 Let Oktyabrya, 117312 Moscow, Russia
buzik@cs.isa.ru

Abstract. A common approach to query log analysis considers any query only as a possible modification of a direct predecessor. The paper considers a branching search. It is shown that up to 20% of sessions containing 3 and more different queries contain combinations which may be interpreted as branchings; a number of branches is a little bigger than two; one of the branches consists of only one query; branching may be realized as both narrowing and broadening.

Keywords: Query reformulation, non-linear search, Web query log.

1 Introduction

The paper considers dependencies between queries submitted by the same user of the Web search engine and is centered on branching dependency. Early conceptual works [1,2,5,9] on algorithmic-like description of information searching behavior do not exclude a possibility of non-linear search: a search process may contain several branches [2] and a complex search task may be decomposed into different chains [9], which converge at the final step. However, following empirical studies of user queries [7,8] use only linear search framework in which a query can be described as dependent only on its direct predecessor. One of the reasons is an absence of a formal language describing non-linear dependencies and tools automatically detecting them in query logs. While [7] and [8] consider user actions in different search contexts and different environments, the works coincide in:

— *a framework*: a current query is considered as a possible modification of only its *direct* predecessor $Q_T = f(Q_{T-1})$. Dependencies on indirect predecessors are neglected;
— *processing*: manual, small datasets (313 sessions in [7], 30 sessions in [8]).

On the contrary, we follow an opposite conceptual framework proposed in [3]:

(1) a query may depend on non-direct predecessor: $Q_T = f(Q_{S<T})$ instead of $Q_T = f(Q_{S=T-1})$. As a result, more than one queries may depend on the same query (a *branching* search: queries $Q_{T1} = f(Q_S)$, … $Q_{T2} = f(Q_S)$ depend on the same Q_S).
(2) a query may be a convergence of *a pair* of other queries $Q_T = f(Q_{S1<T}, Q_{S2<T})$, (a *convergent* search) rather than a modification of a single query.

Interpretations of the same sequence of user queries may significantly vary depending on the query dependencies taken into account. Fig. 1 shows commonly used linear and alternative non-linear interpretations of the same sequences of queries.

C. Tang et al. (Eds.): ADMA 2008, LNAI 5139, pp.717–724, 2008.

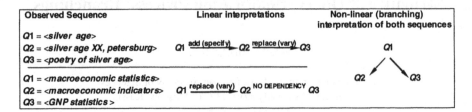

Fig. 1. Observed user queries and their interpretations in linear and non-linear frameworks

Since there is no reason to expect frequent occurrence of non-linear dependencies we need a big collection which may be processed only automatically. An automatic processing may answer the questions on frequencies, patterns and features of each type of search: linear query modification; non-linear modification, in particular branching, convergent and re-convergent search (as a combination of branching and convergence) and occasional non-linear execution of linear dependencies.

We suppose that a non-linear model of query modifications (cf. [6]) more adequately describes a real searching behavior whilst a non-linear search is only partly supported by search tools. Moreover, if a model is adequate, then a direct support of non-linear search may be incorporated into search tools.

This paper is devoted only to the branching search, while convergent and re-convergent structures of query dependency will be considered in a further work, not only due to simplicity reasons but also since a convergent search is less supported by human abilities and obviously needs a psychological explanation. On the contrary, a branching search is not a surprising manner. Searching on the Web comes up against a common situation provoking a branching search: when an initial query retrieves unsatisfactory results but perfectly expresses an information need, a user modifies the query; and if the results of the modified query are also unsatisfactory, a user refines an *initial* query rather than the current modification.

2 Conceptual Framework

This study mainly considers query dependencies on any single predecessor. If several queries depend on the same query ($Q_{T1}=f(Q_S)$, $Q_{T2}=f(Q_S)$,...) we speak about *branching* dependency. We mention but not consider here a *convergent* dependency $Q_T=f(Q_{S1<T}, Q_{S2<T})$ on a pair of predecessors considered as an entity. All dependencies are detected between queries submitted during a short-time period (a *time session* which is a sequence of user transactions with a search engine cut from previous and successive sessions by the gap bigger than the *temporal cutoff*).

Let the dependencies be presented by a graph of a *logical structure* [3], in which each query is presented by one node regardless of a number of occurrences of the query. The connected components of this graph correspond to tasks. Since a real *physical search process* realizing this logical structure is a time-ordered sequence of transactions, different independent tasks or different branches of the same task may alternate and even a linear task may be executed non-linearly if the task is broken by another task (occasional non-linearity of execution). Fig. 2 shows two types of non-linearity in a logical structure and 3 types of non-linearity in a real search.

Type of non-linearity	Sequence of Execution	Dependencies in Execution	Dependencies in Logical structure
Occasional (non-linear execution of linearly-dependent queries)	<cat food> (1) <kitten food> (2) <adma> (3) <adma 2008> (4) <hills cat diet> (5)	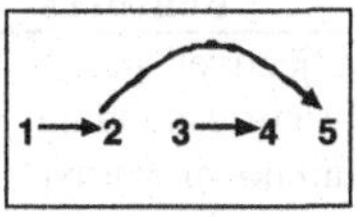 1→2 3→4 5	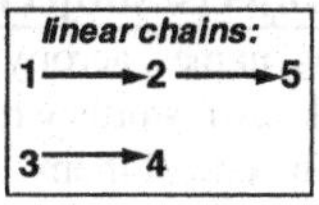 *linear chains:* 1→2→5 3→4
Branching (one query determines several queries)	<cat food> (1) <kitten food> (2) <home for cats> (3) <home for dogs> (4)	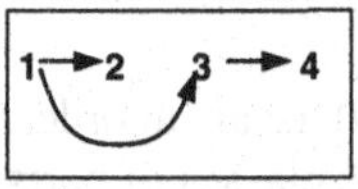 1→2 3→4	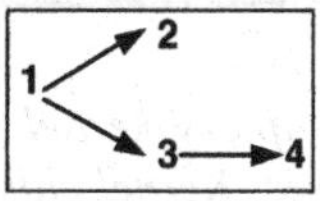 1→2, 1→3→4
Convergence (a query depends on two another queries)	<kitten food> (1) <cat food> (2) <hills> (3) <hills cat diet> (4)	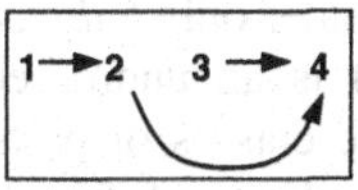 1→2 3→4	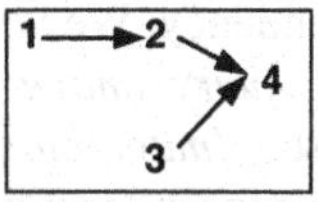 1→2→4, 3→4
Re-convergence (convergence of branched chains)	<cat food> (1) <kitten food> (2) <moscow cats> (3) <cat kitten moscow (4)	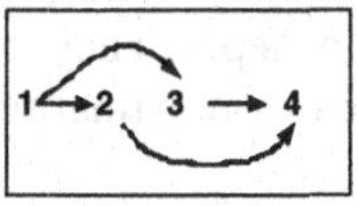 1→2 3→4	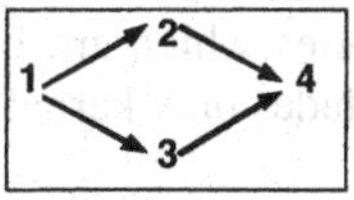 1→2→4, 1→3→4

Fig. 2. Basic non-linearities in logical structure of search and in its physical realization

Different kinds of dependency measures are sound and the best way to detect and to analyze a non-linear search is to use a family of decision rules, which operate with different measures (in particular, combine them) since different rules refine different aspects of a search behavior and may be equally feasible.

3 Partly Layered Query Representation and Processing

Let's begin with an intuitive notion of query dependency (and similarity) Decisions on the fact of query dependency and on the form of dependency are different decisions and take into account different components of queries. For example, among queries Q_1=<*big cat*>, Q_2=<*big brother*> and Q_3=<*cat*> the latter query seems to be more dependent on Q_1 than Q_2. We consider one-word overlap $Q_1 \cap Q_3$ = <*cat*> as more sufficient reason to speak about dependency than one-word overlap $Q_1 \cap Q_2$ = <*big*>. At the same time, we do not ignore <*big*> at all: speaking about dependency of Q_3 on Q_1 we mention that Q_3 differs from Q_1 by <*big*>. Thus, the word ignored in a decision on *dependency* is taken into account in a decision on the *form of dependency*.

We will use two-fold query representations. A narrow class of query terms constitutes *a query kernel* which is used to detect a fact of dependency: a query may depend on another only if the intersection of their kernels is not empty. At the same time we use a broader class of terms as *a query image* which is used to distinct queries and to extract a form of dependency between queries.

Let's consider four classes of words which describe: (1) *Subjects/Objects*, (2) *Features*, (3) *Actions* and (4) *Others* words. The reason to speak about dependency between queries is an overlap of subjects/objects rather than of features or actions of distinct subjects/objects. Table 1 shows what parts of speech are attributed to each class. Non-dictionary words are also heuristically attributed to the classes.

Table 1. Four classes of parts of speech used as basis of Kernels and Images

Objects/Subjects	Features	Actions	Others
nouns, names, acronyms, + unknown words which may be one of them	adjectives, participles, [+ corresponding unknown words] numerals and numbers	verbs, adverbs, adverbial participles [+corresponding unknown words]	all other words (prepositions, articles, etc)

A query kernel Ker(Q) is an unordered set of query terms belonging to kernel classes. *Kernel classes* are classes of parts of speech (Table 1) used to detect a fact of dependency. We will consider only *Subjects/Objects* as the kernel class.

A query image Im(Q) is an unordered set of query terms belonging to image classes. *Image classes* are classes of parts of speech used to distinct queries and to determine *a form* of dependency. A form of dependency is determined only on those queries which are being in dependency by kernels. A minimal set of image classes includes only kernel classes. A maximal set includes all classes and is used by default.

4 Method

We should select a "main" determinant of each dependent query. To do it a certain *decision rule* is applied to the *dependency matrixes* presenting different measures of dependency and to the *precedence matrix* presenting the order of recent occurrences of determining queries before the first occurrence of each dependent query. Term-based dependency measures are used and to calculate them we should detect *"identical" terms* in images of different queries.

Permissible word transformations and identity of terms. The procedure of comparison of two unordered sets is used to reveal the intersection of kernels or images of two considered queries. If two words t_i and T_j are *forms* of the same word they are considered as identical. For example, *cat* is identical to *cats*, *went* is identical to *goes*. If two non-dictionary words may be *a form* of the same word (compatible by endings which may be long in inflecting languages) they also considered as identical.

A trouble in the query log analysis is a lot of query typos. To escape the trouble typos are taken into account in a simple manner: if a long (>5 characters) non-dictionary word from one set may be transformed by one-symbol correction (insertion, deletion or replacement) into a form of a word *from another set* (this word may be either dictionary or non-dictionary), the words are considered as identical.

Two queries is considered as identical if there is a one-to-one mapping of their images $Im(Q_1)=\{t_i,..t_N\}$ and $Im(Q_2)=\{T_i,...T_N\}$ such that any term t_i may be modified into corresponding T_j by the permissible transformation. If there is a one-to-one mapping of subsets of the images these subsets are considered as the intersection.

Dependency measures. Term-based measures of query dependency are used. Query dependency relations are directed (asymmetric). A dependency measure can be constructed as a pair of any similarity metric (which is symmetric) and a direction from a determining query to a dependent one. Proper dependency relations (e.g. narrowing and broadening relations or asymmetric set operations) are originally directed. Table 2 shows two classes of term-based dependency measures.

Table 2. Dependency measures

Derivatives of similarity metrics	Proper dependency measures
— (1) *intersection*: $\lvert\mathrm{Im}(Q) \cap \mathrm{Im}(Q^{\mathrm{Det}})\rvert$ — (2) *symmetric difference*: $\Delta(\mathrm{Im}(Q),\mathrm{Im}(Q^{\mathrm{Det}}))=\lvert\mathrm{Im}(Q)\cup\mathrm{Im}(Q^{\mathrm{Det}}) - \mathrm{Im}(Q)\cap\mathrm{Im}(Q^{\mathrm{Det}})\rvert$ — (1) and (2) normalized by $\lvert\mathrm{Im}(Q)\cup\mathrm{Im}(Q^{\mathrm{Det}})\rvert$ *(Jaccard metrics)*	— *differences*: $\lvert\mathrm{Im}(Q) \setminus \mathrm{Im}(Q)\cap\mathrm{Im}(Q^{\mathrm{Det}})\rvert$, $\lvert\mathrm{Im}(Q^{\mathrm{Det}}) \setminus \mathrm{Im}(Q)\cap\mathrm{Im}(Q^{\mathrm{Det}})\rvert$ — *differences normalized* by $\lvert\mathrm{Im}(Q^{\mathrm{Det}})\rvert$ — binary measures: *narrowing* (expansion by terms); *broadening* (terms exclusion)

A query term is included into a query kernel and a query image as it is. At the first step we check intersection of kernels $\mathrm{Ker}(Q)=\{t_1,\ldots t_n\}$ and $\mathrm{Ker}(Q^{\mathrm{Det}})=\{T_1,\ldots T_m\}$ of a possible dependent query Q and a possible determinant Q^{Det}. Kernel terms $\{t_1,\ldots t_n\}$ and $\{T_1,\ldots T_m\}$ are compared pairwise. If $\mathrm{Ker}(Q)\cap\mathrm{Ker}(Q^{\mathrm{Det}})\neq\varnothing$, the same comparison procedure is applied to *images* $\mathrm{Im}(Q)$, $\mathrm{Im}(Q^{\mathrm{Det}})$ to extract a form of dependency.

We extract dependencies separately *in each time session*. Any query may depend on queries submitted previously during a considered session. Any query may determine queries submitted later during the session.

Dependency matrixes. A dependency matrix is constructed for each dependency measure. Rows present dependent queries and columns present queries-determinants. Only dependencies on queries submitted before the first occurrence of a dependent query are taken into account, i.e. a dependency matrix is a triangle by construction. Elements of a dependency matrix presenting a measure M are "ranks" of the $M(Q_i,Q_j)$ among all $M(Q_i,Q_{j<i})$, i.e. a i-th row contains "ranks" of queries $Q_{j<i}$ submitted earlier in the time session. A row may contain equal "ranks" (in particular, all non-empty scores for binary measures are equal to 1).

Precedence matrix. If a query equally depends on several queries according to a considered measure, one can suppose that the dependency on the most recent among these queries is more significant. To take into account this plausible guess a precedence matrix *Prec* is constructed.

While dependencies between *queries* should be extracted, a search engine query log contains *transactions* (Fig. 3) where (Q, p) denotes a user transaction with p-th page of the results retrieved by query Q.

The procedure of a triangle precedence matrix construction: moving across a time series we detect occurrences of new query Q_i (i.e. a query image of which differs from images of all previously met queries) and rank previous queries $Q_{j<i}$ accordingly to increasing a time distance of their last occurrences to the first occurrence of Q_i. The

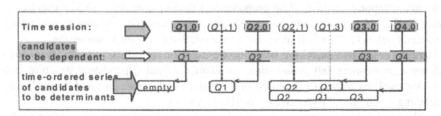

Fig. 3. Constructing a precedence matrix of queries by transactions of a time session

ranks are inserted as i-th row into the matrix of precedence. For example, a precedence matrix for a time session in Fig. 3 is

$$\mathrm{Pr}\,ec = \begin{bmatrix} & Q1 & Q2 & Q3 \\ Q2 & 1 & & \\ Q3 & 1 & 2 & \\ Q4 & 2 & 3 & 1 \end{bmatrix}$$

Decision rules. Decision rules select a "main" determinant of each dependent query among all of its determinants. A decision rule may use one or several measures.

Example. Let $\mathrm{Im}(Q1)=\{A,B\}$, $\mathrm{Im}(Q2)=\{A\}$, $\mathrm{Im}(Q3)=\{B\}$ and $\mathrm{Im}(Q4)=\{B,C\}$ be images of the queries in Fig. 3. Dependency matrixes for *overlap, symmetric difference, narrowing* and *broadening* measures are:

$$M^{\cap} = \begin{bmatrix} & Q1 & Q2 & Q3 \\ Q2 & 1 & & \\ Q3 & 1 & & \\ Q4 & 1 & & 1 \end{bmatrix} \quad M^{\Delta} = \begin{bmatrix} & Q1 & Q2 & Q3 \\ Q2 & 1 & & \\ Q3 & 1 & & \\ Q4 & 2 & & 1 \end{bmatrix} \quad M^{broad} = \begin{bmatrix} & Q1 & Q2 & Q3 \\ Q2 & 1 & & \\ Q3 & 1 & & \\ Q4 & & & \end{bmatrix} \quad M^{narr} = [0]$$

Let a decision rule be used for each measure M and be sound as "select the most recent query among queries maximally influencing the dependent query according to M". The dependency structures extracted by these rules are:

$$R^{\cap} = R^{\Delta} = \begin{bmatrix} & Q1 & Q2 & Q3 \\ Q2 & 1 & & \\ Q3 & 1 & & \\ Q4 & & & 1 \end{bmatrix} \Rightarrow Q1\!<^{Q2}_{Q3\to Q4} \qquad R^{broad} = \begin{bmatrix} & Q1 & Q2 & Q3 \\ Q2 & 1 & & \\ Q3 & 1 & & \\ Q4 & & & \end{bmatrix} \Rightarrow Q1\!<^{Q2}_{Q3}$$

5 Results

A 24-hour fragment of a query log of the major Russian search engine *Yandex* is used. Almost queries are queries in Russian, about 7% of queries are queries in similar Slavonic languages and 10% contain also English words (usually brand names). The *Yandex* log is very preferable since Slavonic languages ultimately simplify a part of speech tagging used to construct kernels and images. The only part of speech corresponds to each dictionary word and non-dictionary words cause no trouble.

The dataset was pre-processed to exclude users who are robots rather than humans. To do it a client discriminator threshold equal to 7 unique queries per 1-hour sliding window was used. 30-min intersession cutoff was used to segment observed transactions into temporal sessions. The preprocessed dataset contains 755,319 users executed 3,272,345 transactions in 1,135,656 time sessions. Sessions containing advanced queries (1.7% of all sessions) were excluded to simplify processing.

Here, *to describe* a searching behavior we use four measures: *overlap, symmetric difference, narrowing* and *broadening*. *To extract* a final dependency structure two rules are used: an *overlap* rule based only on the overlap measure and *"minΔ"* rule combining symmetric difference and overlap measures:

— the most recent among queries which are the most influencing according to the *overlap* measure (*overlap* rule);

— the final determinant is selected among queries which have the minimum symmetric difference with a dependent query: the query which has the biggest overlap with the dependent query among them is selected. If several determinants fulfil this condition, the most recent of them is selected (*"minΔ"* rule).

Binary relations of narrowing/broadening are not used in these rules. However, we use them as features describing a search behavior extracted by these rules.

Table 3 shows similarity of the results of the rules except a fraction of a branching search: the *"min Δ"* rule extracts much more cases of branching. Any non-linearity may occur only if a session contains at least 3 different queries (20.9% of all sessions). We report fractions of branching sessions among these sessions in brackets. We can surely say that a branching search a frequent manner of execution of *several-query* tasks. Branching commonly has a binary form (2.1 branches per branching). One of ~two branches usually contains only one query. Unfortunately, we did not consider time-ordering of long and small branches.

Table 3. Characteristics of different search structures*

Characteristics	*overlap* rule	*"min Δ"* rule
Time sessions containing branching (%)	2.07% (9.90%)	4.33% (20.73%)
Length of linear chains in:		
linearly executed linear chains	1.38	1.28
non-linearly executed linear chains	1.55	1.41
before branching	1.35	1.27
Length of max & min branches in branching	1.63 1,06	1.52 1.04
Number of branches in branching	2.1	2.1

*All lengths are measured in a number of query modifications $Q^{(i)} \rightarrow Q^{(i+1)}$.

Table 4 shows transitions between different kinds of query modifications $Q_i \rightarrow Q_j$ detected in linear chains and presented in terms of narrowing/broadening. A difference between results of two rules application is not significant.

Table 4. Transition matrixes for sequences of modifications in linear chains of 2+ queries

	overlap rule				*"min Δ"* rule			
	final	narrow	broad	other		final	narrow	broad	other
initial	.	.383	.115	.503	initial		.356	.124	.521
narrow	.594	.073	.052	.281	narrow	.753	.075	.042	.130
broaden.	.742	.138	.027	.093	broaden.	.734	.146	.029	.091
other	.653	.076	.046	.225	other	.680	.071	.046	.203

The difference between the rules is huge in pre-branching query modifications and in branches (Table 5). While broadening in pre-branching and narrowing in branching is more expected and confirmed by the *"min Δ"* rule, the *overlap* rule mainly reveals opposite modifications: narrowing in pre-branching and broadening in branching. A common portrait of branching extracted by the *overlap* rule is $AB \rightarrow ABC <^{AC}_{BC}$ while the *"min Δ"* rule also frequently extracts $AB \rightarrow A <^{AC}_{AD}$ combinations.

Table 5. Fractions of operations in pre-branching and in branches

overlap rule				*"min Δ"* rule			
	narrow	broad	other		narrow	broad	other
in pre-branching	47.8	6.8	45.4	in pre-branching	26.3	16.7	57.0
in branches	15.0	27.0	58.0	in branches	49.7	11.7	38.6

6 Conclusion and Further Work

The results are: (1) a branching search is a frequent manner of an execution of several-query tasks; (2) a number of branches is a little bigger than two; (3) one of the branches consists of only one query; (4) not only narrowing but also broadening branching is detected.

This paper is devoted to the branching search. At the next step a convergent and re-convergent search should be extracted and analyzed in terms of a searching behavior. Another, technical task is a complete implementation of the layered representation of a query. Now we use a "semi-layered" representation of a query by a kernel and an image. However, an image includes too different classes of words which should not "have the same rights" in a detection of query dependency (similarity): e.g., a bigger overlap of images mainly based on words belonging to the *Others* class is obviously less valuable than a smaller overlap based on *Subjects* class. This difference should be directly taken into account in a comparison of query images.

References

1. Bates, M.: Information search tactics. J. of American Soc. for Inf. Sci. 30(4), 205–214 (1979)
2. Bates, M.: Idea tactics. J. of American Soc. for Inf. Sci. 30(5), 280–289 (1979)
3. Buzikashvili, N.: The Yandex Study. In: Workshop on Evaluating User Studies in Inf. Access, pp. 48–55. British Computer Society (2005)
4. Buzikashvili, N.: Automatic task detection in Web logs and analysis of multitasking. In: Sugimoto, S., Hunter, J., Rauber, A., Morishima, A. (eds.) ICADL 2006. LNCS, vol. 4312, pp. 131–140. Springer, Heidelberg (2006)
5. Fidel, R.: Moves in online searching. Online Review 9(1), 61–74 (1985)
6. Foster, A.E.: A non-linear model of information seeking behaviour. J. of American Soc. for Inf. Sci. and Tech. 55(3), 228–237 (2004)
7. Rieh, S.Y., Xie, H.: Analysis of multiple query reformulations on the web: The interactive information retrieval context. Inf. Processing & Management 42, 751–768 (2006)
8. Vakkari, P.: eCognition and changes of search terms and tactics during task performance. In: Recherche d'Information Assistée par Ordinateur (RIAO 2000), C.I.D., pp. 894–907 (2000)
9. Wildemuth, B., Jacob, E., Fullington, A., de Blieck, R., Friedman, C.: A detailed analysis of end-user search behaviors. In: 54th American Soc. for Inf. Sci. Meeting, pp. 302–312. ACM, New York (1991)

Mining Top-n Local Outliers in Constrained Spatial Networks

Chongsheng Zhang[1,2], Zhongbo Wu[1,2], Bo Qu[1,2], and Hong Chen[1,2]

[1] School of Information, Renmin University of China, Beijing 100872, China
[2] MOE Key Lab of Data Engineering and Knowledge Engineering, Beijing 100872, China
{rucmaster,rucwzb,qubo,chong}@ruc.edu.cn

Abstract. Outlier mining, also called outlier detection, is a challenging research issue in data mining with important applications as intrusion detection, fraud detection and medical analysis. From the perspective of data, previous work on outlier mining have involved in various types of data such as spatial data, time series data, trajectory data, and sensor data. However, few of them have considered a constrained spatial networks data in which each object must reside or move along a certain edge. In fact, in such special constrained spatial network data environments, previous outlier definitions and the according mining algorithms could work neither properly nor efficiently. In this paper we introduce a new definition of density-based local outlier in constrained spatial networks that considers for each object the outlier-ness with respect to its k nearest neighbors. Moreover , to detect outliers efficiently, we propose a fast cluster-and-bound algorithm that first cluster on each individual edge, then estimate the outlying degree of each cluster and prune those that could not contain top-n outliers, therefore constraining the computation of outliers to only very limited objects. Experiments on synthetic data sets demonstrate the scalability, effectiveness and efficiency of our methods.

1 Introduction

Outlier mining, which aims to find small amount of exceptional objects in a database, is an critical data mining task referred as outlier detection that has lots of practical applications such as telecom or credit card fraud detection, intrusion detection, financial and market analysis, and discovery of criminal activities. To detect outliers, a fundamental issue is how to define an outlier that is meaningful and applicable to the confined problem domains. The issue intuitively leads to the result that different outlying objects may be detected with respect to different outlier views.

Recent researches on outlier mining, viewing from the data perspective, detect outliers in various kinds of data ranging from trajectory database [11], time-series data [12], software engineering data[13], to stream data [14, 15], and RFID data [16]. However, few of them have considered outliers in constrained spatial networks data. While constrained spatial network datasets have distinguished data characteristics, and as existing solutions could not work well such data, we need special definitions and mining algorithms to detect outliers in such datasets. Outlier mining in spatial networks could find applications in traffic analysis on road networks.

C. Tang et al. (Eds.): ADMA 2008, LNAI 5139, pp.725–732, 2008.

The mission of this paper is to discover local outliers efficiently in constrained spatial networks. Constrained spatial networks data are usually modeled as graphs in research, and the data takes several outstanding as well as distinguished characteristics. Firstly, objects in constrained spatial networks behave linearly and sequentially locally on each edge. Neighbors of an object p in the spatial networks can be obtained by just walking along the line. The neighbors will usually distribute sequentially and linearly away from p, instead of surrounding p as the case in traditional data. Secondly, unlike traditional data, we can never know the distance between objects unless we travel around the edges, so in constrained spatial networks the seeking for nearest neighbors would be much more costly than that in traditional data. As can be seen in Figure 1, that though P_1's nearest neighbors seem to be P_2, P_3, P_4 in Euclid Distance, but in fact they are rather far away from P_1 on spatial networks. When we detect outliers in constrained spatial networks data, we should employ such local-linear distribution rules, meanwhile reducing the computation of KNN search on spatial networks.

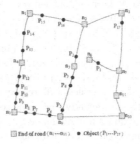

Fig. 1. A spatial network G

In this paper, we introduce a simple and applicable definition of outlier in spatial networks data, and outliers are those who are sparse and isolated with respect to their k nearest neighbors in the spatial networks. In addition, in order to find top-n local outliers efficiently, an efficient cluster-and-bound algorithm is proposed. After clustering individually on each edge, we estimate for each cluster its outlier-ness lower and upper bounds, clusters will be immediately exempt from candidate outlying clusters if they can not contain top-n outliers, thus avoiding the high computation cost of estimating outlier-ness value for each object. In other words, we reduce the computation of outlier-ness values from all the objects to only a small amount of data. Hence, our solution could achieve good performance. Our contributions are as follows:

- We introduce the interesting and applicable problem of local outliers in constrained spatial networks.
- We develop an efficient algorithm for mining top-n local outliers in spatial networks, and perform extensive experiments on synthetic datasets.

The rest of the paper is organized as follows. Session 2 surveys related work. Session 3 gives the definitions of outliers in constrained spatial networks data. An algorithm is provided to efficiently detect outliers in Session 4, and we evaluate the performance of the algorithm in Session 5.

2 Related Work

Existing approaches to outlier mining can be classified into five categories. Distribution-based approaches need some known distribution models be provided and deployed, objects that deviate from the distribution are exposed as outliers [1]. These distributions are usually univariate and would work poorly when the data is multidimensional. In Depth-based approach each object is represented as a point in a k-d space, and is assigned as depth. Those with smaller depth will be in outer layers and be detected as outliers [2].This method can avoid the serious problems of both distribution fillings and poor performance at multidimensional data suffered by distributed-based approaches, however, it does not scale well to high dimensional data. There are generally two notions of distance-based outliers, which are DB (p, D) –outlier [3] and K[th]-Distance based outlier [4] in which outliers are those that are much further away from their K[th] neighbor. In clustering approach each object is usually assigned a degree of membership to each of the clusters, and outliers are those who do not fit to any cluster [5, 6, 7]. Therefore these methods discover outliers as byproducts, are usually not optimized for outlier mining. In density-based approach [8 ,9], each object has a local outlying factor and outliers are those that are isolated or sparse with respect to its k nearest neighbors, but the main drawback is that the computation cost on local reachablility distance is rather expensive.

3 Definitions

Definition 1. Spatial Distance SDist (p,q) is the shortest reachable distance between p and q along the spatial path. If p and q reside on the same edge e, then SDist (p,q) is the direct distance between p and q on edge e. Otherwise, we would have to resort to the ideas like dijkstra to compute SDist (p,q).

Definition 2. $N_K(p)$ is the set of p's k nearest neighbors, which are the most nearest k objects to p in G.

Definition 3. SKDist (p) is the sum of shortest reachable distances between p and each object in $N_K(p)$, which is the set of p's k nearest neighbors.

$$SKDist(p) = \sum_{q \in N_k(p)} SDist(p,q)$$

Definition 4. MaxKDist(p) is the distance between p and its Kth nearest spatial neighbor.

$$MaxKDist(p) = \max\{q \in N_k(p) \mid SDist(p,q)\}$$

Definition 5. MinKDist(p) is the distance between p and its nearest neighbor in the spatial networks.

$$MinKDist(p) = \min\{q \in N_k(p) \mid SDist(p,q)\}$$

Unlike traditional datasets where an object may center at a circle and be surrounded by many neighbors, in constrained road networks, p's nearest neighbors distribute near linearly along the edges, instead of surrounding p. We can know where the next neighbor is just by walking along the edge.

Definition 6. Local sparsity factor LSF(p) is the degree to which p is exceptional, outlying or isolated with respect to its k nearest neighbors.

$$LSF(p) = \frac{|N_k(p)| \cdot MaxKDist(p)}{\sum_{q \in N_k(p)} MaxKDist(q)}$$

The definition is based on the observation and characteristics that, instead of surrounding p, p's neighbors, usually distribute along the edges in a linear-like way. For instance, if p's k nearest neighbors are close to each other, but all of them are rather far way from p, then LSF(p) value would be high, and p would be selected as an outlier. Our definition differs from the LOF definition in [8] in that we take both local density and nearly linear neighborhood distribution features into consideration, meanwhile avoiding the expensive computation cost of reachable distance.

Definition 7. A constrained spatial networks cluster is the set of nearby objects that are close and next to each other. In this paper we represent a cluster as a quad-tuple cluster(cid, e, O, len), with cid being the identifier of the cluster, e being the edge where the cluster resides, O is the set of objects in the cluster, and len is the distance between the first and the last object along the e. In this paper a cluster can only locate on one edge, not across several edges.

Definition 8. $N_K(Cluster_i)$ is a set of clusters that contain the k nearest neighbors of any object in $Cluster_i$.

Definition 9. $MinKDist(Cluster_i)$ is the minimal reachable k-distance of $Cluster_i$, the distance that is equal or lower than $\min(p \in cluster_i | MaxKDist(p))$.

Definition 10. $MaxKDist(Cluster_i)$ is the maximal reachable k-distance of $cluster_i$, the distance that is equal to $\max(p \in cluster_i | MaxKDist(p))$.

Definition 11. $LSF(Cluster_i)$ is the outlying degree of $Cluster_i$, this value is dependent on the LSF value of each object in $Cluster_i$.

Definition 12. $LSF(Cluster_i)_{min}$ is the lower bound of the outlier-ness value of the cluster.

$$LSF(cluster_i)_{min} = \frac{|N_k(p)| \cdot MinKDist(cluster_i)}{\sum_{cluster_q \in N_k(cluster)} MaxKDist(cluster_q)}$$

Definition 13. $LSF(Cluster_i)_{max}$ is the upper bound of the outlier-ness value of the cluster.

$$LSF(cluster_i)_{max} = \frac{|N_k(p)| \bullet MaxKDist(cluster_i)}{\sum\limits_{cluster_q \in N_k(cluster)} MinKDist(cluster_q)}$$

Definition 14. MaxDist(C_i, C_j)is the max spatial distance between any two objects in C_i and C_j; MinDist(C_i, C_j) is the minimum distance for any two objects in C_i and C_j.

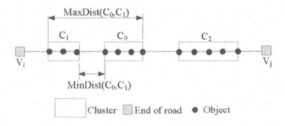

Fig. 2. MaxDist(C_0, C_1) and MinDist(C_0, C_1)

4 Mining Top-n Local Outliers in Constrained Spatial Networks

4.1 A Naive Top-n Outlier Mining Algorithm

For any object p in spatial networks G, we search (and store) its k nearest neighbors, meanwhile we compute the value of MaxKDist(p); Thirdly, we compute LSF value for each object using *Definition 5*; Finally, we sort all the objects in G by their LSF values in descending order, and output the top-n local objects as outliers.

4.2 An Optimized and Efficient Cluster-and-Bound Top-n Local Outlier Mining Algorithm

In this chapter, we first introduce a simple clustering algorithm in spatial networks, followed is a lemma that could help us determine a cluster's k nearest neighbor clusters in a much more precise way, after that we propose an efficient algorithm that estimates the LSF lower and upper bounds given its k nearest neighbor clusters. Thereafter, using the LSF values of the clusters, we prune, meanwhile determine the candidate outlying clusters, finally we compute the LSF values for each object in the candidate clusters and output the top-n objects with the highest LSF values.

In algorithm 1, ξ is a distance threshold that can be an input parameter, as well as a distance determined by the algorithm. It could also be possible that different edges can cluster using different values of ξ . Objects that are within ξ distances will be categorized in the same cluster. We expect to bound each cluster's LSF value, subsequently, we have to determine its k nearest neighbor clusters stated in definition 7. Moreover, in order to involve as less clusters as possible when we are finding a cluster's k nearest neighbor clusters, Theorem 1 is introduced.

Algorithm 1. SpatialCluster

Input: A spatial network graph $G(V, E, W)$, ξ

Output: clusters as described in definition 7.

Begin

1   For each edge in G
2   i = 0, j = 0;
3   while not end of the edge
4   i++, j ++;
5   while len(i+1, i) < | ξ |

6   put Object(i) into Cluster(j);
End

Function 1. CCNE: cluster_compare_and_enqueue

Input: left_cluster, right_cluster, cluster Q

Output: which cluster will be en-queued

Begin

1   left_max_distance = Max_Distance (cluster, left_cluster);
2   right_max_distance = Max_Distance(cluster, right_cluster);
3   left_min_distance = Min_Distance(cluster, left_cluster);
4   right_min_distance = Min_Distance(cluster, right_cluster);
5   if left_max_distance < right_min_distance then
6   en_queue(left_cluster, Q);
7   else if left_min_distance < right_max_distance
8   en_queue(right_cluster, Q);
9   else
10   en_queue(left_cluster, Q);
11   en_queue(right_cluster, Q);
End

Algorithm 2.   K distance-Bound

Input: spatial networks G(V, E, W), k, C,

Output: MinKDist(C,), MaxKDist(C,)

Begin

1    $V_0 V_1$ = find_edge (C,);
2   Q = null;
3   while |Q| + |C,| < k + 1 do
4   lcluster = fetch_nextCluster (RCQ);
5   rcluster = fetch_nextCluster (ACQ);
6   CCNE (C, lcluster, rcluster, Q);
7   MinKDist(C,) =max(len(C,), Min_Distance(C,, Q.tail));
8   while |Q| < k -1 do
9   lcluster = fetch_nextCluster (RCQ);
10   rcluster = fetch_nextCluster (ACQ);
11   CCNE (C,, lcluster, rcluster, Q);
12   MaxKDist(C,) = Max_Distance(C,, Q.tail);
End

Algorithm 3.   Estimation of LSF Bounds

Input: k, C,

Output: C,'s k candidate nearest neighbor clusters

Begin

1   for each cluster C,
2   read its k nearest neighbor clusters;
3   read its k-distance bound MinKDist(C,),
        MaxKDist(C,);
4   compute C,'s LSF bounds
        LSF(Cluster,)_min, LSF(Cluster,)_max based using definition 6,
End

Theorem 1.   Stop conditions for the search of k nearest neighbor clusters. C_i is a cluster on edge e, AQ is the set of C_i's nearest neighbor clusters along the edge, and VQ is that of its nearest neighbor clusters reverse the edge. Clusters in both AQ and VQ are in ascending order according to their network distances to C_i. C_a is the next neighbor cluster of C_i along e, C_v is the next C_{al} neighbor cluster of C_i reverse e , and C_{al} is the last cluster in AQ, C_{vl} is the last cluster in CQ. If the following three conditions are satisfied,

a). $|AQ| + |VQ| \geq k$
b). $\text{MaxDist}(C_i , C_{al}) \leq \text{MinDist}(C_i , C_v)$
c). $\text{MaxDist}(C_i , C_{vl}) \leq \text{MinDist}(C_i , C_{al})$

Then C_i's k nearest neighbor clusters must be in AQ union VQ, and we can stop searching for them.   □

In algorithm 2, we compute, for each cluster C_i, its MinKDist and MaxKDist values, as defined in defintions 9 and 10. Line 3-6 is to make sure that the number of objects in Q and C_i is just equal or larger than k, so we can compute the value of MinKDist (C_i). Similarly, in line 9-12 we compute the value of MaxKDist(C_i).

In algorithm 3, we compute, for each cluster , its $\text{LSF}(C_i)_{min}$ and $\text{LSF}(C_i)_{max}$ values, according to definitions 12 and 13.

After we have $\text{LSF}(C_i)_{min}$ and $\text{LSF}(C_i)_{max}$ values for each cluster C_i, we begin the rank top-n outliers procedure. Initially the candidate sets *CandSet* include all the clusters, firstly we fetch n clusters, sort them in descending order according to their

$LSF(C_i)_{min}$ values, and label the last one as outlier threshold o_t ; for the rest clusters, if its $LSF(C_i)_{max}$ value is smaller than o_t, then we remove it from *CandSet* as it can not contain the top-n outliers; Otherwise, we compare its $LSF(C_i)_{min}$ value with o_t, if it is greater than the latter, then we resort the top-n clusters and update the value of o_t. Once we have scanned all the clusters, we compute $LSF(p)$ for each object p in *Cand-Set*. Finally, we output the top-n objects with the greatest $LSF(p)$ values as outliers.

5   Experimental Results

We evaluate the performance of our proposed cluster-and-bound algorithms on real datasets of sub-networks of the San□Francisco road map, and objects on the road networks are generated by brinkhoff network data generator [17]. Brinkhoff generator has several parameters, as can be seen in figure 3, "Objects agility" is the degree to which the objects are active on the road networks, "cluster queries" is the percentage of the total queries that could be clustered together. "Number of NNs" is completely identical to K in this experiment, that is, how many nearest neighbors we are going to find for the query. "olratio" is the outlier ratio. Both the naive method(we call it N-TOP-N-OD) and cluster-and-bound algorithms for mining outliers are implemented. All algorithms are implemented in Java a on PC with a Pentium 4 CPU of 2.4GHz, a memory of 512Mb.

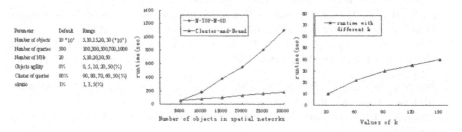

Fig. 3. parameters   **Fig. 4.** runtime compare   **Fig. 5.** runtime with k vlaues

Figure 4 investigates the influences of number of objects (ranging from 10K to 200K) on spatial networks to naive method and cluster-and-bound algorithms. In this experiment, we fixed the values of the parameters. The result is that cluster method outperforms the naïve method. As can be seen in figure 4, while for the cluster-and-bound method runtime increased linearly with the number of points, runtime for the naïve method increased almost exponentially. The reason is that the former method has a much smaller time complexity than the latter as it dismisses most objects that could not possibly become top-n local outliers in batch.

Figure 5 plots the time cost with the changing values of k. We fix number of objects at 5K, Cluster of queries at 40%, and object agility is set to 0. The computation time keeps increasing with k as the greater the k value is, the more traversing and computation are needed when we are targeting the k nearest neighbor clusters and k nearest neighbor objects.One problem exposed is that is our cluster-and-bound algorithm is somewhat vulnerable to value of k.

References

1. Barnett, V., Lewis, T.: Outliers in Statistical Data. John Wiley & Sons, Chichester (1994)
2. Johnson, T., Kwok, I., Ng, R.T.: Fast Computation of 2-Dimensional Depth Contours. In: Proc. SIGKDD, pp. 224–228 (1998)
3. Knorr, E.M., Ng, R.T.: Algorithms for MiningDistance-Based Outliers in Large Datasets. In: Proc. of VLDB, pp. 392–403 (1998)
4. Knorr, E.M., Ng, R.T.: Finding intensional knowledge of distance-based outliers. In: Proc. of VLDB, pp. 211–222 (1999)
5. Ester, M., Kriegel, P., Sander, J., Xu, X.: A density-based algorithm for discovering clusters in large spatial databases. In: Proc. KDD, Portland, Oregon, pp. 226–231 (1996)
6. Guha, S., Rastogi, R., Shim, K.: Cure: An efficient clustering algorithm for large databases. In: Proc. SIGMOD, Seattle, WA, pp. 73–84 (1998)
7. Ng, R., Han, J.: Efficient and effective clustering method for spatial data mining. In: Proc. VLDB, Santiago, Chile, pp. 144–155 (1994)
8. Breunig, M., Kriegel, H., Ng, R.T., Sander, J.: LOF: Identifying Density-Based Local Outliers. In: Proc. of ACM SIGMOD 2000, TX (2000)
9. Jin, W., Tung, A.K.H., Han, J.: Mining top-n local outliers in large databases. In: Proc. ACM SIGKDD, San Francisco, New York, pp. 293–298 (2001)
10. Papadimitriou, S., Kitagawa, H., Gibbons, P.B., Faloutsos, C.: LOCI: Fast outlier detection using the local correlation integral. In: Proc. ICDE, Bangalore, India, pp. 315–326 (2003)
11. Lee, J., Han, J., Li, X.: Trajectory Outlier Detection: A Partition-and-Detect Framework. In: Proc. of IEEE ICDE, Cancun, Mexico (April 2008)
12. Li, X., Han, J.: Mining Approximate Top-K Subspace Anomalies in Multi-Dimensional Time-Series Data. In: Proc. VLDB 2007, Vienna, Austria (September 2007)
13. Yoon, K.-A., Kwon, O.-S., Bae, D.-H.: An Approach to Outlier Detection of Software Measurement Data using the K-means Clustering Method. In: Proc. ESEM 2007, pp. 443–445 (2007)
14. Zhu, Y.Y., Shasha, D.: Efficient elastic burst detection in data streams. In: Proc. SIGKDD 2003, New York, pp. 336–345 (2003)
15. Zhang, X., Shasha, D.: Better Burst Detection. In: Proc. ICDE 2006, Atlanta, GA, USA, p. 146 (2006)
16. Elio Masciari, E.E.: A Framework for Outlier Mining in RFID data. In: Proc. of IDEAS 2007, September 2007, pp. 263–267 (2007)
17. Brinkhoff, T.: A Framework for Generating Network-Based Moving Objects. GeoInformatica 6(2), 153–180 (2002)

Mining Concept-Drifting Data Streams with Multiple Semi-Random Decision Trees[*]

Peipei Li[1], Xuegang Hu[1], and Xindong Wu[1,2]

[1] School of Computer and Information, Hefei University of Technology
Hefei 230009, China
`peipeili_hfut@163.com, jsjxhuxg@hfut.edu.cn`
[2] Department of Computer Science, University of Vermont, Burlington, VT 50405, U.S.A
`xwu@cs.uvm.edu`

Abstract. Classification with concept-drifting data streams has found wide applications. However, many classification algorithms on streaming data have been designed for fixed features of concept drift and cannot deal with the noise impact on concept drift detection. An incremental algorithm with Multiple Semi-Random decision Trees (MSRT) for concept-drifting data streams is presented in this paper, which takes two sliding windows for training and testing, uses the inequality of Hoeffding Bounds to determine the thresholds for distinguishing the true drift from noise, and chooses the classification function to estimate the error rate for periodic concept-drift detection. Our extensive empirical study shows that MSRT has an improved performance in time, accuracy and robustness in comparison with CVFDT, a state-of-the-art decision-tree algorithm for classifying concept-drifting data streams.

Keywords: Data Streams, Concept Drift, Random Decision Trees, Classification.

1 Introduction

Streaming data are widespread along with the rapid development of information technology, such as Internet search requests and telephone call records. Owing to the special characteristics of streaming data, which are continuous, high-volume, open-ended and fast-paced, traditional mining algorithms cannot adapt to mine in real time from these data environments. As concept drift[1] exists widely in data streams, it is a challenge to find the drifting rules and apply them into the drift prediction in real-world applications.

Some mining algorithms for data streams with concept drift have been proposed. For instance, an algorithm for mining decision trees from continuously changing data streams called CVFDT was proposed by Hulten et al[2], which makes use of a sliding window strategy to construct alternative sub-trees for each node, and replaces the old tree with a new tree. An efficient and accurate cross-validation decision tree

---

[*] This research is supported by the National Natural Science Foundation of China (No. 60573174).

C. Tang et al. (Eds.): ADMA 2008, LNAI 5139, pp. 733–740, 2008.

ensembling method was proposed by Wei Fan for improving the accuracy of classification[3]. Another ensemble learning algorithm was proposed by Zhang and Jin, which furnishes training data for basic classifiers and provides effective voting[4]. However, these algorithms classify on certain features of concept drift and ignore the effect of noise on the concept drift detection. Therefore, how to detect different types of concept drift and how to reduce the negative effect from noise are important problems.

To overcome these limitations, an algorithm called MSRT is presented in this paper, which starts with the SRMTDS algorithm (Semi-Random Multiple Decision- Tree algorithm for Data Streams)[5] for the problem of concept-drifting data streams. MSRT takes two sliding windows with pre-defined thresholds, generates different alternative sub-trees for different nodes, uses the inequality of Hoeffding Bounds[6] to distinguish between the true concept drift and the noise, adjusts the training window and test window dynamically to adapt to the concept drift and reduces the effect from noise on concept-drift detection. Our extensive study shows that MSRT outperforms CVFDT on run-time, accuracy and the robustness.

2   Related Work: SRMTDS

SRMTDS is an ensembling algorithm with SRDT (Semi-Random Decision Trees) for the classification of data streams, which creates multiple trees with an initial height of h_0 in a semi-random strategy, uses the inequality of Hoeffding Bounds to determine the split thresholds of nodes with numerical attributes, and introduces a Naïve Bayes method for more accurate class labels.

$$P(e \geq \overline{e} - \varepsilon) = 1 - \delta, \varepsilon = \sqrt{(R^2 \ln(1/\delta))/2n} \tag{1}$$

The inequality of Hoeffding Bounds is given in Eq(1). Consider a real-valued random variable e whose range is E. Suppose we have made n independent observations of this variable and computed their mean $\overline{e}$, which shows that, with probability $1 - \delta$, the true mean of the variable is at least $\overline{e} - \varepsilon$. The value of R is $\log_2(M(c))$, where $M(c)$ is the count of class labels.

The generated trees in SRMTDS satisfy the upper bound on the generalization error of the model of ensemble classifiers, which is given by Breiman[8] as follows,

$$PE \leq \overline{p}(1 - s^2)/s^2 = \overline{p}(1/s^2 - 1) \tag{2}$$

where s is the measure of classification accuracy of a classifier and $\overline{p}$ is the dependence between classifiers. Because the generation of each tree in SRMTDS is independent and there are no interactions between each other when classifying, the value of $\overline{p}$ is small. While the value of s is not fixed due to the randomized method used in SRDT, the probability that the ensemble of SRDT is an optimal model is estimated in Eq(3), i.e., the ensemble model of SRDT is optimal under the circumstances of the confidence of at least $P(M(Att), N, h_0)$.

$$P(M(Att), N, h_0) = 1 - (1-p)^{N \cdot 2^{h_0-1}} = 1 - \left(1 - 1/M(Att)\right)^{N \cdot 2^{h_0-1}} \tag{3}$$

3 The MSRT Algorithm

3.1 Concept Drift

A *concept* in data streams can be a class label or the distribution rules of several attributes in the given instances. The change modes of a concept can be divided into two types of "concept change" and "sampling change" by their different change patterns[9]. Concept change refers to the change of the underlying concept over time, which can be further divided into concept drift and concept shift. Concept drift is about a gradual change of the concept[1] and concept shift describes abrupt changes between different concepts[10]. Sampling change is also called sampling shift[11] or virtual concept drift[1] and refers to the change of a data distribution.

3.2 Algorithm Description

The proposed algorithm of MSRT based on SRMTDS is designed for the classification of concept-drifting data streams, which has three new features. First, it generates diverse alternative sub-trees at decision nodes. Second, it uses two thresholds to distinguish the true concept drift from the noise. Finally, it classifies the test data in a voting mechanism for the majority class. The main process of the algorithm is described as follows.

Algorithm MSRT {*DSTR*, *DSTE*, *A*, *N*, h_0, Δ, τ, n_{min}, *WinSize*, *CheckPeriod*, *TestSize* }

Input: Training set: $DSTR = \{TR_1, TR_2, ..., TR_m\}$; Test set: $DSTE = \{TE_1, TE_2, ..., TE_n\}$; Attribution set: $A = \{A_1, ..., A_{M(Att)}\}$ ($M(Att)$ is the count of attributes in the database); Initial height of tree: h_0; The number of minimum split-examples: n_{min}; Confidence: Δ; Tie threshold: τ; Split estimation function: $G(\bullet)$; The number of SRDT: N; The size of training window: *WinSize*; The checking period for constructing alternative subtrees: *CheckPeriod*; The size of testing window for alternative subtrees: *TestSize*; The class labels of classification in N-SRDT trees: *ClassLabels*;

Output: the class labels of classification on the testing instances

1. for($i = 1$; $i <= N$; i++)
2. {   Create_SRDT(A, T_i, h_0);
3.   for(TR_j $DSTR$, j is from 1 to m)
4.   { Travel tree from the root to the decision node $node_{curi}$;
5.   if(the number of observed instances $n_{curi} >= n_{min}$)
6.   { Update_Estimate(T_i, TR_j, n_{min}, Δ, τ, $G(\bullet)$); }
7.   if(the count of observed training instances at T_i $-count_{Ti}$ % *CheckPeriod* == 0)
8.   { Generate the alternative subtree of $node_{curi}$ };
9.   if($node_{curi}$ has the subtree)
10.   if(n_{curi} % *TestSize* = = 0)
11.   { Adjust the sizes of training and test windows; }
12.   if($count_{Ti} \geq$ *WinSize*)
13.   {   Forget the old data;   }
14.   }

```
15.          for(TE_j DSTE, j is from 1 to n)
16.            ClassLabels[i] = ClassifyTestSet(T_i , TE_j );
17.    }
18.    return FindClassifyingResults(ClassLables);
```

Algorithm MSRT generates N SRDT trees in the semi-random strategy in Step 2 as the same with that of SRMTDS. In Steps 3~6, the information of nodes is updated incrementally. When the statistical count satisfies the threshold of n_{min} at the growing nodes with continuous attributes, the heuristic method of Information Gain combined with the inequality of Hoeffding Bounds is used to compute the split-threshold and the attribute value with the highest information gain will be selected as the final cut-point.

Steps 7~8 construct different alternative sub-trees for different types of nodes when the number of instances at the current node is over the split-threshold. For a node with a numerical attribute, create a sub-tree with the same split-attribute at the root as the node in the original tree; for a node with a discrete attribute, generate a sub-tree and select from the available attributes randomly as the split-attributes. The growing process in the sub-tree follows the method in SRDT and a second new alternative sub-tree could not be generated until the current sub-tree replaces the corresponding branch of the original tree.

The periodic scanning process of the nodes in the tree takes place in Steps 9~11. Compute the error rates of classification of the passed node and the root node in its alternative sub-tree and judge whether the concept drift appears or not. If drifting concepts are detected, some measures are taken to react to this change. The details will be introduced in the Section 3.3.

Steps 12~13 judge whether the size of the current training data is overflowed, and if so, the old data in the current training window are discarded by their "ages", i.e., the principle of "first in, first out" is applied here.

The last step is to classify the testing data by the estimation function of the majority class, since Naïve Bayes is not suitable for databases that have strong dependencies among data attributes. Finally, the class label with the maximum probability classified by the N trees with the voting mechanism is determined as the result of classification for each test instance.

3.3 Dealing with the Concept Drift

The method of two sliding windows presented in this paper is based on the time-window idea for both training and test windows, which seeks to improve the performance by dynamically adjusting the sizes of windows. The sizes of training and test windows are adjusted with two thresholds of p and q and their values are defined with $p = k_1\varepsilon$, $q = k_2\varepsilon$ ($k_1 > k_2$) by the inequality of Hoeffding Bounds, which satisfy the following formula,

$$P(|e-\overline{e}|\geq p)=1-\delta_1, p=k_1\varepsilon, \quad P(|e-\overline{e}|\geq q)=1-\delta_2, q=k_2\varepsilon \qquad (4)$$

where e and $\overline{e}$ are the error rates of classification of the current node in the original tree and the root node in its sub-tree, n is the number of instances at the current node, and the value of ε satisfies Eq(1). If the value of Δe $(=|\overline{e}-e|)$ is not less than that of p, a concept drift appears, the alternative sub-tree replaces the corresponding branch, the size of the training window is shrunk by the size of the test window, and the size of the test window is reduced to a half of the original size, which benefits for a rapid concept drift. If the value of Δe is in the bound of (q, p), it is considered as noise, hence the size of the training window is unchanged, while the size of test window is extended by a half of its original size, which is beneficial to reduce the impact of noise on drift detection. Otherwise, if the value of Δe is less than q, there is no concept drift or the drift rate is very slow so that the size of the training window is increased by the size of the test window and the size of the test window is set to the default value.

3.4 Complexity Analysis

The time cost at nodes with discrete attributes during training is much less and the worst case is $O(M(Att)/(M(Att)-H(node)+1))$ (where $H(node)(\leq h_0 \leq M(Att)/2)$ is the height of the current node), and the main time complexity is on the nodes with numerical attributes, which is $O(m_j^A)$ (m_j^A is the number of distinct values of attribute A_j) in MSRT and SRMTDS, but is up to $O(\Sigma_j m_j^A)$ in CVFDT ($j = 1, ..., M(Att)$. On the whole, the time complexity of each instance is $O(L_s M(CAtt)VM(c))$ for MSRT, $O(L_cM(Att)VM(c))$ for CVFDT and $O(L_tM(Att)VM(c))$ for SRMTDS (L_s and L_c are the maximum path length multiplied by the number of alternative sub-trees in MSRT and CVFDT respectively, L_t is the maximum path length in SRMTDS, $CAtt$ is the number of numerical attributes, and V is the maximum number of attribute values). MSRT performs better on time than CVFDT, especially for discrete databases. However, SRMTDS does not need to construct alternative sub-trees and so the time overhead of training is always less than that of MSRT. With respect to the time complexity of classification, it is $O(M(c))$ of each leaf node for all these algorithms.

The space overhead is relevant to the features of attributes in a given database for these three algorithms, which is $O(T_nM(Att)VC)$ (T_n is the total number of nodes in all trees). Each non-leaf node only keeps the information about the current split attribute in MSRT and SRMTDS, while each node holds the information of all attributes in CVFDT. Therefore, the approximate ratio of their space consumption at each non-leaf node is $1/M(Att)$. However, the space overhead at a leaf node is generally equivalent for MSRT and CVFDT, but is much more than that of SRMTDS.

4 Experimental Evaluations

Experiments are conducted to verify the validity of MSRT in streaming data with different types of concept drift. The parameters are set as follows: $\varepsilon = 10e^{-7}$, $\tau = 0.05$, $n_{min} = 300$, the size of the training window - $WinSize = 50k$ (1k = 1000), the size of test window - $TestSize = 10k$, $N = 5$, $h_0 = 2$, $p = 3\varepsilon$, $q = \varepsilon$ in MSRT, and the size of the sliding window $= 50k$ in CVFDT. All experiments are performed on a P4, 2.66 GHz PC with 512M main memory, running Windows XP Professional. These three algorithms are written in Visual C++. net.

4.1 Databases for Experiments

HyperPlane is a benchmark database for data streams with concept drift, which is denoted by equation: $\sum_d w_i x_i = w_0$ ($d = 50$). Each vector of variables $(x_1, x_2, ..., x_d)$ is a randomly generated instance and is uniformly distributed in the space $[0, 1]^d$. If $\sum w_i x_i = w_0$, the class label is 1, or else 0. The bound value of coefficient w_i is [-10, 10] and each default value is generated at random. The value of w_i increases or decreases continuously by the value of $\triangle w_i$ till it is up or down to the boundary, and then it changes the direction. Noise is introduced randomly by r % and the default value is 5. Besides, the value-changing direction of w_i can be shifted into the opposite direction by the probability of p_w (=10%) after N_e instances are generated. Accordingly the value of w_0 is changed with the change of w_i. In order to simulate the state of concept drift, choose k dimensions of attributes to change their values of w_i and k is initialized as 5.

STAGGER is a standard database to test the classification algorithms' abilities in the concept-shifting data streams[12]. In this database, each instance consists of three attribute values: color {*green, blue, red*}, shape ¶*triangle, circle, rectangle*◇, and size ¶*small, medium, large*◇√ There are three alternative underlying concepts, A: if color = *red* and size = *small*, class = 1; otherwise, class = 0; B: if color = green and shape = *circle*, class =1; otherwise, class = 0; and C: if size = *medium* or *large*, class = 1; Otherwise, class = 0. The randomly generated instances for our experiments contain 4k concepts and each concept generates 1k random instances. The initial concept begins with A, and these three concepts can transfer to each other. The drifting details are as follows: $A \rightarrow B$, $B \rightarrow A$, and $C \rightarrow B$ with a shifting probability of 25%; and $A \rightarrow C$ and $C \rightarrow A$ with a shifting probability of 75%.

The KDDCup99 database[7] is a database for network intrusion detection, which is simulated as streaming data with the sampling change in [9].

4.2 Performance Analysis

Some denotations used are introduced as follows. SRDS_M and SRCD_M indicate the classification strategies of Majority Class (M) used in SRMTDS (SRDS) and MSRT (SRCD). Each database name consists of the name of the database + the size of the training database + the size of the test database + the type of the database (C: numerical, D: discrete, CD: hybrid) + the number of attribute dimensions. **T+C Time** is the training + test time (MSRT runs in a simulated parallel environment of multiple PCs, and the time overhead is computed by the largest one in N trees). **Memo** is the overhead of memory and only the space cost of a single tree is listed in the tables.

The experimental results for the HyperPlane database are listed in Table 1, which demonstrate that the training time of MSRT is only 51.1% of that of CVFDT. Because it generates the alternative root node with the same split attribute as the node with a numerical attribute in the original tree, the time overhead of computation is O(1) while it is up to O($M(Att)$) in CVFDT. There is no difference on the time of classifica- tion between SRMTDS and MSRT, while a little more cost of training time is needed in MSRT (about 0.7 times) than that of SRMTDS. About the space overhead: it is the least in SRMTDS, and in MSRT it changes from a half of that of CVFDT for 100k instances to 0.85 times for 500k instances.

Table 1. The experimental results from the HyperPlane database

Size (10k)	(T+C) Time(s)			Memo (M)		
	CVFDT	SRCD_M	SRDS_M	CVFDT	SRCD_M	SRDS_M
10	72+8	32+8	31+8	67	30	34
30	303+9	132+8	88+8	94	57	24
50	512+8	235+9	154+8	105	89	32

Figures 1 presents the curves of the classification results at every 10k instances for STAGGER database with 4000k instances, which show that the error rate in MSRT is lower than that of CVFDT.

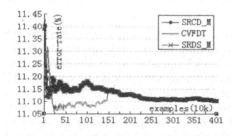

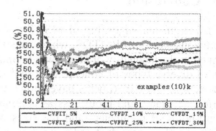

Fig. 1. Classification on STAGGER database

Fig. 2(a). Classification on HyperPlane database in CVFDT

Table 2. The experimental results from KDDCup99 database

Algorithm	CVFDT	SRCD_M	SRDS_M
KddCup99-33w-5.9wCD-41			
Error-rate (%)	5.9236	2.442	2.22
(T+C)Time (s)	90+4	90+4	109+20
Memo (M)	15	12	5

Table 2 lists the experimental results for the KDDCup99 database, which show that the error-rate of classification in SRCD_M is lower than that of CVFDT.

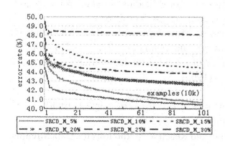

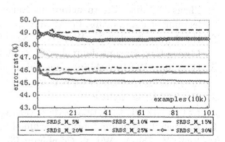

Fig. 2(b). Classification on HyperPlane database in SRCD_M

Fig. 2(c). Classification on HyperPlane database in SRDS_M

In another dimension, our experiments compare the robustness between CVFDT, MSRT and SRMTDS on the HyperPlane database with the noise rate varying from 5% to 30% in Figures 2-(a), (b) and (c), which show that the accuracy of classification in MSRT has improved from 2% to 10% in comparison with both of CVFDT and SRMTDS. One reason for the improvement is that MSRT adopts a semi-random strategy, by which the process of selecting attributes is independent on the distribution of classes. The other reason is that two thresholds are defined to distinguish noise from the concept drift, which are beneficial to weaken the impact of noise on the detection of concept drift.

5 Conclusion

An incremental algorithm of MSRT has been proposed in this paper, based on our previous work of SRMTDS, which uses two sliding windows and two thresholds defined in the inequality of Hoeffding bounds. MSRT can adapt to the data environment with diverse types of concept drift and reduce the impact of noise on concept drift detection. Our experiments have shown that MSRT has an improved performance in time, accuracy, and robustness as compared with CVFDT. How to find the optimal thresholds of parameters and the sizes of windows for distinguishing the different features of concept drift and noise, how to further decrease the overhead of space and how to deal with possible periodic concept drift in streaming data are our future work with MSRT.

References

1. Widmer, G., Kubat, M.: Learning in the presence of concept drift and hidden contexts. Machine Learning 23, 69–101 (1996)
2. Hulten, G., Spencer, L., Domingos, P.: Mining Time-Changing Data Streams. In: ACM KDD Conference on Knowledge Discovery and Data Mining, San Francisco, California, USA, pp. 97–106 (2001)
3. Fan, W.: StreamMiner: A Classifier Ensemble-based Engine to Mine Concept-drifting Data Streams. In: 30th VLDB Conference, Toronto, Canada (2004)
4. Zhang, Y., Jin, X.: An automatic construction and organization strategy for ensemble learning on data streams. In: ACM SIGMOD Record, pp. 28–33 (2006)
5. Hu, X., Li, P., Wu, X., Wu, G.: A Semi-Random Multiple Decision-Tree Algorithm for Mining Data Streams. Journal of Computer Science and Technology 22, 711–724 (2007)
6. Hoeffding, W.: Probability inequalities for sums of bounded random variables. Journal of the American Statistical Association 58, 13–30 (1963)
7. The UCI KDD Archive,
   http://kdd.ics.uci.edu//databases/kddcup99/kddcup99.html
8. Breiman, L.: Random forests. Machine Learning 45, 5–32 (2001)
9. Yang, Y., Zhu, X., Wu, X.: Combining Proactive and Reactive Predictions for Data Streams. In: 11th ACM SIGKDD International Conference on Knowledge Discovery and Data Mining, Chicago, IL, USA, pp. 710–715 (2005)
10. Stanley, K.O.: Learning concept drift with a committee of decision trees. Technical Report AI-03-302, Department of Computer Sciences, University of Texas at Austin (2003)
11. Salganicoff, M.: Tolerating concept and sampling shift in lazy learning using prediction error context switching. Artificial Intelligence 11, 133–155 (1997)
12. Kolrer, J.Z., Marcus, A.: Dynamic Weighted majority: A new Ensemble Method for Tracking Concept Drift. In: 3rd International IEEE Conference on Data Mining, Melbourne, Florida, USA, pp. 123–130 (2003)

Automatic Web Tagging and Person Tagging Using Language Models

Qiaozhu Mei[1] and Yi Zhang[2]

[1] University of Illinois at Urbana-Champaign, USA
qmei2@uiuc.edu
[2] University of California at Santa Cruz, USA
yiz@soe.ucsc.edu

1 Introduction

Social tagging systems, such as Delicious, My Web 2.0, Flickr, YouTube, have been very successful and attracted hundreds of million users. User provided tags of an object/page can be used to help the user re-find the object through search or share the customized object with other people.

Instead of waiting for a user to find and input the appropriate words to tag an object, we propose to automatically recommend tags for user to choose from, a process that requires much less cognitive effort than traditional tagging. In particular, we formalize the tag suggestion problem as a ranking problem and propose a new probabilistic language model to rank meaningful tags, including words or phrases, for bookmarks. Besides, we adapt the probabilistic language model to tag users. The user tags can be viewed as recommended queries for the user to search documents. They can also be used as meta data about the users, which could be beneficial for people search or person recommendation. The effectiveness of the proposed techniques are demonstrated on data collected from del.icio.us.

2 Tag Suggestion by Automatic Labeling Tagging Logs

In this section, we introduce a probabilistic approach to automatically generate tag suggestions by labeling language models estimated from tagging logs. In the rest of this paper, d is a web document, a tag t is a short text segment and V is the vocabulary of all possible tags. A bookmark, r, is a sequence of tags $r[T] = t_1 t_2 ... t_l$, selected by a user $r[U]$ to mark a web document $r[D]$ in a social bookmarking system.

2.1 Candidate Tag Generation

To find a set of candidate tags, the most straight forward way is to use the words and phrases in the web document. However, the vocabulary used in a web document could also be quite different from the tags used by real users. One method is to generate such candidate tags from the tagging logs. We analyzed the tag log

C. Tang et al. (Eds.): ADMA 2008, LNAI 5139, pp. 741–748, 2008.
© Springer-Verlag Berlin Heidelberg 2008

and found that a bookmark has the following characteristics: 1) each bookmark is usually a sequence of tags instead of a single tag; 2) people usually use meaningful phrases rather than single words as tags (e.g., "funny ideas," "learning lessons," "ESL English"); 3) there is usually no explicit segmentation of tags in a bookmark; and 4) the sequence of tags doesn't follow syntax rules. Motivated by this observation, we extract phrases by ranking word ngrams based on statistical T test similar to [8]. Another method is to rely on an outside dictionary to extract candidate tags. Again, we need to guarantee that the candidate tags are likely to be used as tags by real web users. Therefore, it is reasonable to extract tags from a collection of user generated text collection rather than from other sources such as a dictionary. In our experiments, we use the titles of every entry in Wikipedia[1] as candidate tags.

2.2   A Probabilistic Approach to Tag Ranking

To rank the tags based on their relevance to a web document, we borrow the ranking methods in retrieval. In this work, we follow the language modeling retrieval framework, and represent a tag and a web document both with a unigram language model. Formally, we extract a unigram language model, or a multinomial distribution of words from a web document d and a candidate tag t, denoted as $\{p(w|d)\}$ and $\{p(w|t)\}$ respectively. Since we do not rely on the actual content of d, we alternatively estimate $p(w|d)$ based on the social tagging logs. Specifically, we have

$$p(w|d) = \frac{\sum_r c(w, r[T]) \cdot \mathbb{I}[r[D] = d]}{\sum_{w'} \sum_r c(w', r[T]) \cdot \mathbb{I}[r[D] = d]} \tag{1}$$

where $\mathbb{I}[S]$ is an indicator function which is set to 1 if the statement S is true and 0 otherwise, and $c(w, r[T])$ is the occurrence of word w in the tags $r[T]$.

Once we estimated a language model for d, the problem is reduced to selecting tags to label such a multinomial model of words. The easiest way is apparently using words with largest $p(w|d)$. This method may have problem because it is usually hard to interpret the meaning of a distribution of words from just the top words because the top words are usually obscure and only partially captures the information encoded by the whole distribution [11]. Instead, we expect labels that could cover the semantics conveyed by the whole distribution (e.g., a distribution with top words like "tree", "search", "DFS", "prune", "construct" is better to be labeled as "tree algorithms" rather than "tree"). We then follow [11] and present a probabilistic approach to automatically label the document language model $p(w|d)$. The basic idea is that if we can also extract a language model from a tag t, we could use the Kullback-Leibler (KL) divergence to score each candidate tag. Specifically,

$$f(t, d) = -D(d||t) = \sum_w p(w|d) \log \frac{p(w|t)}{p(w|d)}. \tag{2}$$

---

[1] http://en.wikipedia.org

How to estimate $p(w|t)$ is however tricker. The simplest way is to estimate $p(w|t)$ based on the word frequency in a tag. However, a tag is usually too short (e.g., 1 or 2 words) to estimate a reliable language model. If we embed such an estimate in Equation 2, we need to smooth the tag language model so that $\forall w, p(w|t) > 0$ [15]. When a tag is very short, such a smoothed language model would not be trustable. Indeed, in this case $f(t, d)$ will be similar to count the occurrence of t in all bookmarks of d.

We need to find a reliable language model $p(w|t)$ in an alternatively way. One possibility is to approximate $p(w|t)$ from the collection of tagging logs C, and estimate a distribution $p(w|t, C)$ to substitute $p(w|t)$. Similar to [11], we can rewrite Equation 2 as

$$f(t, d) = \sum_w p(w|d) \log \frac{p(w|t, C)}{p(w|C)} - \sum_w p(w|d) \log \frac{p(w|d)}{p(w|C)} - \sum_w p(w|d) \log \frac{p(w|t, C)}{p(w|t)}$$

$$= \sum_w p(w|d) \log \frac{p(w, t|C)}{p(w|C)p(t|C)} - D(d||C) + Bias(t, C). \tag{3}$$

From this rewriting, we see that the scoring function can be decomposed into three components. The second component $D(d||C)$ is irrelevant to t, and can be ignored in ranking. The third component $-\sum_w p(w|d) \log \frac{p(w|t, C)}{p(w|t)}$ can be interpreted as the bias of using C to approximate the unknown language model $p(w|t)$. When the t and C are from the same domain (e.g., if we use C to extract candidate tags), we can fairly assume that such bias is ignorable. Therefore, we have

$$f(t, d) \overset{\text{rank}}{=} \sum_w p(w|d) \log \frac{p(w, t|C)}{p(w|C)p(t|C)} = E_d[PMI(w, t|C)]. \tag{4}$$

Please note that $\log \frac{p(w, t|C)}{p(w|C)p(t|C)}$ is actually the pointwise mutual information of t and w conditional on the tagging logs. $f(t, d)$ can thus be interpreted with the expected mutual information of t and a word in the document language model. Estimating $PMI(w, t|C)$ is straight forward, since we use efficiently find $p(w, t|C), P(w|C)$ and $P(t|C)$ that maximize the likelihood that each word is cooccurring with t in the tagging records. Specifically, we have

$$p(w, t|C) = \frac{\sum_{r \in C} c(w, r[T]) \cdot \mathbb{I}[t \in r[T]]}{\sum_{w'} \sum_{t'} \sum_{r \in C} c(w', r[T]) \cdot \mathbb{I}[t' \in r[T]]} \tag{5}$$

$$p(w|C) = \frac{\sum_{r \in C} c(w, r[T])}{\sum_{w'} \sum_r c(w', r[T])} \tag{6}$$

$$p(t|C) = \frac{\sum_{r \in C} \mathbb{I}[t \in r[T]]}{\sum_{t'} \sum_{r \in C} \mathbb{I}[t' \in r[T]]}. \tag{7}$$

Once the candidate tags are extracted, all the mutual information $PMI(w, t|C)$ can be computed and stored offline. This also improves the efficiency in ranking. Computing the expectation of the mutual information could still be time consuming if the vocabulary is large. To further improve the runtime efficiency, we ignore all the mutual information where $PMI(w, t|C) < 0$. We then select the tags with largest $f(t, d)$ as the suggested tags to a document d.

2.3 Further Discussion: Tagging Users and Beyond

Since eventually we are labeling language models, this method can be applied to suggest tags for users, using the following user language model

$$p(w|u) = \frac{\sum_r c(w, r[T]) \cdot \mathbb{I}[r[U] = u]}{\sum_{w'} \sum_r c(w', r[T]) \cdot \mathbb{I}[r[U] = u]}. \tag{8}$$

The same ranking function can be used to generate labels for this user language model, by replacing $p(w|d)$ with $p(w|u)$ in Equation 4.

3   Experiments

Data. To show the effectiveness of our proposed methods, we collect two weeks (02132007 − 02262007) tagging records from a well known social bookmarking website Del.icio.us[2], There are 579,652 bookmarks, 20,138 users, and 111,381 distinct tagging words.

To test different ways of candidate tag generation, we also collect all the titles of entries in Wikipedia, from the data snapshot of 10/18/2007. There are in total 5,836,166 entries extracted.

Candidate Tags: We explore three different ways of candidate tag generation. For the first method, we simply use single words in the tagging logs as candidate tags. For the second method, we extract significant bigrams from tagging logs using Student's T-Test. This was done using the N-gram Statistics Package [1]. We select the top 15,000 bigrams with the largest T-Score as the candidate tags. The top ranked bigrams are presented in Table 1. For the third method, we use all titles of Wikipedia entries as candidate tags.

Table 1. Top Bigrams from Tagging Logs

Bigrams with Highest T-score			
css design	software tools	web webdesign	mac osx
programming reference	web web2.0	art design	rails ruby
mp3 music	tools web	photo photography	photography photos

It is easy to see that most of the top bigrams extracted from the tagging logs are meaningful. However, they could overfit the log data, where some words are user specific (e.g., webdesign), and some bigrams contain redundant words (e.g., photo photography). Such problem does not show in Wikipedia entries. However, only 48k such entry titles appear in the tagging logs, out of 5,836k.

---

[2] http://del.icio.us/

Tagging Web Documents: The first experiment designed is to suggest tags for web documents. We select web documents with the largest number of bookmarks in the tagging log collection, and automatically suggest tags for them. The results are presented in Table 2. We present the top words in the document language model $p(w|d)$ estimated from the tagging logs in the second column. The right three columns present system generated tag suggestions, using single words, significant bigrams, and wikipedia titles as candidate tags, respectively.

There are several interesting discoveries from Table 2. First, simply using top words in $p(w|d)$ favors frequent terms, such as "web2.0". These are not desirable, because when a user uses it in the future trying to retrieve the documents, he has to spend much extra effort to target the web document from the many documents bookmarked with "web2.0". The labeling based method gives much much better tag suggestions. In column 3, "pipes" seems a better tag than "yahoo" because it captures the meaning of the url "http://pipes.yahoo.com" more precisely. "youtube" seems more precise than all other words in column 2 for the url "http://www.youtube.com/watch?v=6gmP4nk0EOE", which is a video on youtube. "Palette" is a very interesting generalization of the meaning of "http://kuler.adobe.com/," which does not appear in the top words in $p(w|d)$. This is because the method we introduce tries to capture the meaning of the whole language model (i.e., the expectation of similarity of a tag to all the words), which thus generates more precise tags.

However, some tags are obscure or not meaningful. For example, "color," "photo," and "editor" are obscure as tags, and "ajax," "pipes," "feeds" are ambiguous which could mean quite different concepts. Some words are also too domain specific and not so meaningful to the common audience (e.g., "dhtml," "comunidad"). All this is because single words are used as candidate tags. When phrases (significant bigrams, wikipedia entry names) are used as candidate tags, we see that the system generates much more understandable suggestions. Bigrams based tags are much more precise and interpretable. "Ajax code," "mashup pipes," and "api feeds" remove the ambiguity of single words. "Photography tools," "editor flickr," and "color design" are also more precise than "tools," "photo," "editor," and "design". However, some extracted phrases, such as "xml youtube," "adobe color," "color colors," and "css ajax," are good tags but not real phrases. In real life, people may not use such expressions. By using wikipedia entry names as candidate tags, the suggestions are more meaningful and understandable(e.g., "blog feeds, " "javascript library," "internet video," etc).

Tagging Users: We select 10 users with the largest number of bookmarks in the tagging log collection, and automatically suggest tags for them. The results are presented in Table 3.

There are also interesting findings from the tag suggestions for web users. Based on user preference analysis, a suggested tag can help user to find interesting web documents that other people bookmarked with this tag. The preference of a user is presented with a language model estimated from his own tags in column 2. We see that our algorithm suggests interesting tags to the user, pre-

Table 2. Tag Suggestions for Web Documents

URLs	LM $p(w\|d)$	Tag = Word	Tag = Bigram	Tag = Wiki Entry
http://pipes.yahoo.com/ 386 bookmarks	yahoo rss **web2.0** mashup feeds programming pipes	**pipes** **feeds** yahoo mashup rss syndication mashups	**feeds_mashup** **mashup_pipes** web2.0_yahoo rss_web2.0 mashup_rss api_feeds pipes_programming	**pipes** yahoo mashup rss syndication mashups blog_feeds
http://www.miniajax.com/ 349 bookmarks	ajax javascript **web2.0** webdesign programming code webdev	ajax dhtml javascript moo.fx dragdrop phototype autosuggest	**ajax_code** code_javascript javascript_ajax javascript_web2.0 css_ajax programming_web2.0 javascript_programming	ajax dhtml javascript moo.fx **javascript_library** javascript_framework ajax_framework
http://kuler.adobe.com/ 158 bookmarks	color design webdesign tools adobe graphics flash	**color** **colour** **palette** colorscheme colours picker cor	**adobe_color** **color_design** color_colour color_colors colour_desgin inspiration_palette webdesign_color	color colour palette **web_color** colours cor rgb
http://www.youtube.com/ watch?v=6gmP4nk0EOE 157 bookmarks	**web2.0** video youtube web internet xml community	**youtube** **revver** vodcast primer comunidad participation ethnograpy	**xml_youtube** **web2.0_youtube** video_web2.0 web2.0_xml online_presentation social_video youtube_video	**internet_video** youtube **revver** research_video vodcast primer p2p_TV
http://www.picnik.com/ 149 bookmarks	photo photography tools editor online **web2.0** flickr	photo resize flickr editor edit editing crop	**editor_flickr** **editor_online** **online_photo** editor_photo photography_tools photo_tools editor_image	photo resize flickr editor edit editing crop

Table 3. Tag Suggestions for Web Users

Users	LM $p(w\|d)$	Tag = Bigram	Tag = Wiki Entry
User1	photography art portraits tools web design geek	**art_photography** photography_portraits **digital_flickr** photoblog_photography art_photo flickr_photography weblog_wordpress	**art_photography** photoblog portraits photography landscapes flickr **art_contest**
User2	humor programming photography blog webdesign security funny	geek_hack **humor_programming** hack_hacking networking_programming geek_html geek_hacking reference_security	**network_programming** tweak hacking security **geek_humor** sysadmin **digitalcamera**
User3	games arg tools programming sudoku cryptography software	**arg_games** games_puzzles **games_internet** arg_code games_sudoku **code_generator** **community_games**	arg **games_research** games puzzles storytelling **code_generator** **community_games**
User4	web reference css development rubyonrails tools design	rubyonrails_web **css_development** **brower_development** development_editor **development_forum** **development_firefox** **javascript_tools**	javascript css webdev xhtml dhtml css3 dom

sented in column 3 and 4. Tag "art photography" matches user 1's interests. If there's tags like "digital flickr" and "art contest", he is also likely to be interested. This also indicates an opportunity of personalized online advertisements. The interests of user 2 are actually a mixture of several themes. From column 4, we clearly see that "network programming" and "geek humor" are good suggestions to such themes. However, if there is a tag "humor programming" from other users (although looks weird in reality), which perfectly matches different aspects of his interests, he is very likely to explore such a tag. Similarly, we see that user 3 likes games and programming related content, and user 4 likes web development. Our methods suggest very highly relevant and understandable tags to them.

4 Related Work

Recently, researchers have started to realize the importance of social bookmarking. This leads to the exploration of tagging logs in different ways [4,9,3,7,6,14]. Most work are focusing on utilizing social tags, instead of suggesting tags. Folksonomy [9], tagging visualization [3], and spam detection for tagging system [7] are some of such examples. [2] utilizes social tags to help summarization. [6] explores search and ranking in tagging systems. [14] first uses tagging logs to help web search, and [5] gives an empirical justification of helping search with tagging logs. [10] introduced a duality hypothesis of search and tagging, which gives a theoretical justification of using tags to help search tasks. However, none of this work explores the problem of suggesting tags for web documents, or for web users. To the best of our knowledge, automatic bookmark suggestion is not well addressed in existing literature. The only work we are aware of is collaborative tag suggestion described in [13]. They discussed the desirable properties of suggested tags, however their tagging approach is not based on any probabilistic models and rather ad hoc.

The probabilistic language modeling framework for tagging is motivated by the well known language modeling approach in the information retrieval community. In particular, [11] has proposed to assign meaningful labels to multinomial topic models. We adapted the technique to the novel problem of tag suggestion, and generate meaningful tags for web documents and web users.

This paper is also related to early work on suggesting index terms for library documents [12]. However, all such work are based on content of documents, and is not appropriate for social bookmarking systems, where the content of web pages are hard to keep track of but rich tagging log is available.

5 Conclusions

In this work, we formally define the problem of tag suggestion for social bookmarking systems, and present a probabilistic approach to automatically generate and rank meaningful tags for web documents and web users. Empirical experiments show that our proposed methods are effective to extract relevant and meaningful tag suggestions. Such a technique could be applied to other interesting mining problems, such as ad term suggestion for online advertisement systems, and people tagging in social network applications. There are quite a few potential future directions, such as tag suggestion over time, personalized tag suggestion, and collaborative tag suggestion are all among the good examples. Another line of future work is to design a way to quantitative evaluate tag suggestion algorithms.

References

1. Banerjee, S., Pedersen, T.: The design, implementation, and use of the ngram statistics package, pp. 370–381 (2003)
2. Boydell, O., Smyth, B.: From social bookmarking to social summarization: an experiment in community-based summary generation. In: Proceedings of the 12th international conference on Intelligent user interfaces, pp. 42–51 (2007)
3. Dubinko, M., Kumar, R., Magnani, J., Novak, J., Raghavan, P., Tomkins, A.: Visualizing tags over time. In: Proceedings of the 15th international conference on World Wide Web, pp. 193–202 (2006)
4. Golder, S., Huberman, B.A.: The structure of collaborative tagging systems. Journal of Information Science (2006)
5. Heymann, P., Koutrika, G., Garcia-Molina, H.: Can social bookmarking improve web search? In: Proceedings of the international conference on Web search and web data mining, pp. 195–206 (2008)
6. Hotho, A., Jasschke, R., Schmitz, C., Stumme, G.: Information retrieval in folksonomies: Search and ranking. In: Sure, Y., Domingue, J. (eds.) ESWC 2006. LNCS, vol. 4011, pp. 411–426. Springer, Heidelberg (2006)
7. Koutrika, G., Effendi, F.A., Gyöngyi, Z., Heymann, P., Garcia-Molina, H.: Combating spam in tagging systems. In: Proceedings of the 3rd international workshop on Adversarial information retrieval on the web, pp. 57–64 (2007)
8. Manning, C.D., Schtze, H.: Foundations of statistical natural language processing. MIT Press, Cambridge (1999)
9. Marlow, C., Naaman, M., Boyd, D., Davis, M.: Position paper, tagging, taxonomy, ickr, article, toread. In: Proceedings of Hypertext, pp. 31–40 (2006)
10. Mei, Q., Jiang, J., Su, H., Zhai, C.: Search and tagging: Two sides of the same coin? UIUC Technical Report (2007)
11. Mei, Q., Shen, X., Zhai, C.: Automatic labeling of multinomial topic models. In: Proceedings of KDD 2007, pp. 490–499 (2007)
12. Schatz, B.R., Johnson, E.H., Cochrane, P.A., Chen, H.: Interactive term suggestion for users of digital libraries: using subject thesauri and co-occurrence lists for information retrieval. In: Proceedings of the first ACM international conference on Digital libraries, pp. 126–133 (1996)
13. Xu, Z., Fu, Y., Mao, J., Su, D.: Towards the semantic web: Collaborative tag suggestions. In: Proceedings of the Collaborative Web Tagging Workshop at the WWW 2006, Edinburgh, Scotland (May 2006)
14. Yanbe, Y., Jatowt, A., Nakamura, S., Tanaka, K.: Can social bookmarking enhance search in the web? In: JCDL, pp. 107–116 (2007)
15. Zhai, C., Lafferty, J.: A study of smoothing methods for language models applied to ad hoc information retrieval. In: SIGIR 2001: Proceedings of the 24th annual international ACM SIGIR conference on Research and development in information retrieval, pp. 334–342 (2001)

Real-Time Person Tracking Based on Data Field

Shuliang Wang[1, 2], Juebo Wu[2], Feng Cheng[1], and Hong Jin[1]

[1] International School of Software, Wuhan University, Wuhan 430079, China
slwang2005@whu.edu.cn
[2] State Key Laboratory of Information Engineering in Surveying,
Mapping and Remote Sensing, Wuhan University, Wuhan 430079, China
wujuebo@gmail.com

Abstract. In this paper, a novel approach of data field is proposed to discover the action pattern of real-time person tracking, and potential function is presented to find out the power of a person with suspicious action. Firstly, a data field on the first feature is used to find the individual attributes, associated with the velocity, direction changing frequency and appearance frequency respectively. Secondly, the common characteristic of each attribute is obtained by the data field on the main feature from the data field created before. Thirdly, the weighted Euclidean distance classifier is used to identify whether a person is a suspect or not. Finally, the results of the experiment show that the proposed way is feasible and effective in action mining.

1 Introduction

Real-time person tracking in known environments has recently become an active area of research in computer vision. A number of scholars have devoted to such field and lots of successful approaches have investigated to human tracking and modeling, many of them being able to discern pose in addition to differentiating between individuals [1]. Where the images of sufficient quality are available, it is also possible to perform detailed analysis such as face-recognition [2]. Several systems to do this have exploited visual information, particularly for automatic camera control [3]. Other systems have used person tracking to guide biometric acquisition [4]. Calibrated multi-camera systems have been used for person localization and more detailed tracking of heads, hands and full articulated body tracking [5]. However, most contributions are to find and follow people's head, hands and body, not to find the people's action.

As abovementioned, we propose a new way to judge a person whether he/she is a suspect or not in real-time person tracking. The rest of this paper is organized as follows. Data field is presented in section 2. And section 3 gives an overall about person tracking on action mining. Data acquisition is studied in section 4, where the preprocessing and normalization are also introduced. In section 5 a new way is given to describe and measure the features of each person. Two different kinds of data fields are investigated there. Identification and analysis are addressed in section 6. A short conclusion is finally given in section 7.

C. Tang et al. (Eds.): ADMA 2008, LNAI 5139, pp.749–756, 2008.

2 Data Field

Identifying suspect in this paper concerns data field. In this section we provide background on the theory of data field and potential function in the universe of discourse.

Data field is given to describe how the data essentials are diffused from the universe of sample to the universe of discourse. And its potential function is to discover the power of an item in the universe of discourse. It assumes that all observed data in the universe of discourse will radiate their data energies and also be influenced by others. The power of the data field may be measured by its potential with a field function [6]. For a single data field created by sample A, the potential of a point x1 in the universe of discourse can be computed by:

$$f(x) = m \times e^{-(\frac{\|x-x_1\|}{\sigma})^2} \tag{1}$$

Where, $\| x-x_1 \|$ is the distance between A and x_1, m (m≥0) denotes the power of A and σ indicates the influential factors. Usually, $\| x-x_1 \|$ is Euclidean norm. The influential factors σ, e.g. radiation brightness, radiation gene, data amount, space between the neighbor isopotentials, grid density of Descartes coordinate, and so on, all make their contributions to the data field. It is obvious that the potential of point x_1 would become lower if the distance between A and x_1 got further.

In general, there exists more than one sample in the universe of discourse. In such case, to obtain the power of one point, all energies from every sample should be concerned. Because of overlap, the potential of each point in the universe of discourse is the sum of all potentials [6]. Referring to the potential function (1), the potential can be calculated by:

$$f(x) = \sum_{i=1}^{n} (m_i \times e^{-(\frac{\|x-x_1\|}{\sigma})^2}) \tag{2}$$

Where, the sum is over all the sample points.

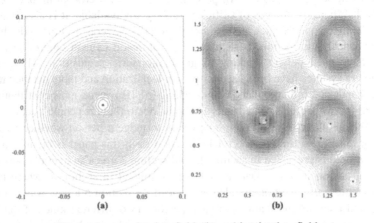

Fig. 1. (a) one-point data field; (b) multi-point data field

In Fig. 1, (a) shows a one-point data field, and (b) shows a multi-point data field.

3 Person Tracking on Action Mining

Data mining is to extract previously unknown, potentially useful, and ultimately understandable patterns from large database or data sets. It is a discovered process from raw data to information, and to interesting knowledge [6, 7].

Action mining has been a field of particular interest with discovering the action pattern of moving objects, and turning the pattern into knowledge. Person tracking, as an application of action mining, is a branch of detecting the moving targets, which is the focus of image understanding and computer vision.

We propose a new method to real-time person tracking using data field. As a whole, Fig. 2 shows the process on how to find a suspicious person. We divide it into two different aspects: one is for training sample while the other is for identifying suspicious object. In the first part, four steps are applied to get sample sets for further classifier, associated with data acquisition, data preprocessing, personality extracting and main feature extracting. After doing so, a suspicious object can be identified by the same steps.

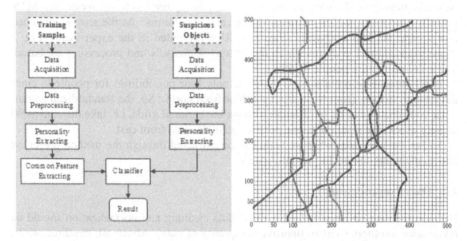

Fig. 2. The process of identification   **Fig. 3.** Background grids by proportion

As the method above, first of all, we will have to choose the attributes of one person that will be analyzed as observed data in data field. Considering all the attributes, we choose three of them as a scale to measure each person.

- The velocity: walking speed of each person. The person's movement is divided into intervals of one second to examine differences in walking speed. In particular, when the person halts, the variance of walking speed tends to grow in proportion to the halt time.
- The direction changing frequency: the number of changes in direction in the linearized walking data of each person. Usually, a person straightly goes to their destination from the current position when acting with a goal in mind, if no obstacle prevents him/her from doing so. In other words, a person will walk back and forth in a certain range, but would exhibit a detour or stop if they are in an unusual state or do not have a specific goal in mind, etc.

- The appearance frequency: the number of each person appearing in monitoring area. Commonly, a person ought not to show up in the same area again and again within a period of time.

In addition to these three attributes, another attributes can be considered, such as category of action, appearing time. The case we will present next is to identify suspicious person in the waiting room at a railway station.

4 Data Acquisition

This section contains two steps: data source and data preprocessing. The tracking data of each walking person were obtained by using a surveillance camera with a video, and preprocessed by using person-tracking system developed at Wuhan University.

4.1 Data Source

At the beginning of the method, the whole area in capture has to be divide into M*N grids by proportion, which contains M rows and N columns. As the area we obtained is a square, the 500*500 grids (Fig. 3) will be presented in the experiment. Fig. 3 shows standardized grids on which the following analysis and processing are based. These color lines are people's paths.

In all observed circumstances, there are only four possibilities for people to enter the area: from east, from west, from south or from north. So, the standardized rectangular coordinates can be set through rotating background grids, i.e. take the canvas 90 degrees clockwise rotation as one person enters the area from east.

So far, the attributes what we want can be extracted through the method presented above, including the positional information.

4.2 Data Preprocessing

Because the data obtained before is dirty, data cleaning and normalization should be taken prior to others so as to improve the quality of data. Above all, the three attributes as describing in section 3 and some other related data will be normalized. Then three normalized data sets will be generated within a period of time in person-tracking system, which will be used for creating data fields.

The data sets of these three attributes will be defined as follows:

$$D_V = \{(x_j, y_j, V_j)\}, j=1, 2, \ldots, m \tag{3}$$

D_V describes the data sets of instantaneous velocity gained at regular intervals. V_j is the instantaneous velocity at the position (x_j, y_j) (see section 4.1).

$$D_{DCF} = \{(x_i, y_i, C_i)\}, i=1, 2, \ldots, n \tag{4}$$

D_{DCF} denotes the data sets of the direction changing frequency. C_i is the total of changing, which is obtained within a spell of time T1. How long the best length is will be depended on the fact, to adjust longer for the festivals and shorter for normal days. 15 minutes are set here.

$$D_{AF} = \{(x_k, y_k, A_k)\}, k=1, 2, \ldots, p \tag{5}$$

D_{AF} indicates the data sets of appearance frequency. A_k is the number of appearing at the point (x_k, y_k) got among a period of time, usually at least twice more than T1. One half hour is considered here.

For the sake of convenience and two people not to make the same path, D_V, D_{DCF}, and D_{AF} should be normalized as follows:

$$X' = \frac{X - X_{min}}{X_{max} - X_{min}} \times 500 \qquad Y' = \frac{Y - Y_{min}}{Y_{max} - Y_{min}} \times 500 \qquad (6)$$

By now, data acquisition has been done and next is to find the feature both in personality and in common.

5 Feature Extracting

To find the different feature, two kinds of data fields will be created here. Data field on the first feature is to describe the three attributes on each person. This kind of data field can just express the personality respectively, because there are not two observed objects to make the same behavior. By extracting the extremum and important isopotentials in the data field on the first feature, the other kind of data field can be created and they express the personality in common. In this section, the feature of real-time people tracking will be found out with isopotentials.

5.1 Personality Extracting

The aim of the data field on the first feature is to find the individual features of each object. Attributes here must have been preprocessed and normalized (section 4). With the velocity, direction changing frequency and appearance frequency, three kinds of data fields are obtained here for each attribute. Take the velocity for example.

First of all, groups of normalized data of three suspects are extracted. $D_V = \{(x_j, y_j , V_j)\}$, a group of the velocities is used to create feature data field. Referring to equation (2), Vj is the value of m and $\| x- x_1 \|$ is the distance between x and the point (x_j, y_j). Considering the potential function, set σ=2 so as to produce a better feature.

For example, in Fig. 4, (a) and (b) show the first feature data field of two suspects (S1, S2) on velocity respectively. And figure (c) shows first feature data field of a valid person on velocity.

The data field on the first feature describes the personality of each person. And the features from such data field can be used to measure each person. However, a kind of people may have some similarities. So it is possible to extract the features in common for these two suspects, from which data field has been obtained in this step.

5.2 Main Feature Extracting

The data field on the main feature is to obtain the feature in common and it can express the similarity of one group. By the data field on the first feature created above, it is necessary to pick up N local maximum potential values and their positions as the main features by:

$$x = \frac{\sum\limits_{i=1}^{N}(P_{V_i} \times x_i)}{\sum\limits_{i=1}^{N}P_{V_i}} \qquad y = \frac{\sum\limits_{i=1}^{N}(P_{V_i} \times y_i)}{\sum\limits_{i=1}^{N}P_{V_i}} \qquad (7)$$

The data field on the main feature for two (S1, S2) of the suspects is illustrated once again by equal potential lines. In Fig. 4, (d) shows the main feature data field of tow suspects on the velocity. The main features of other attributes can be obtained through the same way.

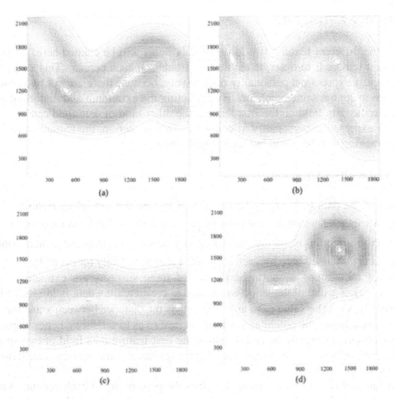

Fig. 4. Data fields: (a) data field on the first feature of S1; (b) data field on the first feature of S2; (c) data field on the first feature of a valid person; (d) Data field on the main feature of two suspects

From Fig. 4, (d) clearly shows that potential value is highly concentrated around the centre in the data radiation context. And the potential in the edge of this area is declined fast to zero, which is suit for expressing the feature in common. All the features above are stored in the feature database and the next work is to identify suspicious object by classifier.

6 Identification and Analysis

Classifier is used for judging a new coming person whether he/she is a suspect or not. By now, essential features on data field have been stored in feature database. The details for distinguishing a suspicious one are as bellow:

Firstly, make sure that the attributes have been preprocessed and then do the data field on the first feature by section 5.1. Three kinds of data fields are obtained here. Secondly, extract the extremum and important isopotentials in the data fields on the first feature and consider them as main features. After that, create a new kind of data field by those main features. All data fields can be acquired and these metrics are the feature fields of person tracking path. Thirdly, combine with the sample features created before and pairs of potentials can be gained. Finally, use WED classifier to fulfil the identification task [8, 9]. The formulation of WED is written as follows:

$$WED = \sum_{i=1}^{6} k_i \times w_i \quad w_i = \sqrt{\frac{f_{i,1}^2 + f_{i,2}^2 + ... + f_{i,n}^2}{n}} \quad (8)$$

Where, i denotes the number of each group, k_i is the weight of group i, $f_{i,j}$ means the potential in the position j of group i. The k_i can be given appropriate weight according to the actual situation. After setting threshold by WED, identification can be done. The object is valid when the threshold is less than that, or others are deemed to suspicious object.

Under the above process on real-time person tracking, 100 samples are used in this experiment, including 15 suspicious people and 85 valid people. The experiment is implemented by a tool developed in C++ (Fig. 2).

The threshold is adjusted in different value by different time in a day. The results show that the precision can achieve 92% when the threshold is set close to WED. On the other hand, the precision is 81% if the threshold is set far away from WED.

7 Conclusion

Data field is proposed to real-time track person's action pattern. A new way in data mining is introduced to describe the metric of attribute according to the essential feature obtained by potential function. The first kind of fields, associated with direction changing frequency, velocity and appearance frequency respectively, are taken to express attributes. Nevertheless, common characteristic of each attribute can be well measured by the data field on the main features. Another important practical issue is classifier. It helps to judge whether a new person is a suspect or not. A better outcome can be obtained by adjusting a proper threshold. The experiment result shows that this new method is feasible and effective.

Furthermore, by adding more valuable features, the accuracy may be improved. The proposed method may analyze the monitoring data automatically and find out the suspicious action intelligently.

Acknowledgements

This paper is supported by National 973 (2006CB701305, 2007CB310804), National Natural Science Fund of China (60743001), Best National Thesis Fund (2005047), and National New Century Excellent Talent Fund (NCET-06-0618).

References

1. Haritaoglu, I., Harwood, D., Davis, L.S.: Real-time surveillance of people and their activities. IEEE Transactions on Pattern Analysis and Machine Intelligence 22(8), 809–830 (2000)
2. Turk, M., Pentland, A.: Face recognition using eigenfaces. In: IEEE Conference on Computer Vision and Pattern Recognition, pp. 586–591 (1991)
3. Pinhanez, C., Bobick, A.: Intelligent studios: Using computer vision to control TV cameras. In: Workshop on Entertainment and AI/Alife, pp. 69–76 (1995)
4. Zhou, X., Collins R.T., Kanade, T., Metes, P.: A master-slave system to acquire biometricimagery of humans at distance. In: First ACM SIGMM International Workshop on Video Surveillance, pp. 113–120 (2003)
5. Bregler, C., Malik, J.: Tracking people with twists and exponential maps. Computer Vision and Pattern Recognition, pp. 8–15 (1998)
6. Li, D.R., Wang, S.L., Li, D.Y.: Spatial Data Mining Theories and Applications. Science Press (2006)
7. Han, J.W.: Micheline Kambr: Data Mining Concepts and Techniques. Higher Education Pre&Morgan Kaufmann Publishers (2001)
8. Li G.L., Chen X.Y.: The discussion on the similarity of cluster analysis. Journal of Computer Engineering and Applications (31), 64–82 (2004)
9. Jain A.K., Murty M.N., Flynn P.J.: Data clustering: a review. ACM Computing Surveys 31(3), 264–323 (1999)

Author Index